EMBRYOLOGY AND GENETICS

VOLUME 2
GENETIC MECHANISMS AND DEVELOPMENTAL SYSTEMS IN EMBRYOGENESIS

Dr. Vijaykumar Deshmukh
and Dr. Jaykumar Deshmukh

ALLIED
HEALTH
PRESS

Embryology and Genetics

Volume 2: Genetic Mechanisms and Developmental Systems in Embryogenesis

Authors: **Dr. Vijaykumar Deshmukh and Dr. Jaykumar Deshmukh**

Allied Health Press
4164 Lakeshore Road
Burlington ON L7L 1A4
Canada
www.alliedhealthpress.com
Email: orders@arclereducation.com

ISBN: 978-1-77956-773-4

Allied Health Press publishes wide variety of books and eBooks. For more information about Allied Health Press and its products, visit our website at www.alliedhealthpress.com

ABOUT THE AUTHORS

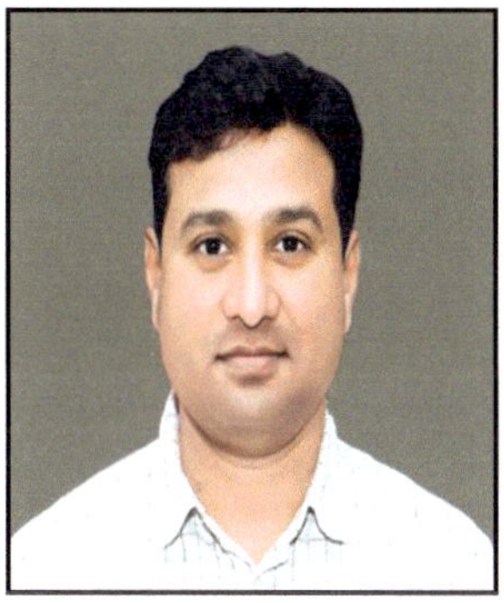

Dr. Vijaykumar D Deshmukh is presently serving as Assistant Professor in Department of Plant Biotechnology, MGM College of Agricultural Biotechnology, Chh. Sambhajinagar (Maharashtra). He obtained his M.Sc. in (Agril. Biotech.) and Ph.D. in (Biotech.). He started his career as an Assistant Professor in 2005. His field of specialisation is Plant Biotechnology and Molecular Biology. He has published Six books and more than 25 research papers in National and international journals. He has participated in International, National and State Level Seminar and Symposiums.

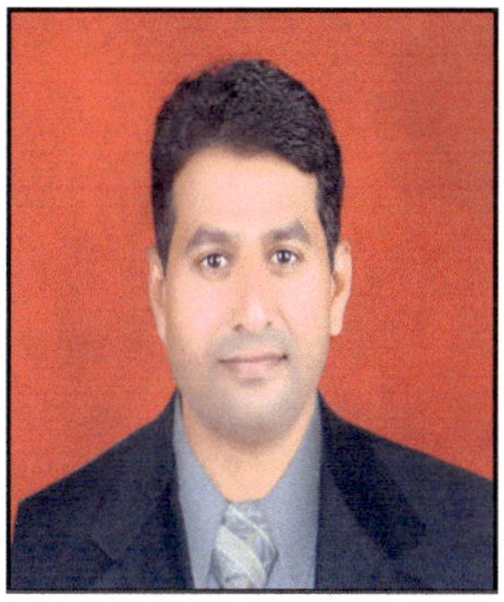

Dr. Jaykumar D. Deshmukh (1981) is presently serving as Assistant Professor in Department of Genetics and Plant Breeding, College of Agriculture Parbhani, Maharashtra, India. He obtained his M.Sc. (GPB) in 2005 and Ph.D. (GPB) in 2013 from Vasantrao Naik Marathwada Krishi Vidyapeeth, Parbhani, Maharashtra. He started his career as an Assistant Professor in 2013. His field of specialisation is Genetics and Plant Breeding. He has published seven books and more than 45 research papers in National and international journals. He has participated in International, National and State Level Seminar and Symposiums.

Brief Table of Contents

Detailed Table of Contents

CHAPTER 2

Axis Formation and Embryonic Patterning 39

CHAPTER 3

Neural Development and Neurogenetics 77

CHAPTER 4

Cardiovascular Embryology and Related Genetic Disorders 115

CHAPTER 9

CHAPTER 10

Prenatal Genetic Diagnosis and Screening 343

CHAPTER 11

Gene Editing and Developmental Research 379

LIST OF FIGURES

PREFACE

Embryology and genetics provide the essential basis of our knowledge of biology, describing how one cell can generate the immense richness of a fully formed organism. The moment sperm and egg combine, a chain of molecular interactions and gene regulatory processes initiates new life. Activation of the embryonic genome, a pivotal process that transfers control from maternal transcripts to the embryo's own DNA, provides the basis for coordinated cell divisions, pattern formation, and lineage determination. Blending classic embryological observations with contemporary genomic and epigenomic strategies, investigators have initiated the challenge of unraveling the succession of events leading cells from totipotency to specialized fate. Advanced imaging technologies, transcriptomic profiling, and single-cell sequencing collectively enhanced the precision of our mapping of early developmental milestones, illustrating how timing, dosage, and spatial context converge at key junctures.

Exploring the relationship between development processes and gene regulation extends beyond scientific curiosity; it provides significant insight into the etiology of congenital malformations. Perturbations in signal pathways, activity of transcription factors, or chromatin behavior can lead to malformations of one or more systems, including the cardiovascular, musculoskeletal, and nervous systems. By studying the genetic underlying bases of normal and abnormal development, the field has begun the process of biomarker discovery for early detection and therapeutic intervention. Epigenetic modifications—DNA methylation and histone modifications—add another level of sophistication to patterns of gene expression and have the capacity to pass environmental influences through cellular lineages. These levels of control ensure embryonic cells to read their positional information correctly and form proper functional tissues. Our understanding of developmental biology and genetics continues to evolve, with growing capacity to predict, diagnose, and ultimately treat developmental disorders previously unknown.

Embryology and Genetics – Volume 2 collects the latest developments in our comprehension of developmental biology from a genetic perspective. The volume, composed of 12 chapters, collects contributions from top developmental biologists, geneticists, and clinicians who have employed the latest methodologies—ranging from CRISPR-based gene editing to live-cell imaging of embryos and integrative bioinformatics—to address basic questions. The effort here is a continuation of the processes laid down in the first volume, further extending the discussion to address later events in embryogenesis, genetics of tissue formation, and translational implications.

Chapter 1 presents detailed analysis of zygotic genome activation that specifies molecular drivers of embryonic transcription and resulting networks controlling early cell divisions. Chapter 1 highlights important experiments and ongoing research that have mapped the enhancers, transcription factors, and chromatin remodeling complexes required for this developmental switch. Chapter 2 presents the formation of the initial body axes—anterior–posterior, dorsal–ventral, and left–right—by following the actions of signaling molecules Wnt, BMP, and Nodal, and their antagonists. The authors address the dynamic interplay between morphogen gradients and cell movements that drive embryonic patterning across species.

Chapter 3 outlines the mechanisms of neural development and neurogenetics, such as the derivation of neural progenitor cells from ectodermal precursors, proneural transcription factor involvement in specifying neuronal subtype, and the genetic basis of neurodevelopmental disease. The chapter outlines advances with single-cell RNA sequencing and organoid models as approaches to unravel the complexity of neural lineages. Chapter 4 presents an integrated review of cardiovascular embryology and related genetic disease, with special stress on the molecular mechanisms that pattern heart tube formation, chamber differentiation, and vascular network organization. Additionally, a thorough review is given of the genetic cause of common congenital heart defects and approaches to reproducing the conditions in animal models.

Chapter 5 covers limb and skeletal development, detailing the signaling centers—e.g., apical ectodermal ridge and zone of polarizing activity—that organize the limb bud and the transcriptional cascades that bring about chondrogenesis and ossification. Genetic mutations underlying skeletal dysplasia's provide examples of how single-gene defects can change bone structure. Chapter 6 covers development of the genital and urinary system, highlighting the genetic and hormonal mechanisms that regulate sexual differentiation, nephron development, and ureter formation. Disorders of sex development and congenital renal malformations are covered both from mechanistic and clinical viewpoints.

Chapter 7 addresses craniofacial development and genetics and the neural crest cell migration that underlies facial skeleton and associated soft tissue formation. The chapter discusses the genetic basis of craniofacial syndromes and how defects in cell migration and differentiation can result in phenotypes such as cleft lip, Pierre Robin sequence, and craniosynostosis. Chapter 8 explores genetic regulation of organogenesis in several systems and themes of lung, liver, pancreas, and gastrointestinal tract development. The chapter emphasizes transcription factors and microRNA networks in regulating tissue-specific differentiation.

Chapter 9 discusses epigenetic control of embryonic development, from how DNA methyltransferases, histone modifiers, and noncoding RNAs orchestrate developmental gene expression programs to how epigenetic dysregulation has just been implicated in imprinting disorders and developmental delay. Chapter 10 discusses prenatal genetic diagnosis and screening, from noninvasive prenatal testing (NIPT) to invasive sampling and chromosomal microarray analysis. Ethical issues and counseling strategies in pregnant parents are also discussed in the chapter.

Chapter 11 discusses gene editing and developmental studies, highlighting CRISPR-based approaches to the study of gene function *in vivo*, disease modeling, and gene correction therapy. Methods, technical issues, and potentialities are described with practical suggestions. Chapter 12 finally connects basic research to clinical practice in genetic counseling and translational embryology. Suggestions for putting developmental discoveries into risk assessment, family planning, and patient care are provided, with emphasis on interdisciplinary communication between the bench scientist and clinician.

This book will be useful to postdoctoral fellows, senior scientists, and graduate students interested in regenerative medicine, genetics, and developmental biology. Clinicians practicing maternal–fetal medicine and genetic counseling units will appreciate detailed descriptions of diagnostic methods and paradigms in counseling. Teachers and senior undergraduate students interested in a treatise on the genetic aspects of embryogenesis will also find the blend of conceptual introductions and experimental protocols useful.

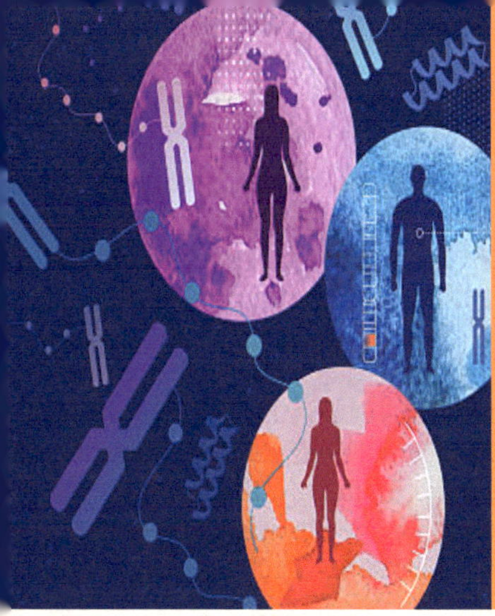

Chapter 1

ZYGOTIC GENOME ACTIVATION AND EARLY EMBRYO DEVELOPMENT

Contents

Introduction

Unraveling the intricate workings of zygotic genome activation (ZGA) is crucial to know the dynamics of early embryo development. ZGA is a milestone in embryogenesis when the process of transforming a fertilized egg, or zygote, to a higher level that can move to the next developmental processes begins. It is during this crucial phase that the embryo makes a transition towards genome-dependent development from maternal to zygotic control. The transition is vital because it lays the foundation for all subsequent cellular divisions and differentiation processes. Experiments have demonstrated that multiple factors and regulatory processes are involved in ZGA, indicating its significance in the promotion of embryonic development success and the establishment of developmental programs governing further development. Notwithstanding the importance of ZGA, mechanisms that govern this process remain far from an understanding, especially in mammalian organisms. Recent studies indicate a sophisticated interaction between maternal and cellular signaling pathways that control the timing of

ZGA. As an example, recent research illustrates the role of TRPS1 as a maternal factor in controlling the 2-cell to 4-cell embryo transition. Loss of TRPS1 has been reported to hinder ZGA by promoting the activation of the AKT/CREB signaling pathway, which is involved in the phosphorylation of essential proteins for genome activation. These findings shed light on the importance of maternal input to embryonic development and highlight the extent to which disruption in these regulatory processes could give rise to developmental anomalies and thus highlight the significance of this field of research in reproductive biology and developmental genetics (Jiang et al., 2025). In addition, the extent to which metabolic processes are intertwined with ZGA cannot be exaggerated. The tricarboxylic acid (TCA) cycle, vital for energy and metabolite supply, is closely linked with the molecular events of ZGA. It has been shown that core TCA cycle enzymes can transiently localize to the nucleus, suggesting direct participation in the initiation of ZGA events such as epigenetic control and chromatin remodeling. Notably, Developmental Pluripotency Associated 2's (DPPA2) role in this direction is revealed through its ability to determine the localization of TCA cycle enzymes and thereby influence the initiation and progression of early embryonic growth. These findings suggest that ZGA not only constitutes a transcriptional process but also a complicated process entangled with metabolic control, advocating for integrative studies that connect cellular metabolism and embryonic developmental changes (Di et al., 2025) (Figure 1.1).

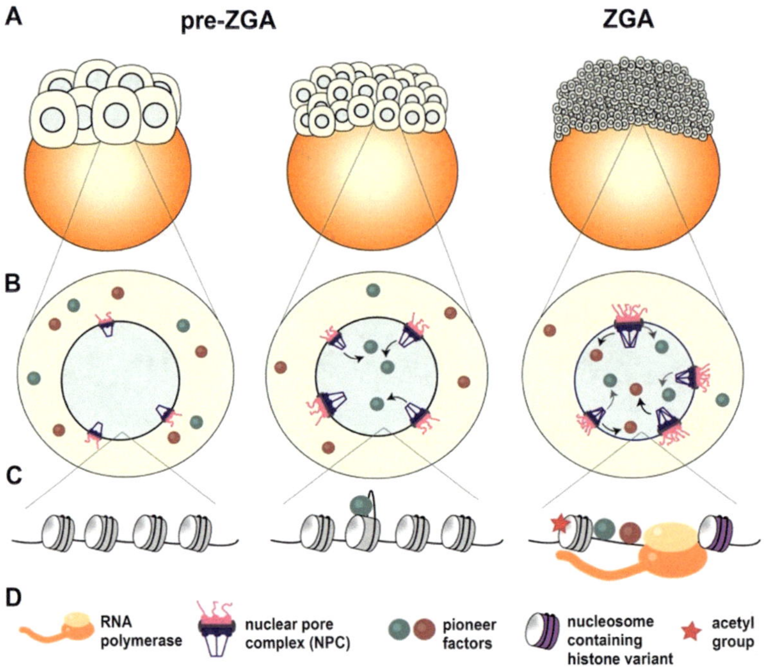

Figure 1.1. Zygotic genome activation and early embryo development.

Source: https://ars.els-cdn.com/content/image/1-s2.0-S0959437X23000424-gr1.jpg.

Definition of Zygotic Genome Activation (ZGA)

ZGA is a turning point process during initial embryo development, where the switch from maternal control to embryonic control of development takes place. In mice, the process commonly happens at the 2-cell stage, while in pigs it happens close to the 4 to 8-cell stage. At ZGA, the embryo starts to express its own genome, allowing it to harness its genetic material well for further developmental procedures. The coordination of this transition is highly important since it sets the stage for cellular differentiation and embryonic identity formation. The timing and regulation of ZGA are also different between species and can affect developmental events. A comprehension of these differences is important since it not only explains normal embryonic development but also sheds some light on developmental disorders that arise because ZGA fails to happen normally. Some recent studies have shown the significant role of certain maternal factors in controlling ZGA. For example, it was shown that the maternal factor TRPS1 was essential for 2-cell to 4-cell transition in mice, which reflects its important role in ZGA. The lack of TRPS1 was found to compromise ZGA by interfering with the AKT/CREB signaling pathway, and this identifies a particular route along which maternal influences affect embryo development at this pivotal point. In addition, research underlines that TRPS1 can influence the transcription of Phosphodiesterase 4D (PDE4D), which can affect the phosphorylation of key regulatory proteins during ZGA. These results highlight the intricacy of ZGA regulation and demonstrate how the interaction between maternal influences and embryonic genome activation is important for normal preimplantation development, important for subsequent embryogenesis stages (Jiang et al., 2025). Aside from maternal influences, long noncoding RNAs (lncRNAs) have also been identified as crucial regulatory components in ZGA, especially in other species like pigs. The lncRNA lncFKBPL is a enhancer-type lncRNA that is responsible for embryonic development in pigs, and the expression of this lncRNA plays a major role in ZGA. The lncRNA interacts with MED8 and CDK9 proteins, thus affecting transcriptional machinery as well as the phosphorylation of RNA polymerase II, an important step for ZGA. If lncFKBPL is disrupted, developmental arrest takes place, especially at the 8-cell stage. These observations shed light on the complex aspects of ZGA, highlighting how maternal elements and molecular elements such as lncRNAs act synergistically to allow early embryo development. These findings open the doors for better comprehension and future investigations into regulatory processes behind ZGA in other vertebrates (Wei et al., 2025) (Figure 1.2).

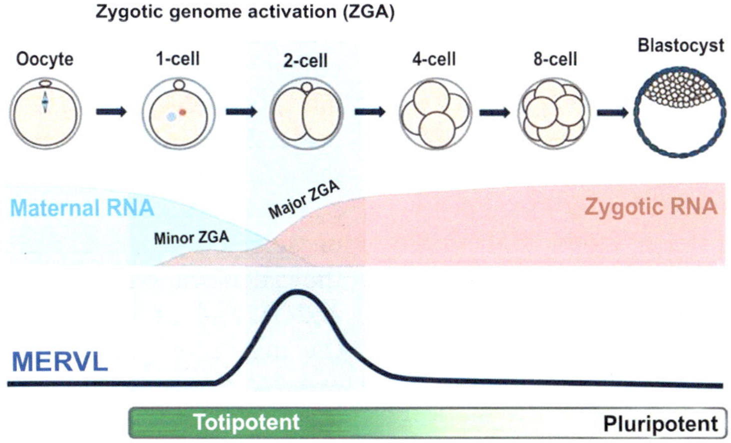

Figure 1.2. Zygotic genome activation (ZGA).

Source: https://www.researchgate.net/publication/386047681/figure/fig1/AS:11431281299813858@1735062560071/Mouse-preimplantation-development-and-zygotic-genome-activation-ZGA-are-accompanied-by.png.

Importance of Zygotic Genome Activation (ZGA) in Embryonic Development

The ZGA process is most critical during embryonic development, which represents a turning point in shifting development control from maternal to zygotic. Following fertilization, the embryo uses maternal mRNAs and proteins for an initial cellular response; however, ZGA represents the stage at which the zygotic genome is activated to be transcriptionally active. The activation is crucial as it is responsible for embryonic autonomy and the regulation of the proper developmental pathways. ZGA disturbances are known to cause developmental abnormalities, emphasizing its importance in ensuring the embryo can navigate major development stages. The transformation caused by ZGA allows the embryos to initiate their genetic programming, which will eventually control cell fate determination and the capacity for additional differentiation and growth. Experiments have revealed that ZGA is not only a transcription process but also directly linked with the metabolic processes that are required for embryonic development. Indeed, studies confirm the involvement of core enzymes of the TCA cycle in initiating ZGA. Reports have it that these metabolic enzymes transiently travel to the nucleus during the process of ZGA, providing developmental processes with requisite metabolites. For instance, Dppa2 significantly impacted the nuclear import of TCA core enzymes and the enhancement of zygotic genome activation. This relationship demonstrates a sophisticated cross-talk between transcriptional activation and metabolism, suggesting that energy supply and metabolic signaling might be involved in the successful execution of ZGA in the earliest seconds of development, as recently reported (Di et al., 2025). Subsequent research has clarified the regulatory process controlling ZGA, demonstrating the roles of particular maternal factors. For example, the maternal protein TRPS1 is recognized as a significant regulator in the process of 2-cell-to-4-cell embryo transition to directly affect ZGA by way of the AKT/CREB signaling pathway. Notably, the absence of TRPS1 interferes with the process of ZGA and induces probable developmental retardation. Further, by controlling Pde4d transcription, TRPS1 appears to be controlling AKT and CREB phosphorylation, which are vital for the successful completion of ZGA. This intricate system of regulation emphasizes the importance of ZGA in guaranteeing accurate embryonic development because any disturbance in these processes can threaten the developmental course, illustrating the delicate balance necessary for effective early embryogenesis (Jiang et al., 2025).

1.1. The Process of Zygotic Genome Activation (ZGA)

The onset of ZGA represents a significant turning point in the developmental course of vertebrate embryos. After fertilization, regulation of gene expression is gradually taken over by the zygotic genome from the maternal mRNAs and proteins. This process is essential for the acquisition of embryonic identity and proper development pathways. The timing and regulation of ZGA are controlled tightly by a number of factors, including transcription factors that allow the genome to react to signaling pathways and turn on selected genes. Current studies emphasize the crucial function of factors like Dux, DPPA2, and DPPA4 in mediating this process. With the increasing transcriptional activity of the zygotic genome, the embryo is set up for further developmental stages, requiring a very orchestrated set of events that lead to gene expression and cellular differentiation. Metabolic activity is crucial in the regulation of ZGA, as energy availability and biochemical resources are the cornerstones of embryonic development. The TCA cycle being involved has been found to be a pivotal player in this role. Specifically, key enzymes of the TCA cycle were demonstrated to move into the nucleus during activation, affecting genome activation and epigenetic modification. Di et al. (2025) describes how these enzymes are involved in essential processes such as opening chromatin and creating a suitable metabolic landscape for gene expression.

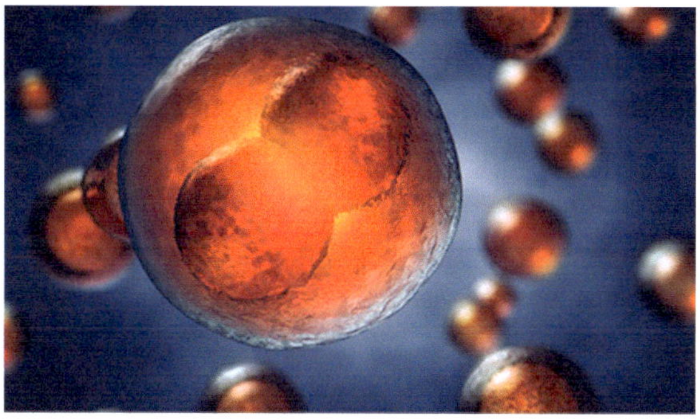

Figure 1.3. Zygotic Genome Activation (ZGA) process.

Source: https://www.activemotif.com/uploads/images/web_site/resources-page/blog/zygotic-genome-activation/zygotic-genome-activation-web.jpg.

In addition, the immediate interaction between TCA cycle enzymes and ZGA factors such as DPPA2 highlights the integrative function of transcriptional activity and metabolism in early stages of development during the embryo. The cross-talk between the two systems not only assists in zygotic genome activation but also supports cellular functions required for embryonic development. Epigenetic changes yet again introduce a level of sophistication to ZGA and embryonic development, determining the expression of genes in the initial stages. Maintaining particular chromatin states from gametes is an important mechanism that guarantees effective ZGA. Previous research has demonstrated that H3K4 methylation marks are required to preserve this epigenetic memory of active chromatin states in embryos, which is essential to help regulate gene expression after and during the ZGA process. Meghana et al. (2025) presents strong evidence from *Xenopus laevis*, showing that such epigenetic modifications are necessary for the expression of essential transcription factors during ZGA. While the embryo moves from transcriptional quiescence to active gene expression, chromatin modification dynamics like H3K4me3 make sure that core developmental programs are efficiently initiated, thereby supporting successful embryogenesis (Figure 1.3).

1.1.1. Timing of Zygotic Genome Activation (ZGA) in Various Species

The timing of ZGA is pivotal during the initial phases of embryonic development in many species. In mammals, ZGA happens comparatively late in life, usually during the 4- to 8-cell stage. The delay is thought to enable the initial dependence on maternal transcripts and proteins that are stored in the oocyte before fertilization. On the other hand, in organisms like zebrafish and amphibians, ZGA happens much earlier, at the 1- to 2-cell stage, facilitating quick developmental transition directly after fertilization. Knowledge about such variations in timing sheds light on the evolutionary innovations that have influenced embryonic development so that researchers can examine how maternal contributions affect ensuing dependence on the zygotic genome. Therefore, the timing of ZGA is not simply of interest but a critical transition that determines the developmental course of many species. Moreover, recent work highlights mechanistic nuances behind ZGA across taxa. For example, research illustrates that in the murine model, zygotic factors like Dux are essential regulators of ZGA, inducing transcriptional cascades required for initial embryogenesis. In humans, new methods have been developed to study ZGA dynamics, showing that modifications of the timing and regulation of the process can have a cascading effect on embryonic development and cause reproductive difficulties, such as early pregnancy loss. New developments employing technology to simulate human embryonic conditions *in vitro* offer new evidence on the processes that occur during ZGA, as scientists seek to understand how the difference in timing of ZGA gives rise to the particular developmental needs of mammals. These investigations gain a better understanding of the genetic and environmental factors during development, which can eventually be used to develop therapeutic interventions for individuals with early pregnancy complications. Additionally, the consequences of these varying ZGA timings go beyond simple developmental biology and impact the research in gene regulatory networks (GRN) and tissue morphogenesis. Since ZGA is the point at which control of gene expression begins to switch from maternal to zygotic levels, knowledge about its timing allows for insights into how embryonic structures arise. The complex interplay between tissue organization and cell fate decisions at this stage is crucial to body plan specification in various species, a theme highlighted by recent studies analyzing how ZGA impacts developmental outcomes. By analyzing the fundamental processes controlling ZGA timing in different species, researchers can establish new hypotheses concerning evolutionary pressures and create interventions that could prevent risks in early embryonic development, thus targeting an important area of reproductive well-being, as emphasized in the newly emerging research (Bentsen et al., 2020; Marta, 2020) (Figure 1.4).

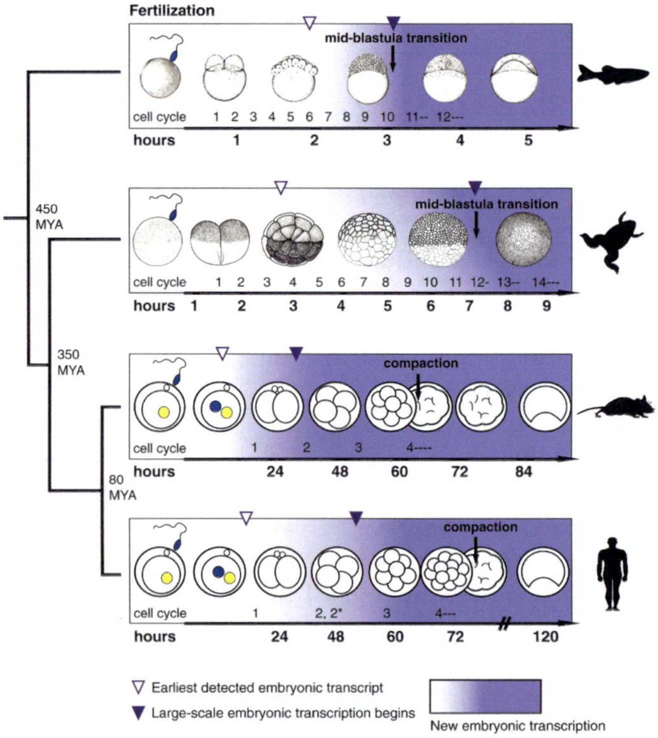

Figure 1.4. Timing of zygotic genome activation (ZGA) in various species.

Source: https://www.cell.com/cms/10.1016/j.devcel.2017.07.026/asset/3955897b-3118-4402-ac6d-f34049af3130/main.assets/gr1_lrg.jpg.

1.1.2. Molecular Mechanisms Involved in Zygotic Genome Activation (ZGA)

The ZGA process is a turning point in early embryonic development, where there is a switch from maternal to zygotic regulation of gene expression. The switch is initiated through sophisticated molecular processes that enable widespread genomic reprogramming of the embryo. Pioneering research has identified key factors responsible for ZGA induction, with emphasis on the functions of DNA-binding proteins and chromatin remodelers to enable ZGA. For example, our knowledge has evolved tremendously through methods such as CRISPR activation, which have been utilized to identify major regulators of ZGA-like transcription in mouse embryonic stem cells (mESCs). These have shown molecular signatures critical for ZGA, citing 24 factors that act together to favor this activation, such as notable players such as DPPA2 and SNF2 Related Chromatin Remodeling ATPase 5 (SMARCA5), emphasizing the complexity of the regulatory network that oversees early embryonic development (Alda-Catalinas et al., 2020).

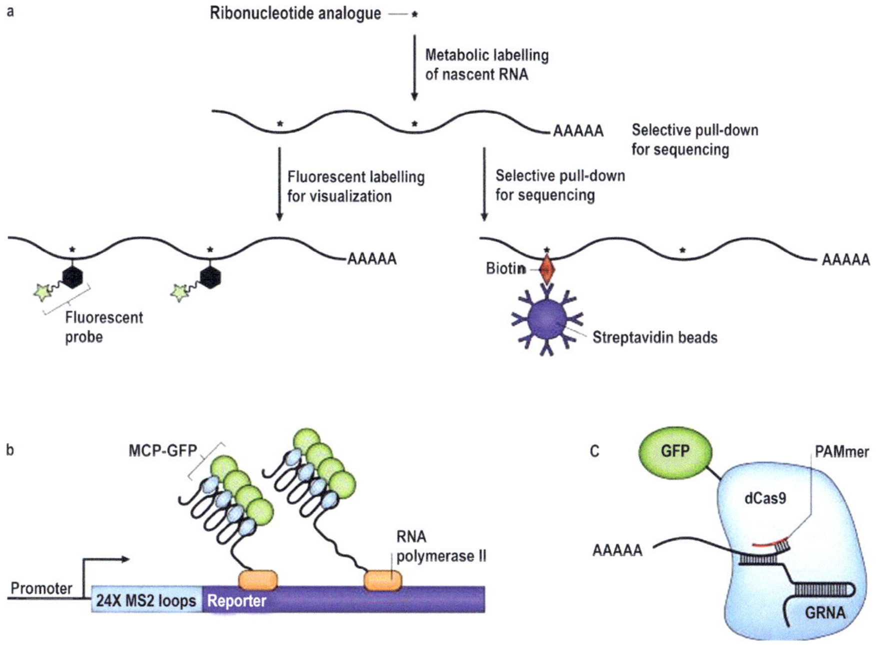

Figure 1.5. Molecular mechanisms involved in zygotic genome activation (ZGA).

Source: https://media.springernature.com/m685/springer-static/image/art%3A10.1038%2Fs41576-018-0087-x/MediaObjects/41576_2018_87_Fig1_HTML.png.

Apart from determining crucial regulators, recent studies have clarified the interactions of different molecular components participating in ZGA. Precisely, Dppa2 and Dppa4 have been defined as being required transcription factors that affect the zygotic transcriptional program. They operate upstream of the double homeobox (Dux), a gene important for determining the embryonic transcription network. These interactions highlight the necessity of particular protein modifications, i.e., sumoylation, in influencing the activity of these transcription factors. The PIAS4 Sumo E3 ligase has been demonstrated to have a negative regulatory effect on DPPA2. Since PIAS4 is repressed during ZGA, removal of this inhibition is essential for enabling the activation of the 2C-like transcriptional program in both ESCs and early embryos (Yan et al., 2019). Furthermore, the proper functioning of ZGA is not only dependent on individual regulatory elements but also on the timely and coordinated execution of these molecular processes. The switch from maternal mRNA dependency to zygotic control entails a finely regulated interplay between transcriptional activation and repression mechanisms. Functional experiments have shown that disruptions in ZGA regulators can significantly impact embryo viability and development. For instance, blocking DPPA2 activity or deregulating PIAS4 impairs early embryonic development in a dramatic manner, which mirrors the sensitivity of the regulatory network in question. The sophisticated layering of transcriptional activation, chromatin remodeling, and epigenetic reprogramming reflects the molecular ballet required in order for ZGA to be successful, which is crucial for later stages of embryo development (Alda-Catalinas et al., 2020) (Figure 1.5).

1.1.3. Role of Transcription Factors in Initiating Zygotic Genome Activation (ZGA)

Transcription factors are central to initiating ZGA, a vital aspect of early embryonic development. ZGA initiates the switch from maternal to zygotic control of embryogenesis and requires a precise coordination of gene expression. Transcription factors like Dorsal and Grainy head are crucial for determining spatial and temporal patterns of gene activity in embryos undergoing development. For example, in *Drosophila* embryos, Dorsal levels form dorsal-ventral gradients necessary for cell fate organization. Recent work has indicated that the activator Grainyhead not only amplifies expression of certain genes but also functions in conjunction with repressors to form sharp gene expression boundaries, enhancing the subtle regulatory networks underlying ZGA. This dynamic interaction between transcription factors highlights their role in laying the groundwork for the rest of the developmental processes necessary for embryogenesis (Jazwinska et al., 2011). In addition, the role of transcription factors is not just limited to the regulation of the zygotic genome activation; they play a crucial role in cell lineage specification and maintaining pluripotency. A good example is the transcription factor POU5F1, which is a master cell pluripotency regulator during early embryo development. It has different roles in different species, but its alteration through CRISPR/Cas9 in cattle has shown important effects on blastocyst formation and embryo viability. In POU5F1-deficient embryos, some development steps are normal, but the loss of this transcription factor results in abnormal expression of essential genes such as CDX2, which underlines its function in lineage specification.

This illustrates how transcription factors not only allow ZGA but also allow proper differentiation of embryonic cells into specialized structures required for successful development (Daigneault et al., 2018). The role of transcription factors in triggering ZGA and controlling downstream developmental programs cannot be overemphasized. They create complex networks that dictate when and how a particular gene is expressed within an embryonic window of critical development. Their capacity to engage with both activators and repressors makes them enable complex regulation of gene expression profiles necessary for proper embryonic morphogenesis. Also, transcription factor function conservation across species, as revealed by mammalian studies, illustrates their underlying role in developmental biology. With continued discovery of these molecular processes, the possibility of manipulating transcription factor pathways offers tantalizing opportunities for advances in reproductive technologies as well as therapeutic intervention in developmental diseases, eventually providing further insight into embryonic development (Daigneault et al., 2018; Jazwinska et al., 2011) (Figure 1.6).

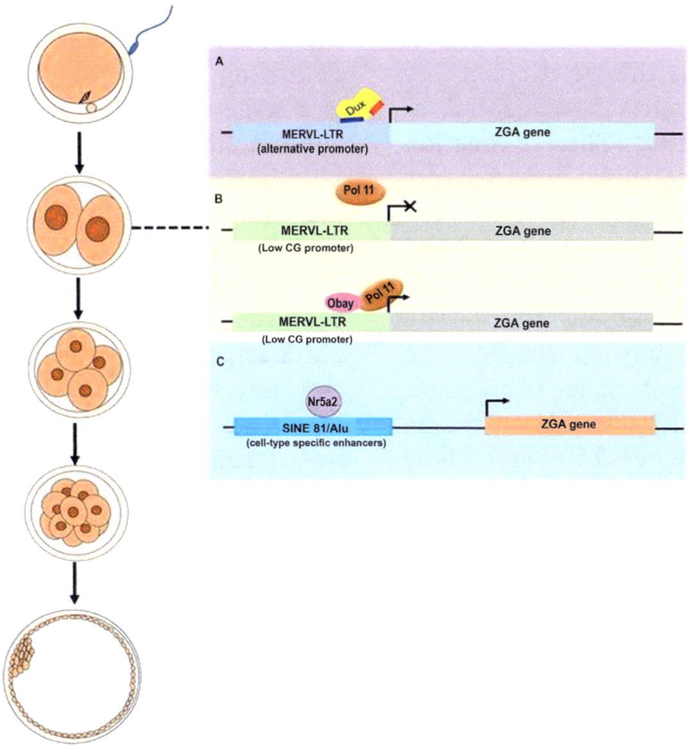

Figure 1.6. Role of transcription factors in initiating zygotic genome activation (ZGA).

Source: https://pub.mdpi-res.com/biomolecules/biomolecules-14-00720/article_deploy/html/images/biomolecules-14-00720-g001-550.jpg?1718699173.

1.2. Significance of Zygotic Genome Activation (ZGA) in Development

ZGA is a critical transition point in early embryonic development when maternal control shifts to zygotic control of gene expression. ZGA triggers the activation of the zygotic genome, enabling the embryo to use its genetic resources to propel further development and differentiation. Interestingly, the transcriptional profile during ZGA is defined by a significant upregulation in the expression of totipotency-related genes, which are fundamental in ensuring the potential of the embryo to give rise to any cell type. Based on recent research, the Dux cluster has an essential role as a master regulator in ZGA, marking its importance in triggering these indispensable genes for normal embryonic development (Lin et al., 2025). In this regulation, ZGA directs several of the genetic programs needed for the proper transition from single-cell zygote to multi-cellular organism. The biochemical conditions at the time of ZGA are also critical, as they must provide embryos with the energy and metabolic building blocks needed to sustain the extensive transcriptional activation that takes place. Recent findings indicate an important interaction between metabolic pathways, specifically the TCA cycle, and ZGA. Enzymes of the TCA cycle have been reported to transiently cross the nuclear membrane, engaging in essential activities like chromatin restructuring and gene activation during this pivotal stage of development. The function of Dppa2, a ZGA factor, also demonstrates this relationship by having an effect on the nuclear localization of the essential TCA enzymes. This connection not only highlights the metabolic requirements during ZGA but also suggests an advanced regulatory network in which metabolism and transcription intersect to promote normal embryo development (Di et al., 2025). The importance of ZGA goes beyond simple gene activation; it provides a platform for subsequent developmental events, which critically depend on the timely and accurate expression of embryonic genes. While ZGA enables the formation of gene networks that guide cell fate decisions as well as differentiation, disruption or delay in this process can have catastrophic effects on the embryo. Experiments using CRISPR-Cas9 technology to genetically modify the Dux gene cluster are a prime example of the significance of this regulatory process. With decreased copies of genes, the corresponding drop in the activation of genes related to totipotency serves to demonstrate the indispensable role these transcriptional regulators play in guaranteeing normal embryonic development. In conclusion, comprehension of ZGA's intricacies not only explains the core concepts of developmental biology but also facilitates better handling of developmental disorders caused by dysregulated gene activation at early life stages (Lin et al., 2025).

1.2.1. Transition from Maternal to Zygotic Control

Maternal to zygotic transition is a key period in early embryo development, representing a shift in control mechanisms as the embryo transitions from maternal gene product dependency to the use of its genomic potential. Early in development, the maternal factors that are deposited into the oocyte by the mother provide initial developmental directions. This maternal regulation offers the biochemical environment necessary for the survival of the embryo and the initiation of cell division. Following growth in embryonic stages, there is a stage called ZGA (ZGA), where the zygotic genome starts to assume the role of regulation. This intricate process is not just a change but includes complex processes of transcriptional activity and maternal mRNA degradation, paving the way for an appropriately functioning embryo that can develop on its own. Research has emphasized the influential role of factors in the maternal-to-zygotic transition. An example is how maternal mRNA and zygotic transcription interact and play an essential part in organizing a functional embryonic environment. When the embryo switches on its genome, some of the maternal transcripts are selectively broken down, and zygotic genes are expressed under controlled conditions. Selective activation and breakdown are tightly regulated, enabling the embryo to achieve specific patterns of gene expression required for proper development. In this stage, the stability factor of Bicoid becomes a critical player by correlating the morphogen gradients with the schedule of zygotic gene activity. This precise coordination demonstrates the embryos flexibility and responsiveness to its developmental environment to ensure it can survive under different conditions. In addition, maternal to zygotic transition is not only essential for proper development but also shows unprecedented plasticity towards environmental cues. Research, for example, performed in *Drosophila melanogaster*, reveals that maternal diet can influence the mRNA content of the egg to orient the developing embryo for possible adverse environments. Nutrient-restricted mothers display alterations in the number of particular transcripts, especially those engaged in energetically expensive functions like translation. Consequently, the eggs laid display a strong adaptation, modifying mRNA deposition in order to better prepare the ensuing embryo for survival. This component of maternal investment emphasizes the evolutionary relevance of the transition since it predicts that maternal conditions have a direct impact on zygotic success, which renders understanding of the transition crucial for the understanding of early embryo development across various species (Arbeitman et al., 2007; Cartwright et al., 2018) (Figure 1.7).

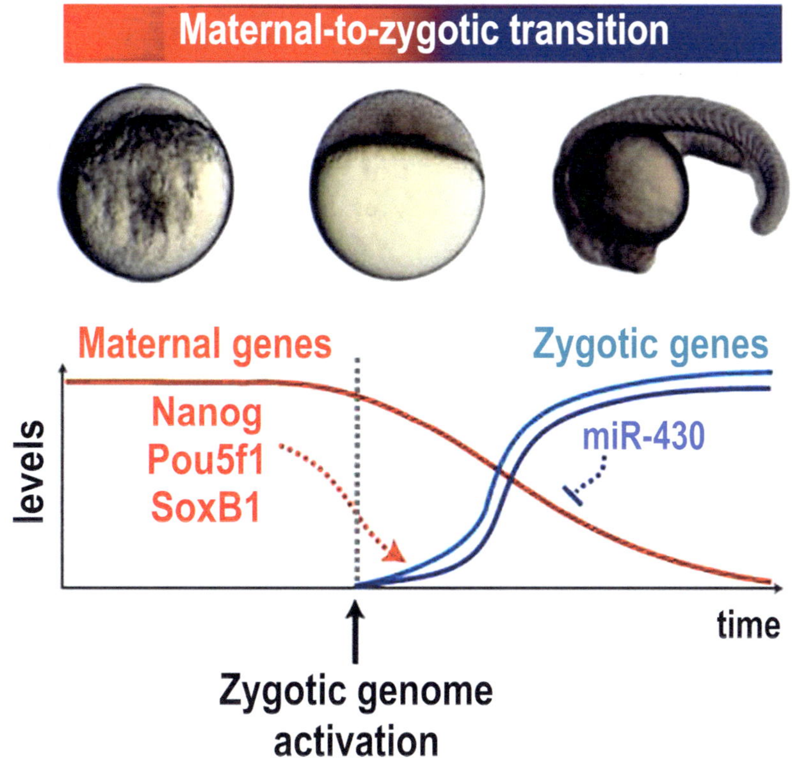

Figure 1.7. Transition from maternal to zygotic control.

Source: https://www.yalescientific.org/wp-content/uploads/2013/12/domino1-500x474.png.

1.2.2. Impact on Cell Differentiation and Development

The ZGA process is a key aspect of embryonic development during early stages since it triggers a cascade of cellular events leading to cell differentiation and maturation. During the late-2-cell stage, ZGA is vital in that it provides the point of shift from maternal control to zygotic control of gene expression. This transition not only begins the expression of hundreds of genes but also affects major developmental pathways that are necessary for the segmentation of embryonic lineage. A key part of this process involves the regulation of diverse chromatin remodeling proteins and transcription factors, which in turn ensure the correct timing and spatial patterns of expression required for successful cell differentiation and development. Appreciation of these dynamics is a key to understanding how deviations in ZGA can result in severe developmental abnormalities, thereby underpinning the significance of the phase in embryo viability and healthy development later on. Recent studies underscore the importance of certain molecules responsible for ZGA and their role in cell differentiation. For example, GATAD2B has been recognized as a central subunit of the Nucleosome Remodeling and Deacetylation (NuRD) complex and is crucial for remodeling chromatin structures to trigger gene activation. Experiments show that GATAD2B depletion causes ZGA defects, with detectable effects like enhanced DNA damage, defective differentiation between inner cell mass and trophectoderm lineages, and changes in the cell cycle. These observations emphasize the subtle balance between chromatin movements at ZGA and ensuing processes that control cell fate choices. Through an understanding of protein function, such as for GATAD2B, we may gain insight into the molecular complexities that regulate embryonic development and which may ultimately guide clinical strategies towards overcoming early developmental flaws. Sperm-derived components also play a role in shaping the initial stages of embryogenesis, adding to the complexity of cell differentiation processes. Recent evidence has shown sperm non-coding RNAs, and more importantly, circRNA-1572 to be key regulators of developmental pathways in the early embryo. Such non-coding RNAs act by mechanisms that include binding and regulating the function of certain microRNAs that, in turn, regulate genes that are responsible for fundamental cellular processes such as the cell cycle. Significantly, perturbations of such RNAs' expression or function can interfere with regular chromosomal structure and F-actin distribution and cause developmental blockage or defective ZGA. The complex interaction between these paternal components and the maternal environment in early development explains the complexity of early embryo development, leading us to think of the general implications of parental contributions on cell fate and organismal health (Cao, 2024; Wu et al., 2025).

1.2.3. Consequences of Disrupted Zygotic Genome Activation (ZGA) on Embryo Viability

The shift of control from the maternal to the zygotic level in the course of embryonic development, termed as zygotic genome activation (ZGA), is a turning point that highly contributes to embryo viability. Interference with ZGA may cause a large array of cellular and developmental abnormalities, which compromise the possibility of normal embryogenesis. It is at this stage that the zygote starts to express its genome, shifting from its dependence on maternal mRNA and proteins to its own genetic coding. Incomplete or interrupted ZGA can lead to a failure to initiate crucial genes necessary for further cleavage divisions, which in turn causes notable developmental delays or even total cessation of emerging embryo growth. Such interference undermines the sophisticated choreography of cellular activities, which leads to less viable embryos that are even unable to move on to implantation. The effects of disturbed ZGA are not limited to outright developmental arrest but can extend to long-term genomic and epigenomic integrity. Recent evidence points toward the pivotal importance of DNA methylation patterns at early embryonic stages in controlling gene expression and guaranteeing cellular differentiation. If ZGA fails to take place in the manner planned, the resulting hypomethylation or aberrant methylation can guide cellular lineage specification astray. As suggested by recent data, proper methylation landscape establishment is necessary for cellular identity maintenance and the avoidance of primordial state regression. The inability of ZGA to appropriately reset the epigenetic environment can therefore result in major deviations of gene expression patterns, ultimately damaging the embryos developmental path and viability (Daniel et al., 2014). In addition, the consequences of compromised ZGA can be further compounded by maternal nutritional status and environmental conditions. Maternal nutritional deficiencies have also been found to permanently influence DNA chemistry in the offspring, as proven in experiments with undernourished pregnant mice. Offspring from such a background showed inappropriate DNA packaging elements and impaired metabolic status, predicting possible embryonic failures due to aberrant ZGA (Elizabeth et al., 2014). Maternal health is therefore closely related to the success of the zygote in meeting the challenges of early development. The synergistic effect of compromised ZGA and pernicious maternal conditions highlights the importance of an integrated comprehension of determinants of embryo viability and calls for continued research in this vital field of developmental biology (Figure 1.8).

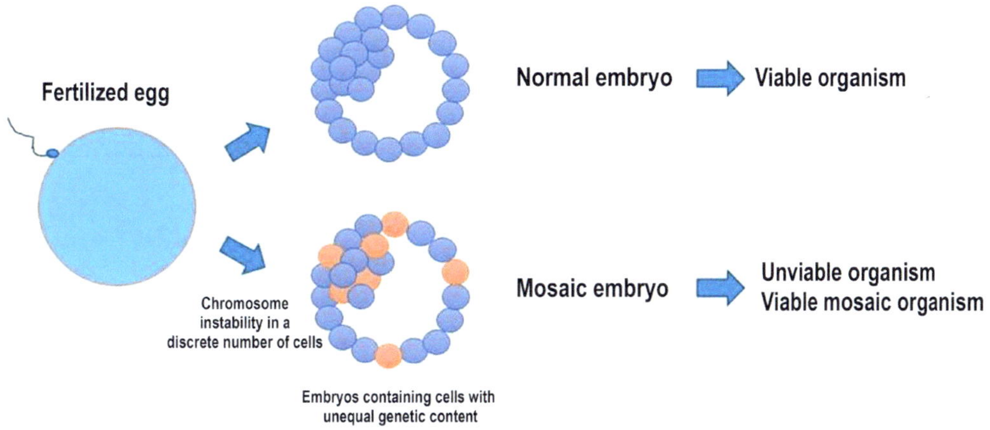

Figure 1.8. Consequences of disrupted zygotic genome activation (ZGA) on embryo viability.

Source: https://www.researchgate.net/publication/333366638/figure/fig4/AS:11431281369782592@1744314566140/Consequences-of-chromosome-abnormalities-in-early-mammalian-embryos-Each-circle.tif.

1.3. Factors Influencing Zygotic Genome Activation (ZGA)

The complex mechanism of ZGA is conditioned by a diversity of factors that are responsible for early embryo development. Among the major determinants, the chromatin structure stands out, which is subject to profound remodeling as the system switches from a transcriptionally silent to a transcriptionally active genomic context. Recent research has shown that the 3D chromatin structure in the nucleus is crucial for gene expression regulation and is responsible for structuring the genomic landscape into topologically associating domains (TADs) and compartments. During ZGA, restoration of these structures helps recruit the transcription factors, such as RNA polymerase II, necessary to initiate transcription. By providing an environment that supports gene activation, chromatin structure significantly influences how developmental programs are implemented during early embryo development (Clemens et al., 2018). Maternal input is also critical to ZGA beyond chromatin structure. Maternally deposited mRNAs and proteins in the oocyte during oogenesis act as the initial regulators before zygotic transcription is initiated. Particularly, the maternal-to-zygotic transition (MZT) is defined by the breakdown of these maternal components and concurrent activation of the zygotic genome. Of one such important maternal component, Stella, it has been determined that it plays an important role in the proper activation of endogenous retroviruses (ERVs), which are known to play a role in controlling embryonic gene expression. Stella's absence causes general transcriptional dysregulation and defective activation of ERVs, indicating the critical role of maternal elements in creating the proper conditions for ZGA (Huang et al., 2017). In addition to this, external environmental components may contribute to the regulation of ZGA, demonstrating the intricacy of this developmental process. Temperature, nutrient level, and hormonal cues could impact embryonic viability and the regulation of ZGA. For example, metabolic condition deviations may change the pathways of signaling that regulate early development gene expression. New findings suggest that the epigenetic landscape, defined by histone and DNA modifications, is dynamic and sensitive to environmental cues. These modifications may be enhancing or suppressing transcriptional activity, thus influencing ZGAs efficiency and timing. The interaction of chromatin remodeling, maternal contributions, and environmental factors ultimately determines the embryonic epigenomic landscape and directs successful maternal-to-zygotic transition during early embryo development (Clemens et al., 2018) (Figure 1.9).

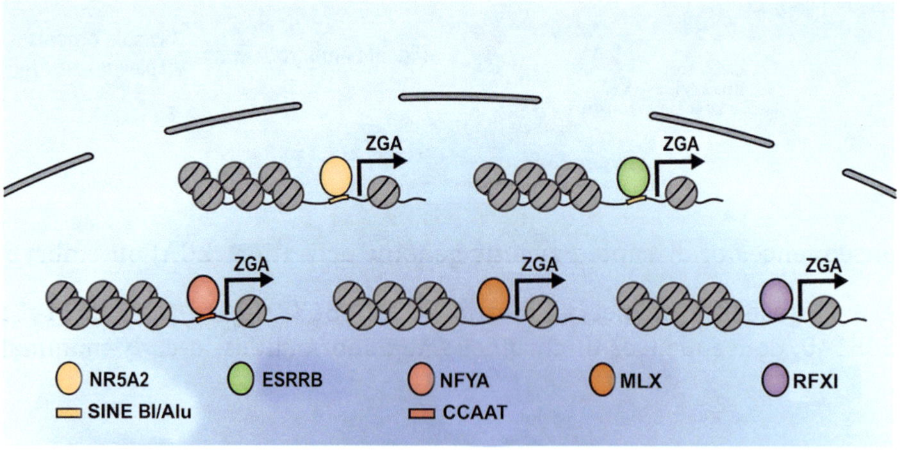

Figure 1.9. Factors influencing zygotic genome activation (ZGA).

Source: https://www.researchgate.net/publication/372964840/figure/fig6/AS:11431281181877903@1692204336287/An-overview-of-pioneer-transcript-factors-important-for-zygotic-genome-activation-ZGA.png.

1.3.1. Environmental Factors Affecting Zygotic Genome Activation (ZGA)

The initiation of ZGA is heavily dependent on environmental conditions, which are instrumental in the development of early embryos. A major determinant includes the metabolic status of the embryo and is directly related to the availability of required nutrients and cellular energy. Under ZGA, the TCA cycle is essential for the provision of reactants and energy required for genomic activation and remodeling of chromatin. Current research establishes the role of central TCA cycle enzymes moving into the nucleus, which in turn facilitates the activation of the zygotic genome. The relationship between DPPA2 and TCA enzymes plays an important role in ZGA and, consequently, early embryonic development. This indicates that environmental factors that affect metabolic pathways can indirectly control ZGA by modifying enzyme localization and activity, thus affecting gene expression and developmental results (Di et al., 2025). Besides metabolic factors, epigenetic signatures inherited from the gametes also have significant roles in controlling ZGA. For example, certain histone marks, e.g., H3K4 methylation, have an epigenetic memory that is essential for the shift from maternal to zygotic control of embryonic gene expression. In organisms such as *Xenopus laevis*, gametic transmission of H3K4 methylation guarantees the maintenance of active chromatin states in the early embryo and thus favorable ZGA. This phenomenon shows that environmental conditions, such as the maternal environment and input into chromatin state, play a pivotal role in influencing epigenetic memory, consequently influencing ZGA efficiency and the correct timing of embryonic development. Therefore, both metabolic and epigenetic environmental conditions play a crucial role in controlling the ZGA dynamics, reflecting the intricacy of early embryogenesis (Meghana et al., 2025). The interaction between external conditions and ZGA is important in understanding developmental biology and the resistance of development to external conditions. For example, stressors like temperature stress or toxin exposure could make metabolic pathways and epigenetic stability vulnerable, causing aberrations of ZGA. These aberrations may be seen as developmental delay or malformations, reflecting the significance of a nurturing environment for successful embryogenesis. New studies point to the promise of environmental interventions, including maximizing maternal health and employing controlled environments in early embryonic life, to maximize ZGA success. These interventions would reduce risks that have been linked to inimical environmental influences, resulting in more effective embryo development. It will be imperative to recognize the complex relationships between environmental factors and ZGA for the development of reproductive technologies and the enhancement of developmental processes in different species (Di et al., 2025; Meghana et al., 2025) (Figure 1.10).

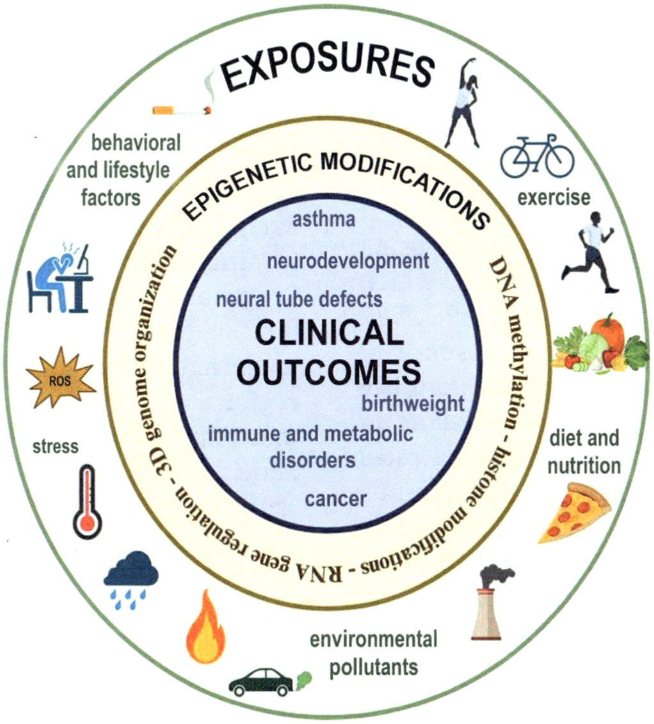

Figure 1.10. Environmental factors affecting zygotic genome activation (ZGA).

Source: https://media.springernature.com/lw685/springer-static/image/art%3A10.1186%2Fs13148-024-01762-3/MediaObjects/13148_2024_1762_Fig2_HTML.png.

1.3.2. Genetic Factors and Their Roles in Zygotic Genome Activation (ZGA)

The ZGA process is important in the development of the early embryo because it is the entry point from a transcriptionally repressed zygote to an active transcribing organism. Genetic components are major regulators of this transition, dictating the timing and degree of ZGA. At this early developmental stage, zygotic transcription activation is stringently regulated by a pool of transcription factors and epigenetic marks that coordinately act to establish correct embryonic gene expression. Research has indicated that the accurate coordination of these genetic components is crucial for the efficient differentiation of embryonic cells because their disruption will result in developmental defects. For example, the coordination of differential gene expression at ZGA not only governs cell fate but also guarantees the integrity of genetic information, making ZGA a gateway checkpoint in embryonic development. A key transcription factor linked to ZGA is POU5F1, which plays a critical role in pluripotency maintenance and early embryo development. The importance of POU5F1 is especially evident in research using gene editing tools, like CRISPR/Cas9, which enable the specific disruption of the POU5F1 gene. In the bovine embryos, the absence of functional POU5F1 causes a total inability to develop blastocysts and instead results in morula stage arrest. Even with identical rates of development and numbers of blastomeres as control embryos by day five, the lack of POU5F1 prevents proper expression patterns of other essential genes, such as CDX2, demonstrating a cascading effect on downstream genetic pathways. These observations identify the complex genetic networks that underlie ZGA and mark the crucial functions of particular transcription factors in guaranteeing proper early embryo development. Genetic stability balance is also crucial for the success of ZGA in embryogenesis. Somatic embryogenesis has been shown through research to pose drastically different genetic integrity in various plant families during the initial developmental stages. In Norway spruce studies, for instance, greater genetic stability in zygotic embryos was found compared to somatic embryos, illustrating inherent variability potentially affecting embryonic ability. Conversely, families with low genetic stability had a higher embryogenic potential at the cellular level. Yet, this seeming strength is mitigated by repressed embryo development in these very same genetically unstable families. The combined impact of genetic influences on both ZGA and total embryo viability highlights the intricate nature of early development, supporting the notion that genetic integrity and transcriptional regulation are inseparable in determining the course of embryonic development (Daigneault et al., 2018; Helmersson et al., 2007).

1.3.3. Epigenetic Modifications During Zygotic Genome Activation (ZGA)

ZGA represents a critical transition during early embryo development from maternal to embryonic regulation of gene expression. Epigenetic marking during this stage allows for the required reorganization of chromatin to permit access to otherwise latent genomic regions. One of the key mechanisms behind these marks is the addition of specific histone marks, like H3K4 methylation, which plays a critical role in defining active chromatin states. Studies reveal that enzymatic activities involved with such modifications, such as from the TCA cycle, are important to facilitate ZGA by offering requisite biochemical substrates that remodel the chromatin environment. This highlights the coordination between metabolic pathways and epigenetic regulation as central contributors to successful embryonic development during ZGA (Di et al., 2025). Furthermore, the transmission of epigenetic memory from gametes to zygotes underlies the regulatory framework controlling

ZGA. Research in model organisms, including *Xenopus laevis*, has revealed the significance of H3K4 methylation as a sign of active transcriptional domains that need to be preserved during the earliest phases of development. This epigenetic memory protects the important transcription factors, such as Pou5f3.2 and Sox3, to be produced at the right time to enable future embryonic differentiation. Interestingly, the activity of H3K4 methyltransferases guarantees the stable transfer of such modifications, yet again highlighting their significance in ensuring the required transcriptional activation at ZGA. Thus, knowing these mechanisms allows us to understand quite a lot regarding early embryos defining their developmental pathways (Meghana et al., 2025). The crosstalk between metabolic enzymes and epigenetic regulators at ZGA further strengthens our understanding of embryonic development at a molecular level. The localization of TCA cycle enzymes, e.g., pyruvate dehydrogenase (PDH), to enzymes emphasizes a new element of metabolic control that is involved in epigenetic alteration. For example, DPPA2 has been recognized as an important factor that guides the localization of these enzymes in the nucleus, thereby affecting the landscape of chromatin and patterns of gene expression necessary for the survival of the embryo. This exchange implies metabolic signals directly communicate with epigenetic modifications to ensure successful ZGA and ensuing developmental stages. Through exploration of these interactions, scientists can better understand the intricate networks that ensure successful embryo development, effectively paving the way for unraveling developmental dysregulation in pathologies (Di et al., 2025) (Figure 1.11).

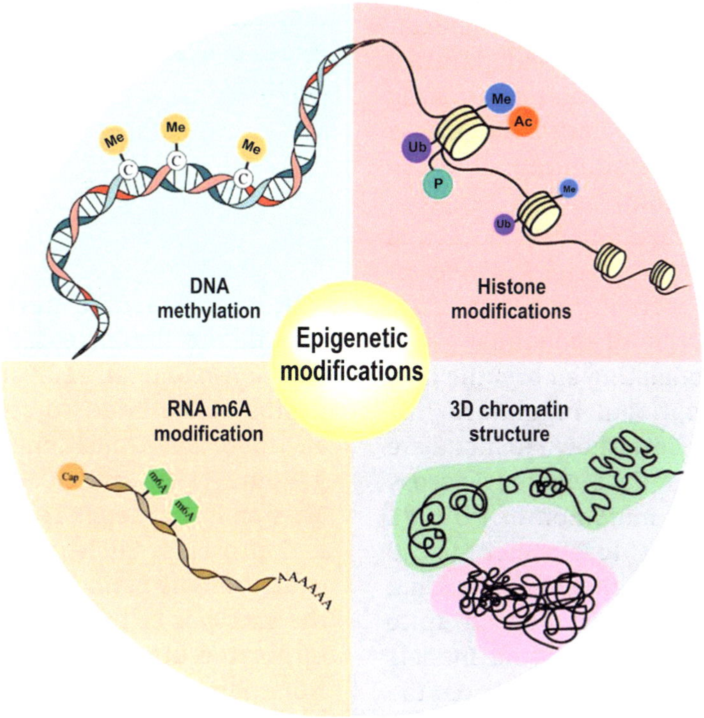

Figure 1.11. Epigenetic modifications during zygotic genome activation (ZGA).

Source: https://onlinelibrary.wiley.com/cms/asset/6d8d34c3-3f5b-4d2b-b31e-d3eb741e6bea/mco2331-fig-0002-m.jpg.

1.4. Comparative Analysis of Zygotic Genome Activation (ZGA) Across Species

The ZGA process represents a critical point in the formation of the early embryo since it is indicative of the shift in control of gene expression from the maternal to embryonic levels. A comparative study of ZGA among different species indicates that the timing and mechanism of activation may significantly vary. In the case of mammals, for example, ZGA is usually at the embryonic cleavage stages and is generally linked with cell fate specification, which then affects blastocyst formation. Experiments in bovine embryos show that genetic control at this stage can be preserved with homologies seen in human embryonic development (Daigneault et al., 2018). Recognizing these comparative dimensions of studying the evolution of early embryonic transcriptional networks allows us to improve our understanding of these mechanisms, and may contribute to progress in reproductive technologies and developmental biology, thus defining the significance of mechanisms being species-specific in ZGA. Species-wide, the function of individual genes at ZGA is critical in modulating embryonic fate. To illustrate, transcriptional regulators like POU5F1 and SOX2 have been shown to modulate pluripotency and early development across different mammals. The inhibition of POU5F1 in bovine embryos stopped development to the blastocyst stage and highlighted a functional conservation with human embryos, in spite of the variations observed in murine models (Daigneault et al., 2018). This underscores the point that although some mechanisms might be conserved, differences in gene control can lead to different phenotypic effects. These differences in gene expression and function as embryos pass through early developmental stages prompt scientists to investigate the implications of these differences, especially as they pertain to cloning and assisted reproductive technologies. In addition, studying ZGA in different taxa uncovers interesting differences in embryogenesis that go beyond mammals. In plant systems, like conifers, early embryo differentiation has a close association with programmed cell death processes, contrasting with animal models in which such processes might differ. An example would be the role of zinc in controlling cell fate during Norway spruce somatic embryogenesis, defining a biochemical involvement in early development that is not present in animal systems. These differences point towards the extent of diversity in embryological approaches taken by various species, and whether and why such adaptations are being promoted by evolutionary pressures. An extensive comparative study of ZGA therefore not only educates us about developmental biology of individual species but also to furthering larger issues of evolutionary development and genetic stability.

1.4.1. Zygotic Genome Activation (ZGA) in Mammals Versus Non-Mammals

ZGA is an essential developmental landmark that differs fundamentally between mammals and non-mammals. ZGA in mammals generally begins at the late two-cell stage, representing an important transition where the embryonic genome takes over control of development after an initial dependence on maternal mRNAs and proteins. Such dependence on maternal contributions defines the pre-ZGA stage, where the embryos cellular machinery is setting itself up for the upcoming activation of its genome. Non-mammalian organisms (e.g., the majority of fish and amphibians) trigger ZGA very early, usually at the blastomere stage. This distinction indicates a profound difference in regulatory mechanisms that control early development, highlighting the evolutionary processes necessary for embryogenesis success in different lineages. The studies point to the plays of paternal factors during early mammalian development, especially through sperm-derived non-coding RNAs. The elements such as circular RNAs (circRNAs) have been known to take a major role in ZGA and early embryonic development, as observed in experiments conducted using porcine models. In particular, circRNA-1572 has been found to be involved in the regulation of essential genes like cyclin B2 (CCNB2), whose disruption causes developmental arrest and defective ZGA.

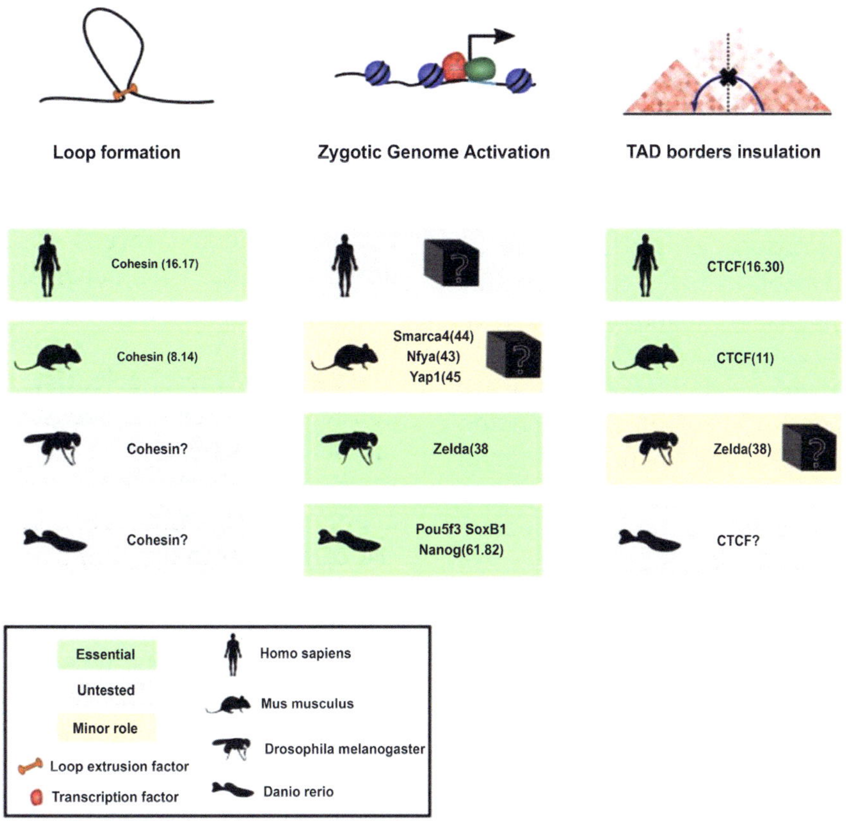

Figure 1.12. Zygotic genome activation (ZGA) in mammals versus non-mammals.

Source: https://ars.els-cdn.com/content/image/1-s2.0-S0955067420300259-gr2.jpg.

This phenomenon highlights that in mammals, maternal as well as paternal contributions are critical in order to establish successful embryogenesis, indicating a more intricate interplay of genetic and epigenetic determinants than in non-mammalian animals, where the contribution of such paternal factors may be less or even non-existent. Another notable difference is found in the replication timing (RT) of DNA in early embryonic development, wherein studies show that mammalian embryos transition from a poorly organized RT to a more organized structure at the four-cell stage. Non-mammals, on the other hand, may have a more stable RT since the beginning of ZGA. It is essential in mammals that transcriptional activation and timing of replication are coordinated, as genome-wide analyses that correlate RNA polymerase II activity with the creation of an orderly nuclear architecture required for fidelity of replication have shown. Such complex timing is likely to contribute to precise regulation of gene expression during the critical period of ZGA. Differences in RT and associated DNA organization between mammals and non-mammals provide evidence of evolutionary adjustments that depend not only on genomic organization but also on the reproductive strategy of each group, thereby illuminating the varied mechanisms controlling early development (Figure 1.12).

1.4.2. Evolutionary significance of Zygotic Genome Activation (ZGA) Variations

The process of ZGA is a central event in early embryo development in many species, and its evolutionary implications have been the focus of extensive discussion in the recent scientific literature. With the evolution of multicellularity, ZGA time and regulation have been found to greatly differ, driving developmental pathways and organismal fitness. The degree of variation in ZGA can be considered to be a powerful regulatory device that enables various species to fine-tune themselves to their respective environmental niches. For example, certain organisms turn on their zygotic genome early on, which could be beneficial in high-speed developmental scenarios, while others do so much later, hence permitting more regulated and gradual shifts from maternal to zygotic control. Comprehension of such variations can help reveal the manner in which evolutionary pressures have influenced embryonic development and reproduction strategies in varied taxa. One of the most important features of ZGA variations is their association with the evolution of small regulatory RNAs, more so microRNAs (miRNAs). These molecules are the basic regulators of gene expression and have co-evolved with the ZGA mechanisms to enable complex developmental processes. The origin of miRNAs predated multicellularity, and their diversification parallels the growing complexity of developmental programs of higher metazoans. During evolution, organisms have been utilizing the power of miRNAs to confer spatiotemporal specificity to gene expression during ZGA, with far-reaching implications for the adaptability and evolutionary success of multicellular organisms. MiRNAs' capacity to modulate the dynamics of gene expression further illustrates how evolutionary developments in mechanisms of ZGA can control developmental pathways, emphasizing the interrelatedness of gene regulation and embryonic development across species. Furthermore, ZGA diversities play an important role in the myriad manifestations of embryonic development affecting traits like tissue differentiation and organ formation. This diversity is not only a function of genetic difference, but is instead an expression of the evolutionary forces that have molded developmental trajectories in order to maximize survival and reproduction. Through investigation of the evolutionary importance of ZGA differences, scientists can learn more about how these processes have resulted in the diversification of life forms and their corresponding developmental strategies. In addition, the significance of ZGA in angiogenesis, a critical process in tissue and organ regeneration, captures the complexity and contextuality of embryonic development. With deeper insight into these fluctuations, it is possible to enjoy the complex networks that regulate early embryo formation, allowing for a wider understanding of multicellular organization and function in biology (Nowak et al., 2018; Philipp et al., 2020).

1.4.3. Implications for Developmental Biology Research

The zygotic genome activation is a critical event in early embryo development with important consequences for developmental biology studies. Elucidating when and how ZGA occurs may provide insight into basic processes including cell differentiation and tissue morphogenesis. As scientists explore the particular regulatory networks controlling ZGA, they might identify new pathways and factors with potential for targeting in therapeutic applications, especially regenerative medicine. The significance is not just within animal models since comparing ZGA processes within and between species provides insights into evolutionary developmental biology. Such cross-study comparisons can clarify environmental pressures' impact on genomic activation, disclosing how organisms change developmentally to respond to their environments, hence expanding our understanding of developmental plasticity in animals and plants (Ikeuchi et al., 2016). In addition, recent improvements in proteomic methods, including the Single-Pot Solid-Phase-enhanced Sample Preparation (SP3), have the capacity to revolutionize developmental biology studies to a large extent. This approach enables the effective analysis of proteomes from small-scale biological samples, enabling the investigation of protein dynamics during ZGA with unprecedented detail and resolution.

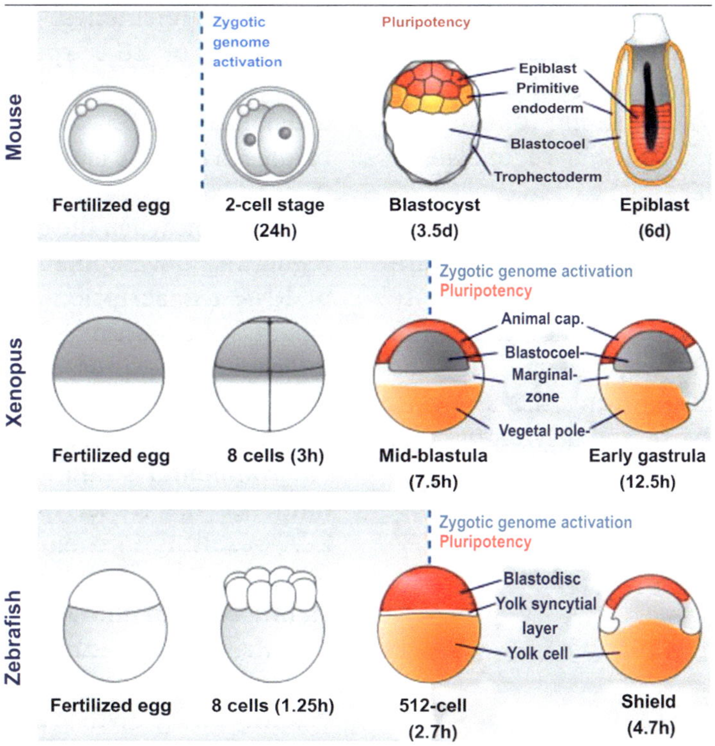

Figure 1.13. Implications for developmental biology research of zygotic genome activation (ZGA).

Source: https://www.researchgate.net/publication/274724374/figure/fig3/AS:267941849595962@1440893723917/Embryonic-development-in-relation-to-zygotic-gene-activation-ZGA-and-pluripotency-in.png.

Analyzing the proteomic landscape at this point can reveal important information about proteins that govern cell processes and morphogenesis in early development. Since SP3 exhibits better performance in the profiling of small amounts of matter, it is able to reveal differences in protein expression between various developmental stages and individuals. Such discoveries may bring advancements in understanding molecular differences that lead to developmental anomalies or disorder, hence improving the accuracy of developmental biology as a field of study aimed at demystifying life's complexities (Christopher et al., 2014). The implications for developmental biology research are also found in the study of regenerative processes, given that the mechanisms of regeneration may present similarities with the regenerative pathways that are triggered during ZGA. Exploring how reprogramming differentiated cells to revert back to a pluripotent state, similar to embryonic stages early in development, could influence tissue engineering and reparative medicine strategies. Furthermore, the involvement of plant hormones in regenerative abilities, as indicated in different studies, can promote cross-disciplinary work where plant biology knowledge will be used to guide animal development. Through the exploration of the interaction between ZGA and regenerative capability, scientists were able to find conserved molecular mechanisms that regulate both processes, thereby paving the way for future therapeutic approaches. Such interdisciplinarity emphasizes the potential to apply developmental knowledge in practical ways to medicine as well as agriculture, highlighting the systemic significance in knowing these early embryonic events (Ikeuchi et al., 2016) (Figure 1.13).

1.5. Experimental Approaches to Study Zygotic Genome Activation (ZGA)

Experimental methods for examining ZGA have come a long way, applying a range of molecular and genetic methodologies to understand the intricate interactions underlying early embryo formation. One promising strategy is the utilization of transgenic models, which enable investigators to visualize and manipulate genetic components linked to ZGA in real-time. With the inclusion of reporter genes attached to ZGA-specific promoters, researchers can monitor the gene expression dynamics at key developmental points. The application of CRISPR-Cas9 technology also allows for the specific disruption of candidate regulatory elements, which is helpful in recognizing pivotal transcription factors and their function in early embryonic transcriptional programs. This multidisciplinary strategy not only better informs our awareness of ZGA but also provides insight into evolutionary divergence and conservation of regulatory processes between species. RNA sequencing (RNA-seq) is another potent experimental method employed in the study of ZGA, specifically in measuring changes in transcription during the critical early divisions of the cell. For example, developmental studies in porcine embryonic development show that ZGA is at the 4-cell stage, representing a critical point when the embryonic genome starts regulating development. Through comparison of RNA transcription profiles under normal and stress conditions, scientists can determine differentially expressed genes (DEGs) that are important for normal embryonic development. Interestingly, RNA-seq experiments revealed that environmental stimuli like high temperatures influence the transcriptome landscape during ZGA, resulting in changes in the expression of essential genes. This revelation emphasizes the significance of knowing how ZGA is affected by intrinsic and extrinsic factors, pointing to its importance in the larger scheme of embryo viability and growth (Sun et al., 2024). In recent research, more emphasis has been placed on the regulatory functions of transposable elements (TEs) in ZGA, which influence the transcriptional structure of early embryos. Using phyloregulatory and transcriptomic strategies, scientists have detected key transcription factors like SRF, which acts as a regulator of MERVL, a prominent family of TEs in mouse development. These TEs are suggested to offer cis-regulatory factors that improve the gene expression landscape during ZGA. Analysis of evolutionary trends of transcription factor binding sites reveals co-evolution among TEs and host genome regulation networks. These observations indicate the sophistication of the gene expression programs triggered at the beginning of development, calling for further studies into how TEs, transcription factors, and ZGA interplay (Hermant et al., 2025).

1.5.1. Techniques for Monitoring Zygotic Genome Activation (ZGA) in Embryos

ZGA's evaluation is key to recognizing the process of early embryo development, since it is where it transitions from maternal to embryonic regulation of gene expression. One such method of tracking ZGA is through fluorescent probes, which are engineered to monitor mRNA splicing and levels of expression in individual embryos.

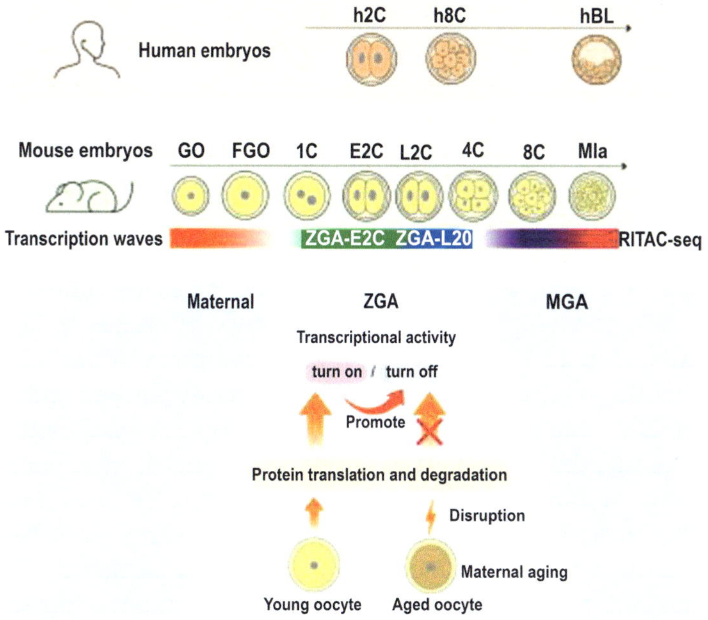

Figure 1.14. Techniques for monitoring zygotic genome activation (ZGA) in embryos.

Source: https://ars.els-cdn.com/content/image/1-s2.0-S2211124724015663-fx1.jpg.

They can be used as markers of the regulatory processes controlling the activation of genes during this developmental stage. Specific constructs, such as a DsRed Express-intron-EGFP, form a visual impression enabling the splicing efficiency to be assessed and consequently the time of ZGA inferred. These methods give important information regarding developmental achievements and the functional condition of the zygotic genome, which can be impaired should splicing activities not work as expected, resulting in adverse effects on embryo viability later (Helmersson et al., 2007). In parallel, the function of zinc ions during embryo differentiation has been an important research area specific to ZGA. Methods through which intracellular zinc can be measured, e.g., through fluorescent probes such as Zinquin, enable investigators to directly view molecular alterations in differentiating embryos. These studies have established a strong correlation between zinc levels and cell fate decision, pointing towards its pivotal role in early embryogenesis. By monitoring zinc levels effectively, scientists will be able to gauge more accurately how differences in the concentration of zinc affect the timing of ZGA and embryonic development. In addition, blocking zinc signaling can provide information on how sustained elevated or depressed levels of zinc can influence the process of normal differentiation, thereby giving rise to disruptive embryonic defects (Helmersson et al., 2007). Further, progress in molecular imaging methods has revolutionized ZGA monitoring by making it possible to view cellular events in real time at the single-cell level. These approaches, in association with genetics, afford a complete system to analyze splicing activity and other regulatory processes in early development. Investigations of splicing factors like SRp38 have unveiled their central functions not only in splicing but also in overall embryonic development. For example, the manipulation of SRp38 levels is sufficient to stop development at numerous points, highlighting the requirement of splicing in efficient ZGA and subsequent embryogenesis. Consequently, the combination of these new monitoring methods opens the door to a better insight into the molecular complexity underlying ZGA, with the ultimate consequence of advances in embryology and reproductive medicine (Siskoglou et al., 2006) (Figure 1.14).

1.5.2. Genetic Manipulation to Study Zygotic Genome Activation (ZGA) Effects

ZGA research is important in the study of early embryo development, especially when viewed from the perspective of genetic manipulation technologies. Species differ with respect to the timeline and mechanism of ZGA, with cattle and pigs showing close similarities to human embryonic development. New genetic modification tools have developed pathways for scientists to explore how manipulation can affect ZGA dynamics (Madeja et al., 2019)). Through the use of methods such as CRISPR-Cas9 and transgenic animal models, it is now possible for scientists to specifically edit genes that are involved in zygotic activation and early embryogenesis. This holds enormous potential for biomedical research, particularly as the scope of what is known about how genetic causes influence developmental pathways continues to grow. As such, this informs a theoretical model for future interventions directed at influencing developmental outputs in both livestock and human models. The applications of gene manipulation to investigate ZGA not only increase our knowledge of early developmental biology but also open doors for useful applications in regenerative medicine and agricultural biotechnology. For example, the development of genetically altered animals can be used as precious models for investigating genetic diseases, understanding the function of individual genes in ZGA processes and early embryonic development (Madeja et al., 2019)). Such investigations may answer fundamental questions about pluripotency and differentiation, showing the mechanisms by which changes in the genomic environment give rise to diverse developmental processes. Furthermore, control over ZGA in animal models can make possible the establishment of directed gene therapies that seek to repair or alleviate genetic defects from the very beginning of embryonic development. This discovery takes advantage of the disruptive power of genetic intervention when applied across developmental biology. Furthermore, novel experimental approaches like transient heat shock have also proven to be strong candidates for probing ZGA. Early studies in zebrafish elucidated an intriguing strategy in which the viability of the embryo and the morphological integrity are determined by the timing of heat shock, which separates DNA and centrosome duplication cycles. These findings accentuate the complex regulatory networks that control concomitant cellular processes in early development. The strategic use of these experimental manipulations enables researchers to analyze the mechanisms behind ZGA in real time, thus determining crucial windows of environmental stress resistance. Through further research into developmental thresholds that reduce teratogenic impact, genetic manipulation methods can be improved, thus making them more effective in exploring ZGA impacts. This complex inquiry not only brings about essential understanding within developmental biology but also underscores the importance of maximal conditions for effective genetic interventions (Figure 1.15).

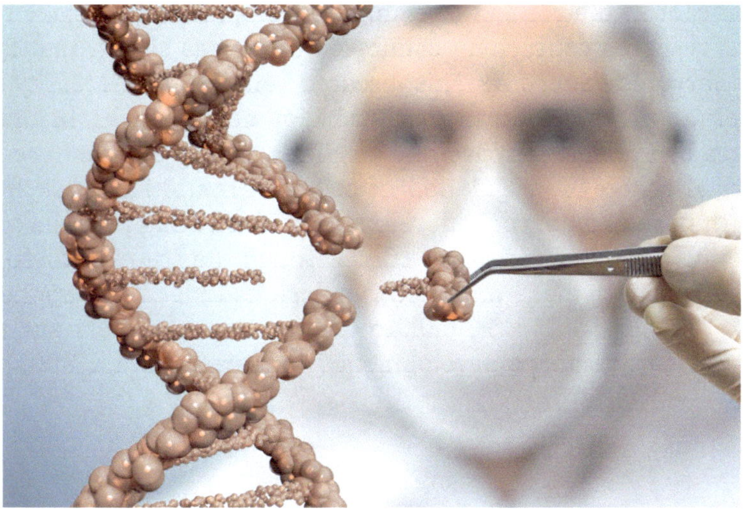

Figure 1.15. Genetic Manipulation.

Source: https://external-content.duckduckgo.com/iu/?u=https%3A%2F%2Fwww.biologyonline.com%2Fwp-content%2Fuploads%2F2020%2F02%2FGenetic-Engineering-Advantages-Disadvantages.jpg&f=1&nofb=1&ipt=afe50ae5fb93c3f9e8d1523f858a0a15600a098c71949113532ca630d46ae450.

1.5.3. Use of Model Organisms in Zygotic Genome Activation (ZGA) Research

The use of model organisms in ZGA research has greatly helped advance knowledge of early development in the embryo. Organisms like zebrafish, mice, and fruit flies have been at the forefront of studies because they have relatively uncomplicated genetics and a short generation time, allowing elaborate experimentation within a reasonable timescale. In zebrafish, for example, the high-speed development from fertilization to visible phenotypes permits scientists to evaluate the timing and process of ZGA, giving insights into the crucial window in which the embryonic genome gains control over development. These model organisms not only enable the investigation of genomic dynamics but also enable the identification of conserved molecular pathways that regulate ZGA processes in different species, which can again be investigated in more complicated organisms, including man, to make comparisons in developmental mechanisms. Further, investigations into ZGA in model organisms show complex interactions between non-coding RNAs and genomic activity in early embryogenesis. Studies highlight the importance of non-coding components, such as long and small non-coding RNAs (sncRNA), in controlling the maternal-to-zygotic transition, which is critical for triggering ZGA. For example, the discovery of transposable elements and their implications in ZGA processes have been reported in other species, which has elucidated how genomic organization can control when ZGA happens. Knowledge of these processes in simpler models provides researchers with tools for constructing high-throughput approaches that analyze the regulatory circuits that control early development. This knowledge can then inform more general studies of reproductive health and infertility because an understanding of ZGA processes in these models has the potential to shed light on the root causes of developmental aberrations in humans (Paloviita et al., 2022). The applicability of model organisms also reaches into research concerning programmed cell death (PCD), which is significant in the context of embryo development, especially during ZGA. In plant systems, for instance, research concerning conifer embryos has shown that PCD is necessary for differentiation and embryonic patterning. This research points to the necessity of balancing cellular processes like proliferation and PCD during early developmental stages. In animal models, the use of synthetic substrates to examine caspase-like activities during early embryo differentiation has yielded crucial information on the regulation of cell fate. Inhibition of such activities has been found to interfere with normal embryonic development, illustrating how the manipulation of gene expression and signaling pathways can affect ZGA. Through the study of these processes in model systems, researchers are able to make informed conclusions that can be applied to both plant and animal developmental biology and, in the end, toward an overall understanding of ZGA and what implications it holds for early embryo development (Helmersson et al., 2007) (Figure 1.16).

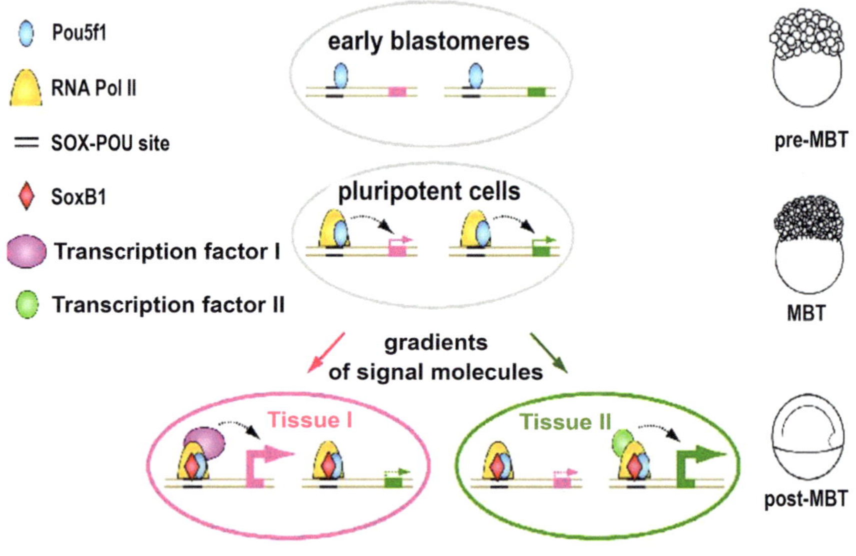

Figure 1.16. Use of model organisms in zygotic genome activation (ZGA) research.

Source: https://external-content.duckduckgo.com/iu/?u=https%3A%2F%2Fwww.researchgate.net%2Fprofile%2FDaria-Onichtchouk%2Fpublication%2F289238919%2Ffigure%2Ffig3%2FAS%3A389124231057414%401469785854323%2FA-hypothetical-model-for-activation-of-the-embryo-genome-ZGA-and-subsequent-event.png&f=1&nofb=1&ipt=b1316988e47b353dcef3c64e77b1c6f2436738177bb3499e2f450f403d3e4d87.

1.6. Clinical Implications of Zygotic Genome Activation (ZGA) Research

The investigation into ZGA has significant clinical implications, particularly concerning early reproductive health and developmental biology. Research highlights the role of transcription factors like TBX3, which is critical for maintaining embryonic pluripotency and histone acetylation levels, essential for successful ZGA. In studies where TBX3 was knocked down, decreased rates of viable embryos at critical early stages were observed, including reduced blastocyst formation and increased apoptosis. Such findings illuminate the potential risks associated with embryo quality in IVF settings, where ZGA efficiency directly correlates with successful implantation and subsequent development into viable pregnancies (Li et al., 2025). Therefore, understanding factors that regulate ZGA might pave the way for improving assisted reproductive technologies and minimizing pregnancy losses. From a clinical perspective, unraveling the molecular mechanisms driving ZGA can lead to better diagnostic and therapeutic interventions for infertility and embryo developmental defects. For instance, the research surrounding GATAD2B underscores its pivotal role in regulating ZGA and early embryonic development. GATAD2B depletion was linked to increased DNA damage and abnormalities during the maternal-to-embryonic transition, leading to compromised embryonic viability. These findings suggest that monitoring levels of GATAD2B and other related proteins may serve as biomarkers for embryo quality assessment in clinical settings. Furthermore, targeted therapies that enhance GATAD2B function or histone modifications could potentially mitigate embryonic developmental challenges, providing critical enhancements to current practices in reproductive healthcare (Cao, 2024). Ultimately, the clinical implications of ZGA research extend beyond therapeutic interventions; they serve to deepen our understanding of the fundamental biological processes underlying human development. Improved knowledge surrounding ZGA not only aids in addressing infertility issues but also informs strategies for preventing congenital anomalies and pregnancy complications. As research collectively delineates the intricate signaling pathways regulating ZGA, clinicians can devise more personalized approaches in reproductive medicine. The advancement *in vitro* fertilization (IVF) techniques will likely evolve in tandem with such knowledge, as the integration of genomic, epigenomic, and transcriptomic data shows promise in optimizing embryo selection and enhancing the overall success rates of assisted reproductive technologies (Cao, 2024; Li et al., 2025).

1.6.1. Zygotic Genome Activation (ZGA) and Its Relevance to Reproductive Technologies

The ZGA process is a critical stage of early embryo development, signaling the shift from dependence on maternal mRNAs to the developing embryo's own genome function. The activation of ZGA takes place shortly after fertilization and is critical to normal development. Abnormalities in ZGA can have profound effects, such as embryonic lethality early in development and heightened vulnerability to genetic disease. Knowledge of the subtleties of ZGA is especially important in the arena of reproductive medicine, including IVF, where embryos are cultured outside the natural uterine space. Any deficiencies in the coordination or performance of ZGA can jeopardize the viability of IVF embryos because the subtle orchestration of genomic activation is critical to successful implantation and further gestation as a healthy fetus. Expanding our knowledge of ZGA ultimately guides attempts to enhance IVF success and overcome frequent failure mechanisms in assisted reproductive technologies. In addition, the importance of ZGA also reaches into the arena of reprogramming chromatin, which is needed to establish totipotency in early embryonic cells. Reprogramming includes complex alterations at the level of the chromatin, such as dynamics of methylation and histone marks, that ensure the embryonic genome activation. Research indicates that any deviation in this reprogramming process can cause chromosomal instability and, by extension, lower embryo viability (Biechele et al., 2015). These findings are important for reproductive technologies because chromosomal abnormalities are a major cause of IVF pregnancy failure. Mitigating these challenges requires expanded investigation into the effects of ZGA on chromatin structure and function, potentially providing avenues for intervention to enhance embryonic health and developmental potential, ultimately increasing success rates for couples seeking assisted reproductive therapy. In addition to the biological intricacies of ZGA and chromatin dynamics, the ethical implications of research in this area must also be considered. Exploration of early embryonic development, particularly regarding ZGA and its associated processes, is fraught with ethical dilemmas, especially in human models. Current research predominantly relies on animal studies to avoid the ethical complications associated with direct human embryo manipulation. However, findings from such studies, such as the link between genomic instability in cattle and its parallels in humans, underscore the pressing need for ethical frameworks that allow for responsible exploration of ZGA in human embryos (Tšuiko et al., 2018). By paving the way for innovative methodologies that respect ethical boundaries, researchers can harness the full potential of reproductive technologies, leading to improved outcomes for individuals and couples facing fertility challenges. Understanding ZGA not only enhances scientific knowledge but also catalyzes advancements in reproductive health practices (Figure 1.17).

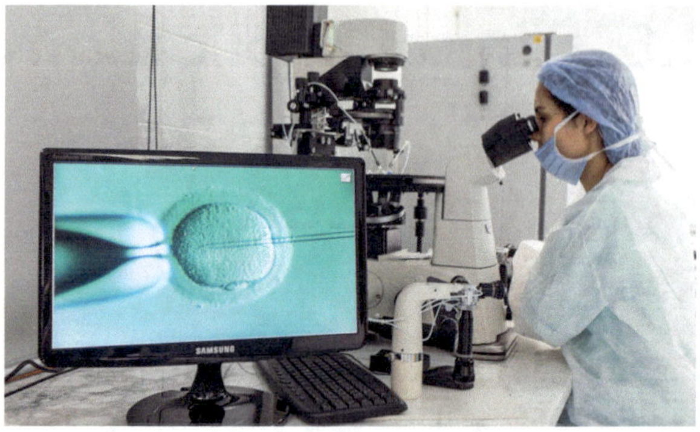

Figure 1.17. ZGA process of early embryo development.

Source: https://external-content.duckduckgo.com/iu/?u=https%3A%2F%2Finsightplus.mja.com.au%2Fwp-content%2Fuploads%2Fassisted-reproductive-technology-reassurance-for-women-677-1024x614.jpg&f=1&nofb=1&ipt=f2bde5565d0d53b5a4ace85194389b25f91634ebca021ca940f29501063544d5.

1.6.2. Potential for Improving Embryo Quality in In Vitro Fertilization (IVF)

The potential for improving embryo quality in IVF is intricately linked to the critical process of ZGA. Early embryo development is contingent upon the proper timing and efficiency of ZGA, whereby transcriptional activity transitions from maternal to embryonic control. This switch is crucial as it marks the onset of the embryos genomes functionality, facilitating the proper expression of genes necessary for development. Understanding the molecular mechanisms governing ZGA can illuminate pathways to enhance embryo viability. Research suggests that aberrations in this process could lead to suboptimal development and increased rates of implantation failure or anomalies, thus underscoring the importance of optimizing ZGA conditions to potentially increase implantation success rates in IVF procedures (Cuthbert et al., 2020). Furthermore, aneuploidy, or the presence of an incorrect number of chromosomes, is particularly problematic during early embryo development. As studies indicate, human embryos exhibit a higher prevalence of chromosomal abnormalities, especially in oocytes from older women, leading to significant challenges in achieving successful pregnancies through IVF. This presents a critical opportunity for interventions, such as preimplantation genetic testing (PGT) and screening techniques, to identify viable embryos with normal karyotypes. By leveraging methodologies like array comparative genomic hybridization and karyomapping, clinicians can better select embryos with higher developmental potential, ultimately improving IVF outcomes. As informed strategies continue to evolve, addressing aneuploidy can enhance our understanding of the early developmental processes during ZGA, thus providing insights into possible interventions that may mitigate the risks associated with chromosomal abnormalities (Ottolini et al., 2015). Additionally, the exploration of sncRNAs provides a promising avenue for augmenting embryo quality in IVF. Emerging research indicates that sncRNAs play a crucial role in regulating gene expression during the critical phases of oocyte maturation and early embryonic development. Abnormal expression patterns of sncRNAs have been correlated with impaired embryo development, suggesting that they may be vital in the mechanisms underlying successful ZGA. By carefully examining the profiles of sncRNAs in both standard and cloned embryos, researchers can pinpoint specific molecular discrepancies that contribute to developmental failure. This information can inform targeted interventions, such as the enhancement of oocyte quality or the manipulation of embryo culture conditions, to optimize the likelihood of achieving viable embryos. Thus, integrating advancements in our understanding of sncRNAs with existing reproductive technologies holds significant potential for enhancing outcomes in IVF practices (Cuthbert et al., 2020) (Figure 1.18).

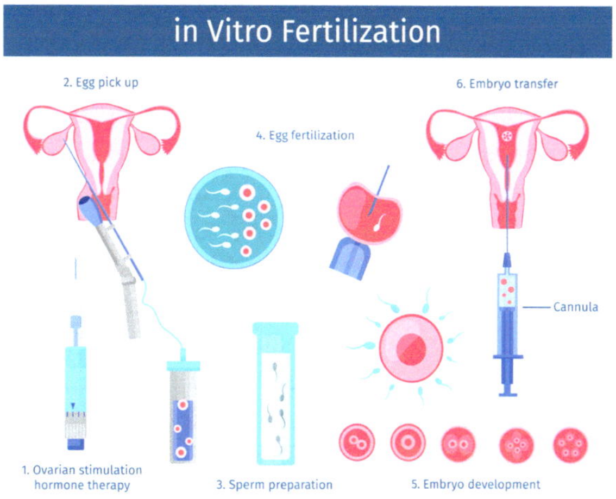

Figure 1.18. Potential for improving embryo quality in IVF.

Source: https://kjkhospital.com/wp-content/uploads/2022/04/37120-1.jpg.

1.6.3. Understanding Developmental Disorders linked to Zygotic Genome Activation (ZGA)

The phenomenon of ZGA is critical for normal embryo development, yet its disruption can lead to significant developmental disorders. During ZGA, the embryo transitions from relying on maternally inherited factors to utilizing its own genomic expression. This transition is pivotal for initiating the complex processes of cell differentiation and morphogenesis. When ZGA is compromised, whether due to environmental factors, genetic mutations, or epigenetic alterations, embryos may experience abnormal development patterns, leading to impaired viability or congenital anomalies. Recent studies have highlighted the role of epigenetic modifications, including histone modifications and DNA methylation, in regulating ZGA, suggesting that disruptions in these processes can result in developmental disorders that manifest early in gestation, thereby underscoring the importance of proper epigenetic programming during this critical phase of embryonic development (Sun et al.,

2021). Furthermore, the interplay between epigenetic factors and external influences can create a fertile ground for developmental disorders linked to ZGA. For instance, certain substances, such as those found in traditional herbal medications, have been shown to induce epigenetic changes that can adversely affect sperm and embryo development. Specifically, a study involving the administration of Wenshen Shengjing Decoction (WSSJD) in mouse models indicated that exposure to such agents could elevate specific histone modifications, such as H3K27me3, leading to developmental arrest in 2-cell embryos. These findings illustrate a potential mechanism for how environmental exposures may interfere with the delicate epigenetic landscape necessary for ZGA, subsequently resulting in impaired embryonic development and increased rates of degeneration (Sun et al., 2021). Such insights call for further investigation into how various external factors influence the epigenetic regulation of ZGA. Moreover, long non-coding RNAs (lncRNAs) have emerged as significant epigenetic regulators during the early stages of embryonic development, particularly concerning ZGA. Research has shown that lncRNAs exhibit a dynamic expression profile that correlates with various developmental stages, contributing to the reprogramming events necessary for ZGA. Disruptions in lncRNA expression can lead to incomplete ZGA, which could contribute to various developmental defects. Notably, studies involving somatic cell nuclear transfer have illustrated how lncRNAs are intricately involved in resetting the epigenetic marks of donor cells, thereby impacting the developmental trajectory of the resultant embryos. This evidence highlights the critical role of lncRNAs in orchestrating the complex processes associated with embryonic development and suggests that aberrations in their expression may be a contributing factor to developmental disorders linked to ZGA. Understanding these multifaceted interactions is essential for unraveling the complexities of embryo development and the etiology of related disorders.

SUMMARY

Investigation of ZGA and embryonic development during the early stages is imperative for progressing our knowledge of developmental biology and reproductive medicine. ZGA constitutes an important transition in which the newly forming embryo commences using its genomic resources to bring about cellular differentiation as well as lineage specification. As new evidence brings into focus the intricacies that surround human embryogenesis, particularly when put in perspective against model organisms such as mice, a complete understanding of these mechanisms is paramount. Recent results highlight the significance of gene dosage compensation after ZGA, exhibiting species-specific differences in X chromosome regulation. This comparative study provides scope for identifying specific regulatory processes that control early human development and thus bridging a pertinent knowledge gap in the area (Petropoulos et al., 2016). The complex interaction of miRNAs during the initial phases of embryonic development cannot be ignored either. These little noncoding RNAs are central to posttranscriptional regulation and play a role in the fine-tuning of gene expression after ZGA. Through translational inhibition and mRNA destabilization, miRNAs orchestrate the subtle ratio necessary for normal cellular outcome during embryogenesis. With their array of functions, miRNA function could offer valuable insights into diseases linked with early development, thereby underscoring their significance in both basic and applied studies in biology. With researchers increasingly shedding light on the functions of different molecular agents throughout ZGA, the prospects for the use of such information in stem cell research and regenerative medicine grow more intense (Bushati et al., 2007). Ultimately, investigating ZGA and early embryo development holds vast potential for scientific advancement. Knowledge of how embryos progress through these embryonic phases educates basic science as well as clinical uses, especially in reproductive biotechnologies and therapeutic treatments. Future research based on detailed transcriptional mappings of human embryos will deepen our knowledge and could also result in advances in the treatment of infertility, genetic diseases, and developmental abnormalities. The conjoining of data from comparative embryology, gene regulation, and miRNA function will lead to a better understanding of the intrinsic processes underlying human development. This multipronged approach promises not just to further developmental biology but also to open the way toward new strategies in regenerative medicine and tailored solutions in personalized healthcare (Bushati et al., 2007; Petropoulos et al., 2016).

The ZGA phenomenon represents a dramatic shift in the development of early embryos towards zygotic control from maternal control in gene expression. The switch ordinarily happens at the mid-blastula transition (MBT) in most model organisms, pointing out how critical timing is when it comes to embryonic development. Pre-MBT, there is a reduction of transcription in early embryonic divisions with the generation of a dependence on maternal mRNA and egg-deposited proteins. Nevertheless, ZGA mechanisms are intricate and include both escape from transcriptional repression and the formation of nascent transcription compartments, which are key to early developmental events. The revelations about ZGA not only contribute to better understanding early developmental biology but also introduce crucial information regarding regulation of gene expression mechanisms that control cellular activities during pivotal stages of development. Furthermore, the contribution of signaling pathways to seed size and growth parallels the complexity of ZGA to zygotic development. Studies have shown that the development of zygotic tissues is controlled by multiple channels of signaling, which are critical for coordinating development of the embryo, endosperm, and seed coat. In particular, HAIKU (IKU) and phytohormone pathways were shown to affect growth parameters, combining maternal and zygotic inputs for coordinated development. This interaction highlights the significance of cross-talk among maternal and zygotic gene regulation in embryonic growth and seed size determination. Similar to the case of ZGA, comprehending these signaling pathways is most important for enhancing agricultural practices and crop yields, offering a practical utility of developmental biology to enhance food security. In addition, improvements in imaging technology have greatly improved our insight into the spatial and temporal pattern of early gene expression during ZGA. The cutting-edge research applying 4D imaging methods has shed light on the structural architecture of transcription compartments, which are part of the gene activation process before MBT. Through the observation of activities of key genes like pri-miR430 and other zinc-finger genes, scientists can now understand better how chromatin architecture modulates the activity of transcription. These compartments, which contain nascent RNAs and active Polymerase II, are prime examples of the complex organization of the embryonic nucleus that aims to accommodate early transcriptional activity. Finally, these discoveries not only augment the basic principles of embryonic development but also lay down a platform for further investigation of the molecular machinery behind early ZGA and its significance towards the entire developmental path in metazoans, hence making noteworthy contributions towards developmental biology.

CLOSER LOOK

ZYGOTIC TRANSCRIPTIONAL PROGRAM

Zygotic transcriptional program is a term given to the activation of the embryo's own genome after fertilization, an important time in early development when regulation of gene expression is switched from maternal to zygotic sources. In the initial stages of embryogenesis, especially in animals such as mammals, frogs, and flies, the developing embryo almost exclusively depends on maternal mRNAs and proteins that were deposited in the egg during oogenesis. These maternal influences impose early cell processes, including cleavage and cell cycle progression, without the zygotic genome being transcriptionally active. The ZGA or maternal-to-zygotic transition (MZT) is the stage at which the embryo starts transcribing its own genes, a developmental shift that is required for subsequent development, differentiation, and embryonic identity formation. This event takes place at species-dependent stages — e.g., at the 2-cell stage in mice, the 8- to 16-cell stage in humans, and the mid-blastula transition in frogs and zebrafish. The initiation of the zygotic gene expression program is marked by the resumption of transcription from previously unscheduled chromatin, resulting in a sudden and coordinated expression of many genes required for embryonic development and cell specialization.

The activation of zygotic transcription involves complex epigenetic remodeling, including changes in chromatin structure, histone modifications, and DNA methylation patterns that enable access to transcriptional machinery. Pioneer transcription factors, such as Nanog, SoxB1, and Pou5f3, play a central role in remodeling chromatin and opening up previously inaccessible genomic regions. These factors bind to specific DNA sequences and help recruit RNA polymerase II, the enzyme responsible for transcribing messenger RNA. The zygotic transcriptional program is tightly regulated and occurs in distinct waves. The minor ZGA, which occurs early, activates a small set of genes and is often considered preparatory, while the major ZGA leads to widespread transcription and signals the full handover of developmental control to the embryo.

In addition to gene activation, the zygotic transcriptional program includes the degradation of maternal mRNAs, a process regulated by both maternal and zygotic factors. This degradation ensures that embryonic development proceeds under the control of zygotic, rather than maternal, gene products. The selective clearance of maternal transcripts and the synthesis of new RNAs establish a new gene expression profile specific to the developing embryo and necessary for tissue specification and organogenesis.

Defects in the zygotic transcriptional program can lead to developmental arrest, abnormal cell differentiation, or embryonic lethality, highlighting its critical role in successful reproduction and embryogenesis. Understanding ZGA is not only fundamental in developmental biology but also has implications in regenerative medicine, reproductive technologies, and stem cell research, where reprogramming of gene expression is a key challenge. In conclusion, the zygotic transcriptional program represents a pivotal developmental milestone where control shifts from maternally inherited instructions to the embryo's own genome, enabling autonomous development and the establishment of organismal identity through precisely regulated gene expression.

REFERENCES

1. Alda-Catalinas, C., Bredikhin, D., Hernando-Herraez, I., Santos, F., Kubinyecz, O., Eckersley-Maslin, M., Stegle, O., et al. (2020). A single-cell transcriptomics CRISPR-activation screen identifies epigenetic regulators of the zygotic genome activation program. *Cell Systems, 11*, 25–41.e9. https://doi.org/10.1016/j.cels.2020.06.004.

2. Arbeitman, M., Baldi, P., Bashirullah, A., Baugh, L., Brand, A., Chen, X., Choe, C., et al. (2007). *Unmasking Activation of The Zygotic Genome Using Chromosomal Deletions in the Drosophila Embryo.* https://journals.plos.org/plosbiology/article?id=10.1371/journal.pbio.0050117.

3. Bentsen, M., Goymann, P., Schultheis, H., Klee, K., Petrova, A., Wiegandt, R., Fust, A., et al. (2020). ATAC-seq foot printing unravels kinetics of transcription factor binding during zygotic genome activation. *Nature Communications, 11.* https://doi.org/10.1038/s41467-020-18035-1.

4. Biechele, S., Lin, C. J., Ramalho-Santos, M., Rinaudo, P., et al. (2015). *Unwind and Transcribe: Chromatin Reprogramming in The Early Mammalian Embryo.* https://core.ac.uk/download/622530005.pdf (accessed on 27 May 2025).

5. Bushati, N., & Cohen, S. M. (2007). microRNA functions. *Annual Review of Cell and Developmental Biology, 23*, 175–205. https://doi.org/10.1146/annurev.cellbio.23.090506.123406.

6. Cao, G. (2024). P-115 GATAD2B is required for pre-implantation embryo development by delaying zygotic genome activation. *Human Reproduction.* https://www.semanticscholar.org/paper/9faa628bac36633a44e273a5864dc2ca65f4f889 (accessed on 27 May 2025).

7. Cartwright, E. L., Crofton, A. E., Feitzinger, A. A., Lott, S. E., et al. (2018). *Effect of Larval Nutrition on Maternal mRNA Contribution to the Drosophila Egg.* https://pmc.ncbi.nlm.nih.gov/articles/PMC5982822/.

8. Cuthbert, J. M. (2020). *Comparative Analysis of Small Non-Coding RNA and Messenger RNA Expression in Somatic Cell Nuclear Transfer And In Vitro-Fertilized Bovine Embryos During Early Development Through the Maternal-To-Embryonic Transition.* https://digitalcommons.usu.edu/cgi/viewcontent.cgi?params=/context/etd/article/8970/&path_info=ADVSetd2020Aug_Cuthbert_Jocelyn.pdf.

9. Daigneault, B. W., Rajput, S., Ross, P. J., Smith, G. W., et al. (2018). *Embryonic POU5F1 is Required for Expanded Bovine Blastocyst Formation.* https://pmc.ncbi.nlm.nih.gov/articles/PMC5958112/.

10. Dexheimer, P. J., & Cochella, L. (2020). MicroRNAs: From mechanism to organism. *Frontiers in Cell and Developmental Biology, 8.* https://doi.org/10.3389/fcell.2020.00409.

11. Di, A., Zhang, X., Song, L., Wang, S., Liu, X., Bai, C., Su, G., et al. (2025). Dppa2 promotes early embryo development through regulating PDH expression pattern during zygotic genome activation. *International Journal of Molecular Sciences, 26.* https://www.semanticscholar.org/paper/1dbb1a4cf032ce2cf1ccc23566e99e98090f4cc4 (accessed on 27 May 2025).

12. Hadzhiev, Y., Qureshi, H. K., Wheatley, L., Cooper, L., Jasiulewicz, A., Nguyen, H. V., Wragg, J. W., et al. (2019). A cell cycle-coordinated Polymerase II transcription compartment encompasses gene expression before global genome activation. *Nature Communications, 10.* https://doi.org/10.1038/s41467-019-08487-5.

13. Helmersson, A. (2007). *Programmed Cell Death and Genetic Stability in Conifer Embryogenesis.* https://core.ac.uk/download/11695235.pdf (accessed on 27 May 2025).

14. Hermant, C., Mourra-Díaz, C. M., Oomen, M. E., Altamirano-Pacheco, L., Pal, M., Nakatani, T., & Torres-Padilla, M. (2025). The transcription factor SRF regulates MERVL retrotransposons and gene expression during zygotic genome activation. *Genes & Development*. https://www.semanticscholar.org/paper/c19557776012bc520b8b5ecf4614f5b4aaa6f641 (accessed on 27 May 2025).
15. Huang, Y., Kim, J., Vinh, D., Lee, C., Penfold, C. A., Żylicz, J. J., Marioni, J. C., et al. (2017). Stella modulates transcriptional and endogenous retrovirus programs during maternal-to-zygotic transition. *eLife, 6*, e22345. https://doi.org/10.7554/elife.22345.
16. Hug, C. B., & Vaquerizas, J. M. (2018). The birth of the 3D genome during early embryonic development. *Trends in Genetics, 34*, 903–914. https://doi.org/10.1016/j.tig.2018.09.002.
17. Hughes, C. S., Föehr, S., Garfield, D., Furlong, E. E. M., Steinmetz, L. M., & Krijgsveld, J. (2014). Ultrasensitive proteome analysis using paramagnetic bead technology. *Molecular Systems Biology, 10*. https://doi.org/10.15252/msb.20145625.
18. Ikeuchi, M., Ogawa, Y., Iwase, A., & Sugimoto, K. (2016). Plant regeneration: Cellular origins and molecular mechanisms. *Development, 143*, 1442–1451. https://doi.org/10.1242/dev.134668.
19. Jazwinska, A., Ozdemir, A., Stathopoulos, A., Stathopoulos, A., Stathopoulos, A., Adryan, B., Biehs, B., et al. (2011). *Lateral Gene Expression in Drosophila Early Embryos Is Supported by Grainy Head-Mediated Activation and Tiers of Dorsally-Localized Repression*. https://journals.plos.org/plosone/article?id=10.1371/journal.pone.0029172.
20. Jiang, X., Xu, W., Sun, J., Lin, J., Lin, Z., Lian, X., Liao, S., et al. (2025). Trps1 regulates mouse zygotic genome activation and preimplantation embryo development via the PDE4D/AKT/CREB signaling pathway. *Cell Biology and Toxicology, 41*. https://www.semanticscholar.org/paper/d81ce5ea5fb56b1ea9b2a67f185ffa26d747a2da (accessed on 27 May 2025).
21. Li, N., Xu, R., & Li, Y. (2019). Molecular networks of seed size control in plants. *Annual Review of Plant Biology, 70*, 435–463. https://doi.org/10.1146/annurev-arplant-050718-095851.
22. Li, X. H., Lee, S. H., Kim, J. D., Lee, G. H., Sim, J. M., & Cui, X. S. (2025). TBX3 is essential for zygotic genome activation and embryonic development in pigs. *Microscopy and Microanalysis*. https://www.semanticscholar.org/paper/0961874a0de8ef7833ef0a01ea3bf62e126b688c (accessed on 27 May 2025).
23. Lin, M., Du, Z., Guo, D., Zhang, Y., & Dan, J. (2025). Dux cluster duplication ensures full activation of totipotent genes. *Proceedings of the National Academy of Sciences, 122*. https://www.semanticscholar.org/paper/acca0bb3d66e33b8750b40eb6d5e775e82302435 (accessed on 27 May 2025).
24. Madeja, Z., Pawlak, P., & Piliszek, A. (2019). Beyond the mouse: Non-rodent animal models for study of early mammalian development and biomedical research. *The International Journal of Developmental Biology, 63*(3–5), 187–201. https://www.semanticscholar.org/paper/9738101d4a6f640c851091d4b8c7790682aa26d1.
25. Menon, T., & Nair, S. (2018). Transient window of resilience during early development minimizes teratogenic effects of heat in zebrafish embryos. *Developmental Dynamics, 247*, 992–1004. https://www.semanticscholar.org/paper/25bae78dec55ea10d197c42f1897ce863d9e6ac6 (accessed on 27 May 2025).

26. Messerschmidt, D. M., Knowles, B. B., & Solter, D. (2014). DNA methylation dynamics during epigenetic reprogramming in the germline and preimplantation embryos. *Genes & Development, 28*, 812–828. https://doi.org/10.1101/gad.234294.113.

27. Nakatani, T., Schauer, T., Altamirano-Pacheco, L., Klein, K. N., Ettinger, A., Pal, M., Gilbert, D. M., et al. (2023). Emergence of replication timing during early mammalian development. *Nature, 625*, 401–409. https://www.semanticscholar.org/paper/f262f8c342e6ba1444555112dee7561117d8ffd6 (accessed on 27 May 2025).

28. Nowak-Sliwinska, P., Alitalo, K., Allen, E., Anisimov, A., Aplin, A. C., Auerbach, R., Augustin, H. G., et al. (2018). Consensus guidelines for the use and interpretation of angiogenesis assays. *Angiogenesis, 21*, 425–532. https://doi.org/10.1007/s10456-018-9613-x.

29. Oak, M. S., Stock, M., Mezes, M., Straub, T., Hynes-Allen, A. M., van den Ameele, J., Forné, I., et al. (2025). H3K4 methylation-promoted transcriptional memory ensures faithful zygotic genome activation and embryonic development. *bioRxiv*. https://www.semanticscholar.org/paper/95eee287be49f3dc09cc1d84c19ec3a5ca60d473 (accessed on 27 May 2025).

30. Ottolini, C. S. (2015). *Chromosome Segregation and Recombination in Human Meiosis: Clinical Applications and Insight into Disjunction Errors*. The Bridge Centre Ltd, UK. https://core.ac.uk/download/30712748.pdf (accessed on 27 May 2025).

31. Paloviita, P., & Vuoristo, S. (2022). *The Non-Coding Genome in Early Human Development—Recent Advancements*. https://www.sciencedirect.com/science/article/pii/S1084952122000490?via%3Dihub.

32. Petropoulos, S., Edsgärd, D., Reinius, B., Deng, Q., Panula, S., Codeluppi, S., Plaza Reyes, Á., et al. (2016). Single-cell RNA-Seq reveals lineage and X chromosome dynamics in human preimplantation embryos. *Cell, 165*, 1012–1026. https://doi.org/10.1016/j.cell.2016.03.023.

33. Radford, E. J., Ito, M., Shi, H., Corish, J. A., Yamazawa, K., Isganaitis, E., Seisenberger, S., et al. (2014). *In utero* undernourishment perturbs the adult sperm methylome and intergenerational metabolism. *Science, 345*. https://doi.org/10.1126/science.1255903.

34. Shahbazi, M. N. (2020). Mechanisms of human embryo development: From cell fate to tissue shape and back. *Development, 147*. https://doi.org/10.1242/dev.190629.

35. Siskoglou, A. (2006). *mRNA Splicing in Early Mammalian Embryos*. https://core.ac.uk/download/29410502.pdf (accessed on 27 May 2025).

36. Sun, M. H., Zhan, C. L., Li, X. H., Lee, S. H., & Cui, X. S. (2024). Transcriptome analysis of the effects of high temperature on zygotic genome activation in porcine embryos. *Scientific Reports, 14*. https://www.semanticscholar.org/paper/9be31ca265e97d7830257311d5b52db15789585e (accessed on 27 May 2025).

37. Sun, Y., Gao, F., Xu, D., Lu, L., Chen, Q., Yang, Z., Wang, X., et al. (2021). Wenshen Shengjing decoction improves early embryo development by maintaining low H3K27me3 levels in sperm and pronuclear embryos of spermatogenesis impaired mice. *Evidence-Based Complementary and Alternative Medicine, 2021*, 1–11. https://doi.org/10.1155/2021/8035997.

38. Tšuiko, O. (2018). *Kromosomaalne Ebastabiilsus Imetajate Varajastes Embrüotes*. https://core.ac.uk/download/187147478.pdf (accessed on 27 May 2025).

39. Wei, R., Yue, Y., Wu, Y., Zhang, C., Jin, J., Liu, Z., & Wang, J. (2025). A long noncoding RNA with enhancer-like function in pig zygotic genome activation. *Journal of Molecular Cell*

Biology. https://www.semanticscholar.org/paper/6d532ca2c5f5d9fadc220c392f65fb09181b1e12 (accessed on 27 May 2025).

40. Wu, F., Liu, Y., Wu, Q., Li, D., Zhang, L., Wu, X., Wang, R., et al. (2018). Long non-coding RNAs potentially function synergistically in the cellular reprogramming of SCNT embryos. *BMC Genomics, 19*. https://doi.org/10.1186/s12864-018-5021-2.

41. Wu, Y., Wei, Y., Li, Y., Dou, Y., Yang, Y., Liu, H., Wang, X., et al. (2025). Sperm-derived CircRNA-1572 regulates embryogenesis and zygotic genome activation by targeting CCNB2 via Bta-miR-2478-L-2. *Advanced Science*. https://www.semanticscholar.org/paper/a99b175b04f6d41e8b378db2a1f3a80dc8dc3adb (accessed on 27 May 2025).

42. Yan, Y., Zhang, C., Hao, J., Wang, X., Jia, M., Li, M., Na, J., et al. (2019). DPPA2/4 and SUMO E3 ligase PIAS4 opposingly regulate zygotic transcriptional program. *PLoS Biology, 17*, e3000324. https://doi.org/10.1371/journal.pbio.3000324.

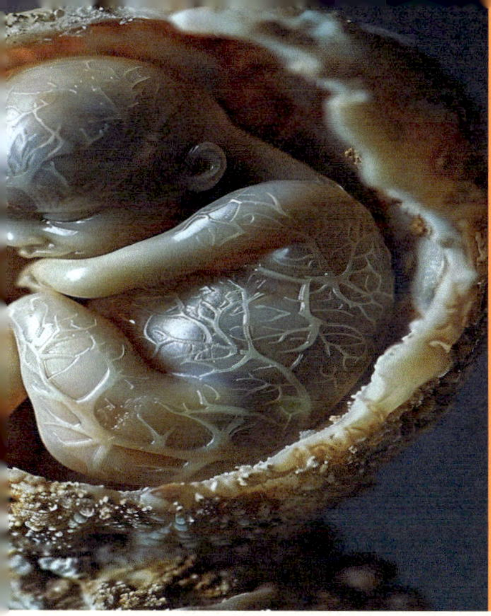

Chapter 2

AXIS FORMATION AND EMBRYONIC PATTERNING

Contents

Introduction

Development of the embryonic axis is a fundamental developmental process in developmental biology that determines the direction and subsequent body plan of an organism. This intricate process comprises a series of finely regulated cell processes and signaling pathways that are responsible for coordinating body structures into spatial relationship. Insights into these dynamics are essential for not only knowing about normal developmental processes but also about pathologic conditions arising due to axis formation defects. Therefore, the majority of studies have been performed on well-characterized model organisms such as *Drosophila melanogaster* and zebrafish, providing insights into evolutionary and conserved developmental pathway evolution. However, sole reliance on a set of restricted species may not be adequate to understand the general mechanisms responsible for animal diversity and embryogenesis evolution. This perspective puts critical questions on what standards are needed for the discovery of novel model organisms to enhance the study of embryonic patterning complexities (Helen et al., 2025). In the past few years, there has been swift development in genomic tools and molecular biology approaches that has rekindled efforts in the study of axis formation and embryonic patterning. High-throughput sequencing and genome editing technologies such as CRISPR/Cas9 have made it possible for researchers to explore non-conventional model organisms, hence expanding our understanding of development in different groups. For instance, studies in zebrafish have shed light on maternally provided proteins, such as Huluwa, in triggering critical signaling pathways necessary for dorsal-ventral axis determination. Most notably, the activation of β-catenin signaling by Huluwa is an illustration of how intricately systems are controlled at the molecular level. However, deconstructing the more intricate regulation processes, for example, post-translational modification like phosphorylation, is an ongoing challenge. This highlights the importance of more sophisticated genetic tools and methods to study these seminal questions in the best possible way (Li et al., 2024). The significance of axis formation also extends to conservation biology and medicine, where insights from developmental studies can inform therapeutic intervention. By resolving the genetic and molecular basis of axis formation, researchers would be able to design new approaches toward the treatment of congenital defects caused by inappropriate embryonic patterning. In addition, as we invest resources in the identification of new model systems, it is all the more critical that we evaluate their potential to the field. This not only requires critical examination of their genetic tractability but also in terms of ecological and evolutionary context. As we embark on this endeavor, the convergence of various biological perspectives will certainly enrich our comprehension of embryonic development, allowing for a more consolidated knowledge of the intricacy of life in various species (Helen et al., 2025) (Figure 2.1).

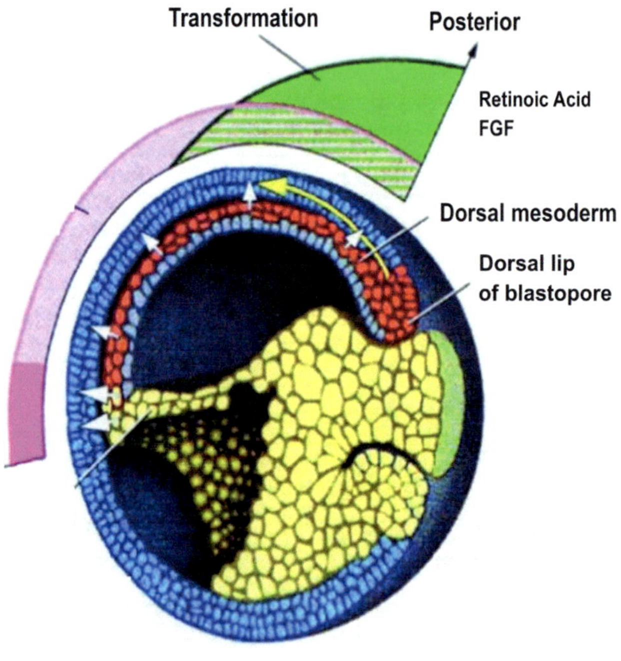

Figure 2.1. Axis formation and embryonic patterning.

Source: https://external-content.duckduckgo.com/iu/?u=https%3A%2F%2Fwww.creative-diagnostics.com%2Fupload%2Fimage%2FMorphogens-Embryonic-Patterning-and-Axis-Formation.png&f=1&nofb=1&ipt=ced30b670da894b2aa65957fb5ed4803fbbe082ca117cfdb592380181015569a.

Definition of Axis Formation

Axis formation is a simple concept that aids in the understanding of embryonic development as well as morphogenesis because it determines the spatial arrangement of an organism. Axis formation is a phenomenon where somebody plans are generated in an embryo that goes on to determine the organization of the organisms as well as the anterior-posterior (head-tail) and dorsal-ventral (back-belly) organization. This intricate process begins with cellular signal transduction pathways that allow embryonic cells to talk to one another, orchestrating their movements and behaviors to achieve optimal alignment and organization. The establishment of the embryonic axis is not just a precursor to organogenesis; it is an active process guided by the local environment and tissue interactions, laying down a foundation for the intricate structures that will develop over developmental trajectories. Research has shown that certain mechanical and biochemical feedback mechanisms are critical in the process of axis formation. An example is the function of the accumulation of interstitial fluid (IF) between embryonic cells to be a critical part of this mechanism. The interaction between cell migration and the movement of IF creates a positive feedback mechanism that regulates morphogenesis during the entire process of early development, particularly in animals such as zebrafish. As described in recent studies, the movement of anterior axial mesendoderm cells drives fluid flow that allows for cellular protrusion and migration, which are necessary for advance of the embryonic axis. This hydraulic feedback system mirrors interaction between physical force and cellular movement, demonstrating the complexity of axis formation process and its implication for successful embryonic patterning (Huljev et al., 2023). In addition, the role of some proteins in axis specification illustrates the molecular complexity that governs embryonic development. For example, the Makorin 1 (Mkrn1) protein is crucial for axis specification and pole plasm assembly in *Drosophila,* a model organism that has been widely utilized in research on developmental biology. Mkrn1 binds to elements of the translational apparatus, efficiently controlling the translation of critical mRNAs that contribute to axis formation, including oskar (osk). Mkrn1 and translational repressors like Bruno1 engage in competitive binding dynamics that provide insight into the mechanistic processes by which molecular interactions drive embryonic patterning. Understanding these molecular interactions is important since it informs how specific embryonic axes are formed and regulated, then go on to determine the growth of structured body forms (Dold et al., 2020).

Importance of Embryonic Patterning

Embryonic patterning is the mechanism that lies at the heart of body plan development in multicellular animals, controlling spatial positioning and tissue differentiation. This is orchestrated through a series of signaling events that define the embryonic axes—anteroposterior and dorsoventral. These embryonic axes, together with the positioning of future organs and structures, also permit the intricate cell-cell interactions leading to specific developmental pathways. Research shows that alterations in the mechanisms regulating embryonic patterning can result in congenital abnormalities, underscoring the importance of maintaining a tight regulation of genetic and environmental factors in development. Understanding such developmental mechanisms can provide insights into not only normal biological function but also the etiology of various developmental disorders caused by mis patterning of the embryo. Moreover, embryonic patterning has a function that goes beyond axis formation; cellular communication that guides further development is part of it. Embryonic cells communicate with the microenvironment through signaling pathways, a critical process for differentiation into specialized cell types.

Cellular crosstalk guarantees transfer of accurate patterning information for proper formation of essential tissues and organs.

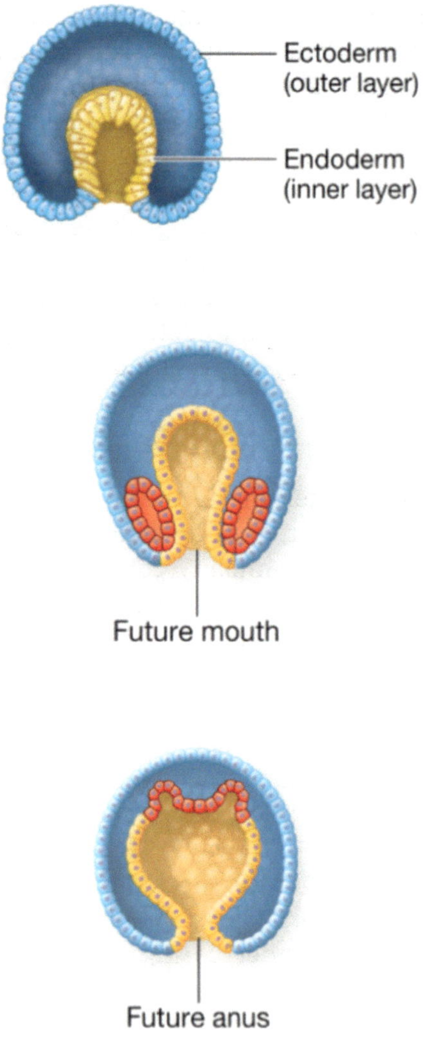

Figure 2.2. Embryonic patterning.

Source: https://lightcat-files.s3.amazonaws.com/problem_images/9d41496beeaff6ea-1677717544267.jpg.

Embryonic patterning has been researched with the use of advanced techniques such as single-cell technologies, which enable scientists to examine cellular heterogeneity and unravel the roles played by stem cells in organogenesis. As it becomes apparent in wound healing research, in which coordination in space and time among multiple cell types regulates efficient healing, so too is it the case with embryonic development, highlighting the intricate dynamics of cell-to-cell interaction underlying mechanisms of patterning (Mélanie Rodrigues et al., 2018). In addition, the interplay between embryonic patterning and environment is an essential focus area in developmental biology. Multiple extrinsic variables such as maternal diet, contaminant exposure, and socio-environmental stressors may be able to compromise the highly regulated signaling pathways that dictate embryonic axis formation. Notably, this interaction occurs in the gut-brain axis because the microbiota affects both host health and embryonic development and, indirectly, can likely influence neurological outcome through metabolic and immune signaling pathways (John et al., 2019). These results point to the significance of embryonic patterning not only in terms of anatomical structure but in broader implications for general organismal health and disease resistance. This realization underlies the cross-disciplinary thrust of developmental biology, as it focuses further investigation on how the extrinsic might alter the intrinsic patterning processes to impact future developmental and regenerative medicine (Figure 2.2).

2.1. Historical Background

The foundation for axis formation and embryonic patterning is historically profound and mirrors the background of developmental biology as a discipline. Early embryological research laid the foundations for current descriptions of how organisms set up body plans. Landmark experiments on model organisms such as frogs (*Xenopus*) and sea urchins demonstrated core principles of gastrulation and the interplay between cell movements that guide developmental processes. This historical trajectory exhibits not only the systematic development of research methods but also the step-by-step unrolling of complexity of genetic and molecular dynamics of development. Therefore, the evolution of model and theory through time mirrors the revolutionary role played by progress in technology in enabling scientists to visualize and palpate developmental processes with unprecedented precision. With increasing years of research, the organism zebrafish, particularly due to its experimental tractability and optical transparency, was utilized as a model organism. The embryo of the zebrafish is optically transparent, which allows for visualization of cell movements and differentiation in real time, transforming vertebrate developmental studies at their essence. Notably, it has been demonstrated in research that the spatial pattern of the tissue progenitors of embryonic shield during early gastrulation.

Such research indicates that progenitor cells of lineages like neural, notochordal, and somitic get incorporated into the embryonic shield domain, displaying a level of radial organization. This zebrafish cell structure observation has not only clarified the complexities of axis formation but also addressed special differences from other vertebrates, increasing our understanding of gastrulation and neural induction morphogenetic motion in zebrafish (Fraser et al., 1995). Similarly, the study of amniote development has also elucidated significantly on the origin of complex structures such as the jaw. The amniote jaw complex illustrates how embryonic cell lineages that are different meet through signaling interaction and movement and combine to give rise to integrated morphological attributes. Experiments reveal the function of cranial neural crest mesenchyme in creating the wide range of the tissues of the jaw, implying the significance of cellular and molecular mechanisms. Moreover, the interaction of biomechanical forces during jaw formation adds another dimension of complexity, showing the adaptive variation that facilitates evolutionary plasticity. Through examining these mechanisms, we are able to better understand both the variability in jaw morphology among species and the risk of defects during jaw formation, highlighting the implication for developmental biology and medicine (Abzhanov et al., 2019).

2.1.1. Early Studies in Embryology

The discipline of embryology has developed enormously in the last century, shedding light on basic processes of axis formation and embryonic patterning. Early observations showed the intricacy of cellular differentiation as embryos progress, with investigations employing model organisms like zebrafish and frog embryos. Recent progress through single-cell RNA sequencing has shown how different cell types arise from pluripotent cells during important developmental periods. For example, scientists such as Wagner et al. examined more than 90,000 cells during zebrafish development, documenting molecular transitions that accompany axis patterning and germ layer formation. Such seminal studies shed light on the complex ballet of transcriptional transitions that regulate vertebrate early development, providing a foundation for interpreting embryonic development, as well as proposed pathologies from developmental defects (Briggs et al., 2018). Aside from vertebrate research, research into invertebrate models has greatly added to our understanding of axis formation. The annelid *Tubifex tubifex*, part of the Spiralia, has traditionally been at the center of research into embryonic axes because its eggs are readily available. Early 1920s classic experiments demonstrated that certain blastomeres at the four-cell stage, specifically the D cell and its progeny, are crucial in axial pattern formation. These studies underscored that the D quadrant acts as an organizer for embryonic axes in various invertebrates. More contemporary research utilizing cell-ablation and restoration techniques has validated the importance of micromeres in determining developmental fates and specifying anteroposterior polarity, thus enhancing the understanding of fundamental mechanisms governing embryonic spatial organization (Shimizu et al., 2014). The amalgamation of data from embryological experiments throughout species has contributed enormously to the overall knowledge of axis formation and embryonic patterning. Through comparative developmental processes among both vertebrates and invertebrates, scientists have elucidated conserved mechanisms and pathways, as well as divergent aspects that shed light on evolutionary biology. These works highlight the significance of early specification events in ensuring appropriate patterning, with transcription factors and signaling molecules playing crucial roles as determinants in cell fate decisions. Additionally, this comparative approach not only expands the knowledge base for embryological development but also has implications for developmental biology and regenerative medicine. As technology advances further, the implication of advanced technologies in genetic and embryological studies will certainly provide greater insights into the intricacies of life from its very beginning (Briggs et al., 2018) (Figure 2.3).

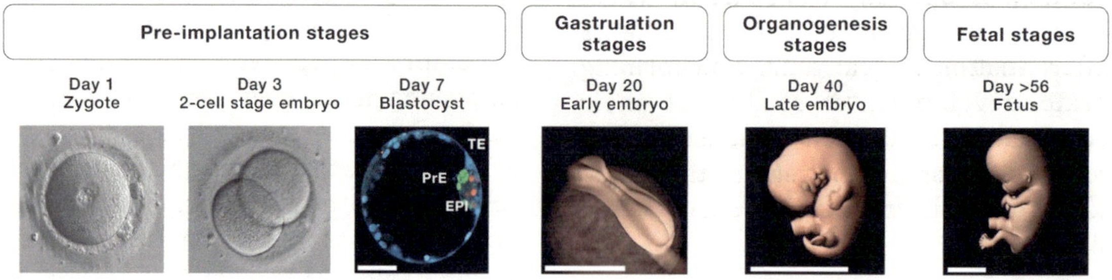

Figure 2.3. Early studies in embryology.

Source: https://www.cell.com/cms/10.1016/j.cell.2023.07.028/asset/2d23b3b4-cc98-48b2-adac-e1707e4db7a9/main.assets/gr1_lrg.jpg.

2.1.2. Key Discoveries in Axis Formation

Axis formation is central to embryonic patterning, as it determines the spatial arrangement of an organism's body plan. The discovery of the function of the Wnt signaling pathway, specifically the Wnt/β-catenin pathway, is one of the key discoveries in axis formation and plays a vital role in the formation of the anteroposterior axis of vertebrates. This pathway also activates transcription factor β-catenin, which migrates to the nucleus and associates with TCF/LEF family proteins to control gene expression vital in axis specification. This cascade of signaling not only coordinates cell fate decisions during early embryogenesis but also affects the further development of definitive structures and organs, finally guiding the formation of body symmetry and orientation. It has become clearer with the understanding of Wnt signaling's complexities how axis formation and its relevance to developmental biology and regenerative medicine have deepened. Another landmark find in axis formation is learning about the function morphogens assume in patterning the embryonic form. Morphogens such as the fibroblast growth factor (FGF) and Sonic Hedgehog (Shh) exert an influence on cells during development by giving them positional information. They diffuse through tissues and form gradients that determine the fate of adjacent cells in proportion to their concentration. It has become apparent through research that these gradients are not simple passive signals but instead include intricate interactions and feedback mechanisms to adjust developmental results.

For instance, Shh is crucial for neural tube formation and limb structure patterning, illustrating the important interaction between morphogen gradients and axis specification. These results emphasize the importance of morphogens as major actors in embryonic patterning, directing tissue organization and function during the developing embryo. Recent progress in our appreciation of the role of liquid-liquid phase separation in cellular biology has also impacted research into axis formation. This phenomenon, wherein biomolecules condense into distinct liquid-like droplets, has been shown to facilitate the formation and maintenance of various cellular structures and processes essential for embryonic development. For example, proteins and RNA can phase separate to form structures that influence gene expression and cellular signaling pathways during axis specification, imitating the physical transitions observed in nonliving matter. The discovery that such phase separation plays a role in organizing embryonic cells highlights a novel aspect of how biochemical processes underlie the structural integrity of developing organisms. As research clarifies the relationships between phase separation, molecular interactions, and developmental outcomes, it becomes apparent that these mechanisms are critical for understanding the nuanced processes involved in axis formation and embryonic patterning, representing a significant frontier in developmental biology research (Dierickx et al., 2017; Shin et al., 2017) (Figure 2.4).

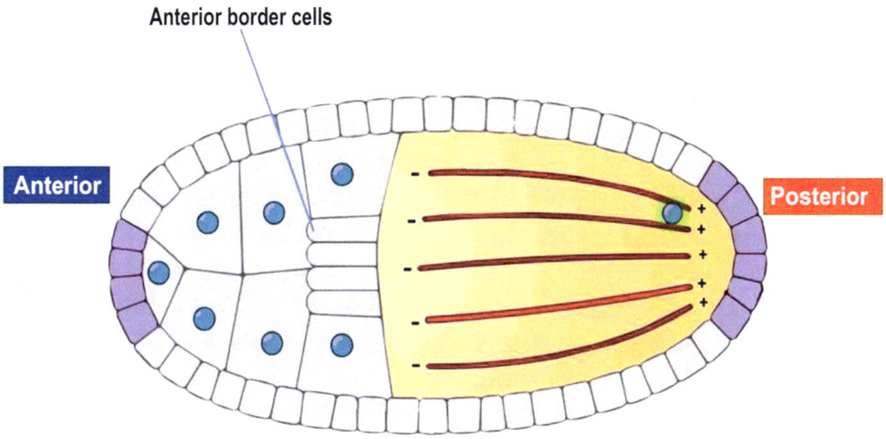

Figure 2.4. Key discoveries in axis formation.

Source: https://i.ytimg.com/vi/371CuIs8icY/maxresdefault.jpg.

2.1.3. Evolution of Research Methodologies

The development of research approaches in developmental biology has revolutionized our current knowledge of axis development and embryonic patterning immensely. Relying mostly on comparative embryology in the past, scientists started incorporating molecular genetics and cellular biology methods to analyze the mechanisms for embryonic development. This was a turning point, as with this method, the scientists were not only able to study the anatomical structures but the molecular signals and pathways that determine development processes as well. Modern methodologies now employ sophisticated imaging methods, high-throughput sequencing, and bioinformatics, allowing for a more in-depth survey of spatial and temporal gene expression patterns throughout embryogenesis. These methods have thus shed light on the subtleties of embryonic development, uncovering the complex interplay between genetic and environmental influences giving rise to correct axis formation and patterning. In recent years, the advent of organoid technology has further revolutionized research methodologies in the study of embryonic development. Brain organoids, for instance, derived from pluripotent stem cells, serve as advanced models that replicate aspects of human brain development, enabling researchers to explore mechanisms of axis formation within the central nervous system (CNS). These three-dimensional constructs recapitulate major aspects of early development, such as cellular heterogeneity and spatial organization, although certain aspects remain to be fine-tuned to reflect embryonic conditions in their entirety. With the use of brain organoids, researchers are able to study developmental processes in a controlled system, test the impact of genetic mutations, and test potential therapeutic strategies for neurodevelopmental disorders (NDD). This novel strategy is representative of the trend towards more advanced experimental paradigms that close the interface between basic and clinical research, bringing us closer to appreciating multicellular organism development. A redefinition of research approaches has also highlighted the need for multidisciplinary efforts in developmental biology. With embryonic patterning and axis formation still being unraveled, classical disciplinary delineations between genetics, developmental biology, and neuroscience are becoming progressively less distinct. Collective endeavors have produced a more inclusive method, integrating discoveries of multiple disciplines to answer tough questions about interactions among genetic and environmental factors on development. Further, as the examination of the microbiota-gut-brain axis, with complex interactions between the host and microbiome, shows, researchers are beginning to realize the need to apply holistic methods. Through collaboration and integration of diverse scientific strengths, the discipline is well positioned to unlock the complex dynamics that dictate axis formation and embryonic patterning to make new contributions and gain a deeper understanding of developmental processes (John et al., 2019; Qian et al., 2019).

2.2. Mechanisms of Axis Formation

The complexity of embryonic development is largely dependent on the processes of axis formation, which determine the initial body plan of the organism. The key mechanisms for these processes are morphogens, signaling molecules that determine cell fate through the establishment of gradients within the embryo. These gradients determine the spatial organization of cellular activities and ultimately contribute to the structural integrity of the organisms. One of the well-known morphogens is the Bone Morphogenetic Proteins (BMPs), which figure prominently in dorsoventral axis patterning. A new perspective in understanding BMP gradients showed that their distribution could be based on a source-sink mechanism, with a dynamic interaction between BMPs and antagonists. Such a finding speaks against earlier models that mostly emphasized counter-gradients, particularly showing the complexity of the signaling pathways for axis specification and embryonic patterning. In addition to signaling by BMP, Hh pathways are essential for oral-aboral axis determination during embryogenesis. Recent studies have shown how Shh and Bmp4 signaling interact to form complementary patterns required for the differentiation of unique cell populations in the mandibular arch. Inactivation of Hh signaling in neural crest-derived mesenchyme results in significant developmental anomalies, including increased BMP activity that alters proper tissue development. Particularly, this perturbation can elicit the replication of frameworks, like the dentary bone, while hindering the formation of functional organs like the tongue. These findings establish the importance of accurate signaling dynamics in becoming proficient in intricate embryonic frameworks, exhibiting how perturbations in such pathways may have far-reaching implications for organismal shape. The work on the mechanisms of axis formation not only increases knowledge of normal developmental processes but also carries fundamental implications for developmental biology and regenerative medicine. By deciphering the interrelationship between different signaling pathways, researchers can possibly develop therapeutic interventions to treat congenital malformations or tissue regeneration. As illustrated by the studies of BMP and Hh signaling, axis formation is characterized by highly regulated interactions between several signaling molecules that need to take place within fixed spatial and temporal contexts. Research into these interactions promises to reveal basic principles that control embryonic patterning. Such information may ultimately create novel strategies in biotechnology and developmental engineering, opening up for positive use in medical science and genetic studies (Figure 2.5).

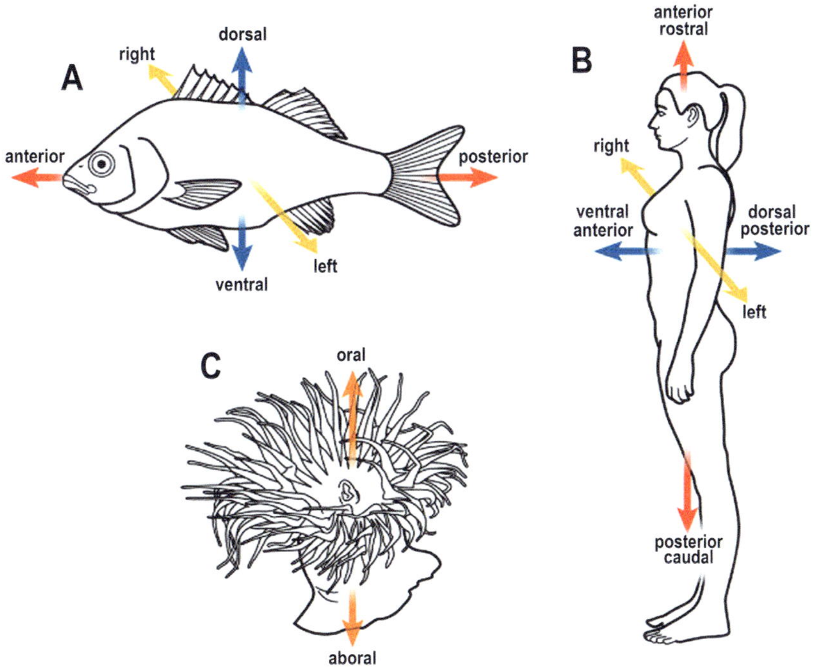

Figure 2.5. Mechanisms of axis formation.

Source: https://external-content.duckduckgo.com/iu/?u=https%3A%2F%2Fembryology.med.unsw.edu.au%2Fembryology%2Fimages%2Fthumb%2F6%2F67%2FAnatomical_axes_comparison.jpg%2F600px-Anatomical_axes_comparison.jpg&f=1&nofb=1&ipt=40d98c73553bf9ced6f4b1335758487265cfc32c8e5945b776a50f9fc24f37f4.

2.2.1. Role of Signaling Pathways

The formation of the primary body axes during embryogenesis is a very complex process that is highly dependent on several signaling pathways. The pathways exist as molecular networks, which are instrumental in transmitting information that is critical to cellular communication and has effects not only on cell fate but also on tissue orientation and organization. In vertebrates, for example, β-catenin-dependent canonical Wnt signaling is essential to establish the dorsoventral, anteroposterior, and left-right axes. Proper activation of these pathways is essential for the preservation of the spatial arrangement of developing structures, since any disruption causes severe morphological defects or developmental disorders. Therefore, the comprehension of how these signaling pathways operate is central to the decoding of the intricacies of embryonic patterning and sheds light on mechanisms that guarantee precise body plan development in vertebrates, pointing to the evolutionary importance and functional conservation among species (Shi, 2024).

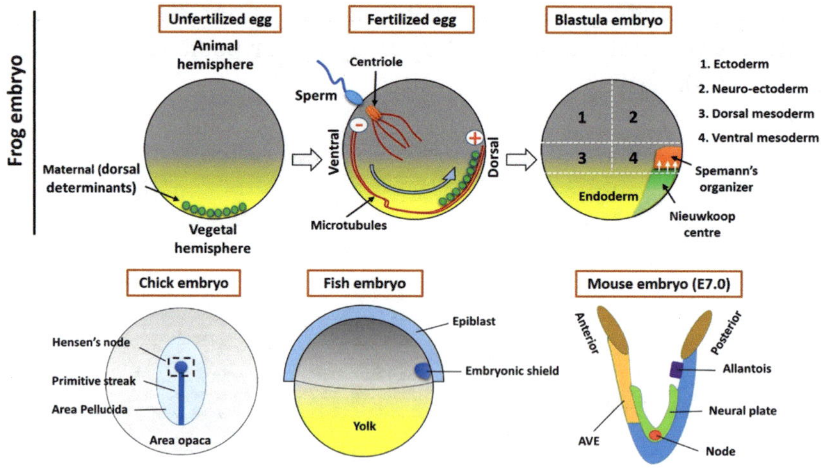

Figure 2.6. Role of signaling pathways.

Source: https://external-content.duckduckgo.com/iu/?u=https%3A%2F%2Fpub.mdpi-res.com%2Fjdb%2Fjdb-09-00047%2Farticle_deploy%2Fhtml%2Fimages%2Fjdb-09-00047-g001.png%3F1635767537&f=1&nofb=1&ipt=a159230242a4e49dc9232fe07cb2d235af82e644f4ee064ef2e915dccf2c9129.

The complex interaction of multiple signaling pathways is critical in mediating the mechanisms of axis formation, leading to a more sharpened understanding of the mechanism of embryo development. Non-canonical Wnt signaling, which is β-catenin independent, demonstrates how more general cellular contexts can modulate local behaviors, including cell polarity and cytoskeletal dynamics. Through regulating asymmetric cell movements and cellular polarization, this signaling pathway plays a role in the creation of an unambiguous embryonic symmetry essential for correct axis specification. In addition, the coordination of signaling pathways such as transforming growth factor β (TGF-β) highlights this complexity further by pointing to the need for accurate regulatory processes directing cell differentiation and organization. All in all, these pathways not only specify body organization but also point to the need for cross-talk between signaling molecules to ensure developmental integrity throughout early embryogenesis (Krishnapati et al., 2024). Investigating the evolutionary history of signaling pathways provides a wider contextual insight into how body plans develop in various metazoan species. Research on ancient organisms such as Hydra illuminates how the pathways originated and why they have remained unchanged over millions of years. In Hydra, elements of the TGF-β signaling pathway, specifically BMPs, were found to be critical in the regulation of body axis formation and organogenesis, much like in higher organisms. The conservation implies that core mechanisms controlling patterning processes are probably the same across species and form the basis of evolutionary importance of these signaling pathways. With scientists learning more about the molecular complexities behind these pathways, implications go beyond simple developmental biology and push forward the understanding of evolutionary biology and the evolution of form and function in multicellular organisms (Krishnapati et al., 2024) (Figure 2.6).

2.2.2. Genetic Regulation of Axis Specification

The genetic control of axis determination is a fundamental feature of embryogenesis that determines tissue and organ structure. It commences with the generation of the three basic germ layers—ectoderm, mesoderm, and endoderm—each giving rise to characteristic body components. Recent findings have also placed emphasis on how signaling pathways, including Wnt, FGF, and Retinoic Acid, manage the spatial and temporal organization of gene expression important for axis determination.

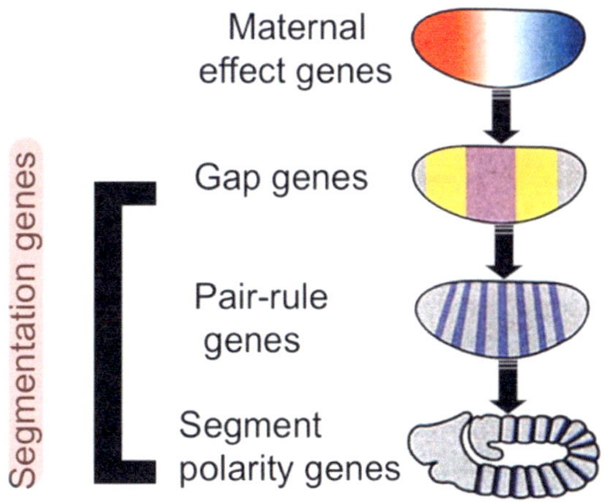

Figure 2.7. Genetic regulation of axis specification.

Source: https://external-content.duckduckgo.com/iu/?u=https%3A%2F%2Fo.quizlet.com%2FxB4VcnIlAqkm8B5utuYQNw.jpg&f=1&nofb=1&ipt=b0e15c89571fd28b2f44d268c25d80cc34c4a599eeb0dbe18e5092882d62f501.

More specifically, these pathways play a cooperative role in regulating major transcription factors that determine anterior-posterior and dorsal-ventral axis development. For example, retinoic acid establishes the anterior-posterior axis through control of the location-specific expression of downstream target genes, illustrating the importance of genetic regulation in ensuring appropriate embryonic patterning. An appreciation of such frameworks not only offers insight into normal developmental events but also reveals mechanisms for congenital anomalies. In addition, different transcription factors act as regulatory hubs within the network of genes that governs axis specification. For example, Sox2 expression has been implicated in the establishment of the prospective gastrointestinal tract and its differentiation into stomach versus intestinal phenotypes. Such factors tend to act in feedback loops, regulating gene expression required to uphold cellular identity and function in development. Evidence also indicates that changes in the levels of these important transcription factors can result in malformation or abnormal development, pointing towards their pivotal role in axis establishment. The interaction between these factors sets up an in vivo system that maximizes proliferation and differentiation so that embryonic tissues can adequately respond to spatial information. Studying these regulating processes provides further insights into embryonic development and its complex biological procedures. With increasing research, the significance of molecular actors like Nrf2 and heme oxygenase-1 (HO-1) has emerged, owing to their role in protection against stress and aging. Nrf2 controls the expression of several genes associated with oxidative stress response, thus building cellular robustness in key periods of development. This suggests that the genetic regulation of axis specification is not only a developmental concern but also a matter of cellular health that could affect aging and longevity. HO-1, a key genetic target of Nrf2, has implications in protective pathways against damage caused by reactive oxygen species. These discoveries highlight evolutionary conservation of genetic processes between phyla, supporting the necessity for broad studies to shed light on multifunctional roles these genes have in early development. Investigating this intersection provides potential avenues for therapeutic approaches and further knowledge of developmental biology (Figure 2.7).

2.2.3. Cellular Interactions During Early Development

Axis formation during embryonic development is underpinned by complex cellular interactions at early stages of development. These are coordinated through signaling pathways allowing communication between cells in close proximity to one another, thus creating necessary gradients and spatial organization. Interestingly, Wnt signaling pathways are implicated as central to mediating these cellular dynamics, with both the canonical and non-canonical branches coordinating the equipartitioning of cell fate choices throughout the developing embryo. Canonical Wnt signaling, dependent on β-catenin, not only plays a role in the patterning of the initial body axes but also helps in the formation of cellular polarity, which is crucial for the bilateral symmetry seen in vertebrates. The two-way nature of these cellular interactions results in a complicated field where successful communication is the key to the formation of the axes, thus underscoring their importance in embryonic development (Shi, 2024). In addition, the formation of specific transcriptional programs is central to early development cell interactions, as in the Drosophila embryos dorsoventral (DV) patterning. This is not only about the interaction between transcriptional enhancers with their specific promoters but also about the effects of chromatin landscapes on gene regulation. Recent research highlights the significance of RNA Polymerase II pausing at DV promoters prior to zygotic genome activation (ZGA), illustrating the way in which this process is utilized for integrating developmental cues before committing to a cell fate. The dynamic nature of transcriptional regulation, modulated by enhancer-dependent histone modification, enables tissue-specific expression of genes, indicating an advanced interplay in which chromatin signatures determine transcriptional outputs. These results clarify the important part cell interactions play in directing developmental programs that result in definitive body structure and functional diversification (Hunt et al., 2024). In conclusion, cellular interactions during early development explain key mechanisms involved in axis formation and embryonic patterning. The intersection of signaling pathways and transcriptional regulation illustrates a very coordinated system in which cells talk and respond to the environment. This complex interaction not only guarantees the proper formation of body plans but also emphasizes the likelihood of disruption in these processes leading to developmental anomalies. With current research delving deeper into the intricacies of these interactions, it is becoming increasingly evident that the integrity of embryonic development depends on the successful coordination of signaling pathways and transcriptional activity. This recognition of cellular interactions as a foundational aspect of developmental biology is essential for advancing our comprehension of normal and pathological developmental processes (Hunt et al., 2024; Shi, 2024) (Figure 2.8).

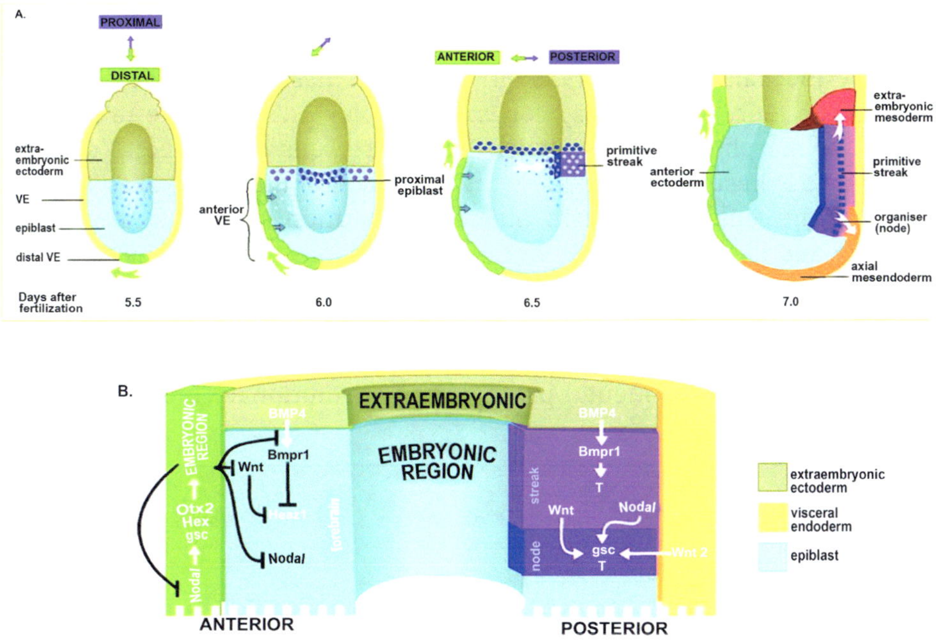

Figure 2.8. Cellular interactions during early development of embryonic axis formation.

Source: https://www.cell.com/cms/10.1016/S0092-8674(00)80560-7/asset/15cb40a5-9113-4127-a6bf-dd63c6e5193c/main.assets/gr2_lrg.jpg.

2.3. Types of Axes in Embryonic Development

The establishment of embryonic axes is a pivotal feature of developmental biology, determining the spatial organization of the developing embryo. The major axes—anterior-posterior, dorsal-ventral, and left-right—are vital in determining the basic body plan of an organism. The anterior-posterior axis determines the head-to-tail orientation, important for the development of differentiated structures like the brain and digestive system, while the dorsal-ventral axis specifies the back-to-belly orientation and the layout of tissue layers and organs. Furthermore, the left-right axis is essential for correct development of asymmetrical structures like the heart and lungs. The interaction of these axes is controlled by intricate signaling pathways and patterns of gene expression that direct cellular differentiation and morphogenesis in the early development stages, highlighting axis formation as central to embryonic patterning. Molecular cues, often in the form of morphogen gradients, are at the core of axis formation and determine the orientation and identity of the embryonic structures.

For instance, the Bicoid protein gradient in *Drosophila* is a model system for the population of anterior-posterior axis, where its concentration is the driving force behind the expression of the genes that ultimately decide the anterior parts of embryos. In vertebrates, similar processes occur through proteins such as Nodal and Wnt, which are integral to the formation of dorsal-ventral axis and determination of left-right asymmetry. Knowing how these gradients interact with transcription factors informs the mechanistic basis of embryonic patterning. The specificity with which these gradients define axes underscores the delicate balance of biochemical and biophysical processes that control early embryonic development and suggests evolutionary innovations that have optimized these systems through time. In addition, the embryonic axis determination pathways are under different regulatory mechanisms that assist in the robustness and diversity of developmental output. Gene regulatory networks (GRNs), for example, play a crucial role in relaying the output of embryonic cells to morphogen signals, such that these cells can respond correctly to spatial information. Not only do these networks allow the formation of the initial axes to happen, but they also allow the rest of the cellular behaviors, including migration, proliferation, and differentiation, to be properly timed and localized. Recent studies have demonstrated that mutations within these GRNs can lead to significantly different patterns of axis formation, which in turn affect overall morphology and phenotypic diversity. By investigating these pathways, researchers can elucidate how embryos adapt to various environmental conditions and genetic backgrounds, further advancing our understanding of both developmental processes and evolutionary biology (James et al., 2015; Schaerli et al., 2018) (Figure 2.9).

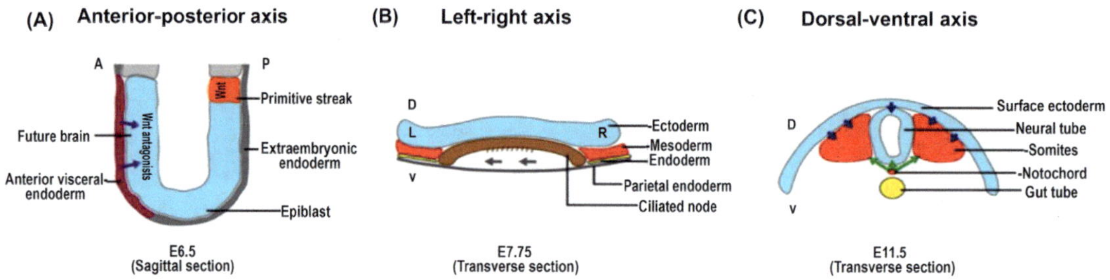

Figure 2.9. Types of axes in embryonic development.

Source: https://www.researchgate.net/publication/353397059/figure/fig1/AS:1048602889691145@1627017819453/Body-axis-formation-in-mouse-embryos-A-Anterior-posterior-establishment-and-brain.png.

2.3.1. Anterior-Posterior Axis

The formation of the anterior-posterior axis is a pivotal event in embryonic development, that sets up the orientation and organization of the developing organism. This axis provides a template upon which the complicated body plan is established, determining the formation of entities like the head and tail in vertebrates. The processes of this specification are vastly different among various organisms and show a complicated interplay between environmental signals and genetic control. For example, the variations in axis development among amphibians, teleosts, and amniotes are a demonstration of evolutionary changes that have taken place, with dorso-ventral polarity acting as a pathway that leads to anterior-posterior positioning. It is not just a matter of academic interest to study these processes; it helps us essentially understand developmental biology and vertebrate evolution. In mammals, cellular interactions and the specification of lineage are necessary for the proper formation of the anterior-posterior axis early in embryogenesis. Lineage segregation at the blastocyst stage produces the inner cell mass and trophectoderm, both serving distinctively in the developmental process. Signaling processes mediated by the visceral endoderm within the inner cell mass are critical in determining the axis.

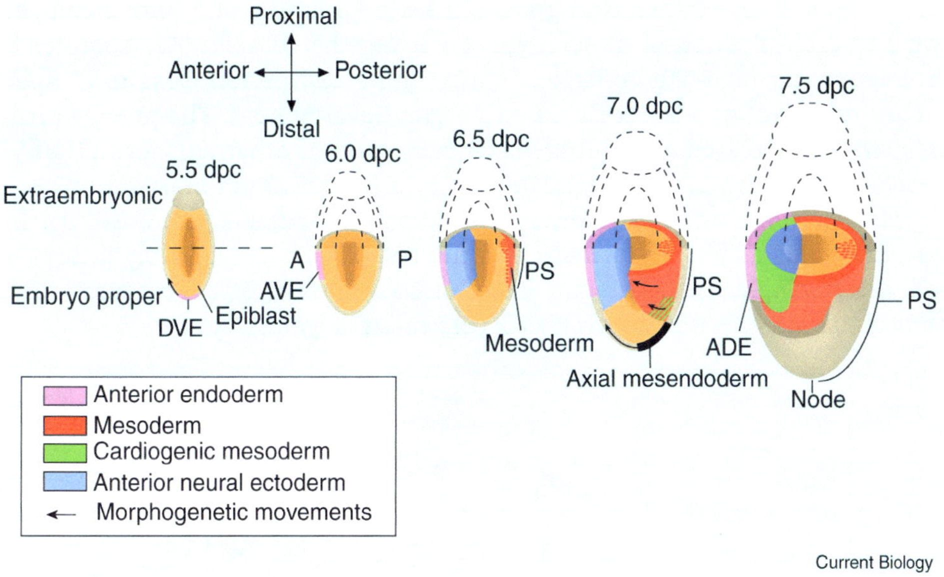

Figure 2.10. Anterior-posterior axis.

Source: https://www.cell.com/cms/10.1016/S0960-9822(01)00417-1/asset/992e6abd-fec3-43db-aa77-e21997b05ec6/main.assets/gr1_lrg.jpg.

These signals coordinate the molecular processes that determine cell fate, which in turn direct the structural organization of the organism. The difficulties involved in researching these interactions, especially the stage of implantation, have necessitated novel procedures like three-dimensional culturing methods. These methods have uncovered heretofore inaccessible knowledge regarding embryonic patterning initiation in response to cellular and signaling dynamics, thus affirming the central position of the anterior-posterior axis in embryonic patterning (Panavaite et al., 2018). Comparative vertebrate lineage studies also shed light on the evolutionary history of anterior-posterior axis specification. Studies probing the ancestral forms of axis development in animals like the dogfish have demonstrated intriguing similarities with amniotes, postulating a common evolutionary origin. The interplay between embryonic and extraembryonic tissues points to the intricacies entailed in the formation of the anterior-posterior axis, with amniotes exhibiting an unparalleled growth of extraembryonic ectoderm allowing for radial symmetry during late stages of the blastula. Finally, these results feed into a general model of axis specification within gnathostomes, integrating results from disparate embryonic systems. Placing the anterior-posterior axis in an evolutionary context enables researchers to appreciate better the similarities and differences within embryonic development, creating an overarching framework that includes biological principles behind the formation of axes and body plan organization (Coolen et al., 2007) (Figure 2.10).

2.3.2. Dorsal-Ventral Axis

The dorsal-ventral (DV) axis is a key determinant of embryonic development in multicellular animals, with implications for body structure and function. The DV axis intersects the anterior-posterior (AP) axis at right angles, imparting vital polarity within the developing embryo. Signaling mechanisms involving morphogens such as the BMPs have an important role to play in defining this axis. BMPs belong to the transforming growth factor-β family and play a central role in cell fate regulation and orchestration of morphogenesis along the DV axis. The complex coordination of these morphogens, through the control of target gene expression, results in specific cellular identities that are required for correct tissue and organ development. The precise formation of the DV axis is not a singular isolated event; it is inextricably part of other axis formations, highlighting the intricacy of vertebrate embryonic patterning mechanisms, as emphasized by the significance of interacting morphogen signaling pathways (Takebayashi-Suzuki et al., 2020). In vertebrate embryogenesis, mechanisms for the formation of the DV axis are inextricably intertwined with AP axis formation. Interestingly, in amphibians like *Xenopus*, embryological research has shown how rotation of the cortex after fertilization plays a role in DV asymmetry.

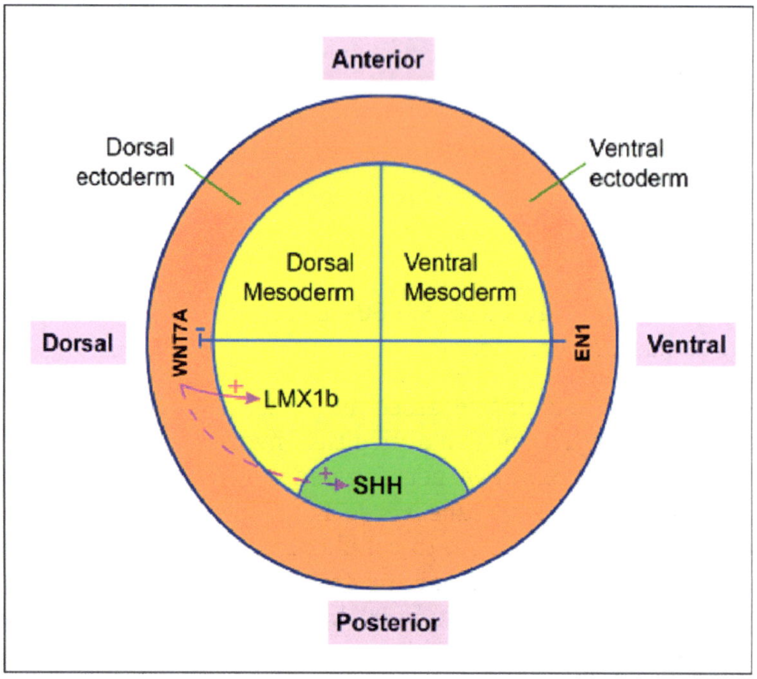

Figure 2.11. Dorsal-ventral axis.

Source: https://www.researchgate.net/profile/Kerby-Oberg/publication/260794228/figure/fig1/AS:669446150557704@1536619808844/The-dorso-ventral-axis-EN-1-is-in-the-ventral-ectoderm-It-supresses-WNT7A-preventing.png.

The rotational movement is accountable for the depositing of maternal determinants to the dorsal side of the embryo, which initiates the molecular interactions needed for forming the Nieuwkoop center. This center is important as it specifies the formation of the Spemann organizer, which is an essential signaling hub in embryonic development. The Spemann organizer not only sets the stage for the DV axis but also gives patterning signals for the later formation of the AP axis. Therefore, the interdependence of these axes reflects the sophisticated regulation mechanisms that control embryonic patterning, and how abnormalities in these processes can result in developmental abnormalities (Carron et al., 2016). The interplay of morphogen signaling pathways further elucidates the complexity of dorsal-ventral axis formation. After the establishment of the Spemann organizer, antagonistic interactions between signals secreted from this region and those from the ventral regions coordinate the differentiation of mesodermal tissues along the DV axis. During gastrulation, this DV information subsequently translates into positional values that aid in organizing the anterior and posterior segments of the embryo. To fully cooperate, an array of signaling factors, including Wnt and FGFs, must work in concert. The regulation of these signals is crucial; for instance, the simultaneous inhibition of Wnt and BMP signaling is necessary to promote the formation of anterior neural tissues. Hence, the synthesis of both DV and AP patterning through coordinated cellular communication underscores the complexity and elegance of embryonic development, showcasing the vital role of the DV axis in shaping the future organism (Carron et al., 2016; Takebayashi-Suzuki et al., 2020) (Figure 2.11).

2.3.3. Left-Right Axis

Left-right axis is a key characteristic of embryonic development that is used in establishing symmetrical body patterns. Patterning on the left-right axis is very important to enable proper organ orientation and function and also systems orientation and function. During early embryogenesis, specialized signaling pathways such as Nodal signaling are important in establishing the initial asymmetry required for left-right patterning. These cues initiate the expression of key transcription factors that drive left-specific and right-specific networks of genes. Understanding the precise mechanisms of left-right axis formation is essential, as perturbation of this process leads to congenital abnormalities and organ malposition's, such as situs inversus totalis, where organs are mirror-reversed of the typical location (Schaerli et al., 2018). Research on the genetic and molecular mechanism of left-right axis determination reveals intricate pathways and interactions among several signaling molecules. For instance, cilia and fluid flow interaction is pivotal in inducing left-right asymmetry in the majority of vertebrates. Cilia create one-way fluid movement that helps in the non-symmetrical patterning of signaling molecules around the embryonic body, which further determines on which side the left and the right sides are developed. Moreover, dysfunction in their activity leads to massive developmental defects, thereby indicating the significance of physical forces in genetic programming in the earliest stages of development (Velten et al., 2015). Thus, any complete understanding of axis formation must include explanation of both genetic regulation and physical forces. The left-right axis is part of the broader field of embryonic patterning, in which there are countless interactions between axes formation, signaling pathways, and cell behavior. The extremely conserved nature of left-right axis mechanisms throughout species attests to evolutionary relevance, proposing an ancestral mechanism that has diversified. Comparative analyses of species including zebrafish, mouse, and human have shed light into molecular discourses that define left-right determination. These details show how conservation and deviation in such processes are able to influence evolutionary paths and developmental routes. Exploring the intricacies of the left-right axis not only serves to advance embryology but also provides new avenues of inquiry into evolutionary biology and congenital anatomy (Schaerli et al., 2018) (Figure 2.12).

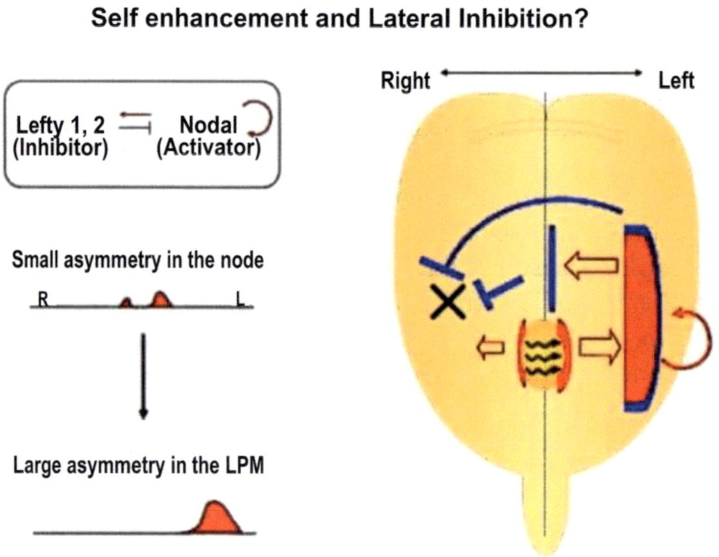

Figure 2.12. Left-right axis.

Source: https://i.ytimg.com/vi/dbJgNa7w_cs/sddefault.jpg.

2.4. Model Organisms in Axis Formation Studies

Axis formation during embryonic development has been richly informed by the use of model organisms, which give us insights into the processes that underlie patterning and body axis formation. Traditional model organisms like *Drosophila melanogaster* and *Xenopus laevis* have been central to an understanding of basic processes in embryogenesis, which exposed the functions of different molecular signals and gene pathways. For example, studies on *Drosophila* have illustrated the process of dorsal-ventral axis formation via sequential complex signaling events during eggshell patterning. Although narrowing the study focus on a few model organisms has led to significant findings, at the same time, it runs the risk of neglecting the wider evolutionary backgrounds and species-specific adaptations that determine axis formation in a variety of organisms. Thus, increasing the repertoire of model organisms might fill gaps in knowledge of intricate developmental processes, such as those that explain animal diversity and speciation (Helen et al., 2025). The latest advances in genetic technology and high-throughput sequencing have also created promising avenues for investigating non-traditional model organisms, which can illuminate the evolutionary foundations of axis formation. These organisms usually have novel cellular and molecular processes that are distinct from the ones found in conventional models. With the help of new genome editing methods like CRISPR/Cas9, one can now manipulate genes in many species that were hitherto neglected because one lacked suitable tools to handle them. This growth is crucial because research in species with different developmental processes can uncover evolutionary innovations that are essential to understanding how different organisms construct body plans. The relationship between genetic information and environmental signals can give greater insight into the processes involved in embryonic patterning and the relevance to evolutionary biology in general (Helen Stott et al., 2025). Additionally, new advances in 3D modeling technologies based on induced pluripotent stem cells (iPSCs) have advanced our comprehension of human axis development, especially concerning somite development. These pluripotent stem cell-derived models allow for the examination of embryonic traits and dynamics that lead researchers further to recapitulate human embryogenesis. The development of axioloids—3D structures that simulate human segmentation and somitogenesis—has proven particularly impactful, as they embody oscillatory dynamics and signaling gradients similar to those found in natural embryonic development. These models reveal significant insights into the critical roles of signaling pathways, such as retinoic acid, in establishing organizational structures during development. Through the ability to study human congenital spine disease, such advances highlight the potential for model organisms to contribute to both basic biological knowledge and clinical practice (Figure 2.13).

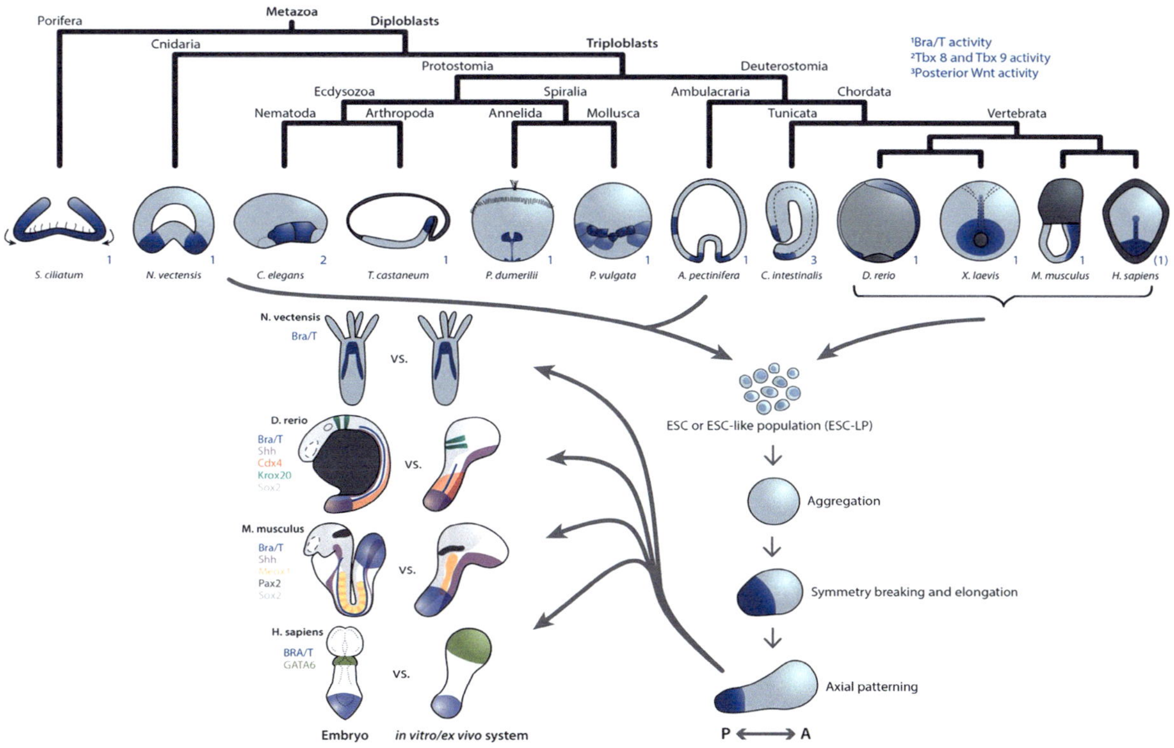

Figure 2.13. Model organisms in axis formation.

Source: https://external-content.duckduckgo.com/iu/?u=https%3A%2F%2Fiiif.elifesciences.org%2Flax%2F69066%2Felife-69066-fig1-v1.tif%2Ffull%2F1500%2C%2F0%2Fdefault.jpg&f=1&nofb=1&ipt=2e99063edbfc2dd6c23e85f1573704a692b359e0b0ccccd6528d9327e6e5410.

2.4.1. Zebrafish as a Model Organism

Zebrafish (*Danio rerio*) have become a leading model system for developmental biology, especially for the analysis of axis formation and embryonic patterning. Their transparent embryo makes it possible to visualize development in real time, and with this, to monitor the dynamics of cellular movements and tissue interactions in a way that has not been possible before. This transparency, combined with the fact that they develop fast—reaching important milestones within days—means that scientists can carry out time-critical experiments at the embryological level. Also, the external fertilization and high fecundity of zebrafish make large-scale genetic screens easy, helping identify genes critical to embryonal axis development. The simplicity of the generation of transgenic lines also extends the usefulness of zebrafish as a model since scientists can modify gene expression and follow the resulting phenotypic changes, thereby determining the molecular mechanisms underlying axis formation in early embryogenesis. In exploring the embryonic patterning in zebrafish, scientists have made great strides in the understanding of evolutionary conservation in developmental processes.

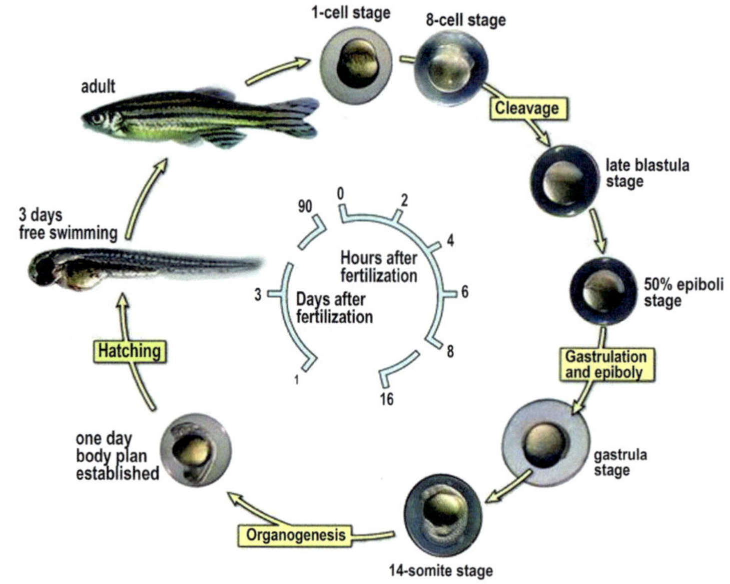

Figure 2.14. Zebrafish as a model organism.

Source: https://veteriankey.com/wp-content/uploads/2016/07/A152551_1_En_14_Fig2_HTML.jpg.

The species has basic similarities with higher vertebrates, humans included, and is therefore an extremely useful resource for comparative genetics and developmental biology. Experiments have shown that these important signaling pathways, including those of Wnt, Hedgehog, and Nodal, that are involved in the determination of body axes and organogenesis are vertebrate-conserved. Scientists have manipulated these pathways using zebrafish as a model organism and been able to view resulting changes in morphology and expression patterns of genes. Such studies not only emphasize the uniqueness of gene function but also demonstrate how disruptions in such pathways can result in developmental abnormalities, thus paving the way for greater insight into congenital conditions in humans (John et al., 2019). In addition, incorporating zebrafish in functional investigations provides means to comprehend intricate relationships, e.g., the gut-brain axis and its role in larger biological contexts, e.g., development and aging. The interactions between the microbiota and embryonic development have only just begun to attract interest, and most notably how microbial metabolites regulate axis formation and neural development. Animal models such as zebrafish are central to understanding these interactions and their relevance to health and disease. For instance, research into the roles of nuclear factor erythroid 2-related factor (Nrf2) in oxidative stress responses has highlighted its involvement in developmental processes and longevity, suggesting broader implications for age-related pathologies (Agnieszka Łoboda et al., 2016). Such findings emphasize the relevance of zebrafish not only for dissecting fundamental developmental biology but also for exploring translational applications related to human health (Figure 2.14).

2.4.2. Mouse Models in Embryonic Research

In embryonic research, mouse models are now priceless vehicles for studying axis formation and embryonic patterning. Using mouse models, one can specifically manipulate genes and check the resultant associated phenotypes and, thereby, interpret molecular events in development. For example, genetic alterations like knockout or transgenic models allow one to ascertain the role of a gene at key phases of development. With reagents like CRISPR-Cas9, scientists can now introduce particular mutations in possible genes to explore their function in embryonic morphology and obtain a richer picture of how various pathways collaborate to build axes and body plans. Mouse models are therefore not simply experimental systems but reflections of developmental biology's complexity as well, allowing for outcomes translatable to human congenital disorder therapeutic regimens. Furthermore, the use of mouse models does not confine itself to easy genetic manipulation but permits also the investigation of environmental effects on embryonic development. The work of some authors demonstrated that the input from external sources, for example, maternal nutrition and teratogen exposure, could radically alter the course of normal embryonic patterning. By subjecting pregnant mice to various conditions, scientists can track resulting developmental malformations in offspring that provide hints about gene-environment interactions.

These experiments are critical in assessing how developmental disruptions might eventually have long-term health outcomes, including NDDs and other birth abnormalities. Consequently, the application of mouse models offers a more holistic view of embryonic development, both uniting genetic and environmental factors to offer insight into how these factors interact early in life to govern later health. Finally, the technology innovations in mouse models, such as *in vivo* imaging and embryonic stem cell (ESC) manipulation, have considerably improved our understanding of embryonic patterning. These approaches enable real-time observation of embryonic tissues and their dynamic evolution through development.

For instance, scientists can use advanced imaging techniques to monitor cell motion and molecular interactions in live embryos, obtaining an unprecedented insight into the processes of axis formation. In addition, derivation of organoids from mouse ESCs has provided new opportunities for modeling complex tissue interactions and developmental processes. By integrating *in vitro* results with *in vivo* information, scientists can construct comprehensive maps of developmental processes that reflect both environmental and genetic inputs. Ongoing development of mouse models is therefore a characteristic of contemporary embryonic science and drives our understanding of fundamental biological processes for axis formation and embryonic patterning (Figure 2.15).

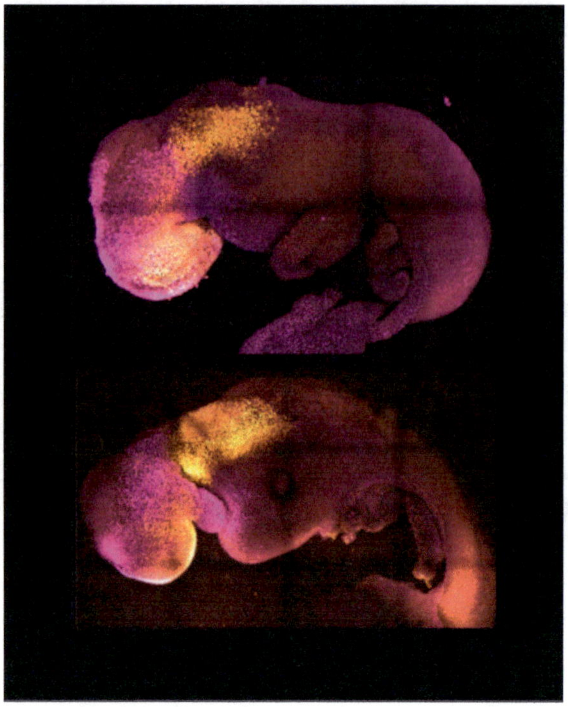

Figure 2.15. Mouse Models in Embryonic Research.

Source: https://www.nih.gov/sites/default/files/news-events/research-matters/2022/20220913-heart-formation.png.

2.4.3. Drosophila and Its Contributions to Understanding Patterning

Drosophila melanogaster has greatly influenced our understanding of axis formation and patterning of the embryo. As a primary model system, *Drosophila* offers a simple yet highly relevant system to examine complex developmental processes. The most significant contribution may be finding mechanisms for dorsal-ventral axis formation. It has been found through research that the formation of this axis is directly associated with the spatial distribution of morphogens, such as the Bicoid protein, responsible for causing proper cell fate determination along the anteroposterior axis. These studies emphasize the importance of gradient formation in development, thereby establishing a basis for principles of morphogen action and cellular response applicable beyond *Drosophila* to mammalian and other biological systems, including therapeutic potential. In addition, recent advances in genetic engineering, and particularly CRISPR/Cas9, have renewed interest in *Drosophila*, providing scientists with the ability to dissect the genetic mechanisms of embryonic patterning with unprecedented precision. Helen et al. (2025) points out that while *Drosophila* is a model organism for many embryogenic pathways, the complexities of development seen across organisms require an expanded tool kit that includes genetic tools for less-studied organisms. Such cross-species understanding of the genetic processes of pattern formation can reveal something about the evolution of developmental processes and the diversity of body plans of the animal kingdom. In so doing, *Drosophila* explains its own development but, equally importantly, acts as a point of reference for the explanation of the evolutionary paths of other species. In light of these contributions, it becomes evident that ongoing research into *Drosophila* is both timely and critical for enhancing our understanding of developmental biology. The lessons learned from this model organism about morphogen gradients, signaling pathways, and genetic interactions have provided a framework for analyzing similar processes in more complex organisms. In addition, Schroeter et al. (1996) emphasizes that interrogation of the underlying biochemical signals that control tissue organization can provide new insights into developmental disorders in man. This synthesis of *Drosophila* research with knowledge from other organisms deepens our understanding and encourages questions of the basic questions of embryogenesis and patterning. With these studies, *Drosophila* remains a cornerstone of developmental biology, bridging the gaps between basic science and applied uses in medicine and biotechnology (Figure 2.16).

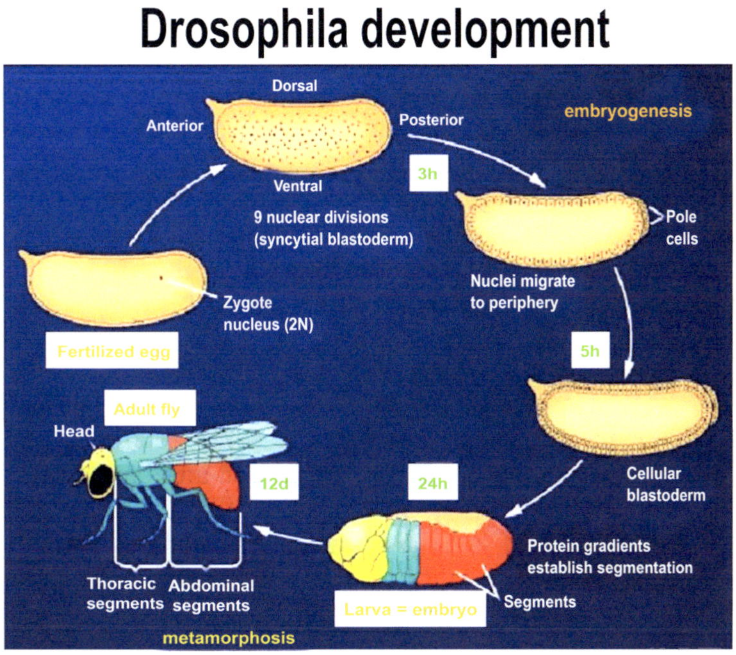

Figure 2.16. Pattern formation in *Drosophila*.

Source: https://external-content.duckduckgo.com/iu/?u=https%3A%2F%2Fimage1.slideserve.com%2F2117927%2Fslide3-l.jpg&f=1&nofb=1&ipt=83d9448b23bd390de98c8199af333986af12c2aa494d73e7e699dea423740e11.

2.5. Experimental Techniques

Research on axis formation and embryonic patterning requires powerful experimental approaches to unravel the molecular mechanisms involved. One such approach involves manipulation and observation of embryos *in vitro*, as seen from studies with squid embryos. Through the culturing of embryos in a controlled environment, scientists can treat embryos in an organized manner, for instance, using lithium chloride (LiCl), to determine its effect on developmental processes. The dose-dependent reaction to LiCl treatment provides valuable understanding into how changes in signaling pathways can yield variable embryonic phenotypes, especially influencing ectodermal structures. This carefully regulated environment allows for precise assessments of how modifications in chemical exposure influence axis orientation and ultimately contribute to our understanding of developmental biology and evolutionary conservation insights across species (Crawford, 2003). In addition to the application of chemical agents, experimental techniques such as phase-averaging velocity field measurements can elucidate complex biological systems and processes. For instance, using techniques analogous to those employed in engineering fluid dynamics, researchers can quantify the dynamics of embryonic patterning by investigating flow structures analogous to those seen in rotating axial fans. By synchronized velocity field measurements around forming embryos, researchers are able to see patterns of vortex generation and turbulence that are potentially connected with developmental windows for the formation of the axis and for the differentiation of cells. Such methods not only confirm numerical models but also form the basis for an appreciation of the mechanical influences on axis development during early embryogenesis (Choi et al., 2000). In addition, the merging of classical embryological methods with sophisticated imaging and analytical tools increases the ability to investigate axis formation in detail. In particular, the use of imaging methods together with experimental manipulation enables the real-time observation of developmental alterations under different stimuli. Such approaches can make the subtle motion and interaction of cells visible, allowing the development's spatial and temporal dynamics to be interpreted. Eventually, the ongoing improvement of these experimental methods will enable further breakthroughs in the area of axis formation and embryonic patterning, further elucidating the underlying principles controlling organismal development (Crawford, 2003).

2.5.1. In Situ Hybridization (ISH)

The method of *in situ* hybridization (ISH) has become a key technology in the study of gene expression in early development, especially in axis formation and embryonic patterning. Through the localization of particular RNA transcripts in embedded tissue sections, ISH offers a vital look into the spatial-temporal regulation of gene expression. This ability comes into play particularly when examining the roles played by different genes in determining body axes and the subsequent morphogenetic movements. For example, through the study of cadherin expression patterns using ISH, scientists can determine the extent to which differential adhesion properties of cells affect their organization during embryo development. These discoveries unveil complex interplay among gene expression, adhesion of cells, and the global organization of embryonic bodies, which are crucial for axis development to occur properly. ISH also plays a crucial role in understanding the molecular mechanisms driving important processes such as gastrulation. As the developing embryo undergoes this extremely important stage, proximal-distal axis formation is central to driving the fate determination of pluripotent stem cells.

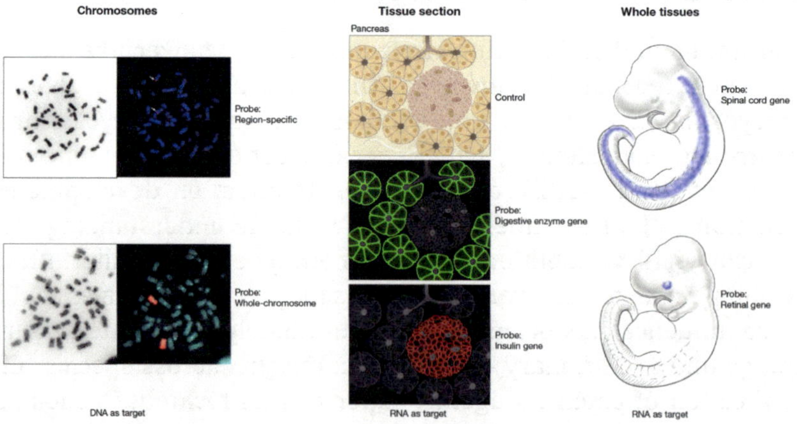

Figure 2.17. *In situ* hybridization (ISH).

Source: https://external-content.duckduckgo.com/iu/?u=https%3A%2F%2Fwww.genome.gov%2Fsites%2Fdefault%2Ffiles%2Fmedia%2Fimages%2Ftg%2FIn-Situ-Hybridization.jpg&f=1&nofb=1&ipt=fad8e5e3d0caa460ed3c04306cf8c0e52e792059fd818de5ad2f688a3295483f.

Experiments involving ISH have revealed that although the initial axis formation in developmental mutants is preserved, the later stages are disrupted, pointing to a complex interaction of signaling pathways. For instance, in Lmbrd1 deficient mice, the early embryonic stages remain undisturbed because initial axis formation signals are present. Nonetheless, as observed by ISH of pertinent genes like FGF 8, gastrulation initiation is unsuccessful, demonstrating the sensitivity of nodal signaling pathways for successful embryonic patterning (Buers et al., 2016). Incorporating ISH data into overall knowledge of embryonic development is an indication of the significance of this technique in modern developmental biology. Together with improvements in imaging methods and computer analysis software, ISH can provide detailed gene-expression profiles that guide the planning of gene manipulation experiments as well as targeted gene therapies. For example, cadherin expression patterns not only demonstrate their dynamic function in cell sorting and separation of tissues but also show how differential adhesion plays a role in segmentation of neuronal pools along the anterior-posterior axis (Polanco et al., 2021). This link highlights the complex role of gene expression in embryonic axis establishment and path, proving the importance of ISH as a cornerstone method in investigating the roots of embryonic patterning (Figure 2.17).

2.5.2. CRISPR-Cas9 Gene Editing

The CRISPR-Cas9 gene editing tool has transformed research into axis formation and embryonic patterning through the ability to make precise changes in specific genes in different organisms. By the careful use of CRISPR, scientists can explore the functions of key signaling pathways, including Wnt signaling, which plays a key role in anterior-posterior patterning of developing embryos. The potential to knock out pivotal genes, for example, DpWnt-1 in the pine caterpillar moth, demonstrates how CRISPR helps define the underlying biological mechanisms influencing embryonic mortality and developmental defects. Importantly, this kind of research shows that the outcomes of gene editing go beyond plain mutagenesis; they allow for further clarification of intricate biological events, being both methodological innovation and conceptual model for the analysis of functional gene function in non-model organisms (Huang et al., 2017). Additionally, the examination of gene modification consequences by means of CRISPR-Cas9 focuses on the mechanisms of neural patterning controlled by Wnt signaling pathways. The selective regulation of downstream target genes by the Wnt protein is important during the formation of particular neural fates, which is not yet fully comprehended. Target genes like sp5a and sp5l, which are important in the Wnt-dependent mediation of neural plate patterning in zebrafish, have been the focus of attention. Through the application of CRISPR technology to target these genes for editing, scientists can investigate their function in embryonic development *in vivo* and obtain fundamental information regarding how Wnt signaling regulates axis formation in vertebrates. The area of research indicates the importance of CRISPR-Cas9 in resolving basic questions in biology that are central to understanding embryonic development and the conservation of organismal diversity (Mohanty et al., 2019). Lastly, the incorporation of CRISPR-Cas9 in developmental biology is the potential for the research to translate to therapeutic treatments and applied biology. Gene editing to the highest level of accuracy not only enhances our understanding of gene function but also portends the development of new pest control measures, as seen with the manipulation of *D. punctatus*, which are among the major defoliators of forest ecosystems. By finding gene function through targeted editing, the possibility of developing eco-friendly methods of agriculture turns into reality. With increasing research taking up the CRISPR-Cas9 technology, its dual role in investigation and real-world applications reflects the revolutionary impact it has on understanding complex biological issues concerning axis formation and embryonic patterning. It highlights the critical function of gene editing in both expanding our current knowledge of key processes as well as informing future biological interventions across various fields (Huang et al., 2017; Mohanty et al., 2019) (Figure 2.18).

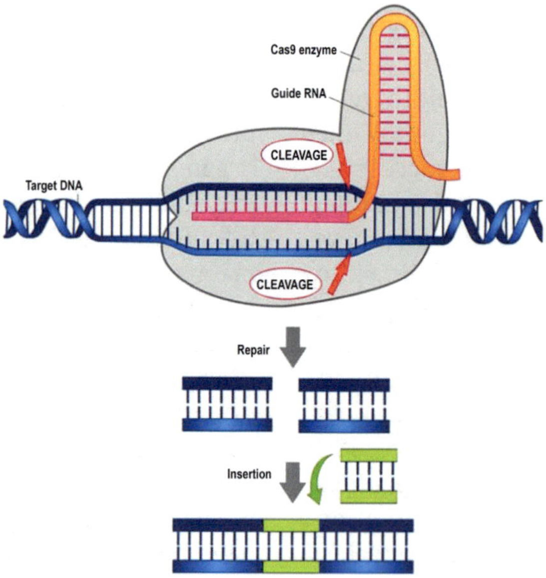

Figure 2.18. CRISPR-Cas9 gene editing.

Source: https://external-content.duckduckgo.com/iu/?u=https%3A%2F%2Fwww.labiotech.eu%2Fwp-content%2Fuploads%2F2017%2F05%2Fcrispr-cas9-drug-discovery2-1.jpg&f=1&nofb=1&ipt=74ef00144f1b156941f10cdddba89127646088a84e19248076f1dd7e1ba66c07.

2.5.3. Live Imaging of Embryonic Development

Live imaging tools have transformed our insights into embryonic development, with the new level of detailed observations into the dynamic processes controlling axis formation and patterning in early embryos. By employing cutting-edge microscopy techniques, scientists can now observe cellular behavior in real time, describing how cells communicate and adapt to each other during the fundamental phases of development. This light recording not only captures the morphogenetic events taking place but also makes it possible to analyze cellular movement, including migration, division, and differentiation. Using fluorescent labeling and time-lapse imaging, researchers have been able to follow spatiotemporal patterns of gene expression, which are critical to the formation of body axes and organ placement, respectively. These methods have shed light on the intricate dance of cell-cell interactions, uncovering how embryonic bodies are arranged and how fate is decided throughout development. The impact of microbiota on embryonic development has been a high-profile research area, bringing focus to the boundary between environmental factors and biological processes. These studies highlight the importance of gut microbiota as an agent of developmental effect, with effects not just on physiological function but also with the capacity to regulate embryonic axis formation and patterning via multiple signaling pathways. Microbial metabolites, for instance, can regulate host cellular response and thereby condition the microenvironment in which embryonic cells operate. Current research has demonstrated how different microbial content in early life—birth mode, diet, and pathogens—can program developmental trajectories. Understanding the microbiota-gut-brain axis, as highlighted in current studies, is central to illuminating the complexities of environmental influences in sensitive periods of development leading to long-term health in the developing organism (John et al., 2019).

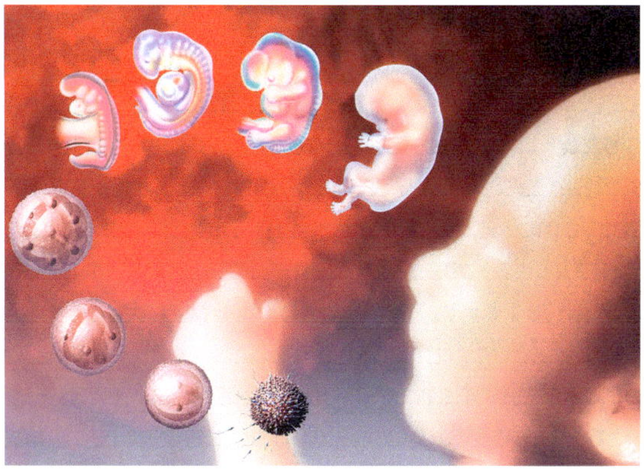

Figure 2.19. Live imaging of embryonic development.

Source: https://external-content.duckduckgo.com/iu/?u=https%3A%2F%2Fimages.fineartamerica.com%2Fimages-medium-large%2Fembryo-development-hans-ulrich-osterwalder.jpg&f=1&nofb=1&ipt=d7d488f42cf75f40834c55ec6d538d0d758fe99511757b975b3967d898367ff9.

Besides, axis formation mechanisms are greatly interconnected with cellular crystallization processes that make traditional models of development complicated. New evidence shows that, like in artificial systems' nonclassical pathways, embryonic cells may also involve particle-attachment mechanisms when they form organized structures. This analogy suggests that cell aggregation and differentiation forces may be more complex than ever previously envisioned, and therefore may be a function of interfacial force and cell-cell interaction variations. Investigations into these interactions could give rise to our understanding of how different cellular behaviors blend to give rise to stable, functionally ordered embryonic tissues. By integrating knowledge from both crystallization dynamics and embryology, scientists can design models of axis formation and unveil novel strategies in investigating developmental abnormalities (James et al., 2015) (Figure 2.19).

2.6. Implications of Axis Formation Research

The significance of axis formation research far transcends embryonic growth, since grasping the complex signaling pathways at work can inform other areas of biology. The development of embryonic axes is an essential process upon which accurate organogenesis and tissue differentiation depend. Perturbations in these processes can cause congenital malformations and developmental disorders. Experiments on the molecular mechanisms that control axis formation illustrate the interconnected nature of various biological systems, with disruption at early phases of development having long-term implications throughout the life of an organism. Such realization not only emphasizes the processes involved in normal developmental biology but also sets a course for the investigation of the etiology of numerous diseases associated with disturbance of development and thereby encourages further research in this direction. Also, recent findings in axis formation studies indicate its relevance to shedding light on complex environmental factors that guide development. Such external factors as maternal nutrition, exposure to toxins, or stress, for instance, may alter the expression of key developmental genes, leading to altered axis formation. Such genetic versus environmental dynamics is especially relevant to the study areas of evolutionary biology and ecology. The repercussions are extensive, as they suggest that environmental stress can create dramatic effects on developmental paths, potentially creating evolutionary change. By exploring the sensitivity of axis formation to environmental signals, scientists can clarify the mechanisms of phenotypic variation and adaptation, thereby leading towards a more cohesive understanding of development and evolution. Additionally, axis formation research holds promising therapeutic implications, especially in regenerative medicine and the treatment of disorders arising from aberrant development. Insights gleaned from this research may inform strategies for manipulating stem cell differentiation and enhancing tissue regeneration. For instance, understanding the role of signaling molecules in axis formation can lead to the development of targeted therapies that guide stem cells toward desired phenotypes. Moreover, as research increasingly highlights the role of the microbiota in developmental processes, as demonstrated in the context of the microbiota-gut-brain axis, therapeutic interventions could be designed to optimize microbial composition for better health outcomes (John et al., 2019). The potential to translate basic research on axis formation into clinical applications signifies a crucial intersection between developmental biology and medical science, indicating a wealth of opportunities for future investigations.

2.6.1. Understanding Congenital Disorders

The intricate processes governing axis formation and embryonic patterning have significant implications for understanding congenital disorders. During early embryonic development, precise signaling pathways dictate the spatial organization and differentiation of cells. Disruptions in these pathways can lead to abnormal axis formation, resulting in congenital conditions such as holoprosencephaly or spina bifida. By studying the molecular mechanisms that underpin these processes, researchers can identify potential genetic and environmental contributors to congenital disorders. Importantly, the identification of critical genes and proteins involved in signaling pathways not only enhances our understanding of embryonic development but also offers insights into the etiology of specific congenital disorders that arise from aberrations in these processes. Critical advancements in model organism research have further illuminated the link between axis formation and congenital disorders. It is essential to explore a broader array of model organisms to fully comprehend the diversity of embryonic patterning in both vertebrates and invertebrates. By expanding our research beyond traditional models like *Drosophila melanogaster*, we can investigate the unique embryonic signaling mechanisms that contribute to different forms of congenital disorders. As highlighted by recent findings on dorsal-ventral axis regulation in zebrafish and *Xenopus*, these species exhibit diverse patterns of signaling that can influence body axis development. Enhanced understanding of these non-traditional model organisms provides a richer framework for examining the role of maternal contributions in embryogenesis and the consequent risk factors for congenital disorders, thereby expanding the scientific community's capacity to develop targeted interventions and therapies. Significantly, the interplay between genetic and environmental factors during the early stages of development is crucial for understanding the origins of congenital disorders. The phosphorylation of proteins such as Huluwa underscores the intricate regulation involved in axis formation, as shown by its impact on β-catenin signaling pathways. Mutations or dysregulations in these signaling cascades can prevent proper axis formation, leading to congenital disorders characterized by severe morphological abnormalities. Understanding the specific roles of proteins and their regulatory mechanisms provides valuable insights into the pathophysiology of these conditions. By elucidating the critical factors involved in embryonic axis determination, researchers can establish important connections between developmental biology and clinical outcomes, paving the way for more effective strategies to prevent and treat congenital disorders through informed therapeutic interventions (Figure 2.20).

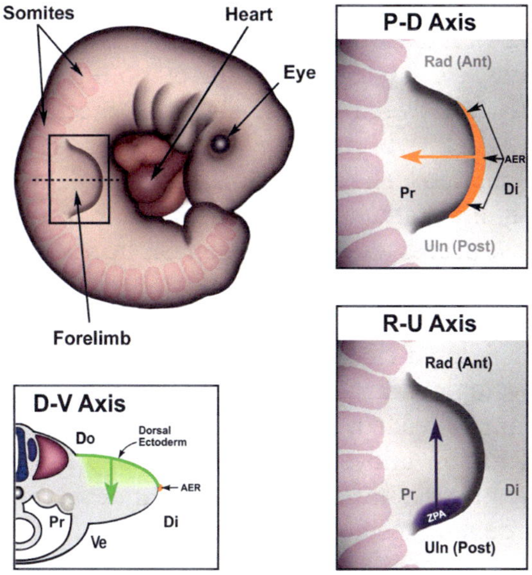

Figure 2.20. Congenital disorders in axis formation.

Source: https://journals.sagepub.com/cms/10.1177/1753193418801280/asset/3b80e1d9-137e-4456-94b4-838f1dc786ca/assets/images/large/10.1177_1753193418801280-fig1.jpg.

2.6.2. Applications in Regenerative Medicine

The integration of advanced materials in regenerative medicine is transforming therapeutic strategies, particularly through innovative approaches such as electrospinning. This technique enables the production of nanofibers from various materials, which can be tailored in terms of diameter, composition, and surface properties to emulate the extracellular matrix (ECM). By designing scaffolds that mimic native tissue architecture, researchers can effectively manipulate cell behavior, promoting cell adhesion and growth crucial for tissue engineering. For instance, aligned nanofibers can direct cellular migration and proliferation, enhancing the regeneration of tendons and peripheral nerves. Such scaffolds not only support cellular activities but also facilitate nutrient transport, signaling, and waste removal, thus creating an optimal microenvironment for healing and regenerative processes in damaged tissues. The development of these tailored scaffolds signifies a pivotal advancement in regenerative strategies, providing hope for more effective treatments in tissue repair and regeneration (Xue et al., 2017). Moreover, smart biomimetic devices represent a cutting-edge frontier in the realm of regenerative medicine, combining mechanical adaptivity with sophisticated microelectronics. These devices can self-assemble and attach to biological tissues, allowing for real-time monitoring and guidance of cellular behaviors during regeneration. Their design draws inspiration from natural processes, enabling them to interact dynamically with their environment. For instance, these devices can facilitate neuronal growth by gently enclosing nervous fibers and delivering localized stimulation, promoting recovery after injury. Their ability to integrate electronic components within soft, biocompatible materials presents novel opportunities for developing intelligent prosthetics and implants that respond to physiological changes. This advancement not only enhances tissue communication but also offers potential for improved interaction between implanted devices and surrounding tissues, leading to better integration and functionality in regenerative applications (Karnaushenko et al., 2015). The intersection of electrospun nanofibers and smart biomimetic devices illustrates the significance of interdisciplinary approaches in regenerative medicine. By leveraging nanotechnology and advanced materials, this field is making strides towards improving clinical outcomes in tissue regeneration. Research into these artificial ECMs reveals promising findings in various applications, from nerve repair to wound healing. For instance, the ability to engineer scaffolds that replicate the complex hierarchical structures of natural tissues ensures that these materials can provide mechanical support while promoting cellular responses that mimic natural healing processes. As the understanding of biological patterns and axis formation advances, the potential to create more effective regenerative solutions becomes increasingly viable, paving the way for therapies that can significantly enhance recovery experiences for patients at various stages of tissue damage and healing (Karnaushenko et al., 2015; Xue et al., 2017).

2.6.3. Insights into Evolutionary Biology

The concept of body axis formation has substantial implications for understanding evolutionary biology, particularly concerning the evolution of body plans throughout the animal kingdom. A critical exploration of cnidarians, such as Hydra, offers valuable insights into primitive signaling mechanisms that govern cellular organization. The TGF-β signaling pathway, which includes essential BMPs, is vital for the maintenance of the Organizer region in Hydra. This pathway exemplifies the conserved nature of certain biological processes across disparate organisms (Krishnapati et al., 2024). By analyzing how these molecular signaling networks function in cnidarians, researchers can glean information about the evolutionary transitions that led to more complex metazoans, as well as their developmental processes. Thus, the study of cnidarian axis formation not only enhances our comprehension of embryological patterns but also contributes to a broader understanding of evolutionary developmental biology. Investigations into Wnt signaling pathways further illustrate the intricate relationships between embryonic axis formation and evolutionary biology. The canonical Wnt pathways, dependent on β-catenin, play a crucial role in determining the dorsoventral, anteroposterior, and left-right axes during early embryonic development. Meanwhile, non-canonical Wnt signaling influences cellular movements and the establishment of polarity, both essential for proper patterning (Shi, 2024). It is through the understanding of these pathways that significant correlations have been drawn between genetic signaling mechanisms and the evolutionary adaptations seen in vertebrates. The disruption of Wnt signaling not only highlights the fundamental importance of these processes in embryogenesis but also raises pertinent questions about the evolutionary consequences of molecular signaling changes, providing a rich context for future research in developmental biology and evolutionary theory. Ultimately, uncovering the parallels between axis formation and evolutionary biology reshapes our understanding of organismal development throughout geological time. The conservation of critical signaling pathways, such as TGF-β and Wnt, underscores the evolutionary relationships across various species and provides insight into how complex structures and systems have emerged. In tracing the lineage of these signaling mechanisms from simpler organisms like cnidarians to more sophisticated vertebrates, scientists can piece together the evolutionary narrative that governs biological form and function. The integration of findings from these diverse fields reinforces the idea that embryonic patterning not only shapes organisms but also reflects the underlying evolutionary history that has contributed to the rich diversity of life observed today. This intersection of axis formation and evolutionary biology is essential for a comprehensive understanding of how embryonic processes have shaped the development of species over millions of years.

SUMMARY

The study of axis formation and embryonic patterning exposes the complex interplay between cellular movements and development signals. As presented in recent research, including zebrafish explant experiments, embryonic cells still possess the ability to organize and develop mesodermal structures, highlighting an impressive robustness against cell mixing perturbations (Timothy et al., 2020). This robustness suggests that the underlying mechanisms of axis specification are evolutionarily conserved and that similar processes can offer insights into how they might work in other species. Also, such discoveries highlight the importance of morphological signals and how deviations from normal morphogenetic processes can interfere with neural tissue patterning, with far-reaching implications for developmental anomalies. Advances in organoid development and stem cell technology immensely improve our knowledge of organogenesis, reflecting the rules of axis formation in an artificial setting (Xinaris et al., 2015). Utilizing three-dimensional culture systems, scientists are able to see how stem cells organize themselves to mimic embryonic structures. This ability to control cellular milieus creates new opportunities for modeling both normal developmental pathways and disease states. In addition, these advancements enable researchers to investigate the complex interactions between cellular organization and external signals with important nodes in the developmental story that could represent general principles of biology across different systems. Finally, the interaction between embryonic patterning and axis formation is a unifying theme in developmental biology that relates cellular communication, spatial orientation, and genetic regulation. The strong mechanisms that underlie these processes are critical in guaranteeing the proper establishment of body plans in multicellular life. While research continues, the discussion between basic science and translational medical practice becomes more evident, with implications in regenerative medicine and therapeutic intervention. Comprehension of the intricate biology of axis establishment and its ramifications not only further our basic knowledge but also sets the stage for revolutionizing innovations in tissue engineering and disease modeling, in the end closing the divide between embryology and clinical practice.

The complex mechanisms of axis development and embryonic pattern formation are highlighted by a range of molecular interactions and developmental signals that determine the formation of body structures. One of the notable observations is the melanin distribution gradient seen along the dorsal-ventral axis, especially among domestic geese. Of particular interest, studies at various stages of embryogenesis indicated the expression of major melanin synthesis genes like TYR, TYRP1, and EDNRB2 that were very high in dorsal skin at early embryogenesis but showed decreased expression by subsequent stages. In addition, the ASIP gene showed increased expression in distal foot compared to dorsal skin after E22, suggesting an intricate regulatory process involved in pigmentation patterns. The discovery of eight gene ontology terms involved in melanin biosynthesis emphasizes the significance of these molecular processes in axis formation and embryonic development as a whole (Yang et al., 2024). In another concurrent line of research, mammalian tooth development offers another window into embryonic patterning on the anterior-posterior axis. The unambiguous demarcation in heterodonty, with simpler teeth anteriorly and more elaborate structures posteriorly, underscores the importance of certain signaling pathways during jaw differentiation. An evaluation of gene expression across early odontogenesis highlighted region-specific expression patterns for key signaling molecules, such as BMP and FGF. Interestingly, the identification of an as-yet uncharacterized gene, SATB2, that is differentially expressed in incisor and molar developing areas highlights its significant role in the formation of anterior teeth. SATB2 manipulation has shown its essential function not only in incisors but also in the modulation of patterns in molar region, demonstrating the intricate relationships responsible for embryonic tooth development (Nevoránková et al., 2024). Collectively, these studies shed light on basic mechanisms of axis formation and embryonic patterning, revealing the subtle interplay between genetic determinants and developmental signals. The implications of melanin distribution indicate that gene expression profiles for pigmentation are rigorously controlled throughout embryonic development, informing our understanding of morphological variation. Concurrently, determination of the genetic determinants of dental development illustrates how unique expression patterns are responsible for regional specialization along the jaw. The lessons learned from these forays not only deepen our view of the biological basis of axis formation but also set the stage for continuing research efforts intended to unveil the intricacies of embryonic development in different species. The synthesis of these findings consolidates the idea that embryonic patterning and axis formation are essential to grasping organismal diversity and evolution.

CLOSER LOOK

ORAL-ABORAL AXIS

The oral-aboral axis is a fundamental body axis observed in radially symmetrical animals, particularly cnidarians (like jellyfish, sea anemones, and corals) and echinoderms (such as sea stars and sea urchins). This axis runs from the mouth (oral end) to the side opposite the mouth (aboral end) and is a key organizer of body structure and orientation in these animals. Unlike the bilateral symmetry seen in humans and other vertebrates, where there are distinct left-right and head-tail (anterior-posterior) orientations, radially symmetrical animals rely primarily on the oral-aboral axis to establish their body plan. In cnidarians, for example, the oral end typically contains the mouth and tentacles used for feeding, while the aboral end may be attached to a substrate or free-floating in the water. This axis defines how cells, tissues, and organs are spatially organized during development and regeneration, influencing how the organism interacts with its environment.

In embryonic development, the establishment of the oral-aboral axis is a crucial early event that influences morphogenesis and differentiation. In cnidarians, such as the model organism *Nematostella vectensis* (a sea anemone), the oral pole is usually defined first, often through localized gene expression or maternal determinants in the egg. The aboral pole is established later, creating a polarity that guides the formation of structures like the gastrodermis, epidermis, nerve net, and tentacles. Molecular studies have shown that the Wnt signaling pathway plays a central role in defining the oral end, similar to its role in anterior-posterior axis formation in bilaterians. This suggests a deep evolutionary link between the body axis systems of radially and bilaterally symmetrical animals.

In echinoderms, which undergo a transformation from bilateral larvae to radially symmetrical adults, the oral-aboral axis also plays a key role in development. During larval stages, echinoderms like sea urchins exhibit bilateral features, but as they metamorphose into adults, they reorganize around the oral-aboral axis. The mouth, located on the underside of the adult body, becomes the oral side, while the opposite side becomes the aboral surface, often containing structures like the anus and the madreporite (a part of the water vascular system). This metamorphosis and reorientation underscore the plasticity and evolutionary adaptability of the oral-aboral axis in different lineages.

Understanding the oral-aboral axis provides important insights into evolutionary developmental biology (evo-devo). It helps researchers trace the origins of body patterning mechanisms and how they may have evolved into the more complex body plans of bilaterians. Moreover, the study of this axis informs us about axis specification, regeneration, and even stem cell behavior in simple animals, many of which can regenerate entire bodies from small fragments. In summary, the oral-aboral axis is a central organizing principle in radially symmetrical animals, guiding embryonic development, body structure, and regeneration. It not only defines how these organisms grow and function but also provides a vital comparative model for understanding the evolution of body axes across the animal kingdom.

REFERENCES

1. Abzhanov, A., Baggiolini, A., Baroffio, A., Beverdam, A., Chevallier, A., et al. (2019). *Molecular and Cellular Mechanisms Underlying the Evolution of Form and Function in The Amniote Jaw.* https://core.ac.uk/download/323079229.pdf.
2. Briggs, J. A., Weinreb, C., Wagner, D. E., Megason, S. G., Peshkin, L., Kirschner, M., & Klein, A. M. (2018). The dynamics of gene expression in vertebrate embryogenesis at single-cell resolution. *Science, 360.* https://www.semanticscholar.org/paper/b873726bc2d62d83bb23641958072dcd9dbcc29a (accessed on 27 May 2025).
3. Buers, I., Pennekamp, P., Nitschke, Y., Lowe, C., Skryabin, B. V., & Rutsch, F. (2016). *Lmbrd1* expression is essential for the initiation of gastrulation. *Journal of Cellular and Molecular Medicine, 20*, 1523–1533. https://doi.org/10.1111/jcmm.12844.
4. Carron, C., & Shi, D. (2016). Specification of anteroposterior axis by combinatorial signaling during *Xenopus* development. *Wiley Interdisciplinary Reviews: Developmental Biology, 5.* https://www.semanticscholar.org/paper/457a38c2168214be094763502af8b6f474b583a4 (accessed on 27 May 2025).
5. Choi, J. H., Kim, H. B., Lee, S., & Lee, I. (2000). Velocity field measurement of flow around an axial fan using a phase-averaged 2-frame PTV technique. *Transactions of The Korean Society of Mechanical Engineers B, 24*, 114–123. https://www.semanticscholar.org/paper/9c57c8a44169cefaf85e64260e2ac0a6d1a9e9e4 (accessed on 27 May 2025).
6. Coolen, M., Da Silva, C., Lallemand, Y., et al. (2007). *Evolution of Axis Specification Mechanisms in Jawed Vertebrates: Insights from A Chondrichthyan.* https://core.ac.uk/download/4877499.pdf.
7. Crawford, K. (2003). Lithium chloride inhibits development along the animal vegetal axis and anterior midline of the squid embryo. *The Biological Bulletin, 205*(2), 181–182. https://www.semanticscholar.org/paper/c3f92e7264c8b2a801a91ab5e78b3306b896566d (accessed on 27 May 2025).
8. Cryan, J. F., O'Riordan, K. J., Cowan, C. S. M., Sandhu, K. V., Bastiaanssen, T. F. S., Boehme, M., Codagnone, M. G., et al. (2019). The microbiota-gut-brain axis. *Physiological Reviews, 99*, 1877–2013. https://doi.org/10.1152/physrev.00018.2018.
9. De Yoreo, J. J., Gilbert, B., Sommerdijk, N. A. J. M., Penn, R. L., Whitelam, S., Joester, D., Zhang, H., et al. (2015). Crystallization by particle attachment in synthetic, biogenic, and geologic environments. *Science, 349.* https://doi.org/10.1126/science.aaa6760.
10. Dierickx, P., van Laake, L. W., & Geijsen, N. (2017). Circadian clocks: From stem cells to tissue homeostasis and regeneration. *EMBO Reports, 19*(1), 18–28. https://doi.org/10.15252/embr.201745130.
11. Dold, A., Han, H., Liu, N., Hildebrandt, A., Brüggemann, M., Rücklé, C., Hänel, H., et al. (2020). Makorin 1 controls embryonic patterning by alleviating Bruno1-mediated repression of oskar translation. *PLoS Genetics, 16.* https://www.semanticscholar.org/paper/8e206479e2779643a6b828c3b831b17ee7062042 (accessed on 27 May 2025).
12. Fraser, S. E., & Shih, J. (1995). *Distribution of Tissue Progenitors Within the Shield Region of The Zebrafish Gastrula.* https://core.ac.uk/download/4893795.pdf.
13. Fulton, T. J., Trivedi, V., Attardi, A., Anlaş, K., Dingare, C., Martínez Arias, A., & Steventon, B. (2020). Axis specification in zebrafish is robust to cell mixing and reveals a regulation

of pattern formation by morphogenesis. *Current Biology, 30*(15), 3063–3064. https://doi.org/10.1016/j.cub.2020.07.022.

14. Huang, Y., Liu, H., Liu, Q., Zhang, et al. (2017). Genome editing of *Wnt-1*, a gene associated with segmentation, via CRISPR/Cas9 in the pine caterpillar moth, *Dendrolimus punctatus*. https://core.ac.uk/download/232589608.pdf (accessed on 27 May 2025).
15. Huljev, K., Shamipour, S., Pinheiro, D., Preusser, F., Steccari, I., Sommer, C., Naik, S., et al. (2023). A hydraulic feedback loop between mesendoderm cell migration and interstitial fluid relocalization promotes embryonic axis formation in zebrafish. *Developmental Cell*. https://www.semanticscholar.org/paper/4621a52719cc46c370cc6f82c4d6a8aaba28ec07 (accessed on 27 May 2025).
16. Hunt, G., Vaid, R., Pirogov, S., Pfab, A., Ziegenhain, C., Sandberg, R., Reimegård, J., et al. (2024). Tissue-specific RNA polymerase II promoter-proximal pause release and burst kinetics in a *Drosophila* embryonic patterning network. *Genome Biology, 25*. https://www.semanticscholar.org/paper/b0ebbb29e2f5299dda7f2c97cdc992c2a5809e8e (accessed on 27 May 2025).
17. Karnaushenko, D., Münzenrieder, N., Karnaushenko, D. D., Koch, B., Meyer, A. K., Baunack, S., Petti, L., et al. (2015). Biomimetic microelectronics for regenerative neuronal cuff implants. *Advanced Materials, 27*, 6797–6805. https://doi.org/10.1002/adma.201503696.
18. Krishnapati, L., & Ghaskadbi, S. (2024). TGF-β signaling molecules in Hydra: Role of BMP and BMP inhibitors during pattern formation. *The International Journal of Developmental Biology*. https://www.semanticscholar.org/paper/e51bdddd1848d1959ae0cce866e7685ee859d560 (accessed on 27 May 2025).
19. Li, Y., Yan, Y., Gong, B., Zheng, Q., Zhou, H., Sun, J., Li, M., et al. (2024). A Huluwa phosphorylation switch regulates embryonic axis induction. *Nature Communications, 15*, 2057. https://www.semanticscholar.org/paper/0ede7219bd0f6fb76629ae715d671c565c51a535 (accessed on 27 May 2025).
20. Łoboda, A., Damulewicz, M., Pyza, E., Józkowicz, A., & Dulak, J. (2016). Role of Nrf2/HO-1 system in development, oxidative stress response and diseases: An evolutionarily conserved mechanism. *Cellular and Molecular Life Sciences, 73*, 3221–3247. https://doi.org/10.1007/s00018-016-2223-0.
21. Mohanty, S. (2019). *The Role of Sp1 Family Genes in Wnt Mediated Neural Plate Patterning* [Master's thesis, University of Ottawa]. CORE. https://core.ac.uk/download/186711803.pdf (accessed on 27 May 2025).
22. Nevoránková, P., Šulcová, M., Kavková, M., Zimčík, D., Balková, S., Peléšková, K., Kristeková, D., et al. (2024). Region-specific gene expression profiling of early mouse mandible uncovered SATB2 as a key molecule for teeth patterning. *Scientific Reports, 14*, 4847. https://www.semanticscholar.org/paper/7fdc8c2c4640d177e08288095042a61ab05ea536 (accessed on 27 May 2025).
23. Panavaite, L. (2018). *Emergence of Cellular Heterogeneity and Body Plan in Early Mammalian Development* [Doctoral dissertation, University of Cambridge]. CORE. https://core.ac.uk/download/160442148.pdf.
24. Polanco, J., Reyes-Vigil, F., Weisberg, S. D., Dhimitruka, I., & Brusés, J. L. (2021). Differential spatiotemporal expression of type I and type II cadherins associated with the segmentation of the central nervous system and formation of brain nuclei in the developing mouse. *Frontiers in Molecular Neuroscience, 14*, 633719. https://doi.org/10.3389/fnmol.2021.633719.

25. Qian, X., Song, H., & Ming, G.-L. (2019). Brain organoids: Advances, applications and challenges. *Development, 146*, dev166074. https://doi.org/10.1242/dev.166074.

26. Riley, J. S., & Tait, S. W. G. (2020). Mitochondrial DNA in inflammation and immunity. *EMBO Reports, 21*. https://doi.org/10.15252/embr.201949799.

27. Rodrigues, M., Kosaric, N., Bonham, C. A., & Gurtner, G. C. (2018). Wound healing: A cellular perspective. *Physiological Reviews, 99*, 665–706. https://doi.org/10.1152/physrev.00067.2017.

28. Schaerli, Y., Jiménez, A., Duarte, J. M., Mihajlovic, L., Renggli, J., Isalan, M., Sharpe, J., et al. (2018). Synthetic circuits reveal how mechanisms of gene regulatory networks constrain evolution. *Molecular Systems Biology, 14*, e78102. https://doi.org/10.15252/msb.20178102.

29. Schroeter, S., & Blakely, R. (1996). Drug targets in the embryo. *Annals of the New York Academy of Sciences, 801*, 1–12. https://www.semanticscholar.org/paper/a80d39ced20ce81276746fe3e6b5474a44f8b6f0 (accessed on 27 May 2025).

30. Shi, D. L. (2024). Canonical and non-canonical Wnt signaling generates molecular and cellular asymmetries to establish embryonic axes. *Journal of Developmental Biology, 12*. https://www.semanticscholar.org/paper/b11029b499ab3d5b70da9111f9817aff9194d1f1 (accessed on 27 May 2025).

31. Shimizu, T., & Nakamoto, A. (2014). Developmental significance of D quadrant micromeres 2d and 4d in the oligochaete annelid Tubifex tubifex. *The International Journal of Developmental Biology, 58*(6–8), 445–456. https://www.semanticscholar.org/paper/84c5019bdcc16274ced57a8c55c2f509d67ee853 (accessed on 27 May 2025).

32. Shin, Y., & Brangwynne, C. P. (2017). Liquid phase condensation in cell physiology and disease. *Science, 357*, eaaf4382. https://doi.org/10.1126/science.aaf4382.

33. Stott, H. L., & Yakoby, N. (2025). Diversity of *Drosophila* egg patterning: The missing tools to explore embryonic axis formation. *Frontiers in Cell and Developmental Biology, 13*. https://www.semanticscholar.org/paper/a5ff28d14da83c4915357f48874ca232c271d14c (accessed on 27 May 2025).

34. Takebayashi-Suzuki, K., & Suzuki, A. (2020). Intracellular communication among morphogen signaling pathways during vertebrate body plan formation. *Genes, 11*, 864. https://www.semanticscholar.org/paper/2c0e72f4d12a7b5db29af4d6fd3cc9ca7d899d87 (accessed on 27 May 2025).

35. Velten, L., Anders, S., Pękowska, A., Järvelin, A. I., Huber, W., Pelechano, V., & Steinmetz, L. M. (2015). Single-cell polyadenylation site mapping reveals 3′ isoform choice variability. *Molecular Systems Biology, 11*, 812. https://doi.org/10.15252/msb.20156198.

36. Willet, S. G., & Mills, J. C. (2016). Stomach organ and cell lineage differentiation: From embryogenesis to adult homeostasis. *Cellular and Molecular Gastroenterology and Hepatology, 2*(5), 546–559. https://doi.org/10.1016/j.jcmgh.2016.05.006.

37. Xinaris, C., Brizi, V., & Remuzzi, G. (2015). Organoid models and applications in biomedical research. *Nephron, 130*, 191–199. https://doi.org/10.1159/000433566.

38. Xu, J., Liu, H., Lan, Y., Adam, M., Clouthier, D. E., Potter, S. S., & Jiang, R. (2019). Hedgehog signaling patterns the oral-aboral axis of the mandibular arch. *eLife, 8*. https://doi.org/10.7554/elife.40315.

39. Xue, J., Xie, J., Liu, W., & Xia, Y. (2017). Electrospun nanofibers: new concepts, materials, and applications. *Accounts of Chemical Research, 50*, 1976–1987. https://doi.org/10.1021/acs.accounts.7b00218.

40. Yamanaka, Y., Yoshioka-Kobayashi, K., Hamidi, S., Munira, S., Sunadome, K., Zhang, Y., Kurokawa, Y., et al. (2022). Reconstituting human somitogenesis *in vitro*. *Nature, 614*, 509–520. https://www.semanticscholar.org/paper/5f837f12bc7b2351802f9d4e9a7197fed36cb016 (accessed on 27 May 2025).

41. Yang, Y., Wang, C., Liu, Y., Li, G., Wang, X., Wang, H., & He, D. (2024). Comparative transcriptomic analyses reveal key genes underlying melanin distribution during embryonic development in geese (*Anser anser*). *British Poultry Science*. https://www.semanticscholar.org/paper/28840b718888c5539c07c62f097ab056208db64d (accessed on 27 May 2025).

42. Zinski, J., Bu, Y., Wang, X., Dou, W., Umulis, D. M., & Mullins, M. C. (2017). Systems biology derived source-sink mechanism of BMP gradient formation. *eLife, 6*, e22199. https://doi.org/10.7554/elife.22199.

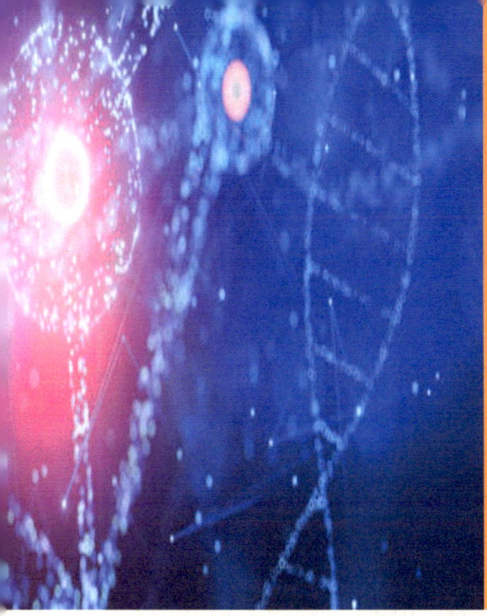

Chapter 3

NEURAL DEVELOPMENT AND NEUROGENETICS

Contents

Introduction

In the emerging and dynamic field of neuroscience, understanding neural development and neurogenetics is important to unravel the complexities of the human brain. Neural development involves processes through which nerve cells or neurons form, migrate, differentiate, and make synaptic connections. Neurogenetics, on the other hand, investigates the genetic processes underlying such developmental processes and provides insight into normal as well as pathological brain function. The interaction between environmental forces and genetic factors is the essence of neurodevelopmental research, focusing on the contribution of both heredity and environment to the patterning of neural structures. Through such analysis, researchers expect to enlighten the pathways to neurodevelopmental disorders (NDDs), guiding therapeutic interventions. Unambiguous comprehension of such interactions is paramount not only for scientific research but also for clinical utility. Neuroscience techniques have significantly enhanced our understanding of neurogenetics and neural development. Novel innovation in image tools and gene manipulation has provided an unprecedented degree of access to the anatomy of neural circuits and the function of specific genes in the behavior of neurons. Techniques such as CRISPR-Cas9 gene editing make it possible for precise changes in genetic material, and scientists can utilize them to investigate the nuances of neurodevelopmental processes. At the same time, non-invasive imaging techniques, including functional MRI and diffusion tensor imaging, enable the visualization of brain structure and function in living organisms. These innovations have made it possible for scientists to investigate complex phenomena such as synaptic plasticity and neural network development. By integrating findings across methodologies, researchers are better able to overcome the constraints inherent to brain disorder research, allowing for the creation of more targeted and effective interventions. The implications of neurogenetics and neurodevelopment are far-reaching beyond academia, affecting medicine, psychology, and education. Knowledge and understanding derived from neurogenetic study feed into early intervention and diagnosis approaches for NDDs, improving the overall quality of life for those affected in the end. What's more, knowing the genetic mechanisms behind the disorders can shape personal treatment, with therapies being designed to suit individuals. In the classroom, knowledge of neural development can influence curricula that develop cognitive abilities and support a variety of learning styles. The crossing of neural development with neurogenetics, therefore, not only enhances our theoretical basis but also equips practical applications that confront actual issues. Through this interdisciplinary investigation, the subject keeps evolving, playing up the role of genetic and developmental science in individual and societal health (Figure 3.1).

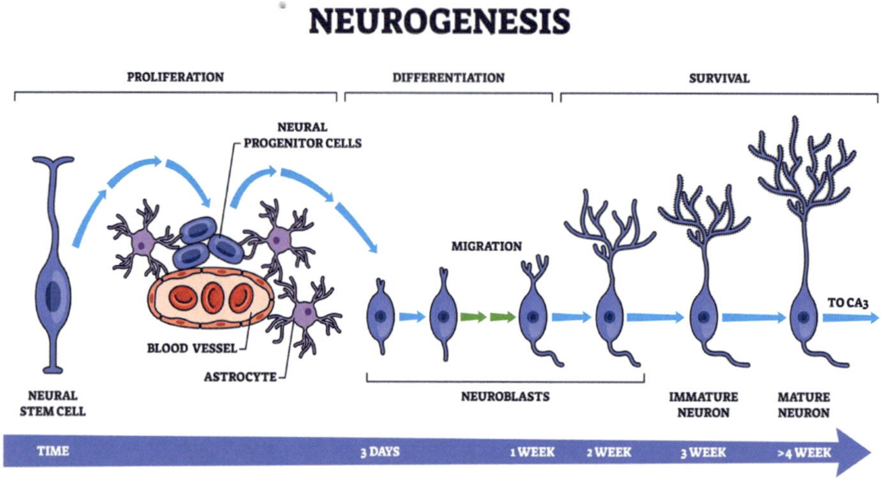

Figure 3.1. Neurogenesis.

Source: https://www.simplypsychology.org/wp-content/uploads/neurogenesis.jpeg.

Definition of Neural Development

Neural development refers to the intricate processes by which the nervous system develops, grows, and becomes organized during embryonic and postnatal life. It is characterized by a chain of highly coordinated events that involve neural induction, neuronal differentiation, and synaptogenesis. Neural development is triggered initially by the development of the neural tube from the ectoderm, which differentiates to form the brain and spinal cord. Through this, various types of cells differentiate from neural progenitor cells (NPC), one of which is the glial cells and the neurons that are essential to maximal performance. There are extrinsic signals in the environment managing all stages of development, including molecular cues from surrounding cells, in a bid to migrate and synapse neurons. The complexity of such a process underscores the inter-dependent nature between environmental stimulus and genetic factors, a challenge at the center of deciphering neural development and its relevance to neurogenetics. The theory of neural development is also immediately associated with the understanding of various NDDs that emerge when such processes fail. Environmental toxins, genetic mutations, and fetal exposure to toxic substances could potentially destroy the typical pattern of neural development to induce autism spectrum disorder (ASD) and schizophrenia. Braun et al. (2016) demonstrates the connection by demonstrating how changes in glutamate signaling and network dynamics can act as indicators of genetic risk for schizophrenia. Moreover, the interaction between genetic susceptibility and the environment highlights the function of neuroplasticity, where the capacity of the brain to reorganize and adapt itself can hamper or facilitate developmental challenges. The comprehension of the neural development concept in such a setting provides evidence for the preventive measures and therapeutic interventions that enhance the outcome in subjects suffering from these disorders. In addition, developments in neurogenetics increase our understanding of brain development since they lay out the complex genetic foundations that govern these processes. The brain-gut axis and how microbiome interactions in the gut influence neural development and behavior are emphasized as key in contemporary research, as seen in irritable bowel syndrome research (Emeran et al., 2023). This complex association attests to the complex nature of brain development, which is not solely gene sequence determined but by environmental and psychosocial conditions as well. Emergent theory of such connections gives a more holistic view of brain development and function across a lifetime. With researchers still unraveling the genetic and epigenetic processes involved, the pathway to neural development will increasingly be more and more elucidated in the context of these dynamic interactions, laying the foundation for novel avenues in neurodevelopmental research and clinical practice (Figure 3.2).

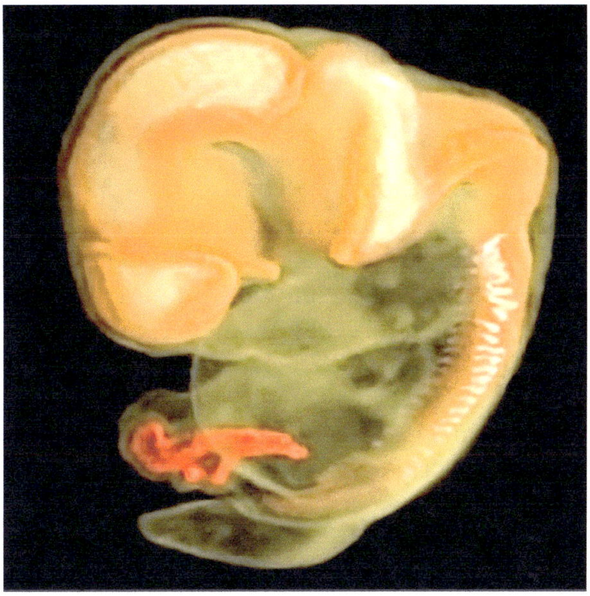

Figure 3.2. Neural development.

Source: https://cdn.storymd.com/optimized/NpA7MOIld9/original.jpg.

Overview of Neurogenetics

The field of neurogenetics is a core interdiscipline, which combines genetics and neuroscience to study the genetic processes of neural development and associated disorders. The study depicts the influence of genetic variation on processes of neurobiology like the differentiation, migration, and connectivity of the neurons. The knowledge of these genetic processes is valuable, as it could possibly shed light on the processes of a number of NDDs such as autism and schizophrenia. Research has also identified a number of important genes that are involved in the positioning and function of the neurons and, as such, control cognitive and affective outcomes. Through the study of genetic contributions to the neural processes involved, neurogenetics elucidates the ways in which variations from normal neural development give rise to psychopathologies, deepening our understanding of behavior biology. Neurogenetics also investigates how genetic susceptibility and environmental factors have complex interactions, a determinant significant in the development of a wide variety of behavioral and psychiatric disorders. Gene-environment interaction therefore has enabled scientists to understand how specific genetic variants can predispose a person to certain environmental stimuli that, subsequently, can exacerbate NDDs. For instance, it has been hypothesized through research that gene-by-environment interactions (G × E) effects are key in the explanation of psychopathy and antisocial behavior since, if their genotype, some individuals would be more vulnerable to environmental factors such as trauma or socio-economic status (Murray et al., 2018). The framework thus shifts away from the individual genetic or environmental account to a more integrative view and emphasizes the complexity of neurodevelopmental pathways. Also, the identification of causative genes underlying abnormal neuronal positioning is another critical advance in neurogenetics. Abnormal migration of neurons during brain development has been identified to be implicated with a range of NDDs, including intellectual disability and autism (Jeffrey et al., 2015). With identification of specific genetic determinants involved in such processes, researchers are able to introduce more targeted therapeutic interventions. For example, an understanding of the genetic processes by which neurons are positioned during development can uncover new means of preventing neuronal malformations. With continued study of neurogenetics, it not only holds the potential to decipher the fundamental mechanisms of neural development but also to create new avenues for therapeutic intervention that will aid in preventing the disabling consequences of NDDs on individuals and society.

Importance of Studying Neural Development and Neurogenetics

Studying neural growth and neurogenetics is crucial to elucidate the complex mechanisms that control nervous system development and function. In the course of developing the brain, neurogenesis and synaptogenesis take place in definite temporal and spatial contexts that profoundly affect cognitive and behavioral processes. From studies on neural stem/progenitor cells (NSPCs), investigators reveal how NSPCs are controlled by the production of metabolites playing a critical function in the development of the brain. Interestingly, purines are crucial elements of this metabolic equilibrium as central components of nucleic acids and vectors of energy within the cell. Disturbance in purine metabolism may result in abnormal development of the nervous system, such as in certain forebrain malformations if the de novo synthetic pathway is inhibited. Through the research on these mechanisms, researchers can inform us regarding NDDs and possible lines of therapy on which they may be alleviated (Yamada et al., 2024). Additionally, the study of neurogenetics carries through to the realm of personalized medicine beyond the specific conditions listed above. One's mental capacity, susceptibility to neurological disease, and treatment outcome can be greatly affected by genetic variation. In examining such genetic factors, researchers are able to determine biomarkers for predictive susceptibility to conditions like ASD or schizophrenia. Such a genetic focus broadens the field of knowledge not only on the etiology of such conditions but also on their complex patterns of inheritance. As genetics is increasingly understood in an attempt to inform the development of the brain, so too grows the capability of modeling intervention to the patient's personal genetic makeup. This union of neurogenetics and clinical care is an example of the significance that an appreciation for neural development must hold for the development of therapeutic interventions in a number of neurodevelopmental disorders (Kartal, 2024). Aside from its clinical applications, the study of neurogenetics and neural development provides deep insight into evolutionary biology. An understanding of how neural structures and genetic processes evolved adds meaning to an understanding of diversity in cognitive function between species. Examination of comparisons of processes of neural development between organisms allows scientists to observe shared pathways and species-specific innovations underlying species-specific behavior. This comparative framework not only promotes our understanding of brain evolution but also illuminates the forces of evolution acting on neural systems. Scientific inquiry in neural development and neurogenetics thus links basic scientific inquiry to valuable applications across disciplines, making it valuable both inside and outside research fields. The coming together of the developmental, genetic, and evolutionary studies gives life to the controversy in neural science by showing the importance of universal studies in these intertwined disciplines (Kartal, 2024).

3.1. The Basics of Neural Development

Neural development is a sophisticated, highly orchestrated process that starts early during embryogenesis and extends into postnatal life. It is necessary for the creation of the complex neuron networks that make up the brain and spinal cord. Major events in neural development involve neural induction, in which the ectoderm is differentiated into neural tissue, followed by neural proliferation, migration, and differentiation of neural precursor cells into distinct types of neurons and glial cells. At this time, highly controlled gene expression patterns are important in these events to direct cell fate and proper neuron specification, which is essential for proper neural circuit function. Knowledge of these stages provides the basis for investigating other aspects of neurogenetics, which is concerned with the interaction between genes and nervous system development, explaining how genetic considerations can have an effect on normal and abnormal neural pathways in the individual. The compartmentalization of the brain into different areas is also vital to its functionality and is the result of the exacting development that occurs during embryogenesis. For example, recent research has targeted segmentation of neural tissue into prosomeres in the diencephalon. The Max Planck Zebrafish Brain atlas, which made possible the mapping of gene expression in zebrafish, shows how molecular methods can demystify the limits of these brain areas. Research has pinpointed a number of marker genes which define regions like the thalamus and prethalamus, pointing to neurochemical domains that are key to the functionality of the brain. This research emphasizes the significance of neuroanatomy when taking into account the overall structure and function of the brain within the context of development and evolution, demonstrating the significant role played by such mapping in depicting our comprehension of neural structure. Finally, the interplay between neural development and genetic factors-inflamed neurogenetics-shows up in several studies regarding language acquisition and infant neural circuits. Emerging theories suggest infants utilize integrative models to map phonology via motor-auditory interaction, essential for speech development. The mechanism relies on the intercommunication of motor and sensory mechanisms that regulate the fine-tuning of neural pathways engaged in speech. The role of dopaminergic signaling in regulating successful attempts at speaking production further shows the convergence of genetic and neurodevelopmental forces during early childhood. Clarification of these correlations is central to using knowledge into probable developmental disorders, finally heading to interventions that have the ability to reverse the impact of genetic factors on neural and behavioral outcomes (Figure 3.3).

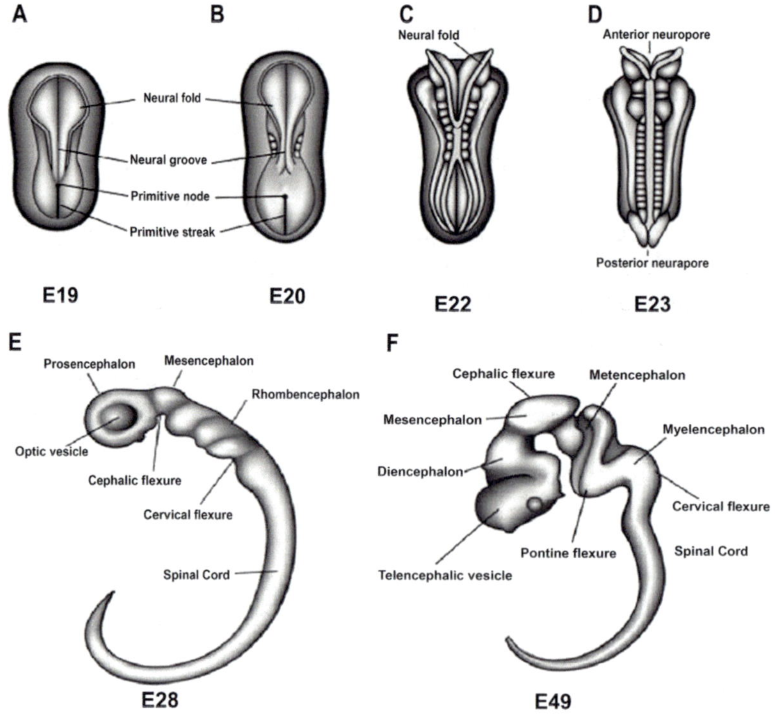

Figure 3.3. The basics of neural development.

Source: https://media.springernature.com/lw685/springer-static/image/art%3A10.1007%2Fs11065-010-9148-4/MediaObjects/11065_2010_9148_Fig6_HTML.gif.

3.1.1. Stages of Neural Development

The stages of development of the neural process are very important for the development of the central nervous system (CNS) with the initiation of the process called neurogenesis, where neuronal progenitors proliferate and give rise to neurons. The process is strictly regulated by several genetic and environmental factors to generate neurons in sufficient numbers and types necessary for the functionality of circuits. Recent developments have shown that the application of neural organoids from human-induced pluripotent stem cells (iPSCs) represent strong models for investigating these initial stages, where researchers can witness neurogenesis in person. Nonetheless, although such organoids yield very precious information, their inability to meet the intricate interaction of support tissues, including the meninges, calls for new coculture systems that improve mature neuronal features and developmental precision (Hannah et al., 2025). This puts a high value on introducing environmental and genetic predispositions into the neurodevelopmental account. After neurogenesis, neural differentiation takes place where progenitor cells give rise to varied neuronal and glial cell populations. This is regulated by a broad array of signaling pathways and transcription factors determining cell fate. Cell type characterization is important since everyone has unique functions in the nervous system, ranging from functions in neurotransmission, support, and neuroprotection. This increased availability of very powerful imaging tools coupled with deep learning algorithms further improved insights into this stage with the capability of viewing cell dynamics that were never before observed. For example, deep learning techniques have been used to great success to study the interactions at different levels of development and provide evidence regarding target identification for NDDs (Mgbole et al., 2024). This achievement shows the intricacy of not just neuronal identity formation but heterotypic cell type integration into neural circuits as well. The last phase of neural development is synaptogenesis and the pruning of synaptic connections that are required for functional neural networks. Cells develop axons and dendrites during this phase, which synapse and conduct cell-to-cell communication. Both intrinsic genetic and extrinsic environmental factors shape this phase, placing importance on experience-dependent formation of neural circuits. In addition, the role of supporting cells, such as astrocytes and microglia, is essential for synaptic refinement since they help eliminate unnecessary synapses and allow efficient signaling to take place. The relationship between genetic programming and everyday experiences continues to be a topic of active interest, especially the understanding of NDDs brought about by disruptions to these essential processes. Thus, the study of neural development phases not only helps us understand normal brain development but also informs strategies for prevention and treatment of related disorders (Figure 3.4).

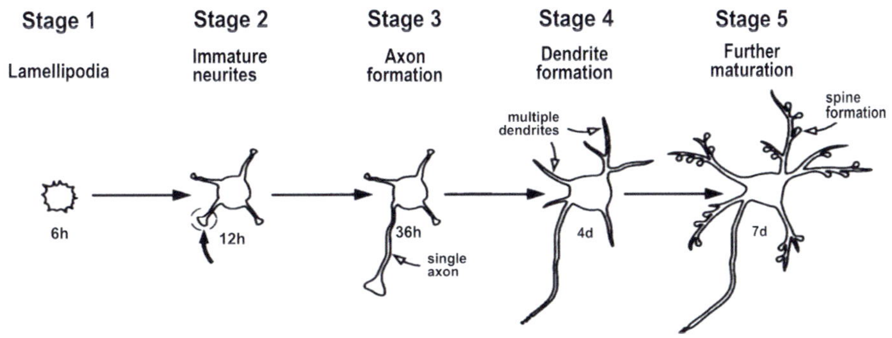

Figure 3.4. Stages of neural development.

Source: https://www.researchgate.net/profile/Sarah-Newey/publication/8101025/figure/fig2/AS:669154151505929@1536550190723/Establishment-of-polarity-and-stages-of-neuronal-development-in-hippocampal-neurons.png.

3.1.2. Key Processes Involved in Neural Development

The mechanisms of neural development are complex and of critical importance to the formation of CNS architecture and function. Underlying all of these mechanisms is neurogenesis, which is the creation of new neurons from NPCs. This process begins early during embryonic development, where the neuroepithelium is the subject of a series of tightly controlled divisions that produce diverse neuronal populations. Later, these new neurons migrate radially along scaffolding radial glial cells, which give both structural support and directional instruction. The accuracy of the migration patterns is critical since misplacement of neurons during development causes disorders and functional impairments in the mature brain circuits, pointing to the significance of deciphering these processes not only in biological but also in clinical terms. In addition, the construction of neural circuits involves intricate interactions among heterogeneous cell types and extracellular matrix components. Cell adhesion and repulsion mechanisms specify the ultimate location of the neurons in cerebral organization.

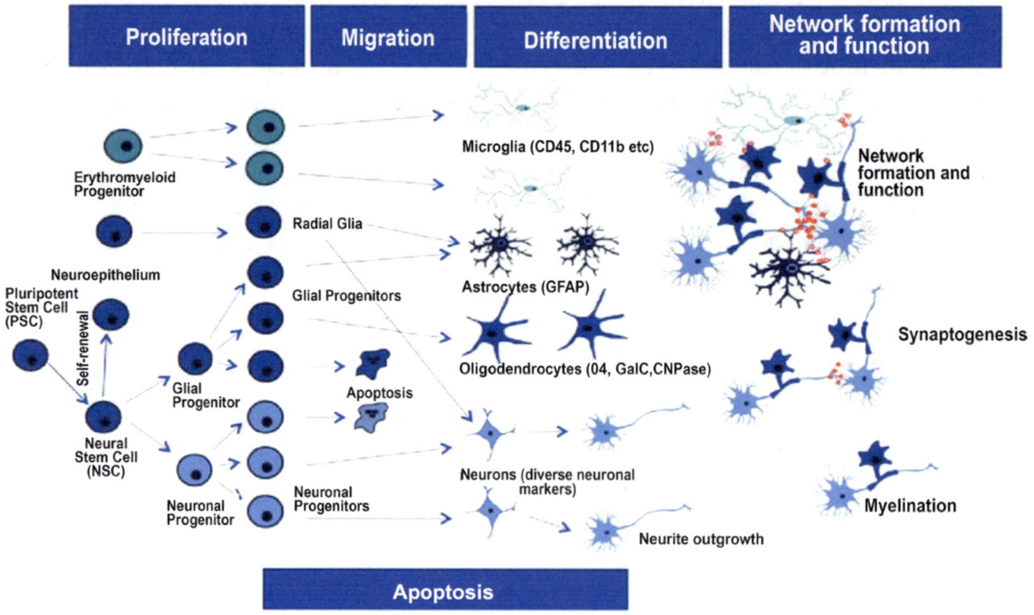

Figure 3.5. Key processes involved in neural development.

Source: https://www.researchgate.net/profile/Ellen-Fritsche/publication/326301658/figure/fig1/AS:676970518036481@1538413757884/Neurodevelopmental-processes-essential-for-nervous-system-development-It-is-assumed-that.png.

During this phase, the neurons project their axons and dendrites, forming synapses and integrating with prevailing networks. The process of formation of radial histogenetic units, wherein neurons with similar molecular profiles are organized into groups, is yet another illustration of the structured process of brain development. The differentiating layer-specific character gives rise to the varied functional regions of the brain upon formation of these units. Recent studies have assisted in clarifying the significance of these radial units, showing their usefulness in describing the overall morphology and function of the CNS, as in cases such as the radial model of the mouse pallial amygdala as an example of such concepts being implemented in practice (Garc et al., 2020). In addition to the structural and migrational components of neural development, genetic and neurochemical factors regulate the course of neuronal differentiation and function. Increasing study carries with it the integration of genetic backgrounds, cognitive, and environmental factors in providing the more holistic understanding of brain development. For example, the developmental model points to early traumatic events and the establishment of maladaptive beliefs as important factors which make an individual susceptible to later neurological and psychiatric disorders. Such an interaction between genetic and cognitive factors can help explain more complicated conditions such as depression, in which particular genetic polymorphisms have been shown to interact with neurobiological and cognitive mechanisms to enhance the symptoms. Current research focuses on uncovering these complex interactions, which not only enhance our knowledge of the development of the brain but also lead to the development of novel therapeutic approaches targeting neurogenetic pathways across a range of psychiatric disorders (Aaron, 2008) (Figure 3.5).

3.1.3. Role of Environmental Factors in Neural Development

The intricate interplay between environmental influences and neural growth has garnered extensive attention in neurogenetics research. Ranging from prenatal exposure to toxins to social conditions after birth, varied environmental inputs can heavily influence neurodevelopmental trajectories. For instance, maternal well-being and pregnancy life decisions have been identified as critical determinants that could restructure fetal neural development and networking. Studies have established that some teratogens, like alcohol and other drugs, can cause congenital anomalies, but more importantly those that involve cardiovascular structures, further impacting overall brain function and health. Besides, gestational problems have been discovered to be frequently linked with NDDs, and this supports the significance of comprehensive prenatal care aimed at the genetic vulnerabilities as well as environmental exposure, as both combined can lead to permanent changes to neural structure and cognitive processes, which could be expressed later in life (Zubrzycki et al., 2024). After birth, environmental factors remain to be expressed, particularly during the periods of neural plasticity. During childhood and adolescence, exposure to certain environmental factors—pollution, socio-economic status, and neighborhood safety—has been proven to affect cognitive and brain development. New findings from the Adolescent Brain and Cognitive Development (ABCD) study illustrate how neighborhood violence and air pollution are linked to measurable alterations in the brain, which alter gray matter density and patterns of connectivity. In particular, the evidence of accelerated brain aging found among some teens appears to be connected with exposure to adverse environmental conditions, suggesting an interactive dynamics between neural and extrinsic determinants. These associations highlight the absolute significance of environmental context in establishing neural pathways—proving that brain development is not simply an outcome of genetics but is significantly driven by conditions surrounding them, which can best support or obfuscate neurodevelopment (Ray et al., 2024). In addition, an understanding of the interdependence between the environment and neural development has significant implications for interventions targeted at healthy brain outcomes. Interventions that increase exposure to healthy settings—such as reducing pollution, community safety, and socio-economic status—might not only enhance better cognitive functioning but also diminish the risk of negative outcomes associated with harmful environments. Interventions early on in life for susceptible populations might enhance resilience and provide opportunities for best learning and emotional health, essentially planting seeds for better neurological destinies. Synthesis of neurogenetic information with environmental factors is pertinent to devising integrated policies that address not only the genetic vulnerability but also the imperative environmental determinants affecting brain formation. Emphasizing multi-dimensional approaches will clarify the process of neural development and pave the way for new strategies in assisting populations with cognitive growth (Ray et al., 2024) (Figure 3.6).

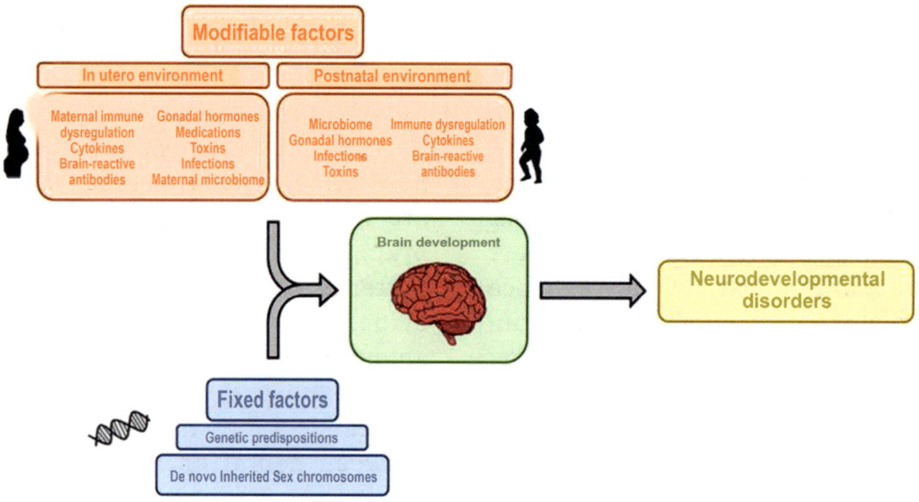

Figure 3.6. Role of environmental factors in neural development.

Source: https://www.researchgate.net/publication/333439866/figure/fig1/AS:11431281250331770@1717813209972/Genetic-and-environmental-factors-that-influence-brain-development-and-contribute-to-the.tif.

3.2. Genetic Influences on Neural Development

The complex interaction between genetics and neural development is highlighted by several studies into how genetic variations influence the structure and function of the brains. In particular, genetic influences can determine not just the overall structure of neural circuits but also the timing of neuronal differentiation and maturation. These are important in developing cognitive and emotional abilities later in life. For example, recent studies suggest that specific genetic mutations can cause structural defects in brain areas related to emotional control and thus cause behavioral disorders like psychopathy. This underlines the need for comprehensively understanding genetic impacts, including interactions of genetic tendencies and environmental influences shaping neural development and resulting behavioral consequences as illustrated through new G × E interaction models (Murray et al., 2018). In addition, research involving the application of iPSCs has also transformed our comprehension of the genetic basis for neural development. Through the differentiation of patient-specific cells, researchers are able to reproduce the pathophysiologic conditions behind different neurological diseases in a dish. Through this, one is able to study neural lineage differentiation and the effects of particular genetic mutations on neural phenotypes. For example, research has indicated that mutations associated with neurodegenerative disorders exhibit unique cellular behavior during differentiation, which can inform on early developmental defects and subsequent expressions in neurodegeneration (Ethan et al., 2017). The capacity to define these alterations at a cellular level not only deepens our knowledge of developmental biology but also hastens the discovery of promising therapeutic targets for the treatment of various neurological disorders. Aside from single gene contributions, the combined effect of many genetic factors also adds complexity to understanding neural development. Polygenic traits, which are those that regulate cognitive function or vulnerability to psychiatric illness, for example, are typically influenced by many genes. This polygenic structure makes it difficult to identify discrete genetic contributions to neural development. In addition, gene expression variations can be caused by both genetic context and environmental exposures, with consequent phenotypic variations. The convergence of genomic information with data from cellular and animal models remains central to unraveling the genetic makeup of neural development. Hence, a continuous effort at collaborative research and the use of sophisticated genomic tools is imperative in further defining the intricate network of genetic controls on neurogenesis (Murray et al., 2018) (Figure 3.7).

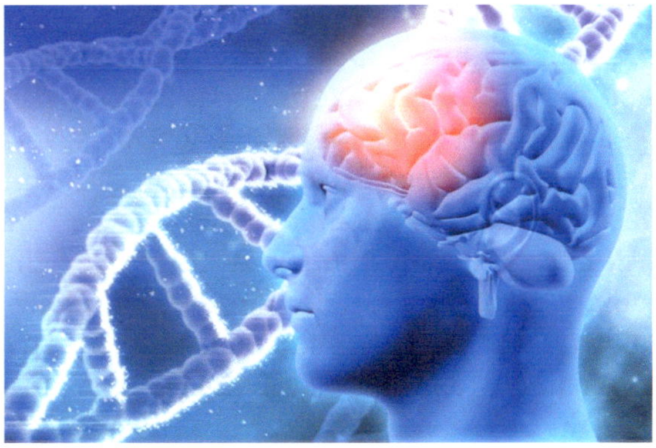

Figure 3.7. Genetic influences on neural development.

Source: https://www.psypost.org/wp-content/uploads/2018/10/genetics-brain-dna.jpg.

3.2.1. Genes Involved in Neural Differentiation

Neural differentiation is an important process that determines the pattern of nervous system development, and it is strongly determined by an extensive group of genes. These genes direct the development of pluripotent stem cells to specialized neural cells, such as neurons and glial cells. Among different genetic regulators, histone variants are important in controlling chromatin structure and accessibility, thus affecting gene expression patterns during neural differentiation. For example, types like H3-3A and H3-3B, associated with NDDs like Bryant-Li-Bhoj syndrome, interfere with normal processes of neuronal maturation and activity. Dysregulation of gene expression patterns influencing neuronal fate brings into focus the role of these histone variants in the larger context of neurogenetics, suggesting their possible contribution to developmental delay and intellectual disabilities (Annabel et al., 2024). Aside from histones, recent genomic studies have also deepened our knowledge of the genetic underpinning of neural differentiation by dissecting the many loci implicated in brain structure and function. Genome-wide association study (GWAS) of close to 75,000 participants revealed 254 independent loci that were associated with subcortical brain volumes, indicative of the role of certain genes in the development and structuring of neural circuitry. These observations demonstrate a complex interaction of genetic variants with neurodevelopment, such that genes act in a permissive manner in the growth and morphology of the brain. The expression of these genes is particularly observed in numerous neural cell types and differentiation phases, providing explanations of how genetic propensities can shape individual neurodevelopmental trajectories and make individuals susceptible to Parkinsons disease and attention-deficit/hyperactivity disorder (García-Marín et al., 2024). The study that demonstrates the role played by these genetic factors in the differentiation of nerves carries broad implications for NDD understanding. As an illustration, the gene expression changes that are associated with H3.3 variants uncover an important interplay between chromatin structure and neuronal function, as deformations have the potential to produce serious neurological effects. Further, since polygenic scores from GWAS studies have been shown to possess predictive value in various populations, it highlights the complex relationship between genetic predisposition, brain structure, and individual risk for neuropsychiatric disorders. By clarifying these genetic processes of neural differentiation, scientists not only further our understanding of brain development but also lay the ground for specific therapeutic methods that can counteract the effects of NDDs resulting from certain genetic variants (Annabel et al., 2024; García-Marín et al., 2024) (Figure 3.8).

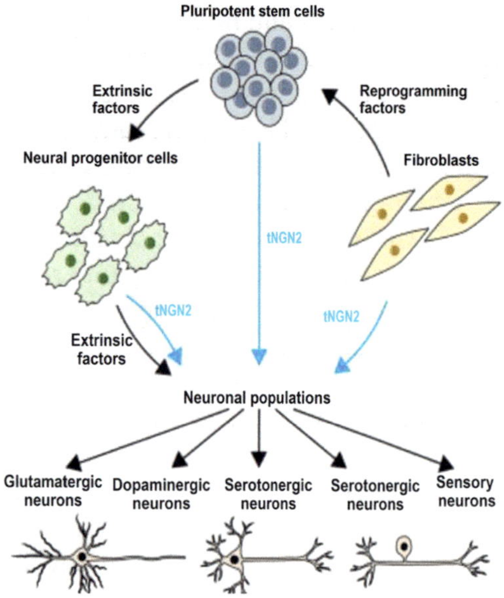

Figure 3.8. Genes involved in neural differentiation.

Source: https://ars.els-cdn.com/content/image/1-s2.0-S2213671121005968-fx1.jpg.

3.2.2. Genetic Mutations and Their Impact on Neural Development

The intricacies in neural development are significantly influenced by genetic mutation, which can possibly disrupt the precision tuning orchestration of signaling cascades required in proper brain development. Genetic mutations also lead to deficiency in the function of essential proteins involved in processes related to neurodevelopment. For instance, mutations of the Sonic hedgehog (Shh) pathway can cause interference with the morphogenetic signals needed for neural tube development. Recent evidence shows that Fuz, a protein required for ciliary function, biochemically interacts with Gpr161, a Shh signaling negative modulator. Disruption of this interaction results in gross phenotypic malformations in the mouse model, uncovering the role of such genetic factors in controlling neural outcomes during embryonic development (Kim et al., 2024). Identification of such genetic interactions sheds light on the broader implications that mutations have for neural development and associated disorders. In addition to Shh signaling, there are other genetic pathways that play crucial roles in neural development and in producing variations in brain structure and function. Cell proliferation and differentiation processes can be interrupted by genetic mutations to result in neural tube defects or disorders such as ASD and schizophrenia. Studies have revealed that the cumulative effect of several mutations can become so robust as to deeply affect neurodevelopmental processes. As a point of illustration, mutations in those genes that regulate synaptic plasticity can generate altered neuronal connection and resultant cognitive impairment (Kim et al., 2024). This helps highlight an essential aspect of neurogenetics: the interplay between the genetic makeup of an individual and the environmental factors that sculpt neural networks and behavior. Thus, untangling the role of genetic mutations in these cases becomes key to decoding the etiology of hundreds of thousands of NDDs. Moreover, gaining deeper understanding of the effects of genetic mutations on brain development has the potential to translate into therapy. As research continues, interventions designed to repair or substitute for single mutations are being found. For example, genetic engineering technologies, like CRISPR-Cas9, offer routes for directed intervention that could restore normal function to deleterious mutation in genes responsible for neurodevelopmental pathology. Furthermore, continued exploration of genetic networks, like Fuz and Gpr161 interaction during neural tube development, offers opportunities for novel therapeutic targets (Kim et al., 2024). With the increasing knowledge of these genetic models, it can potentially lead to more powerful diagnosis and tailored treatments based on the individual's specific genetic pattern for NDDs, thereby improving the prognosis for this at-risk group (Figure 3.9).

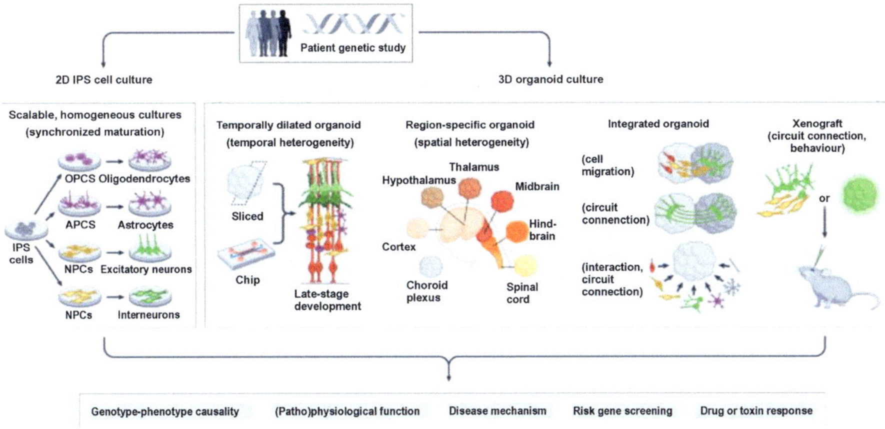

Figure 3.9. Genetic mutations and their impact on neural development.

Source: https://media.springernature.com/lw685/springer-static/image/art%3A10.1038%2Fs41576-023-00626-5/MediaObjects/41576_2023_626_Fig2_HTML.png.

3.2.3. Epigenetics and Its Role in Neural Development

Epigenetics plays a crucial role in brain development, influencing the expression of genetic information in the complex processes of brain morphogenesis and maturation. DNA methylation, histone modification, and non-coding RNA are elementary mechanisms that play a part in regulating gene expression in response to intrinsic as well as extrinsic stimuli. These epigenetic modifications are not always fixed; rather, they may be dynamically regulated by environmental influences such as stress, diet, and toxin exposure. For instance, it has been revealed by studies that adverse conditions during periods of neural development are able to cause long-lasting persistent epigenetic modifications that affect brain function. It is comprehending such mechanisms that is important, for they elucidate how environmental environments interface with genetic tendencies to affect the brain's neural environment that can predispose a person towards neurological disorders and disabilities (Do, 2024). Studies on the interaction between epigenetics and neurodevelopment have shed much light on the pathogenesis of mental illnesses. Bipolar illness is just one illustration of environmental factors, including exposure in utero of the mother and trauma in early life, influencing genetic risk to modulate expression via epigenetic modification. One specific area of focus has been the discovery of specific epigenetic marks, such as 5-hydroxymethylcytosine, associated with neuronal differentiation and cognition. This underlines the importance of epigenetic regulation in early brain development and its influence on longer-term psychiatric outcome. The distinction of these processes allows researchers to uncover future biomarkers and therapeutic targets, leading to new interventions that could reverse the effects of detrimental environmental exposures on mental health (Kumar et al., 2023). In addition, the transgenerational effects of epigenetics as they relate to neural development need keen examination since they explain how exposures and experiences can impact generations to come. The effects of epigenetic changes have the potential to be inherited, hence linking environmental conditions in one generation to the neurobiological effects in subsequent generations. The effects are passed on through altered gene expression that influences various neurodevelopmental processes. For example, research shows that exposures to chemicals during key developmental windows can trigger permanent epigenetic modifications that influence not just the exposed person but even their progeny, increasing susceptibilities for disorders like addiction and mood disorders. These findings underscore the necessity of considering epigenetic processes as integral components of neurodevelopmental research, as they demonstrate a range of effects on neural pathways through generations (Do, 2024; Kumar et al., 2023) (Figure 3.10).

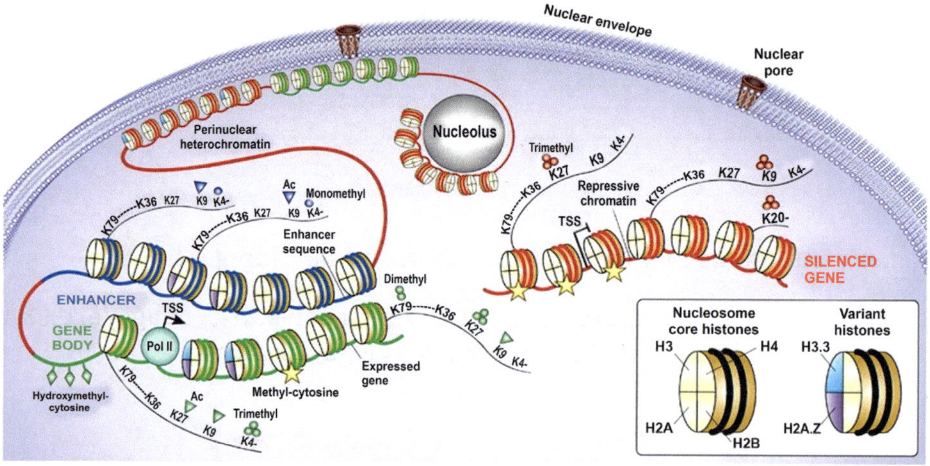

Figure 3.10. Epigenetics and its role in neural development.

Source: https://media.springernature.com/m685/springer-static/image/art%3A10.1038%2Fnpp.2012.78/MediaObjects/41386_2013_Article_BFnpp201278_Fig1_HTML.jpg.

3.3. Neurogenesis: The Formation of Neurons

Neurogenesis is fundamental to the development of the neural system, which represents the generation of neurons from precursor cells. This complex biological process starts at the stage of embryonic development when NPCs are stimulated to divide and then become mature neurons. The coordination of these processes is tightly controlled by internal genetic stimuli and external environmental influences. Current research highlights the need to study model organisms like zebrafish, which have become the promising tools used to decipher the mechanisms of neurogenesis. These creatures enable the study of embryonic and adult neurogenesis and the dynamic processes involved in neuronal development and preservation throughout life (Schmidt et al., 2013). Deciphering these mechanisms holds great promise for furthering therapeutic approaches to neurological diseases and trauma. Whereas a lot of early emphasis on neurogenesis has been placed on embryonic growth, studies have more and more put the spotlight on the role of neural stem cells (NSCs) within the adult mammalian CNS. More recent discoveries indicate that neurogenesis does not end in early years but rather continues in certain areas of the adult brain, particularly the subventricular zone of the forebrain. This region acts as a reservoir for NSCs and offers a steady supply of newly generated neurons to areas like the olfactory bulb. Research demonstrates that these NSCs are highly plastic, being able to differentiate into different types of neuronal and glial cells both *in vivo* and *in vitro*. Such findings not only dispute the belief that neurogenesis occurs only during developmental processes but also open new avenues for creative strategies to leverage the promise of NSCs in regenerative medicine (Galli et al., 2003). The concept of neurogenesis has far-reaching implications for a vast variety of neurological disorders. Since NSCs have the ability to grow indefinitely and preserve stable functional characteristics, scientists are investigating their potential for therapy in the repair of neuronal functions in neurodegenerative diseases and brain damage. The investigation is aimed at understanding the elements that affect NSC differentiation and integration into pre-existing neural circuits, which is essential for successful intervention measures. In addition, the investigation of external stimuli, including exercise and environmental enrichment, shows how to stimulate neurogenesis in adults, pointing to the brains impressive plasticity. By dissecting the intricate interactions of genetic and epigenetic mechanisms of neurogenesis, researchers are making considerable progress toward the creation of specific therapies that might dramatically change cognitive impairment treatment and other neurological diseases (Figure 3.11).

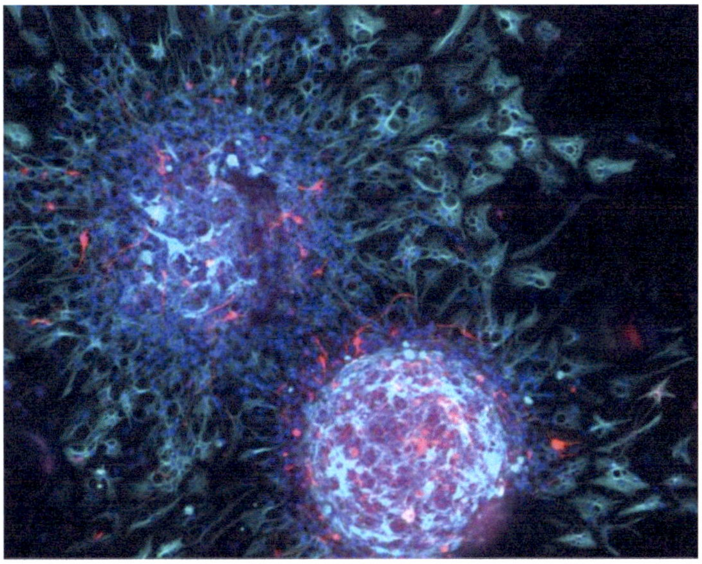

Figure 3.11. Neurogenesis: The formation of neurons.

Source: https://qbi.uq.edu.au/files/3715/Neural-stem-cell-QBI-brain-physiology-neurogenesis.jpg.

3.3.1. Definition and Significance of Neurogenesis

Neurogenesis, the formation of new neurons from neural stem and progenitor cells, is a built-in process of both nervous system formation and ongoing nervous system plasticity. The process mostly takes place during embryogenesis, laying the groundwork for the complex neural circuits that underlie a range of cognitive and sensory capabilities. However, neurogenesis is not only restricted to embryogenesis; it has been shown in adult organisms too, for example, in certain brain regions like the hippocampus, where it is involved in memory and learning. Neurogenesis is important because disruption of it has been linked with several neurodevelopmental and psychiatric conditions, thus defining its importance in health and disease. The importance of neurogenesis is not in the production of neurons alone, but in making neural circuit function and plasticity appropriate. For example, in sensory neural circuit formation, proper specification and differentiation of the neurons matter, as shown in experiments on the nociceptive class IV dendritic arborization neurons of *Drosophila.* These studies imply the manner in which signal pathways like Hedgehog and Epithelial growth factor receptor are directly involved in regulating neurogenesis with accurate neuronal placement and connectivity.

Therefore, neurogenesis is a vital connection between the genetic predispositions and functional outcomes within the nervous system, where both the generation and integration of new neurons partake in the ability of the organisms to adapt to responses in the environment as well as to adjust to experiences, hence determining behavior and survival (Karim et al., 2011). In addition, neurogenesis is also thought to have been accountable for brain asymmetry and evolutionary changes, according to research in the habenular. The nucleus of the epithalamus that links different areas of the brain shows left–right size and neural circuit asymmetries among vertebrates and may be a result of differences in neurogenetic mechanisms. The differential regulation of the duration of neurogenesis accounts for these asymmetries based on the study, demonstrating not only that neurogenesis specifies individual neural structures but also gives evidence of overall evolutionary trends. Appreciation of the importance of these neurogenetic events clarifies the ability for neural development to be both internally influenced by genetic factors and externally influenced by pressures, and how this sheds light on the complex interaction between neurogenesis, neurodevelopment, and evolutionary adaptation in complex behavior (Aizawa et al., 2011).

3.3.2. Neurogenesis in Different Stages of Life

Neurogenesis, the creation of new neurons, differs dramatically at every phase of life, each characterized by distinct developmental features and functional consequences. In fetal development, neurogenesis is widespread, with the brain creating more than 100 billion neurons. This neuron explosion is essential for the formation of the fundamental architecture of the brain to support eventual cognitive activities and emotional control. As humans move into childhood, neurogenesis persists but at a slower rate, culminating in adolescence. It is a time of dramatic structural changes in the brain, notably areas like the hippocampus that play a critical role in learning and memory. But these phases too are vulnerable; there are extrinsic factors like malnutrition, stress, and toxin exposure, which negatively influence neurogenesis and ensuing mental capacities, illustrating the fine balance that defines neural formation in early life. In adults, neurogenesis continues, though at a lower rate than in earlier stages of life. Adult hippocampal neurogenesis (AHN) is especially noteworthy since it is thought to be involved in memory creation as well as emotional control. Evidence from research reveals that lifestyle decisions, including physical activity and mental stimulation, are capable of triggering AHN, enabling ongoing brain plasticity and resistance to neurodegeneration. Additionally, the ability for neurogenesis in adulthood gains importance in the setting of numerous health disorders. For example, cancer therapies like chemotherapy and radiotherapy indiscriminately suppress the proliferation of cells, leading to adult NSC impairment and resulting cognitive deficits, especially in memory and emotional states. Knowledge of these dynamics points to the central role of neurogenesis as a key mediator of cognitive and psychological well-being in adult samples, thus making it both central in clinical neuroscience and rehabilitation. As one ages into older adulthood, neurogenesis alters once more, typically being accompanied by marked cognitive decline and mental health difficulties. Aging is generally characterized by a reduction of neurogenesis, especially in the hippocampus, where new neurons are essential for the preservation of cognitive functions. It has been found in research that activities of daily life contribute a great deal to cushioning the cognitive decrease seen in late life. Participation in social, cognitive, and physical activities has been associated with maintaining cognitive function, implying that lifestyle factors can drive neurogenesis and promote cognitive resistance even in old age. Also, evidence indicates that decreases in cognitive activities are inseparable from losses of verbal speed and memory, meaning that active participation counteracts neuropsychological decline. In this way, the inclusion of interventions to promote neurogenesis as a result of lifestyle changes could represent an effective method for the increase of mental health benefits and cognitive functioning in elderly individuals, such as the interaction between neurogenetics and lifestyle influences throughout life (Brent et al., 2011) (Figure 3.12).

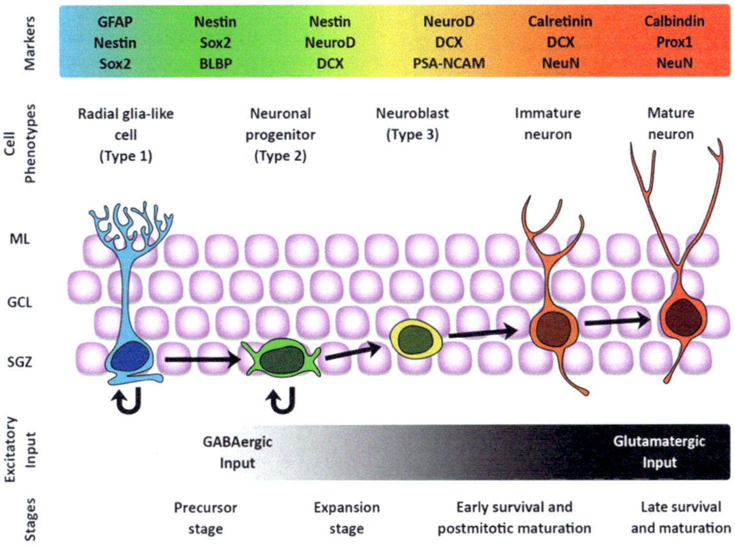

Figure 3.12. Neurogenesis in different stages of life.

Source: https://www.researchgate.net/publication/334428578/figure/fig1/AS:11431281182196434@1692326605337/Stages-of-hippocampal-neurogenesis-Depiction-of-the-stages-of-the-neurogenic-process-in.png.

3.3.3. Factors Influencing Neurogenesis

Neurogenesis is a complicated process that is highly affected by biological and environmental factors, which have been gaining more interest in the study of neural development. Sensory experience is one of the most important factors to contribute to neurogenesis, especially during the early postnatal critical period. It has been found that the olfactory bulb, which is one of the central regions for smelling, has a high rate of neurogenesis dependent on sensory experiences. In particular, the transcription factor Npas4 is seen to have a central function in the survival and integration of newly formed interneurons within the olfactory bulb, showing the influence external stimuli can have on the formation of neural circuits. Sensory deprivation, on the other hand, has been shown to decrease both the volume of the olfactory bulb and the number of interneurons, showing how crucial sensory input is for supporting the process of neurogenesis throughout key development stages (Kwon et al., 2024). Moreover, interactions between neurogenesis and systemic conditions like inflammation and neurotrophic signaling also make it more difficult to understand neural development. The nerve growth factor (NGF) has now proven to be a vital agent in mediating cellular interactions between neural cells and many of the body's systems, including cancer. High levels of neurotrophins such as NGF are not only able to facilitate survival and proliferation of neurons but could even impact the tumor microenvironment, pointing towards dual functions in both neural and cancer biology. For example, the dialogue between nerve and cancer cells has implications for the understanding of the regulatory processes involved in tumorigenesis. This intricate relationship highlights how the same molecular components can function differently within different contexts and influence neurogenesis, behavior, and even disease development (Benzaquen et al., 2024). Environmental aspects also play a crucial role in modulating neurogenesis, at many different levels, ranging from genetic predisposition to daily life choices. Physical exercise has been extensively reported to increase neurogenesis, especially in the hippocampus, a region of the brain important for learning and memory. Exercise induces the release of neurotrophic factors, which stimulate the growth and differentiation of NPCs into mature neurons. In addition, nutrients, including omega-3 fatty acids and antioxidants, are thought to foster neurogenic activity through the reduction of oxidative stress and enhancement of brain health in general. As a result, these lifestyle elements can result in dramatic alterations in rates of neurogenesis, which may impact cognitive performance and resistance to neurodegenerative disease in turn. The complex interplay of these influences underlines the multidisciplinary nature of neurogenesis, which ties genetic, environmental, and lifestyle factors to broader neural development (Kwon et al., 2024).

3.4. The Role of Stem Cells in Neural Development

The complex interaction between stem cells and neural development is essential in understanding normal brain function as well as the underlying pathogenesis of NDDs. NSCs, with the special capacity to differentiate into different types of neuronal and glial cells, have pivotal functions in the development and maintenance of neural networks within the CNS. In embryonic development, these stem cells play a vital role in the complex layering and patterning of the brain and a supporting scaffold upon which future neural connections will form. In addition, dysregulation of proliferation or differentiation in NSCs can give rise to severe developmental disorders, underscoring the necessity of neurogenesis—a procedure regulated by the complicated interaction between genetic and environmental influences. Explorations of how NSCs react to pathological states can provide insights that are critical not just in fundamental neurobiology but also in possible therapeutic strategies for NDDs. Adult neurogenesis has been indicated to have potential, and neurogenic areas of the adult brain, including the hippocampus, have been found to produce new neurons throughout life. This continuous process, while limited in many age-related and neurodegenerative disorders, testifies to the brain's plasticity and self-repair ability. It should be particularly noted that knowing the determinants of the fate of NSCs in adulthood is crucial for designing strategies for exploiting their regenerative capacity. The gliogenesis process, which produces glial cells that nourish and support neuronal function, is no less significant. The equilibrium between neurogenesis and gliogenesis is important for keeping the brain functioning optimally and treating diseases like Multiple Sclerosis (MS), whose pathologies are caused by interruptions in these processes, leading to cognitive deficits and neuroinflammation (Hijal et al., 2024). Recent advancements in stem cell research, specifically the application of methods like photobiomodulation (PBM), have been promising in improving the differentiation of stem cells into neuronal cell lines *in vitro*. PBM, an aversive photo treatment, has also been shown to modulate stem cell behavior, inducing proliferation and positive differentiation effects. Current data show that some wavelengths can improve the development of NEBs from adipose-derived stem cells, which are key intermediates in the generation of functional neurons (Mulaudzi et al., 2024). The differential regulation of essential markers characteristic of neural progenitors and mature neurons highlights the therapeutic promise of such approaches. Therefore, the comprehension and optimization of these pathways of differentiation have far-reaching implications for regenerative medicine, providing revolutionary means to treat neurodegenerative diseases and injuries by possibly recapturing lost neural functions (Figure 3.13).

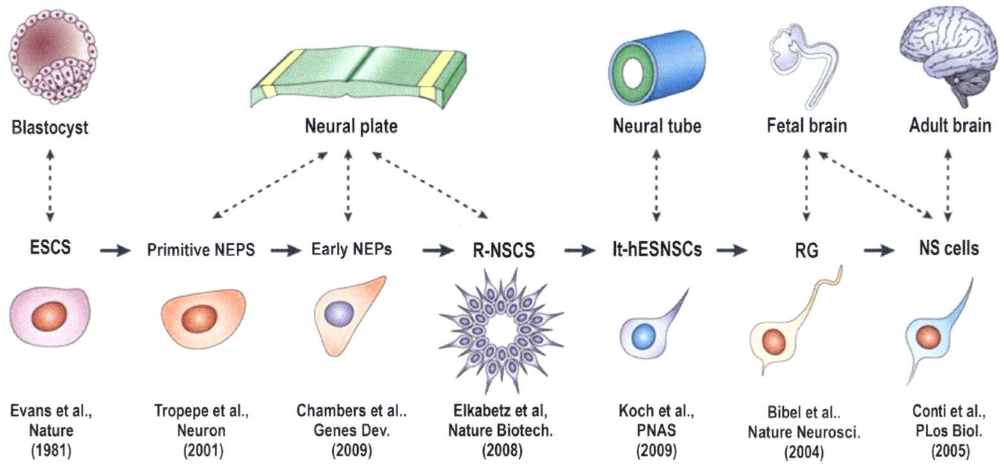

Figure 3.13. The role of stem cells in neural development.

Source: https://media.springernature.com/full/springer-static/image/art%3A10.1038%2Fnrn2761/MediaObjects/41583_2010_Article_BFnrn2761_Fig1_HTML.jpg.

3.4.1. Types of Stem Cells Involved in Neural Development

The world of neural development is heavily influenced by a number of stem cells, the most prominent of which are NSCs and embryonic stem cells (ESCs). NSCs are able to self-renew and differentiate into neurons, astrocytes, and oligodendrocytes and are vital in brain development. They contribute to the intricacy of the CNS structure so that different neural populations can grow. ESCs, formed from the inner cell mass of the blastocyst, possess a pluripotency to differentiate into any type of cell, such as neural progenitors. Such inherent malleability renders ESCs an effective tool for the study of neural development and prospective therapeutic application. The interaction between ESCs and NSCs underlines the complex regulatory mechanisms that govern the specification of neural lineage, at the core of studies addressing NDDs and designing appropriate interventions. *In vitro* studies have unraveled the potential application of a variety of different methods to enhance stem cell differentiation into neural lineages. Advances in methodology, such as the production of NEBs from stem cells, offer a means to mimic early phases of neurodevelopment and enable the study of complex neural interactions. The technique of inducing NEBs has exhibited promise in initiating the efficient differentiation of stem cells into functional neural precursors. For instance, PBM, a penetrating light treatment, has been discovered to optimize the induction of NEBs, with higher cell viability and higher differentiation yields.

The findings confirm that environmental factor modulation significantly influences stem cell fate decisions in neural development and is therefore a potential area of study and clinical value in regenerative medicine, such as in the instance of neurogenesis (Mulaudzi et al., 2024). Further, exposure to the environment has not to be downplayed as it has the ability to influence NSCs that impact neural development significantly. For instance, research on the mechanism of neonicotinoid insecticides shows the potential neurotoxic impacts on NSCs that play a critical function during early brain development. Inhibition by compound exposure such as 6-chloronicotinic acid (6-ClNA) has been reported to disrupt NSC proliferation and differentiation, reporting extreme modifications in the gene expression networks related to apoptosis and inflammation. These findings emphasize the need to study the environmental factors capable of altering NSC behavior since environmental toxins are also bound to play a role in the etiology of NDDs. The study of the interplay between environmental factors and stem cells is a crucial step in developing means of preventing neurodevelopmental risk and advancing our knowledge of neural plasticity in neurogenetics (He et al., 2024) (Figure 3.14).

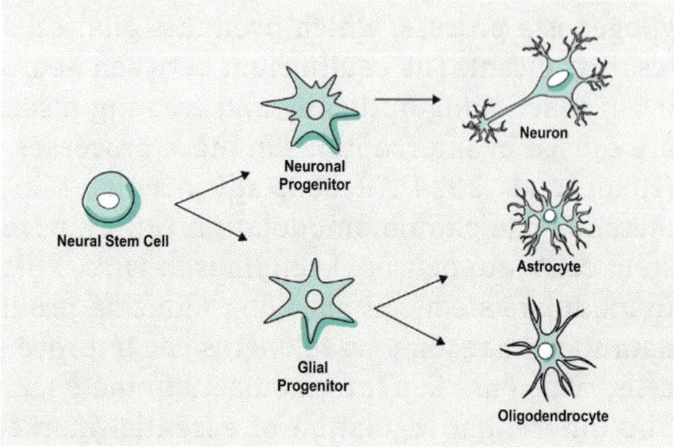

Figure 3.14. Types of stem cells involved in neural development.

Source: https://captivatebio.com/wp-content/uploads/2023/01/captivate-bio-neural-stem-cells-illustration-1024x638.png.

3.4.2. Mechanisms of Stem Cell Differentiation

The processes of stem cell differentiation are central to the comprehension of neural development and neurogenetics, as they provide the basis for the construction of particular neural cell types from a universal stem cell progenitor. Differentiation is initiated by a multifaceted interaction between extrinsic signals and intrinsic regulatory programs. Extracellular molecules, including growth factors and morphogens, trigger signaling cascades that activate transcription factors central to lineage specification. For example, the differentiation of pluripotent stem cells into NPCs is mediated by gradients of signaling factors such as fibroblast growth factor (FGF) and transforming growth factor-beta (TGF-β), which eventually control patterns of gene expression. This serves to highlight the need for spatial and temporal regulation of stem cell fate decisions such that resulting populations of cells have the appropriate characteristics for healthy functional outcomes in neural circuits. In addition, mutations in genes can deeply affect stem cell differentiation pathways to cause NDDs. A strong example is the neurogenetic disorder Bryolt-Li-Bhoj syndrome (BLBS), where mutations in the H3-3B gene interfere with regular neural development. With the use of iPSCs differentiated into NPCs, studies have identified mutations having the potential to induce dysregulated gene expression and changed chromatin accessibility, ultimately influencing neuronal fate and function. In particular, H3-3B p.Leu48Arg variant was detected to enhance H3.3 expression, enabling hyper-deposition into nucleosomes that changed gene regulatory networks (GRN). As noted in this example, insights into mechanistic specifics of stem cell differentiation can reveal wider implications for the etiology of NDDs and guide therapeutic interventions to correct these dysregulations. Moreover, the interaction between genetic influences and stem cell differentiation also poses important questions about differences between individuals in the development of the brain across different populations. Dyslexia, for example, is 44 to 75% heritable, suggesting a high degree of genetic influence. Various genes, like KIAA0319, have been found to be linked with reading disability, but the mechanisms behind them are not well understood. Experimental strategies using human embryonic stem cells (hESCs) make it possible to knock down a particular gene and see its effect on neural differentiation. Knockdown of KIAA0319 impacts early stages of differentiation of neuroepithelial cells, ultimately impacting subsequent neuronal migration and cortical layer formation. Such observations emphasize the critical function of genetic regulation in stem cell differentiation in the nervous system and show how disturbances can result in functional deficiencies characteristic of NDDs (Figure 3.15).

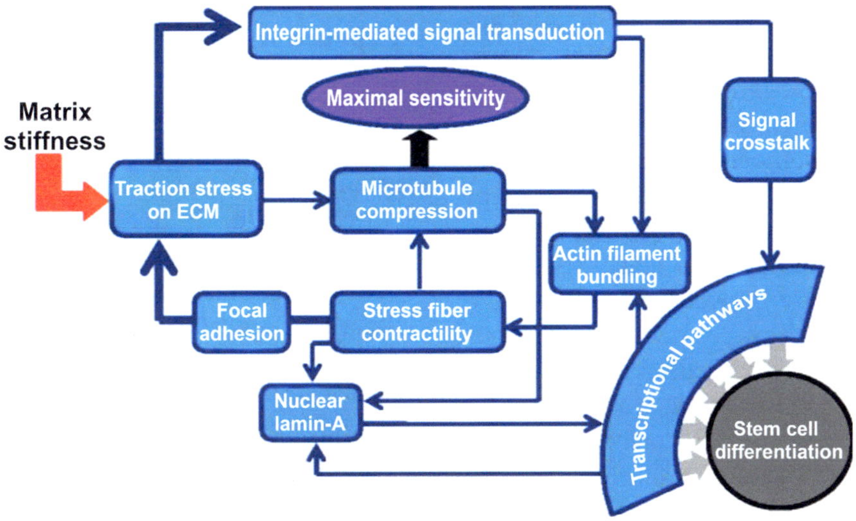

Figure 3.15. Mechanisms of stem cell differentiation.

Source: https://media.springernature.com/lw685/springer-static/image/art%3A10.1186%2Fs13287-015-0083-4/MediaObjects/13287_2015_83_Fig1_HTML.gif.

3.4.3. Potential Therapeutic Applications of Stem Cells

Stem cells are of extraordinary promise in the arena of neural development and neurogenetics, especially in terms of their potential therapeutic roles in the management of neurological disease. Available evidence suggests that stem cells have specialized regenerative capacity, which enables them to differentiate into distinct cell types such as neurons and glial cells. This inherent potential places them at the center of promising candidates for therapeutic interventions in diseases like Parkinsons disease, amyotrophic lateral sclerosis (ALS), and spinal cord injury. Through the use of stem cells, researchers seek to restore the lost function of neurons and induce tissue repair. An in-depth understanding of the molecular mechanisms governing neuronal differentiation, survival, and integration is still imperative to effectively tapping the potential of stem cells in the clinic. As these pathways are continually being clarified by ongoing studies, the basis for new stem cell-based treatments is being established with the potential to enhance neurological disease patient outcomes. The use of NSCs reaches beyond simple regenerative therapy; it also includes the management of highly malignant tumors like glioblastoma (GBM). GBM, or highly proliferative and highly resistant GBM, poses many of the challenges in neurogenetics and neural development research. Evidence is pointing towards a bipotential role for NSCs in the case of GBM, where they can promote tumor development or be a possible method of inhibiting tumor growth, based on their microenvironment. Therefore, it is important to learn about the intricate relationship between NSCs and GBM to design proper therapeutic interventions. By hitting specific molecular mechanisms controlled by NSCs, for example, Notch and SHH, scientists could change treatment strategies from conventional treatments to more creative ones that involve stem cells in a focused way. Such developments could eventually result in individualized therapies taking into account the distinct biology of each patient's tumor and the nearby neural tissue (Singh et al., 2025). Apart from their potential in neurodegenerative disorders and tumors, stem cells have also been found to have great potential in treating other neurological disorders that feature tissue damage and scarring. Damage to the nervous system tends to result in the development of scar tissue, which tends to hinder recovery and healing. Recent studies have highlighted the role of adipose-derived stem cells (ADSCs) in mediating inflammation and promoting tissue regeneration, thus providing a promising avenue for mitigating pathological scarring. By employing ADSCs, researchers aim to induce favorable healing responses while minimizing the adverse effects associated with abnormal scar formation. The advancement of techniques that utilize these stem cells, including innovative applications like cell-free therapies, is rapidly evolving. Knowledge of ADSCs' interactions with the damaged neural environment has the potential to give insights into their therapeutic potential in avoiding and healing scarring, thus promoting the recovery of patients with neurological injuries (Wang et al., 2024).

3.5. Neurodevelopmental Disorders (NDDs)

Neurodevelopmental Disorders (NDDs) constitute a heterogeneous group of conditions resulting from aberrant brain development, which frequently present as a continuum of behavioral, cognitive, and emotional difficulties. Comprising ASD, attention-deficit/hyperactivity disorder, and intellectual disability, these disorders tend to have a profound impact on the life of an individual with NDD, affecting education, occupational function, and social relationships. The multifactorial etiology of NDDs is responsible for their complexity, including genetic mutations, environmental factors, and neurobiologic underpinnings. Current research has started to shed light on the exact cellular and molecular pathways responsible for the pathogenesis of these disorders, especially in relation to the involvement of genetic factors such as mutations in BCL11A and BCL11B, both being transcription factors involved in neural development, that have been linked to other NDDs, such as delays in development and brain structural changes (Seigfried et al., 2024). There is increasing evidence to establish the importance of pregnancy maternal health in the pathogenesis of NDDs, especially that due to maternal immune activation (MIA). From epidemiological reports, it is clear that infection exposure in early pregnancy significantly elevates risks for neurodevelopmental outcomes among the offspring, a connection that highlights the convergence of environmental stress and genetic vulnerability in NDDs. The maternal immune response can interfere with neurodevelopmental processes required for normal fetal development, with the possibility of resulting in behavioral phenotypes specific to many NDDs. Rodent models have facilitated the study of this phenomenon, enabling scientists to examine the neural processes that are disrupted as a result of immune activation. Rodent models offer information on the possible pathways that connect early-life immune adversity and subsequent neurodevelopmental outcomes (Hall et al., 2023). The knowledge acquired through both genetic and environmental influences highlights the imperative for a holistic knowledge of NDDs in improving therapeutic interventions. Treatment strategies available today primarily treat symptoms and not the etiopathogenesis, emphasizing an important lacuna in clinical practice. By drawing on the understanding gained from investigations into mutations like those which occur in BCL11A and BCL11B, together with the insights of maternal immune activation studies, there is scope to guide the formulation of focused interventions. Subsequent research needs to give high priority to clarifying the molecular connections between genetic predisposition, environmental factors, and neurodevelopmental pathways towards the ultimate goal of applying these to specific therapeutic approaches. This integrated strategy holds the potential to improve our knowledge of NDDs and lead to improved treatments, ultimately resulting in improved outcomes for those living with these intricate conditions (Seigfried et al., 2024) (Figure 3.16).

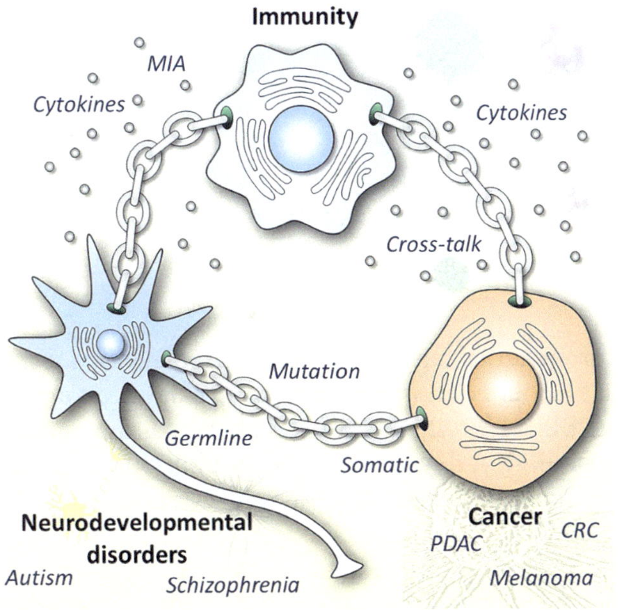

Figure 3.16. Neurodevelopmental disorders (NDDs).

Source: https://www.cell.com/cms/10.1016/j.isci.2022.104492/asset/f400cc35-07b3-42bd-b5d6-70ca1f91200b/main.assets/fx1_lrg.jpg.

3.5.1. Overview of Common Neurodevelopmental Disorders (NDDs)

NDDs represent a broad range of conditions that disrupt the usual development of the brain and nervous system in children. Disorders such as ASD, ID, ADHD, and developmental delay share a range of neuropsychiatric symptoms. Generally emerging at key windows of development, NDDs have the potential to affect cognitive, emotional, and social functioning, which can present high levels of difficulty for affected individuals and their families. Their etiology is multifactorial, typically being the result of an interaction between genetic vulnerabilities and environmental factors that intervene in the highly involved processes of neural development. Knowledge of these etiological determinants is crucial for the establishment of targeted therapeutic plans that are capable of enhancing the quality of life of those afflicted by these disorders, as existing therapy is largely aimed at the management of symptoms and not the correction of underlying pathophysiological processes (Seigfried et al., 2024).

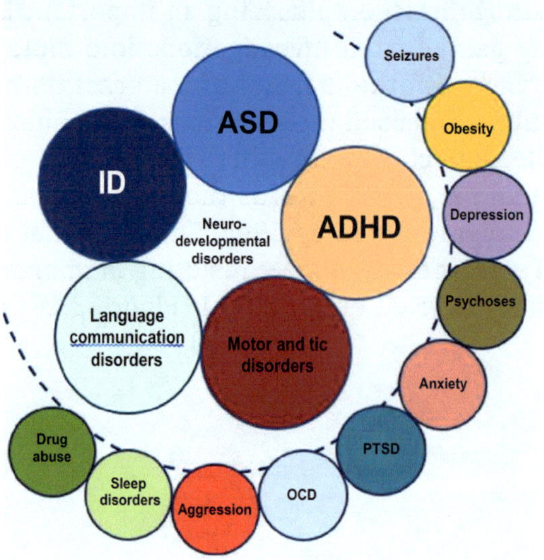

Figure 3.17. Common neurodevelopmental disorders.

Source: https://ik.imagekit.io/f4mmquslgy/31-Figure1-1__1__2p-xS39aB.png?ik-sdk-version=javascript-1.4.3&updatedAt=1658914994923.

The recent progress in neurogenetics has elucidated the molecular mechanisms behind NDDs and has explained how certain mutations in genes disrupt the development of the brain. Importantly, mutations in BCL11A and BCL11B, which are key transcription factors, have been associated with a variety of NDDs, including ASD and ID. Studies employing model organisms have shown that changes in Bcl11 function can result in profound disruptions in NPC dynamics, ultimately influencing processes like neurogenesis, neuronal migration, and synaptic integration. These findings highlight the significance of learning about genetic contributions to neurodevelopment because they may give us vital insight into possible paths for therapeutic intervention. By uncovering the particular cellular and molecular processes involved, scientists can lay the groundwork for novel, targeted therapies that treat the underlying causes of these disorders instead of merely providing symptom relief (Seigfried et al., 2024). Additionally, the thalamocortical system's function in NDDs has come to receive more attention, specifically through examining sleep spindles. Sleep spindles, oscillatory patterns of brain activity seen during NREM sleep, reflect thalamocortical connectivity and maturation of neural networks. Emerging evidence underscores the presence of spindle abnormalities as potential biomarkers for a number of NDDs, such as ADHD, ID, and ASD. Through the investigation of spindle activity in animal models as well as human subjects, investigators are gaining mechanistic insights that can elucidate the pathophysiological characteristics of these disorders. These observations suggest that sleep spindle pattern monitoring may have important future implications for early detection and effective treatment regimens and is an exciting lead for neurodevelopmental and neurogenetic research (Figure 3.17).

3.5.2. Genetic and Environmental Risk Factors

It is vital to comprehend the complex interaction between genetic and environmental risk factors in order to deconstruct the mystique of neural development and neurogenetics. Genetic tendencies are responsible for a variety of NDDs, with specific alleles indicating heightened susceptibility. Variations in genes with synaptic function, for instance, have been implicated in disorders like ASD and schizophrenia. Nonetheless, it is not solely genetic factors that present the full picture; environmental factors, including prenatal toxin exposure, nutritional inadequacies, and psychosocial stressors, combine with genetic susceptibility to create neural outcomes. The interplay between these factors can result in differences in neural circuitry and behavior, highlighting the necessity of an integrated approach to the study of the etiology of NDDs. Recent progress in knowledge of neural mechanisms and their genetic basis has underscored the need to explore how different factors converge and affect behavior. The problem here is to break down complicated behavioral phenotypes into molecular and genetic processes that mediate them. To fulfill this purpose, scientists have begun constructing models that connect between neural calculations and the biochemical pathways affected by genetic components. In particular, methods that consider regulation of gene expression across various neurodevelopmental stages during decision-making are promising in explaining and explaining the neurogenetic processes underpinning certain behaviors, as noted in the value-based decision-making work. These integrative models are crucial in enabling the augmentation of scientific knowledge regarding how genetic and environmental factors jointly shape neural development (Hsu et al., 2014). The application of human NPCs is a promising route to analyze the transcriptional programs that regulate neurodevelopment while simulating the effects of genetic risk factors related to neuropsychiatric disorders. Examining how the progenitor cells get differentiated into mature neurons provides insight into the molecular characteristics associated with disorders like autism. For example, during differentiation, there are specific patterns of gene expression for ASD susceptibility genes, which reflect possible dysregulation associated with environmental exposures during key windows of neurodevelopment. Through weighted gene co-expression network analysis, scientists are able to map the regulatory networks controlling these interactions between genes and inform studies of how mutations in candidate genes influence neuronal differentiation. Therefore, NHNPs not only enable the investigation of genetic effects but also provide information on therapeutic approaches for improving disruptions in neural development due to different environmental factors (Chen et al., 2012).

3.5.3. Current Research and Treatment Options

Recent advances in neurogenetics have made important contributions toward our knowledge of neural development, especially concerning early life stress (ELS) and its psychological consequences. The most recent research indicates that the ventral striatum (VS), a brain area that plays a key role in reward processing, moderates the impact of ELS on anhedonic symptomatology. Using blood oxygen level-dependent functional magnetic resonance imaging (fMRI), current research, including that in the Duke Neurogenetics Study, has identified that reduced VS reactivity is associated with increased susceptibility to anhedonia in patients with a history of ELS. This line of research offers important information, suggesting that lower reactivity to reward can increase the risk of developing depression and alcohol problems and that there is a call for specific interventions in at-risk populations (Baranger et al., 2015). As a matter of treatment, a shift in paradigm is being witnessed whereby the idea of personalized medicine is gaining ground in the field of neurology. Personalized medicine customizes medical interventions according to genetic profiles, combining clinical data with individual genetic data to enhance patient care. Utilizing advances in neurogenetics, clinicians are able to more precisely predict disease susceptibility and age of onset, enabling them to detect disease earlier and tailor therapeutic interventions. Such integration not only supports the greater clarity of individual differences in response to treatment but also increases the efficacy of interventions for depression and anxiety disorders. In addition, the blending of personalized approaches with overarching clinical understanding heralds new treatment innovations, a tangible example of the potential for enhanced outcomes in a range of neurological disorders (Zavoreo et al., 2014). Aside from personalized medicine, taking a person-focused approach in patient care is also essential for promoting therapeutic relationships. This involves stressing a comprehensive approach to the patient, accepting the physical, psychological, social, and spiritual aspects of health. Through empathy, trust, and responsiveness between patients and healthcare professionals, treatment effectiveness can be maximized. For example, collaborative partnerships facilitate further investigation into the biological and psychosocial determinants of mental health, thus culminating in more specialized and efficacious intervention strategies. While research endeavors to deconstruct the enigmas of neural development as well as neurogenetics, adopting both personalized and person-oriented approaches can go a long way towards more humanized care in addressing the specific needs of those afflicted with neurodevelopmental and psychiatric conditions (Zavoreo et al., 2014).

3.6. Advances in Neurogenetics

The field of neurogenetics has undergone significant advancements in recent years, fundamentally altering our understanding of neural development. These developments encompass the integration of genetic information and molecular pathways that govern neuronal differentiation and synaptogenesis. For instance, the identification of specific genes involved in neurogenesis, such as those regulating NPC proliferation, has highlighted the intricate genetic underpinnings that contribute to brain morphology and function. Moreover, the use of advanced genome-editing technologies, like CRISPR-Cas9, enables researchers to manipulate these genes in experimental models. Such interventions allow for the exploration of not just the developmental processes but also their implications in NDDs. As a result, we gain deeper insights into how genetic variations influence susceptibility to conditions such as ASDs, which has critical repercussions for identifying biomarkers and potential therapeutic targets in neurogenetics. Advancements in neurogenetics also shed light on the implications of genetic mutations in neurodegenerative diseases. For example, studies have shown that specific genetic variants can affect the trajectory of diseases such as Alzheimer's and Huntingtons. The identification of genes linked to amyloid-beta processing and tau phosphorylation enhances our understanding of the pathophysiology associated with Alzheimer's disease, opening avenues for innovative treatment modalities. Additionally, neurogenetics research highlights the role of neuroinflammation and its genetic correlates in neurodegeneration. By elucidating the genetic factors involved, researchers can better understand individual variability in disease progression and therapeutic response, promoting a more personalized medicine approach in neurology. Such comprehensive insights into how genetic factors intersect with environmental influences further stress the importance of neurogenetics in developing effective interventions for neurodegenerative disorders. The clinical applications of neurogenetics are expanding, particularly in areas such as neuromodulation and personalized treatment strategies. Techniques such as deep brain stimulation (DBS) have gained prominence in treating movement disorders, notably Parkinson's disease, by modulating dysfunctional brain circuits. Recent advancements in DBS technology now enable simultaneous monitoring of brain activity while delivering targeted stimulation, a step forward in understanding complex neural circuits associated with movement disorders (Kim et al., 2021). Similarly, integrating neurogenetic information with neuromodulation approaches can lead to groundbreaking strategies that address the underlying genetic abnormalities contributing to various neurological conditions. This fusion of genetic insights and therapeutic interventions holds promise for enhancing clinical outcomes and tailoring treatment plans to each patient's unique genetic makeup. As the field progresses, the interplay between neurogenetics and neuromodulation is likely to reveal novel pathways for intervention, reflecting the transformative potential of this integrated approach in the realm of neural development and neurogenetics (Figure 3.18).

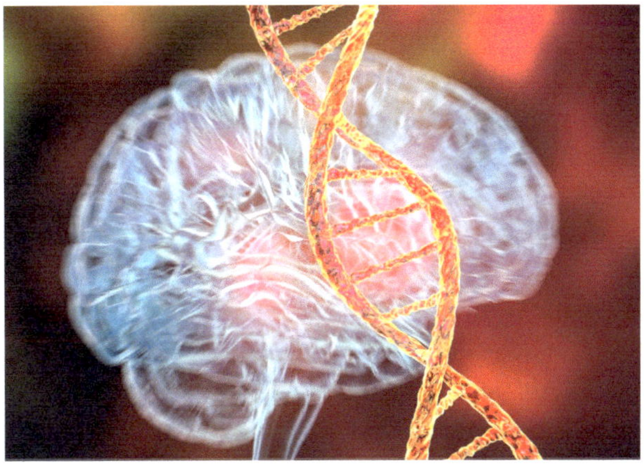

Figure 3.18. Neurogenetics.

Source: https://scontent.fdel27-5.fna.fbcdn.net/v/t39.30808-6/481703612_119 437 6172249418_352080417862763118_n.jpg?_nc_cat=103&ccb=1-7&_nc_sid=127cfc&_nc_ohc=xiukL3 uVN2MQ7kN vwHTiGoz&_nc_oc=Ad nf9d ofM kL7Ru ykS 2eGG AN4 l1Ad1aAt1Jyn z7g3PR6U 7BP mc4RWCfrUpC hS6G3 X DpDd xcErq_j7j SfN0ze48-Np&_nc_zt=23&_nc_ht=sco ntent.fdel27-5.fna&_nc_gid=hF3OEa Mn E0T6 NA1TCbi RRg&oh=00_AfKWs dKfZ ILGVdkx-sE-40E52d uzmT3exaB B751YQL7vGw&oe=6828ECFA.

3.6.1. Techniques Used in Neurogenetic Research

The study of neurogenetics has witnessed a dramatic shift with the discovery of iPSC technology. iPSCs have emerged as central to the modeling of neurodevelopmental and neurodegenerative disorders by enabling researchers to obtain patient-specific cell lines. The derivation of these cells comes through the reprogramming of somatic cells, which maintains the epigenetic information important for understanding the resultant pathophysiology while allowing for the study of phenotypes in an *in vitro* context. As shown by scientists, this method has enabled the study of phenogenetic correlations, permitting more profound analysis of how genetic mutations occur in neurological disorders. By documenting iPSC-generated phenotypes, researchers can monitor disease presentation variability and investigate possible therapy avenues that attack these precise cellular differences (Ethan et al., 2017). The versatility of iPSCs in neurogenetics is evidence of their potential to bridge basic research and clinical uses. Another key method in neurogenetic studies is genome editing, specifically utilizing the CRISPR-Cas9 system. This approach allows for precise modifications to the genetic code and offers researchers the power to create particular gene knockouts or insertions to illuminate the functional positions of target genes in neural contexts. For example, scientists can trigger mutations pertaining to disorders like Alzheimer's and Parkinsons disease and thus recapitulate the conditions in a controlled laboratory environment. Utilizing the technique of CRISPR, researchers can identify how specific genetic variations lead to disease phenotypes, providing a means for discovering likely biomarkers and therapeutic targets. Additionally, the capability to modify gene expression levels with precision allows examining epigenetic processes that might affect neurodevelopment. This has major implications for comprehending not only genetic disorders but also the dynamics of gene-environment interactions that underlie neural development (Stormy et al., 2010). Furthermore, high-throughput sequencing technologies have transformed the field of neurogenetics by making genome-wide association studies (GWAS) possible on a large scale. Using these methods, researchers can find genetic variants connected with different neurological conditions and thereby comprehend the better architecture of genes underlying these disorders. By examining large datasets across different populations, GWAS assist in identifying new risk factors, pointing to the polygenic basis of most neurodevelopmental disorders. Combining these observations with transcriptomic and proteomic data can shed light on how certain genes affect neural development and function. Furthermore, these technologies allow for the discovery of rare variants that could be disease-conducive. As the field evolves, such integrative strategies will improve knowledge regarding complex traits and strengthen the therapeutic interventions designed to correct abnormal genetic effects (Ethan et al., 2017).

3.6.2. Recent Discoveries in Neurogenetics

Recent improvements in neurogenetics have opened up a new generation of research on neural development and the nuances thereof. Among the core areas of current investigation is the understanding of the genetic basis of NDDs like schizophrenia. This complex investigation is premised on the dysconnection hypothesis, which states that schizophrenia occurs as a result of disorganized neural connectivity. Recent research has utilized non-invasive imaging methods and computational neuroimaging tools to demystify the intricacies of such dysconnections. These technologies allow researchers to map the dynamic workings of neural networks, thereby strengthening the theoretical basis of the dysconnection hypothesis as explicated in different studies, for instance, the integration of molecular biology and genetics with systems biology, for more comprehensive elucidation of the neurobiological underpinnings of schizophrenia (Friston et al., 2016). The Enhancing NeuroImaging Genetics through Meta-Analysis (ENIGMA) Consortium is a prime example of a concerted effort to refine our understanding of neurogenetic processes and their effects on brain structure. By sharing information from more than 24,000 participants, ENIGMAs overarching strategy enables the detection of genetic variants affecting key brain areas including the hippocampus and white matter microstructure. This meta-analysis as a collaboration generates a scale of power not adequate in separate studies, thus uncovering associations otherwise potentially invisible. The results on genetic contributions to variations in subcortical volume have far-reaching implications for the understanding of neurodevelopmental disorders, especially how they develop structurally in the brain. As research continues to unfold, the consortium's projects are set to intensify understanding of the genetic contributions to neurological disorders, enlarging the platform for therapeutic interventions (Paul et al., 2014).

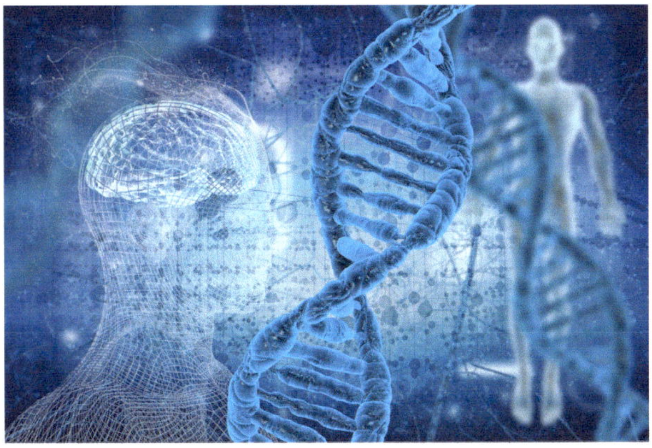

Figure 3.19. Discoveries in Neurogenetics.

Source: https://dromicslabs.com/wp-content/uploads/2024/08/20220412-dna.jpg.

In addition, as neurogenetic science evolves, developing methodologies are unearthing the dynamic interaction between genetic and environmental factors to shape brain development. Gene-environment interaction studies have demonstrated epigenetic modifications as powerful influences on neural plasticity and resistance to psychiatric disease. For example, stressors experienced at important developmental windows have the potential to induce epigenetic alterations that modulate gene expression such that it confers risk for depression or ADHD. These findings emphasize the importance of joining genetic research with psychological and environmental theories because it provides a richer picture of how pathology in the brain unfolds. The richer, multidimensional perspective of neural development offered by recent neurogenetic breakthroughs not only enriches theories but also informs clinical practice, suggesting novel early intervention strategies and treatment methods for NDDs (Figure 3.19).

3.6.3. Implications of Neurogenetic Research For Understanding Brain Function

Neurogenetic studies are central to understanding the complex interactions between genes, neural circuitry, and behavior. The recent developments in linking the neural mechanisms of behavior to their molecular and genetic foundations have highlighted the importance of grasping these relationships. Even though there has been significant progress in the discovery of neural circuits playing specific roles in behavior, relatively fewer advances have been observed in linking these circuits with their genetic basis. The difficulty is to break down multifaceted behavioral phenotypes into quantifiable molecular and physiological parameters so that it is easier to see how genetic forces influence brain function. Through the use of analytical approaches bridging neural mechanisms and genetic information, scientists are in a position to develop a more integrative model bringing value-based decision-making into play with the pertinent genetic processes, leading to new insights into the neurogenetic forces driving behavior (Hsu et al., 2014). *In vitro* systems using human neural progenitors provide new avenues for the study of NDDs and their genetic etiology. Such models provide the prospect to manipulate human genetic backgrounds with the maintenance of relevant physiological properties of human neural systems. This can allow scientists to identify the transcriptional programs used for neural differentiation, thus allowing further insight into the molecular properties implicated in disorders like autism. By examining the gene expression patterns of differentiating neuronal progenitors, important regulatory relationships among autism susceptibility genes can be revealed. As a result, the use of human neuronal cultures enables scientists to explore the functional effects of genetic mutations during brain development, eventually leading to the development of targeted therapeutic approaches (Chen et al., 2012). The findings of neurogenetic studies have broader than scientific implications, affecting the way neuropsychiatric disorders are treated therapeutically. By understanding the specific molecular pathways that lead to brain development and function, it becomes easier to craft precision medicine approaches targeted to an individual's genetic background. Additionally, understanding how genetic variations interact with environmental inputs can contribute to more effective prevention and treatment strategies for NDDs. While scientists persist in untangling the intricate dynamics of neural and genetic networks, the prospects for our understanding of brain function expand rapidly. Not only do these discoveries enhance scientific understanding but also contribute to real-world impacts on clinical interventions focused on managing the numerous issues posed by neuropsychiatric disorders, guaranteeing that what is learned from neurogenetic research finds its way into practical intervention (Chen et al., 2012; Hsu et al., 2014).

SUMMARY

In short, the complex interaction between neurogenetics and neural development profoundly influences cognitive processes and learning mechanisms. As seen in recent research, children exhibit high degrees of adaptive ability in acquiring multisensory integration, which changes their learning outcomes. Evidence from research shows that older children process information with higher and faster speed and efficiency, utilizing more powerfully cognitive control and memory retrieval neural resources. This development unveils a key developmental pathway that highlights the changing character of neural networks essential for multisensory learning. Therefore, knowledge of how these neural pathways develop can guide learning strategies and interventions based on different stages of development, eventually enhancing learning opportunities in children and adolescents during their developmental stages (Raduner et al., 2025). In addition, the neural processes involved in the perception of tonal contrasts illustrate the complexity of language acquisition as a human aspect of neural development. The differences revealed in mismatch negativity (MMN) responses in different age groups reflect the steady improvement in neural sensitivity required for language processing. Importantly, although children exhibit less mature tonal perception capabilities, adolescence constitutes a critical turning point towards more adult-like neural outcomes. These results demonstrate how neurogenetic processes impact linguistic abilities, indicating that the interaction among environment, genetics, and timing of development plays a central role in achieving optimal cognitive performance. This study paves the way for further investigation into how time-dependent language-specific neural adaptations occur, highlighting the importance of situating educational provision within developmental neuroplasticity (Wu et al., 2025). Together, the findings of varied research on neural development and neurogenetics identify fundamental inroads into the course of cognitive and perceptual abilities through childhood and adolescence. Conjoining behavioral data with neuroimaging evidence explains how age factors affect multisensory learning and language perception, supporting the notion that maturation is a complex process determined by genetic and environmental factors. As researchers continue to tease out these intricate associations, it increasingly becomes apparent that enriching learning environments at periods of critical developmental windows can profoundly influence cognitive trajectories. As such, ongoing research in this field will not only further the understanding of neural processes but will also be central to informing successful educational practices within an increasingly complex and interconnected world.

The complex interplay between neurogenetics and neural development is highlighted by the important part played by genetic and environmental influences in the development and maturation of the nervous system. It has been proven that genetic code dictates behavior in NSCs, how they differentiate and multiply within embryonic development. The significance of such processes is best highlighted through conditions like GBM, wherein genetic markers such as CD133 have been correlated with resistance in tumors and a negative prognosis. Using liquid biopsies to examine the patient serum protein profiles, investigators were able to identify biomarkers that not only demonstrate the mechanisms behind GBM but also assist in stratifying patients based on their survival outcomes. This novel strategy connects basic neuroscience and clinical translation, emphasizing an important crossroads in understanding neural development and neurogenetics (Joyce et al., 2024). In addition, the use of cutting-edge proteomic and machine learning techniques has given a new window of opportunity for examining the intricacies of neurogenetics. Specifically targeting proteins in association with neural function, these approaches have discovered a group of 24 proteins associated with CD133 that are predictive of 12-month overall survival rates in GBM patients. This discovery has broad significance in the context of understanding tumor biology, presenting a potential diagnostic model that uses non-invasive monitoring methods over classical tissue sampling. These developments put neurogenetics in a position to change clinical outcomes profoundly, allowing for more effective monitoring and treatment protocols that are personalized to patient profiles. The convergence of high-throughput methodologies with neurogenetic studies is thus a critical breakthrough in handling lethal brain tumors and raising a more sophisticated understanding of neural pathologies (Joyce et al., 2024). Looking forward, there is an urgent necessity for ongoing research into how neurogenetics and stem cell-based approaches cross-talk in different pathological conditions. As observed in the field of cardiovascular disease, with stem cell therapy as a novel area of promise for regeneration, the science of neurogenetics could also become a key in developing therapeutic mechanisms for neurological disorders. The conformity of different stem cell types highlights tissue-specific progenitors and multipotent mesenchymal cells as pivotal in healing as well as preventing damage. The future work should center on the enhancement of methods for determining the effectiveness of these cellular therapies as well as proposing standardized measures for their deployment. Therefore, the promotion of interdisciplinary research may shed light on pathways that bridge the root elements of neural development with new treatment paradigms in regenerative medicine.

CLOSER LOOK

NEURAL STEM/PROGENITOR CELLS (NSPCS)

NSPCs constitute a population of cells residing in the CNS that have the capacity to self-renew and differentiate into the predominant cell types of the nervous system, such as neurons, astrocytes, and oligodendrocytes. NSPCs are of prime importance in embryonic brain development and, to some extent, in adult neurogenesis. Throughout embryogenesis, NSPCs are highly prevalent and mitotically active to generate the extensive cellular diversity and intricate architecture of the embryonic brain and spinal cord. They are present initially in the neural tube, the embryonic precursor for the CNS, and subsequently in specialized regions such as the ventricular zone and subventricular zone, where they remain mitotically active and form neural lineage cells in a highly regulated fashion.

In the adult brain, NSPCs are mainly found in two established neurogenic niches: the subgranular zone (SGZ) of the hippocampal dentate gyrus and the subventricular zone (SVZ) lining the lateral ventricles. Within these locations, they are responsible for adult neurogenesis, giving rise to new neurons that become incorporated into mature neural circuits. For instance, in the hippocampus, new neurons are engaged in learning, memory, and mood regulation. While adult NSPCs are far less active than in development, their existence underlies brain plasticity and provides an arena for regeneration when the brain is injured or diseased.

NSPCs can be generally grouped into NSCs, which possess long-term self-renewal capability and the ability to give rise to all major CNS cell types, and NPCs, which are more limited in their potential and proliferation capability. NSPCs' behavior is also governed by intrinsic genetic instructions as well as extrinsic cues from their microenvironment, such as growth factors such as FGF and EGF, cell-cell interactions, and extracellular matrix components. The interplay between self-renewal and differentiation is important to determine appropriate CNS formation and avoid disease like tumor growth or neurodevelopmental abnormalities.

With respect to neurodegenerative conditions and brain injuries, NSPCs are of high interest owing to their possible application in cell replacement therapy and regenerative medicine. Investigative methods seek to activate intrinsic NSPCs or transplant extrinsic NSPCs for repair of injured neural tissue. It has been found that NSPCs are able to respond to brain injury by enhanced proliferation and migration towards the injury site, even though their ability to integrate functionally is still an issue. Additionally, NSPCs are being investigated as a means to model disease states and test drugs, particularly with patient-derived iPSCs used to generate disease-relevant NSPCs *in vitro*.

Overall, NSPCs are a multifaceted and vital element of the CNS, tasked with producing and sustaining neural cell populations throughout life. Their special characteristics render them central to brain development, plasticity, and potential therapeutic options, providing promise for the treatment of a variety of neurological diseases and injuries using stem cell-based interventions.

REFERENCES

1. Aizawa, H., Amo, R., & Okamoto, H. (2011). Phylogeny and ontogeny of the habenular structure. *Frontiers in Neuroscience, 5.* https://www.semanticscholar.org/paper/324afd23dcac9bdcd047ffe853d068ce5d633f82 (accessed on 27 May 2025).
2. Baranger, D. A. A., Bogdan, R., Corral-Frías, N. S., Hariri, A. R., et al. (2015). Stress-related anhedonia is associated with ventral striatum reactivity to reward and transdiagnostic psychiatric symptomatology. https://core.ac.uk/download/70381945.pdf (accessed on 27 May 2025).
3. Beck, A. T. (2008). The evolution of the cognitive model of depression and its neurobiological correlates. *American Journal of Psychiatry, 165*(8), 969–977. https://doi.org/10.1176/appi.ajp.2008.08050721.
4. Benzaquen, D., Lawrence, Y. R., Taussky, D., Zwahlen, D., Oehler, C., & Champion, A. (2024). The crosstalk between nerves and cancer—A poorly understood phenomenon and new possibilities. *Cancers, 16.* https://www.semanticscholar.org/paper/2ba68e040be897e733ba0c182ff96a21d7d27c5d (accessed on 27 May 2025).
5. Braun, U., Schäfer, A., Bassett, D. S., Rausch, F., Schweiger, J. I., Bilek, E., Erk, S., et al. (2016). Dynamic brain network reconfiguration as a potential schizophrenia genetic risk mechanism modulated by NMDA receptor function. *Proceedings of the National Academy of Sciences, 113*(44), 12568–12573. https://doi.org/10.1073/pnas.1608819113.
6. Chamberlain, S. J., Chen, P. F., Ng, K. Y., Bourgois-Rocha, F., Lemtiri-Chlieh, F., Levine, E. S., & Lalande, M. (2010). Induced pluripotent stem cell models of the genomic imprinting disorders Angelman and Prader–Willi syndromes. *Proceedings of the National Academy of Sciences, 107*(41), 17668–17673. https://doi.org/10.1073/pnas.1004487107.
7. Chen, L., Gao, F., Gao, K., Geschwind, D. H., et al. (2012). Modeling the functional genomics of autism using human neurons. https://core.ac.uk/download/323078500.pdf.
8. Dias, G. P., Hollywood, R., Bevilaqua, M. C. do N., da Luz, A. C. D. S., Hindges, R., Nardi, A. E., & Thuret, S. (2014). Consequences of cancer treatments on adult hippocampal neurogenesis: Implications for cognitive function and depressive symptoms. *Neuro-Oncology, 16*(4), 476–492. https://doi.org/10.1093/neuonc/not321.
9. Do, J. (2024). The role of epigenetics and contributing impact of stress, multigenerational, and developmental factors in opiate addiction. *Cureus, 16.* https://www.semanticscholar.org/paper/4f5c59a58906804d215493a5ce25d83ce453df69 (accessed on 27 May 2025).
10. Ekström, A. G. (2022). Motor constellation theory: A model of infants' phonological development. *Frontiers in Psychology, 13.* https://doi.org/10.3389/fpsyg.2022.996894.
11. Friston, K., Brown, H. R., Siemerkus, J., & Stephan, K. E. (2016). The disconnection hypothesis. *Schizophrenia Research, 176,* 83–94. https://doi.org/10.1016/j.schres.2016.07.014.
12. Galli, R., Gritti, A., Bonfanti, L., & Vescovi, A. L. (2003). Neural stem cells. *Circulation Research, 92,* 598–608. https://doi.org/10.1161/01.res.0000065580.02404.f4.
13. García-Calero, E., & Puelles, L. (2020). Histogenetic radial models as aids to understanding complex brain structures: The amygdalar radial model as a recent example. *Frontiers in Neuroanatomy, 14.* https://doi.org/10.3389/fnana.2020.590011.

14. García-Marín, L., Campos, A., Diaz-Torres, S., Rabinowitz, J. A., Ceja, Z., Mitchell, B. L., Grasby, K. L., et al. (2024). Genomic analysis of intracranial and subcortical brain volumes yields polygenic scores accounting for variation across ancestries. *medRxiv*. https://www.semanticscholar.org/paper/848999cb2ad63dc3f9fd988f549800bc8129d814 (accessed on 27 May 2025).

15. Gutierrez Herrera, C., & Tarokh, L. (2024). A thalamocortical perspective on sleep spindle alterations in neurodevelopmental disorders. *Current Sleep Medicine Reports, 10*, 103–118. https://www.semanticscholar.org/paper/1a1dcaf38d802cda895a412e94862e7bd906b6b1 (accessed on 27 May 2025).

16. Hall, M., Willis, D. E., Rodriguez, E. L., & Schwarz, J. (2023). Maternal immune activation as an epidemiological risk factor for neurodevelopmental disorders: Considerations of timing, severity, individual differences, and sex in human and rodent studies. *Frontiers in Neuroscience, 17*. https://www.semanticscholar.org/paper/c65366b922e1c14aaa3204066b183966bd628509 (accessed on 27 May 2025).

17. He, M., Lin, Y., Zhang, X., Wang, S., Yang, X., Cui, F., & Sheng, X. (2024). 6-Chloronicotinic acid induces toxicity in mouse neural stem cells via the C3ar1 signaling. *Journal of Applied Toxicology, 45*(5), 783–794. https://www.semanticscholar.org/paper/66ad1e4b20366df165ff349c494bbed1e0791028 (accessed on 27 May 2025).

18. Hijal, N., Fouani, M., & Awada, B. (2024). Unveiling the fate and potential neuroprotective role of neural stem/progenitor cells in multiple sclerosis. *Frontiers in Neurology, 15*. https://www.semanticscholar.org/paper/b91a4b737177f94261942d7ad463c0c4ca745b37 (accessed on 27 May 2025).

19. Hollingsworth, E. W., Vaughn, J., Orack, J. C., Skinner, C., Khouri, J., Lizarraga, S. B., Hester, M. E., et al. (2017). iPhemap: An atlas of phenotype to genotype relationships of human iPSC models of neurological diseases. *EMBO Molecular Medicine, 9*(12), 1742–1762. https://doi.org/10.15252/emmm.201708191.

20. Hsu, M., Saez, I., & Set, E. (2014). *From Genes to Behavior: Placing Cognitive Models in The Context of Biological Pathways*. https://core.ac.uk/download/323081372.pdf.

21. Jones, H. E., Robertson, G. L., Bodnya, C., Romero-Morales, A. I., O'Rourke, R., Gama, V., & Siegenthaler, J. (2025). Leptomeningeal neural organoid fusions as models to study meninges-brain signaling. *Stem Cells and Development*. https://www.semanticscholar.org/paper/666346b73b198a16d703e9bb79242221b4017c46 (accessed on 27 May 2025).

22. Joyce, T., Tasci, E., Jagasia, S., Shephard, J., Chappidi, S., Zhuge, Y., Zhang, L., et al. (2024). Serum CD133-associated proteins identified by machine learning are connected to neural development, cancer pathways, and 12-month survival in glioblastoma. *Cancers, 16*. https://www.semanticscholar.org/paper/978966e174b3f1fc5a284f5ad7eb61a861cb5631 (accessed on 27 May 2025).

23. Karim, M., & Moore, A. (2011). Convergent local identity and topographic projection of sensory neurons. *The Journal of Neuroscience, 31*, 17017–17027. https://www.semanticscholar.org/paper/98cd0d75bd4e9c06c8b1821aed8fe4a13992b777 (accessed on 27 May 2025).

24. Kartal, V. (2024). Prediction of monthly evapotranspiration by artificial neural network model development with Levenberg–Marquardt method in Elazig, Turkey. *Environmental Science and Pollution Research International, 31*, 20953–20969. https://www.semanticscholar.org/paper/9d1b48a5ec7e58693ce6b4077c9dca5e4741edac (accessed on 27 May 2025).

25. Kim, S. E., Kim, H. Y., Wlodarczyk, B. J., & Finnell, R. H. (2024). Linkage between Fuz and Gpr161 genes regulates sonic hedgehog signaling during mouse neural tube development. *Development, 151*(19). https://www.semanticscholar.org/paper/0dc6d1ad69262294f77a6608e0c4d50e8b085d39 (accessed on 27 May 2025).

26. Kim, S., Kang, S., Kim, J., Lee, D., Kim, S. H., Lee, J., Jang, K. I., et al. (2021). Closed-loop neuromodulation for Parkinson's disease: Current state and future directions. *IEEE Transactions on Molecular, Biological and Multi-Scale Communications, 7*, 209–223. https://www.semanticscholar.org/paper/9e0b85742cf5a768c74e53baa143ebb5a764c211 (accessed on 27 May 2025).

27. Kumar, A., Kos, M., Roybal, D., & Carless, M. (2023). A pilot investigation of differential hydroxy methylation levels in patient-derived neural stem cells implicates altered cortical development in bipolar disorder. *Frontiers in Psychiatry, 14.* https://www.semanticscholar.org/paper/06d4958a1cb811a7e4bab64298bb1e0f380375d3 (accessed on 27 May 2025).

28. Kwon, O. H., Choe, J., Kim, D., Kim, S., & Moon, C. (2024). Sensory stimulation-dependent Npas4 expression in the olfactory bulb during early postnatal development. *Experimental Neurobiology, 33*, 77–98. https://www.semanticscholar.org/paper/6f73f154c27f37c2b0f7a8cc1db960d74e2e748d (accessed on 27 May 2025).

29. Kyryk, V. (2024). Stem cell therapy for cardiac regeneration: Key points. *Cell and Organ Transplantology.* https://www.semanticscholar.org/paper/6a1b536f3691ad0d162e4187a4a2e2ffd1507b5f (accessed on 27 May 2025).

30. Lukić, B. (2025). Applied machine learning methods with long-short term memory based recurrent neural networks for multivariate temperature prediction. *arXiv, abs/2503.06278.* https://www.semanticscholar.org/paper/69d6d0925430f37bd273a0899af82999eced62ce (accessed on 27 May 2025).

31. Mayer, E. A., Ryu, H. J., & Bhatt, R. R. (2023). The neurobiology of irritable bowel syndrome. *Molecular Psychiatry, 28*(6), 1451–1465. https://doi.org/10.1038/s41380-023-01972-w.

32. Mgbole, T. J., & Olayanju, A. Z. (2024). Evaluating deep neural networks in optimizing drug discovery and precision medicine: A review. *World Journal of Advanced Research and Reviews.* https://www.semanticscholar.org/paper/9414915042cd4be8d8dbe81cbb49ab5e633d5a97 (accessed on 27 May 2025).

33. Moffat, J. J., Ka, M., Jung, E. M., & Kim, W. Y. (2015). Genes and brain malformations associated with abnormal neuron positioning. *Molecular Brain, 8*, Article 72. https://doi.org/10.1186/s13041-015-0164-4.

34. Mulaudzi, P. E., Abrahamse, H., & Crous, A. (2024). Impact of photo biomodulation on neural embryoid body formation from immortalized adipose-derived stem cells. *Stem Cell Research & Therapy, 15.* https://www.semanticscholar.org/paper/67be22437f58ac7a3dc1cd45394775c420553cea (accessed on 27 May 2025).

35. Murray, L., Dotterer, H. L., Waller, R., & Hyde, L. W. (2018). Neurogenetics approaches to understanding psychopathy. In *Routledge eBooks.* https://doi.org/10.4324/9781315111476-7.

36. Noh, I. B., Lee, J., & Lee, S. W. (2024). Development of situation awareness model in robotic spot-welding (RSW) system based on sensor data visualization. *International Journal of Precision Engineering and Manufacturing-Smart Technology.* https://www.semanticscholar.org/paper/bb7650aabcb67bb1f993a14881375570196be02a (accessed on 27 May 2025).

37. Paniagua, S., Cakir, B., Hu, Y., Kiral, F. R., Tanaka, Y., Xiang, Y., Patterson, B., et al. (2022). Dyslexia associated gene KIAA0319 regulates cell cycle during human neuroepithelial cell development. *Frontiers in Cell and Developmental Biology, 10.* https://www.semanticscholar.org/paper/80c1fab22adfab5888065b14c5145ceb62bde238 (accessed on 27 May 2025).

38. Raduner, N., Providoli, C., Di Pietro, S. D., Schneebeli, M., Karipidis, I. I., Casimiro, E., Bedi, S., et al. (2025). Growing minds, integrating senses: Neural and computational insights into age-related changes in audio-visual and tactile-visual learning in children. *bioRxiv*. https://www.semanticscholar.org/paper/2c9a1ec800aa1e75cad023d446ba09ab30973cc2 (accessed on 27 May 2025).

39. Ray, B., Jensen, D. M., Suresh, P., Thapaliya, B., Sapkota, R., Farahdel, B., Fu, Z., et al. (2024). Adolescent brain maturation associated with environmental factors: A multivariate analysis. *Frontiers in Neuroimaging, 3.* https://www.semanticscholar.org/paper/ab567950d337b4ecda330161816fd2f73fd74529 (accessed on 27 May 2025).

40. Sangree, A. K., Angireddy, R., Bryant, L. M., Layo-Carris, D. E., Lubin, E. E., Wang, X. M., Clark, K. J., et al. (2024). A novel iPSC model of Bryant-Li-Bhoj neurodevelopmental syndrome demonstrates the role of histone H3.3 in neuronal differentiation and maturation. *bioRxiv.* https://www.semanticscholar.org/paper/97e3e86be649d7b40bab7b37fc9db0a599c902dc (accessed on 27 May 2025).

41. Schmidt, R., Strähle, U., & Scholpp, S. (2013). Neurogenesis in zebrafish–from embryo to adult. *Neural Development, 8,* Article 3. https://doi.org/10.1186/1749-8104-8-3.

42. Seigfried, F. A., & Britsch, S. (2024). The role of Bcl11 transcription factors in neurodevelopmental disorders. *Biology, 13.* https://www.semanticscholar.org/paper/2d36680255c6af2d103c8a40ebc86aa5f77ea4e1 (accessed on 27 May 2025).

43. Singh, K., Sethi, P., Gupta, J. K., Dubey, A., Sharma, M. C., Jain, D., Bhatt, A., et al. (2025). Exploring the dual roles of neural stem cells in glioblastoma: Therapeutic implications and opportunities. *Current Stem Cell Research & Therapy*. https://www.semanticscholar.org/paper/4bfcd1cf806a9b9752978bdd3f38c886fa2d3ade (accessed on 27 May 2025).

44. Small, B. J., Dixon, R. A., McArdle, J. J., & Grimm, K. J. (2011). Do changes in lifestyle engagement moderate cognitive decline in normal aging? Evidence from the Victoria Longitudinal Study. *Neuropsychology, 26*(2), 144–155. https://doi.org/10.1037/a0026579.

45. Terven, J. R. (2025). Deep reinforcement learning: A chronological overview and methods. *AI.* https://www.semanticscholar.org/paper/40d1e0a1e8a861305f9354be747620782fc203ce (accessed on 27 May 2025).

46. Thompson, P. M., Stein, J. L., Medland, S. E., Hibar, D. P., Arias Väsquez, A., Rentería, M. E., Toro, R., et al. (2014). The ENIGMA Consortium: Large-scale collaborative analyses of neuroimaging and genetic data. *Brain Imaging and Behavior, 8,* 153–182. https://doi.org/10.1007/s11682-013-9269-5.

47. Wang, M., Zhao, J., Li, J., Meng, M., & Zhu, M. (2024). Insights into the role of adipose-derived stem cells and secretome: Potential biology and clinical applications in hypertrophic scarring. *Stem Cell Research & Therapy, 15.* https://www.semanticscholar.org/paper/4c4fd022cfa765c5be3f20907ce7457207f4c9e0 (accessed on 27 May 2025).

48. Wu, H., Zhang, Y., Liu, Y., Zhang, S., Zhang, L., Shu, H., & Zhang, Y. (2025). The neural development of Chinese lexical tone perception: A mismatch negativity study across childhood,

adolescence, and adulthood. *Brain Sciences, 15.* https://www.semanticscholar.org/paper/c2900594e0b79a481e63a02272a9553f843ef8a3 (accessed on 27 May 2025).

49. Wu, P., & Li, Z. (2024). Optimized wind power prediction and energy storage scheduling using genetic algorithm and backpropagation neural network. *International Journal of Renewable Energy Development*. https://www.semanticscholar.org/paper/a98dd61135b93281cc2e220758deb41b23edce9d (accessed on 27 May 2025).

50. Wullimann, M. F., Mokayes, N., Shainer, I., Kuehn, E., & Baier, H. (2023). Geno architectonics of the larval zebrafish diencephalon. *The Journal of Comparative Neurology, 532*, 901–919. https://doi.org/10.1002/cne.25549.

51. Yamada, S., Mizukoshi, T., Sato, A., & Sakakibara, S. I. (2024). Phrynosoma's and purine metabolism in mammalian neural development: A review. *Acta Histochemical et Cytochemical, 57*, 89–100. https://www.semanticscholar.org/paper/28a612bfd0a4354422d29be259b085c04145226e (accessed on 27 May 2025).

52. Zavoreo, I., Lisak, M., Bašić Kes, V., Demarin, V., & Trkanjec, Z. (2014). Perspektive medicine usmjerene prema osobi u neurologiji. https://core.ac.uk/download/33277130.pdf (accessed on 27 May 2025).

53. Zubrzycki, M., Schramm, R., Costard-Jäckle, A., Grohmann, J., Gummert, J. F., & Zubrzycka, M. (2024). Cardiac development and factors influencing the development of congenital heart defects (CHDs): Part I. *International Journal of Molecular Sciences, 25*. https://www.semanticscholar.org/paper/d6c8289029804e400856237a6d1d1c7a76cde199 (accessed on 27 May 2025).

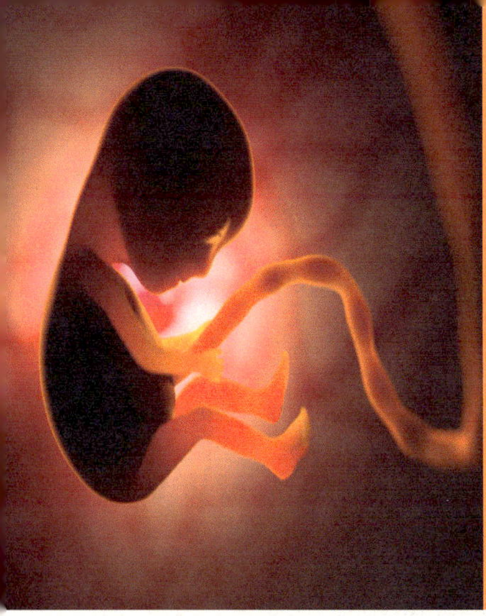

Chapter 4

CARDIOVASCULAR EMBRYOLOGY AND RELATED GENETIC DISORDERS

Contents

Introduction

Cardiovascular embryology is important to investigate because it helps explain the formation of the heart and vasculature, and the genetic abnormalities that may develop along the way with this intricate process. Development of the cardiovascular system involves a cascade of precisely coordinated events starting from the heart tube formation and continuing through the multiplexed cellular differentiation and morphogenesis stages. Interruptions during any stage of this development can result in congenital heart defects (CHD), which account for a major public health issue worldwide. Investigating the complex mechanisms of cardiovascular embryology has the goal of determining the genetic, environmental, and molecular factors responsible for these defects, thus providing the avenue for novel therapeutic interventions and preventive strategies that can prevent these risks as far as such congenital conditions are involved. Along with embryonic growth, the study of associated genetic disorders reveals the intricate interrelation between genetic susceptibility and environmental factors on cardiovascular well-being. New findings emphasize how maternal well-being as well as external stressors can impact not only the mother but also her child's cardiovascular system. For example, hypertensive pregnancy diseases and gestational diabetes are major risk factors with established correlations to long-term cardiovascular issues in women, especially as they pass through various stages of life. Knowledge of these associations offers crucial information on the general implications of maternal health on fetal growth as well as long-term cardiovascular outcomes. Therefore, the study of cardiovascular embryology within the context of genetic disorders brings out the complexity of heart development and the variables that affect its integrity. Additionally, the importance of epigenetic mechanisms is better appreciated as central to linking environmental exposures with genetic susceptibility to cardiovascular diseases. Epigenetic modifications may arise from stressors encountered across vulnerable developmental windows, influencing gene expression without modifying the underlying DNA sequence. These changes can be transmitted through generations, as indicated by the increasing number of studies on intergenerational transmission of the effects of trauma. Through the emphasis on the role played by both developmental and epigenetic influences, scientists can reveal pathways contributing to cardiovascular disease, leading to a well-rounded understanding of such complexities. The interaction of genetic, environmental, and epigenetic factors ultimately highlights the need to view cardiovascular health from a multidisciplinary point of view, which is crucial to formulate individualized prevention and treatment strategies in line with individual and family health profiles (Figure 4.1).

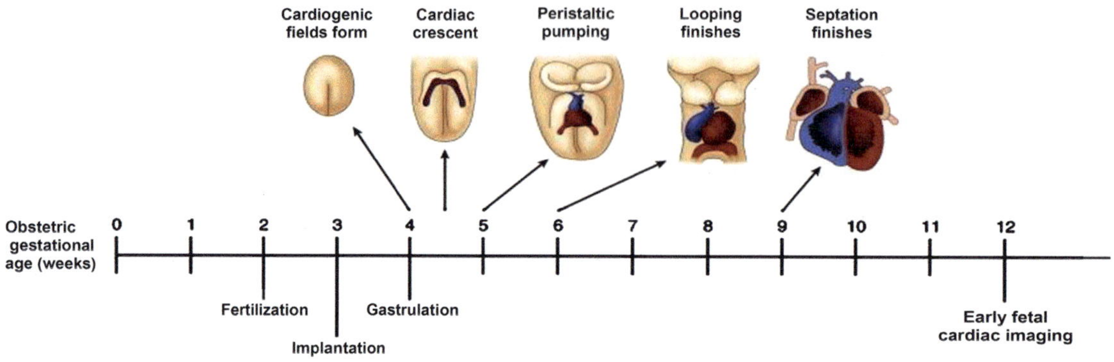

Figure 4.1. Embryology of the cardiovascular system.

Source: https://radiologykey.com/wp-content/uploads/2019/09/f002-001-9781416031727.jpg.

Definition of Cardiovascular Embryology

The phrase cardiovascular embryology is used to describe the specialized discipline of embryology that studies the development of the cardiovascular system in embryos. This is the highly complex process that leads to the establishment of the heart, blood vessels, and related structures early in development from initial cardiac fields to the fully formed circulatory system. Knowledge of cardiovascular embryology is essential because it exposes the biological processes involved in normal cardiovascular development and the possible deviations that may result in congenital heart disease. Such diseases, which become apparent early in life, result from disruptions in the process of embryonic development and account for a large part of infant mortality and morbidity over the long term, which necessitates wide research within this field. The embryological development of cardiovascular systems starts with mesodermal formation, resulting in the formation of primary heart fields. These domains converge to form an embryonic heart tube that loops, partitions, and remodels. Signaling pathways, particularly Wnt and Notch, play a crucial role in guiding this process to form correctly and orient cardiac structures appropriately. Abnormalities in these pathways can lead to numerous genetic disorders related to structural heart defects. Current research has elucidated the intricate interaction of genetic factors with environmental factors during embryonic development, wherein the multifactorial etiology of such conditions has been underscored. Elucidating the fine points of these interactions is crucial for formulating effective prevention and treatment strategies for cardiovascular diseases stemming from embryonic defects. Further, progress in genetic research has greatly facilitated our knowledge regarding cardiovascular embryology. With the use of methods such as genome-wide association studies and functional genomics, various loci associated with cardiovascular development and susceptibility to disease have been identified. For example, genetic changes involving proteins such as ACE2 have been highly associated with cardiovascular disease and health, showing the relationship between predisposition and clinical presentation. Such discoveries open up the possibility for potential interventions that could prevent developmental abnormalities in cardiovascular disorders. Differentiating how the genetic factors impact the embryological processes enables clinicians and researchers to formulate improved screening techniques and therapeutic strategies, eventually enhancing outcomes for those predisposed towards cardiovascular genetic disorders, as illustrated in the larger picture of integration of cardiovascular embryology and associated genetic disorders.

Importance of Studying Cardiovascular Development

Cardiovascular development is central to unraveling the subtleties of congenital heart disease and accompanying genetic disorders. As one of the first functional organ systems to develop in the embryonic organism, the cardiovascular system is especially susceptible to disturbances, which can lead to severe health consequences. Cardiovascular embryology research is used to elucidate the intricate signaling cascades and gene pathways guiding heart development, including malformation resulting from genetic mutation or environmental factors. Clarification of the more subtle points of developmental sequences enables enhanced diagnosis and treatment methods for CHDs, which continue to be a significant neonatal cause of death. Moreover, fetal cardiovascular development analysis offers the foundation for studying potential interventions that may avoid the impact of adverse maternal conditions or environmental stimuli, under a preventive model for cardiovascular health. The role of epigenetics in cardiovascular development constitutes another priority line of research because it shows toward the manner in which extrinsic factors influence gene expression during embryonic development. Epigenetic modifications, such as DNA methylation and histone methylation, are required for the proper development and function of the heart. Evidence indicates that disturbance of these epigenetic processes may cause irreversible cardiac phenotypic changes and predispose the individual to enhanced vulnerability in the future to developing various cardiac diseases. For instance, certain imprinted genes are involved in the regulation of fetal development and placental development, which are important for cardiovascular function. Within the domain of assisted reproductive technologies, understanding how such epigenetic changes may be influenced is essential, as it could explain the higher incidence of cardiovascular abnormalities in children born of IVF (Huntriss et al., 2018). Consequently, an investigation of the relationship between epigenetics and cardiovascular development presents new possibilities for therapeutic intervention. Furthermore, the potential for applications of cardiovascular developmental studies is vast beyond embryology, now extending to genetics and maternal-fetal medicine. How fetal cardiovascular outcomes are influenced by maternal disease conditions, such as polycystic ovary syndrome, is representative of overlap. These women are likely to have systemic metabolic dysfunction which can interfere with normal embryonic development, accounting for environmental-genetic interaction (Daniel et al., 2015). As complications in maternal health on the rise, additional understanding of the part they play in influencing cardiovascular development becomes more and more important. Such holistic practice therefore results in improved clinical recommendations for maximizing maternal health and thereby fetal cardiovascular function. By outlining these associations, studies of cardiovascular development not only enhance our knowledge of congenital disease, but they also directly influence public health policy as means of limiting the morbidity of cardiovascular disease in the offspring generation (Figure 4.2).

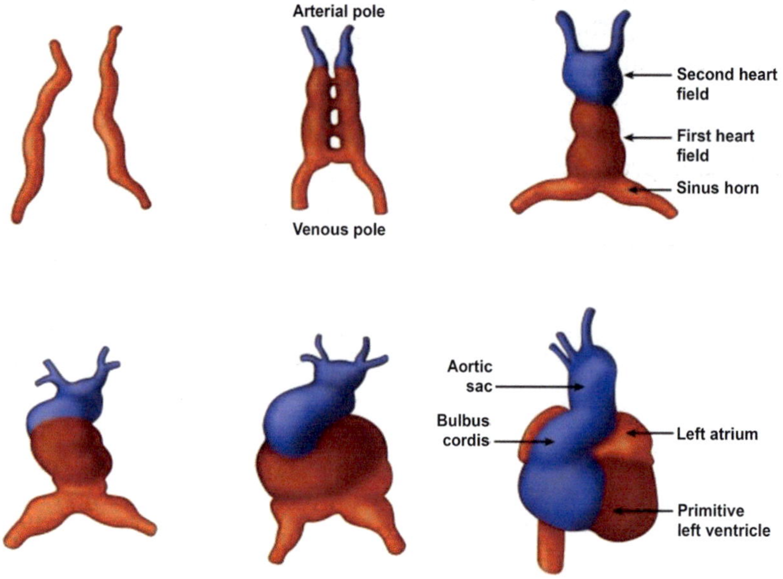

Figure 4.2. Cardiovascular development.

Source: https://radiologykey.com/wp-content/uploads/2019/09/f002-003-9781416031727.jpg.

Overview of Genetic Disorders Related to Cardiovascular Embryology

A consideration of cardiovascular embryonic genetic disorders reveals a complex interplay between genetic predispositions and the development of cardiovascular structures. These disorders can arise as a result of mutations in significant developmental genes that have a central role to play in embryogenesis. For instance, CHDs represent one of the most common birth defects, typically caused by genetic defects which disrupt normal cardiac development. Research has indicated that genetic differences that are involved in cardiogenesis have the ability to result in structural anomalies of the heart, such as ventricular septal defects and atrial septal defects. The multifactorial nature of these conditions suggests that environmental influences and genes have important roles in the causation of CHDs at susceptible stages of development. This emphasizes the necessity of genetic screening and counseling to determine the individual risk factors of cardiovascular anomalies among children. Further, recent studies have put a focus on the application of polygenic risk scores (PRS) to ascertain the risk of cardiovascular disease development, revealing sex-specific associations that are of concern. Remarkably, genetic susceptibility to major depression has been associated with a heightened risk of cardiovascular diseases, especially among females. For instance, an increase in the polygenic score for major depression by one standard deviation was associated with an increased risk of atrial fibrillation and coronary artery disease among women, regardless of previous psychiatric diagnoses. This indicates that genetic determinants affecting cardiovascular health might differ uniquely between genders, emphasizing the need for gender-specific risk assessment models. These findings not only enhance the knowledge of cardiovascular embryology but also present possible directions for intervention and prevention strategies focusing on the reduction of risks in genetically predisposed individuals (Jiang et al., 2024). The relationship between hypertensive disorders of pregnancy (HDPs) and genetic predispositions is another important feature in cardiovascular embryology. Hypertensive disorders are major causes of maternal morbidity and mortality and have long-term cardiovascular implications for women with affected conditions. Recent studies using Mendelian randomization have determined certain proteins related to gestational hypertension and preeclampsia that demonstrate complex associations between genetic markers and cardiovascular risk factors in pregnancy. For example, some proteins like NT-proBNP and HSP27 demonstrate strong correlations with increased risks of HDPs. Since such proteins are critical to cardiovascular function, knowing their underlying genetics could pave the way to major advances in risk stratification and management of pregnant women. Such an integrative path with emphasis on genetic considerations and implications for cardiovascular embryology is therefore still vital to tackling these major health issues (Schuermans et al., 2024).

4.1. Basic Principles of Embryology

The early development of the embryo is of great importance for setting up the cardiovascular system, a system which is essential for general embryonic survival and growth. The heart starts to develop shortly after the onset of fertilization, with a mechanism referred to as cardiogenesis. This is tightly regulated by a cascade of genetic and molecular signals that tell mesodermal cells to differentiate into cardiac progenitor cells. These progenitor cells continue to develop into the heart tube, which serves as the basis for the mature heart. The principles of embryology highlight that alterations in this complex process can result in CHDs, which are among the most prevalent types of birth abnormalities and frequently result from genetic and environmental influences. Inspection of these embryonic mechanisms brings with it important information pertinent to cardiovascular health and disease, most notably the vulnerability to genetic diseases that influence heart development. The importance of embryonic stem cells (ESCs) and their differentiation routes cannot be overstated in cardiovascular embryology. Stem cells possess the capacity to give rise to all heart and vascular cell types, which lays a foundation to comprehend how individual cardiac lineages form. Differentiation occurs in coordination with vascular structure formation, which is crucial for supplying developing tissues with nutrients and oxygen. Aberrations in this process of differentiation, specifically caused by genetic abnormalities or environmental stressors during embryogenesis, have the potential to result in life-threatening cardiovascular diseases. Understanding the interactions between genetic processes and embryonic milieus is important, particularly as research progresses with the vision to exploit stem cell technology for regenerative treatments in cardiovascular medicine, promising to cure genetic diseases resulting from embryological mistakes (Alekseev et al., 2022).

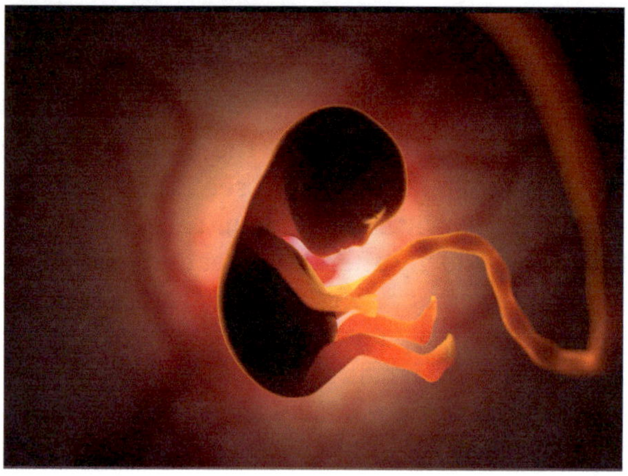

Figure 4.3. The embryo.

Source: https://external-content.duckduckgo.com/iu/?u=https%3A%2F%2Fwww.verywellhealth.com%2Fthmb%2FyASDI6MGFEOcpNLZkFC3MmsV1f8%3D%2F2133x1406%2Ffilters%3Afill(87E3EF%2C1)%2FGettyImages-1288913695-230c3b035bce4442b29e1598a492022d.jpg&f=1&nofb=1&ipt=00b9128f67cc778c201052b3761038b192b57079f7724dbcd64faacabd892b20.

Increased research has brought into focus the role of exogenous influences, such as maternal nutrition and health, on cardiovascular development in the embryo. Maternal conditions of diabetes or obesity may cause oxidative stress and inflammation, which negatively impact endothelial function and embryonic heart development (Shulga, 2022). Both stresses can disrupt the balance of signaling mechanisms that control cellular differentiation and organogenesis, resulting in increased congenital cardiovascular malformations. The appreciation of these relationships reinforces early intervention and lifestyle changes to reduce the risk related to maternal health. In addition, these findings open up avenues for designing preventive measures and therapeutic targets that can ensure fetal cardiovascular protection and prevent the development of genetic diseases and lay the groundwork for a healthy life after birth (Figure 4.3).

4.1.1. Stages of Embryonic Development

The embryonic development stages are important for comprehending not only the patterns of normal growth but also for the mechanisms involved that could give rise to cardiovascular defects. Fertilization initiates this process, and it results in the zygote, which then undergoes cleavage, forming a blastocyst. Through further development, ESCs start to differentiate into different lineages such as mesoderm, which is cardinal for cardiovascular forms. The formation of the heart is especially prone to disruptions at this point in development since it is one of the first organs to be formed. Knowledge of these initial development timetables enables researchers to pinpoint times of vulnerability in which environmental influences or gene mutations can have a dramatic effect on cardiovascular formation, thus establishing the potential for future disorders. The role of outside factors during embryonic formation cannot be overemphasized. Teratogens, some drugs, chemicals, and even maternal illnesses included, cause harm to organogenesis, specifically that of the heart. The chicken embryo (CE) model has been especially useful for understanding these teratogenic effects, particularly with respect to nervous system defects, which often negatively co-correlate with those of the cardiovascular system. As also described in recent studies, microcomputed tomography (μCT) offers a novel method for imaging and analyzing these developmental processes. Through the use of μCT, scientists are able to quantify the structural alterations in the cardiovascular system as they progress over time, offering valuable data to learn about how disruptions in embryonic development may result in CHDs and other genetic afflictions related to cardiovascular anomalies (Rzhepakovsky et al., 2024). In addition, gene mutations also contribute considerably to the integrity of cardiovascular formation during embryonic development. Cardiomyopathies, like left ventricular non-compaction (LVNC), have been associated with certain hereditary disorders that impair the structural and functional integrity of the heart. Studies of affected pedigrees have revealed new genetic mutations that cause defective development and function of cardiac myocytes, including MYH7 gene mutations. These findings emphasize the significance of whole-genome screening early in embryogenesis, since alterations in myocardial formation can significantly affect cardiovascular health. The linkage between genes and cardiovascular outcomes emphasizes the significance of a good understanding of the process of embryonic development, which can help to identify populations at risk for genetic disorders presenting in the cardiovascular system (Hesaraki et al., 2022) (Figure 4.4).

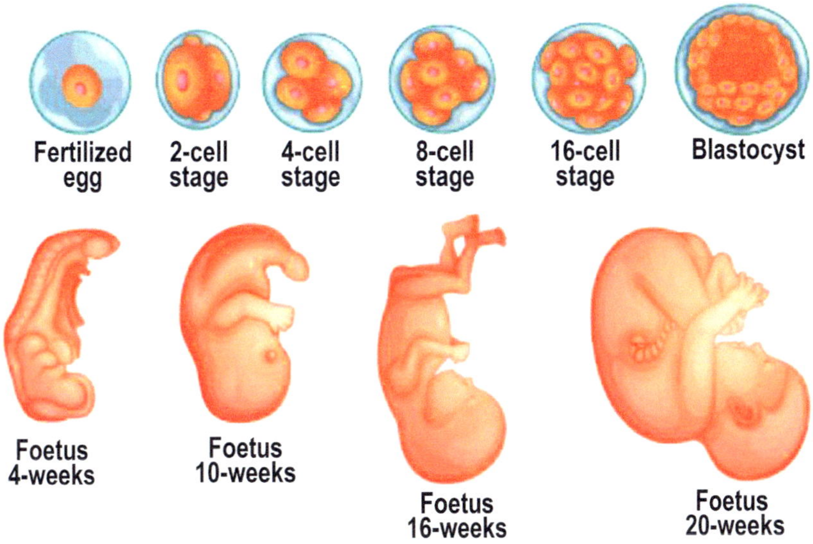

Figure 4.4. Stages of embryonic development.

Source: https://zivafertility.com/wp-content/uploads/2022/01/image2-2.png.

4.1.2. Key Processes in Cardiovascular Development

Cardiovascular development is an extremely well-coordinated process that begins early in embryogenesis, involving local signaling mechanisms, gene expression, and cell differentiation. Among the most fundamental processes is the formation of the heart tube, which is the precursor of the adult heart organ. This initial step relies on the interaction between various transcription factors and signaling molecules that specify cell fate and lineage. Growth factors such as vascular endothelial growth factor (VEGF) are also implicated in the process of angiogenesis to help ensure that the new cardiovascular system is able to respond to the embryos increasing metabolic demands. Also, the development of the endothelial layer covering blood vessels is a stage that is most important in helping establish a working circulatory system, forming a foundation for subsequent cardiogenic events crucial for further development and efficient operation of the heart (Rossignol et al., 2025).

The advancement of cardiac embryogenesis sees emerging as important milestones key processes like septation and heart looping. Heart looping consists of the spatial reorganization of the heart tube, enabling the formation of differentiated cardiac chambers. This intricate morphogenetic process is controlled by numerous signaling pathways, such as Notch and Wnt, that control the differentiation and growth of cardiomyocytes. Septation further segments the heart into left and right chambers, a development that is necessary for separation of oxygenated and deoxygenated blood flow. Mutations in gene networks that are responsible for such processes can result in CHDs, which are some of the most common genetic disorders in humans. The mechanisms behind these developmental processes are essential to understand since they guide potential therapeutic targets for the management of congenital cardiovascular diseases (Richard et al., 2024). The function of lipid signaling in cardiovascular development has been the focus of much interest, most importantly of phosphoinositide's that modulate cellular processes. Phosphoinositide's, such as phosphatidylinositol 4,5-bisphosphate, play a crucial role in organelle identity and cellular signaling, which is involved in cellular trafficking that is necessary for cardiovascular development. Recent studies propose that aberrations in phosphatidylinositol metabolism may be associated with heterogeneous genetic disorders affecting cardiovascular health. For example, certain variants in metabolic pathways have been found to cause disease such as Tetralogy of Fallot and lymphatic diseases, emphasizing the pleiotropic nature of genetic variants. These observations highlight the complex relationships between lipid signaling, cardiogenesis, and the susceptibility of hereditary malformations in the cardiovascular system, thus determining the course of diagnostics and therapeutic strategies in congenital heart diseases (Rossignol et al., 2025) (Figure 4.5).

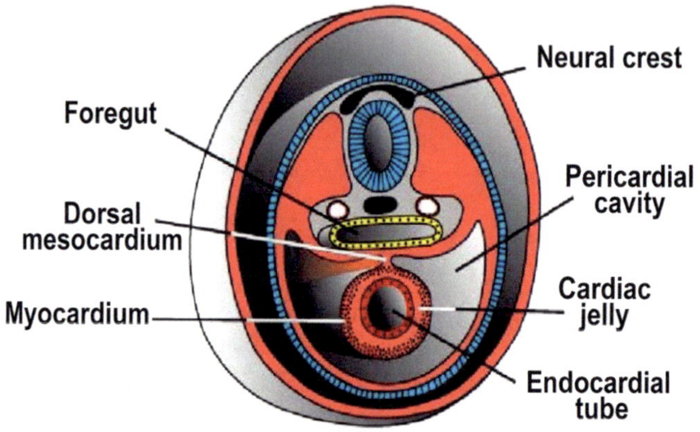

Figure 4.5. Embryology cardiovascular system (heart development).

Source: https://external-content.duckduckgo.com/iu/?u=https%3A%2F%2Fimage.slidesharecdn.com%2Fembryology-cardiovascularsystemheartdevelopment-100612045438-phpapp01%2F95%2Fslide-20-1024.jpg&f=1&nofb=1&ipt=c3551d736afd6d2a4842a3682809a0fae9218d65d162ecfa25115ad6f3fc9133.

4.1.3. Role of Signaling Pathways in Heart Formation

The complex process of heart development is controlled by a set of signaling pathways that regulate the initial phases of cardiac development. Some of the key pathways used are the Hedgehog (Hh) signaling pathway and the Wnt signaling pathway, both of which control cardiac cell fate and morphogenesis. The Hh pathway, for instance, has been demonstrated to regulate facets of left-right lateralization and cardiovascular growth necessary for the development of structures such as the atrioventricular canal to be properly formed. Abnormalities in these signaling pathways result in CHDs, which illustrates the causal relationship between these molecular signals and heart development. Deciphering the subtleties of these signaling cascades can yield clues to the etiology of several genetic disorders that manifest with cardiac abnormalities and thus open the door to novel therapeutic approaches.

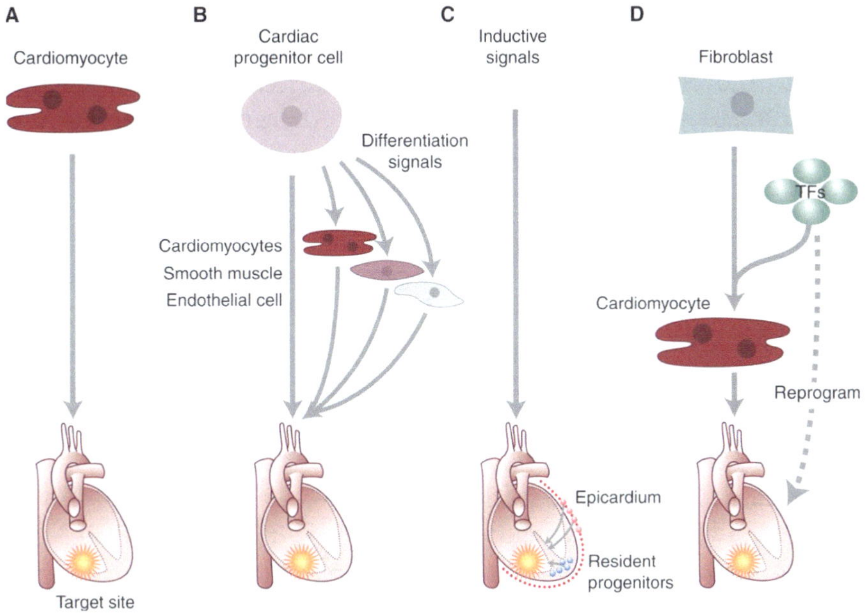

Figure 4.6. Signaling and transcriptional networks in heart development.

Source: https://external-content.duckduckgo.com/iu/?u=https%3A%2F%2Fcshperspectives.cshlp.org%2Fcontent%2F5%2F3%2Fa008292%2FF6.large.jpg&f=1&nofb=1&ipt=72c9eaa0ef986887174917b080907c1f3aa2e1c1530a230a05dc0ea413bc5392.

In probing the possible effect of external factors on cardiac development, it has been demonstrated through research that deprivation of folate and exposure to environmental toxins during the critical stages of pregnancy can have a major impact on the formation of the heart. Studies in avian and mouse models have shown that these factors modulate Wnt signaling pathways critical to gene expression required for proper cardiomyocyte migration and cardiogenesis. Interference with Wnt-mediated gene expression has the potential to cause delays in development related to CHDs. This statistical correlation between environmental risk factors and reliance upon sufficient folate levels provides a multifactorial model of heart development bridging the fields of genetics and environmental factors. These observations are especially relevant considering that most pregnancies in this period of embryonic development are unplanned and thus warrant greater public awareness toward prenatal health. In addition, the fact that signaling pathways are central to cardiac development further underscores the necessity of a field of development-based understanding in the study of CHDs. From this school of thought, malformations can occur because of aberrations in the very signaling cascades that are critical for normal organogenesis. The relationship between atrioventricular canal defect (AVCD) and other genetic disorders is an exemplification of this phenomenon because, according to studies, alterations in Hh signaling can lead to AVCD pathogenesis. These conditions, which usually occur in combination with other genetic anomalies, highlight the interrelatedness of signaling pathways of cardiogenesis and their contribution to multifactorial genetic disorders. Through the application of a developmental field approach, researchers are able to further examine the complexities of cardiac development and the causes of CHDs in developmental biology and genetic studies ultimately to guide future therapeutic interventions toward effectively treating these conditions (Baban et al., 2019; Linask et al., 2013) (Figure 4.6).

4.2. Anatomy of the Developing Heart

The embryological morphology of the forming heart is an interesting and fertile area of study that is essential to the study of cardiovascular embryology and the genetic defects that can influence cardiac development. In early embryogenesis, the heart begins to develop between the third week of gestation, the first step in a series of highly complex morphogenetic events.

First, the heart itself is merely a simple tube that forms through looping and chamber development into its eventual four-chambered form. Through this, there are interactions between various embryonic tissues that are significant, including the endocardial cushion formation, which is critical for septation, and outflow tract morphogenesis. This developmental sequence not only forms the basis for a cardiac functional system but also preconditions understanding of CHDs that arise from deviations in these process sequences. In addition, the anatomical organization of the developing heart is closely associated with genetic determinants that can cause a variety of cardiovascular diseases. Genetic predispositions can give rise to vulnerabilities during the critical developmental stages of the heart, indicating that some CHDs may be brought about by a mix of genetic mutations and environmental factors. Advances in recent bioengineering methodologies, including the use of human induced pluripotent stem cells (iPSCs), have enabled researchers to create patient-specific cardiac models reproducing these genetic variations. Such models allow for examination of cardiac anomaly expression and permit therapeutic interventions to be tested *in vitro,* highlighting the promise of personalized medicine in the therapy of genetic cardiac diseases (Jin et al., 2025).

Combining genetic and environmental information could greatly improve our comprehension of the pathogenic mechanisms of cardiovascular malformations. Moreover, it is necessary to consider the growing incidence of cardiovascular diseases among the young, which is increasingly acknowledged in the field of contemporary medical studies. Thorough evaluation of risk factors, especially in the case of people in the initial phases of heart development, is needed for early diagnostic procedures.

Working with young medical students for research has thrown into relief the role of lifestyle options and genetic vulnerabilities, and presented shocking figures about high stress, poor nutrition, and physical inactivity playing a part in this (Popov et al., 2024). Therefore, learning the anatomy of the developing heart cannot just involve cutting open morphogenetic processes but assessing how social and genetic inputs overlap to create outcomes. With ongoing research to unveil the intricacies of cardiovascular embryology, preventive actions and individualized therapy might enhance the quality of life in individuals who are genetically susceptible to cardiovascular diseases (Figure 4.7).

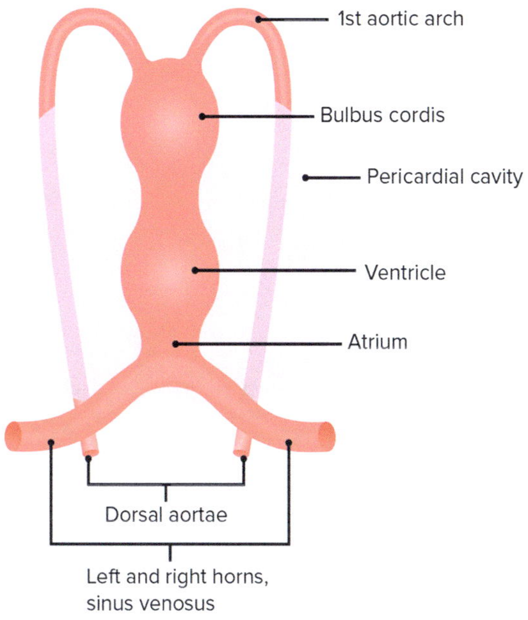

Figure 4.7. Development of the heart.

Source: https://cdn.lecturio.com/assets/Early-Development-of-the-Heart-Diagram.png.

4.2.1. Structure of the Embryonic Heart

The embryonic heart develops in a dynamic and intricate way, initially as a basic tube that differentiates into a multi-chambered heart with the ability to sustain circulation. Development of the heart begins in the third week of pregnancy, when mesodermal cells differentiate into cardiomyocytes. This primary heart tube subsequently goes through a series of morphogenetic transformations, such as looping and septation, which serve to form the four chambers: right and left atria, and right and left ventricles. All of these chambers are important in the circulatory system due to their ability to facilitate separation between oxygenated and deoxygenated blood. It is important to learn about this intricate process because structural formation errors in the heart can lead to CHDs, which are also genetically determined, and thus it is important to learn about embryonic cardiac structure in cardiovascular embryology and genetics (Vaishnav et al., 2025). While the embryonic heart develops, various structures form that aid in keeping it functional and intact. They encompass such important components as the atrioventricular valves and outflow tracts to pulmonary and systemic circulation. The heart in its early stage consists of a rudimentary tube for blood flow through a simple left-to-right flow.

This one tube, however, gets reorganized into a sophisticated architecture in the process of remodeling. The septa that form between chambers have the function of separating the flow of blood, thereby making oxygen transport more efficient. Abnormalities in such a septation process can be seriously clinically related, such as congenital heart diseases in their various forms. The critical analysis of such structural formation, thus, provides valuable insights into likely genetic determinants that could be responsible for these conditions (Paolini et al., 2025). The structural composition of the embryonic hearts is not only specified by mechanical considerations; it is also partly specified by genetic considerations. New techniques in studying genes have shown that heart malformations during development can result from mutations in certain genes, with an effect on the structure and function of the organs.

Examples include single nucleotide polymorphisms and grosser chromosomal abnormalities in association with certain CHDs. These genetic differences can interfere with regular signaling pathways that take part in heart morphogenesis during the crucial embryonic development stages. The examination of the interaction between genetic components and structural defects of the heart offers a complete knowledge of congenital heart diseases, showing the significance of dealing with both genetic and structural aspects in researching cardiovascular embryology and its associated disorders (Vaishnav et al., 2025) (Figure 4.8).

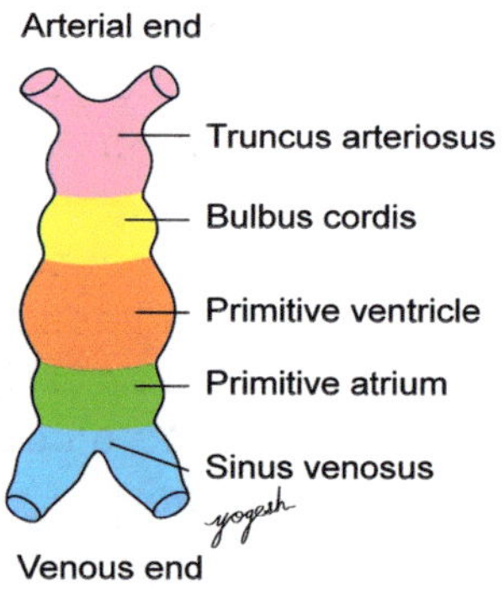

Figure 4.8. Formation of heart-embryo.

Source: https://medfoxes.com/wp-content/uploads/2022/01/image.png.

4.2.2. Formation of Major Blood Vessels

Development of large blood vessels, vasculogenesis and angiogenesis, is essential in the development of the cardiovascular system during embryonic development. Vasculogenesis is the development of new blood vessels from mesodermal cells, mainly endothelial progenitor cells, and happens mainly in early embryogenesis.

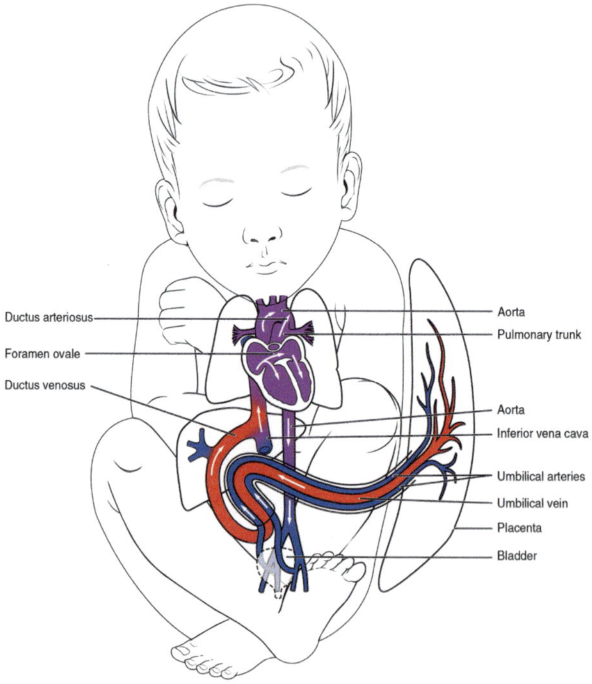

Figure 4.9. Formation of major blood vessels.

Source: https://s3-us-west-2.amazonaws.com/courses-images-archive-read-only/wp-content/uploads/sites/403/2015/04/21031527/2139_Fetal_Circulation.jpg.

This serves as the background for the development of a viable circulatory system. After vasculogenesis, angiogenesis is accountable for remodeling and enlargement of already formed vessels into a network. This adaptive process is vital for adequate blood supply, as it enables the emerging tissues to fulfill their metabolic needs. Therefore, discovery of molecular mechanisms of these processes is essential, particularly because genetic elements controlling vascular formation may result in congenital heart malformations and other vascular abnormalities. Regulation of large vessel formation engages a complex array of signaling pathways and gene factors. Central among these are the vascular endothelial growth factor (VEGF) and its receptors that control endothelial cell growth and migration and consequently vessel sprouting and branching. Transcription factors like basic helix-loop-helix (bHLH) proteins also play important roles in the endothelial progenitor cell differentiation. Notably, current research has identified genetic polymorphisms that affect collateral vessel formation, indicating that personal genetic makeup could explain differences in vascular formation and function (James, 2025). These insights pave the way to therapeutic treatments that have the potential to modulate these pathways to treat cardiovascular disease caused by flawed vessel development or function. Further, the result of dysregulation in blood vessel formation is critical, leading to a variety of cardiovascular diseases. Atherosclerosis represents a severe pathological condition related to dysregulation of vascular growth resulting in the accumulation of plaques and narrowing of the arterial lumen, ultimately causing ischemia and organ damage (Kie Kłbowski et al., 2024). Smooth muscle cell growth and inflammatory mechanisms, which are regulated by genetic determinants, play a role in the pathogenesis of atherosclerosis, emphasizing the importance of genetic predisposition for the manifestation of cardiovascular conditions. While we continue to unravel the intricacies of genetic and large vessel development interaction, innovative ideas on prevention and treatment of related disorders will ensue, further enlightening us on cardiovascular health throughout life (Figure 4.9).

4.2.3. Transition from Embryonic to Fetal Circulation

Transition from embryonic to fetal circulation is a pivotal developmental phenomenon marking the alteration in the functional organization of the cardiovascular system. Throughout embryogenesis, the embryo depends predominantly upon an early vascular system, such that oxygenated yolk sac and maternal circulation blood is channeled to the incipient tissues. As gestation advances into the fetal period, numerous consequential alterations take place. The three significant embryonic shunts—ductus venosus, foramen ovale, and ductus arteriosus—are critical to adapting to the fetal state by shunting blood past non-performing pulmonary and hepatic circuits. This allows for proper oxygenation and delivery of nutrients to the developing fetus and directs total development of essential organs required for postnatal existence. As the fetus is preparing for an effective independent circulatory system, a number of anatomical and physiological changes take place. Closing of the ductus venosus after birth signals the beginning of the fetal circulations definitive stage. This closure is followed by the change in patterns of blood flow in that the right atrium's pressure decreases as a result of the onset of lung function, making the foramen ovale to close and blood flow freely from the right atrium to the right ventricle, then to the lungs to be oxygenated. After birth, the ductus arteriosus connecting the pulmonary artery to the aorta also closes with increased oxygen levels and decreased prostaglandins. These processes are not only important for the establishment of a functional postnatal circulatory system but also provide the basis for understanding congenital cardiovascular maladies, as defective closure or operation of these structures can result in severe health problems in neonates (Caitlin et al., 2022). The role of genetic influences on the transition between embryonic and fetal circulation has received significant attention in recent research. Mutations in genes involved in heart and large vessel development can result in CHDs, potentially impairing the normal postnatal adjustment of blood flow. Certain fetal cardiovascular abnormalities can be identified prenatally using sophisticated imaging modalities, and this allows for early prevention and treatment. Congenital heart disease diagnosis commonly leads to a thorough evaluation for related genetic disorders and extracardiac abnormalities, as evidenced by new discoveries emphasizing the value of early prenatal diagnosis (Savirón-Cornudella et al., 2022). As a result, knowledge about normal cardiovascular development and the identification of potential disruptions can decrease risks related to congenital disorders, ultimately enhancing neonatal outcomes and informing future healthcare policy (Figure 4.10).

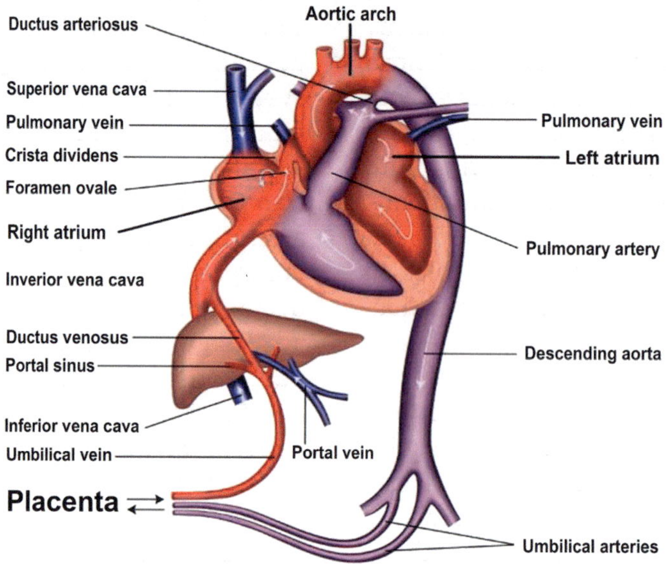

Figure 4.10. Transition from embryonic to fetal circulation.

Source: https://www.openanesthesia.org/wp-content/uploads/2023/06/13/Fetal-Circulation-Transition-at-Birth-and-Persistent-Fetal-Circulation_figure-1-vq7um8.png.

4.3. Genetic Factors in Cardiovascular Development

Understanding of genetic factors in cardiovascular development is at the heart of explaining mechanisms of various heart diseases. Genetic mutations are at the heart of causation of hereditary cardiovascular diseases (HCDs), which are a collection of diseases that have an influence on cardiac structure and function. Diseases such as hypertrophic cardiomyopathy (HCM) and dilated cardiomyopathy (DCM) are not merely prevalent but also linked to established genetic mutations that disrupt typical embryologic development of the heart. Improvements in genomic technologies over the past few years have rendered it easier to detect these mutations, thereby achieving better diagnosis and facilitating the creation of targeted interventions. As scientists uncover deeper into the genetic origins of such conditions, they stress the importance of the integration of genetic testing into everyday clinical practice, which will ultimately rechanneled patient management strategies in cardiovascular treatment (Vaishnav et al., 2025).

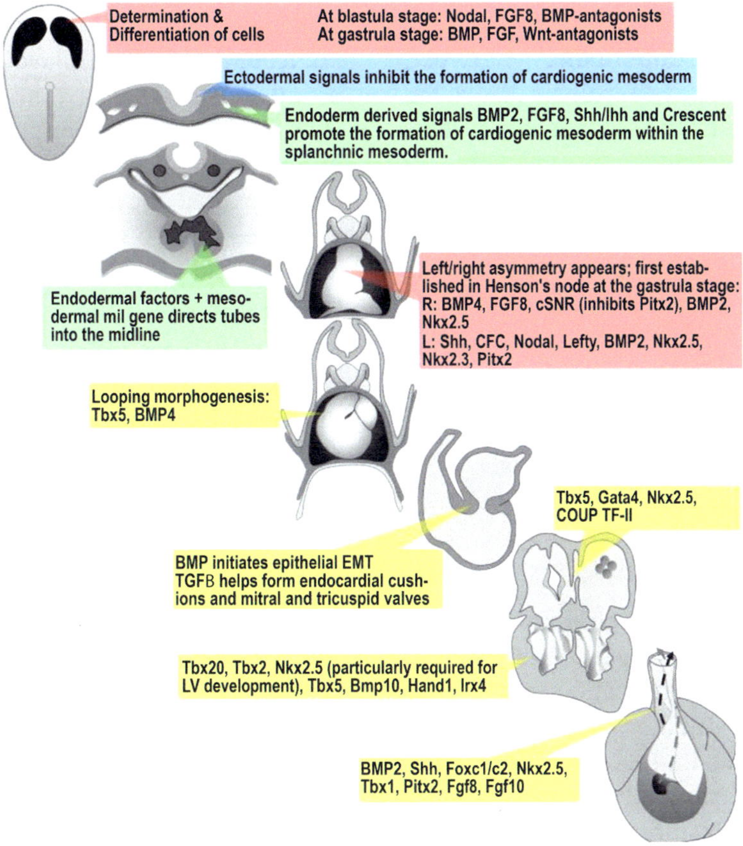

Figure 4.11. Genetic factors in cardiovascular development.

Source: https://embryology.med.unsw.edu.au/embryology/images/4/41/Molecular_%26_Genetic_Cardiac_Development_Factors.jpg.

The intersection of genetic predisposition and environmental factors places another dimension on the complexity of cardiovascular conditions. Evidence indicates that both lifestyle and genetic contributions, such as diet and physical activity, influence susceptibility to cardiovascular diseases among individuals. Identification of the polygenic nature of the diseases indicates the ways in which different genetic variants may interact to influence environmentally linked effects to lead to disparate phenotypic presentations. This complexity highlights the need to quantify an individual's PRS in thinking about cardiovascular well-being and interventions. Such multivariate analysis may not only predict disease risk but also enhance prevention strategies tailored to genetic susceptibility, emphasizing the impact of personalized medicine on the treatment of cardiovascular diseases (Paolini et al., 2025). With ongoing studies, therapeutic value in unraveling the contribution of genetics to cardiogenesis becomes increasingly obvious. The promise held by gene editing technologies such as CRISPR/Cas9 may fix specific instances of established genetic mutations linked to HCDs. These developments may, eventually, lead to revolutionary interventions that address the root cause of cardiovascular abnormalities rather than merely managing signs. Also, determination of interdependency between cardiovascular disease and neurologic disorders, such as treatment-resistant depression, reveals the complex implications of the influence of genetic factors. The shared pathophysiological pathways that connect cardiac well-being and mental health emphasize the need for an integrative modality of intervention, promoting cardiovascular risk intervention as a part of comprehensive care for psychologically disturbed patients (Paolini et al., 2025; Vaishnav et al., 2025) (Figure 4.11).

4.3.1. Role of Genes in Heart Morphogenesis

Cardiac morphogenesis is a complex process that is orchestrated by a gene network to produce the precise formation and arrangement of cardiac tissue during embryogenesis. These genes regulate important events such as mesoderm formation and primary heart tube formation, which are essential for the establishment of a functional cardiovascular system. Disruption in the expression of these genes has been reported to result in various CHDs, revealing their significant contribution towards normal heart development. Genetical studies have revealed many transcription factors and signaling pathways, including the Notch and Wnt pathways, as necessary for cardiac cell differentiation and proliferation. For instance, the Craniofacial Development Protein 1 (CFDP1) has been found to play an important role in coronary artery disease, highlighting how certain gene activities during morphogenesis have long-lasting impacts on cardiac health (Panagiota et al., 2022). The function of particular genes involved in heart development goes far beyond simply initiating morphogenic events; they are also fundamental in the regulation of cell fate and lineage determination. During embryonic development, cardiomyocytes are differentiated from mesodermal progenitors, a process regulated by finely controlled gene expression. Major advances in deciphering these intricate interactions have been made possible by advanced genetic tools, including CRISPR-Cas9, which enable scientists to manipulate gene function in model organisms, including zebrafish. Research has shown that genes like HOPX play key roles in cardiomyocyte maturation and cell division, indicating that their regulation plays a role in not just primary heart development but also the heart's functional potential (Clayton, 2020). The implications are significant, as these findings shed light on possible therapeutic targets for the treatment of genetic conditions that involve cardiovascular development. In addition, studying the genetic mechanisms of heart morphogenesis reveals depth of regulatory sophistication that can speak to developmental biology and to the clinic as well. For example, dysregulation of gene networks that participate in myocardial trabeculation and valve formation, functions intimately related to global cardiac function, can result from disruptions to these networks. Genomics, with its ability to make use of comparative methodologies such as single-cell RNA sequencing, has been able to uncover the dynamic gene expression patterns of cardiac differentiation. These methods enable the research community to identify the interactions among various cell types involved in heart development and pin-point potential gene candidates that may be manipulated to augment cardiac healing processes after injury. Ultimately, the knowledge of the genetic basis of heart morphogenesis not only progresses the field of cardiovascular embryology but also achieves imperative insights into mechanisms behind numerous genetic conditions influencing heart structure and function (Panagiota et al., 2022) (Figure 4.12).

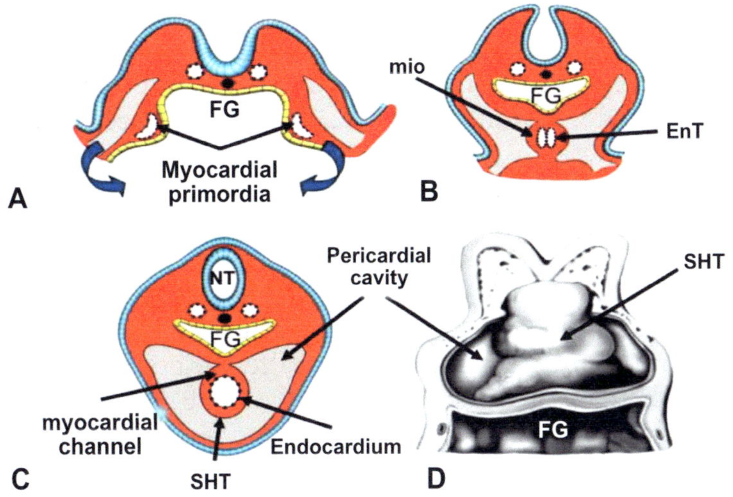

Figure 4.12. Role of genes in heart morphogenesis.

Source: https://pub.mdpi-res.com/life/life-13-00165/article_deploy/html/images/life-13-00165-g003.png?1672968209.

4.3.2. Common Genetic Mutations Affecting Cardiovascular Development

Identification of the genetic mutations responsible for affecting cardiovascular development is pivotal to elucidating the causation of CHDs. One such noteworthy genetic component is the mutation in the FLT4 gene that has been strongly linked with conditions such as Tetralogy of Fallot (TOF). Research highlights the fact that FLT4 mutations, while primarily accountable for lymphatic conditions such as Milroy disease, do possess a singular contribution towards cardiac abnormalities. Specifically, FLT4 mutations involved in TOF result in abnormal protein accumulation within endothelial cells, thus triggering proteostatic and metabolic signaling processes that are essential for normal cardiogenesis. This dual function mirrors the compounding pleiotropic effect of genetic mutations, requiring merging of developmental biology with genetics in order to adequately grasp mechanisms of congenital heart disease (Richard et al., 2024). Additionally, the connection between predisposition of genes and pregnancy-related hypertensive disorders underscores the multifaceted interdependence of cardiovascular health and genetic predispositions. A recent genome-wide association analysis uncovered novel loci involved in preeclampsia and other hypertensive disorders of pregnancy, including genes critical to placental development and blood pressure maintenance. Mutations within such loci individually have high concordance with altered vascular remodeling and kidney function, implicating their role in the cardiovascular system's adaptation in pregnancy. These findings emphasize the multifaceted nature of genetic impact on heart development, underscoring the possibility that maternal genetics could actually play a strong role in determining both maternal and fetal health conditions (Tyrmi et al., 2023). Notably, research into differences in genetics as they apply to heart development is not limited to individual conditions, with broader use for public health. The identification of common genetic mutations that are the cause of heterogeneous cardiovascular anomalies will direct screening regimes and potential therapies for affected subjects. Also, this information promotes a multidisciplinary approach with the collaboration of genetics, developmental biology, and public health programs to offset the effects of hereditary disorders on cardiovascular function. With research continuously mapping the intricate genetic underpinnings of cardiovascular development, there is a pressing need to foster interprofessional collaboration among researchers, clinicians, and geneticists to enhance diagnostic accuracy and develop patient-specific therapies for congenital heart malformations as well as associated conditions. Such collaborative efforts can open doors towards significant advances in early detection and management methods in clinical practice (Richard et al., 2024; Tyrmi et al., 2023) (Figure 4.13).

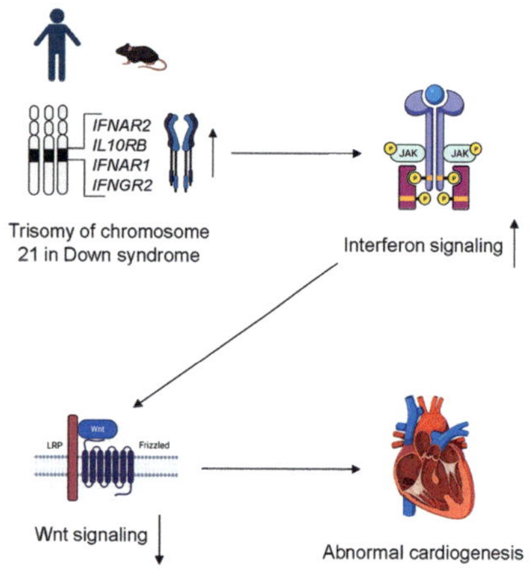

Figure 4.13. Genetic mutations affecting cardiovascular development.

Source: https://external-content.duckduckgo.com/iu/?u=https%3A%2F%2Fscx1.b-cdn.net%2Fcsz%2Fnews%2F800a%2F2023%2Fscientists-discover-me-1.jpg&f=1&nofb=1&ipt=f76608ababba76248aeb164ee3c79540e37c7138c909443cb4ba57da56346274.

4.3.3. Interaction Between Genetic and Environmental Factors

The interaction between genetic and environmental factors is a critical area of consideration in the realm of cardiovascular embryology and related genetic disorders. Genetic predispositions can influence an individual's susceptibility to various cardiovascular abnormalities, yet these susceptibilities are often manifested only under specific environmental conditions. For instance, environmental exposure to pollutants, such as those found in coke oven emissions (COEs), has been shown to exacerbate cardiovascular conditions in genetically predisposed individuals. A notable study demonstrated that genetic variations in PINK1, particularly the SNP rs3738136, significantly affected blood pressure responses in workers exposed to COEs, suggesting a clear interaction where genetic factors modify the impact of environmental exposures on cardiovascular health (Sun et al., 2024). This illustrates that the development of cardiovascular disorders is not solely reliant on genetic inheritance but is heavily influenced by environmental interactions. In the context of genetic disorders, understanding how environmental factors interplay with genetic predispositions can illuminate complex pathways that contribute to disease manifestations. For example, research into autism spectrum disorders (ASD) has uncovered how specific lipid profiles, influenced by environmental conditions such as diet and sleep disturbances, correlate with genetic variations affecting neurodevelopment (Yap et al., 2023). Such findings indicate that the lipidomes composition can serve as a mediating factor between genetic susceptibility and environmental exposures, with implications that extend to cardiovascular health. Since lipid metabolism is integral to cardiovascular function, disruptions in lipid profiles could also be reflective of underlying genetic vulnerabilities paired with environmental stressors. Thus, examining these relationships not only aids in understanding ASD but also provides insight into potential cardiovascular implications stemming from these combined influences. Understanding these interactions lays the groundwork for targeted interventions and personalized medicine approaches aimed at mitigating cardiovascular risks. By appreciating how genetic and environmental factors converge, healthcare practitioners can devise strategies tailored to individual risk profiles. For instance, patients exhibiting certain genetic markers related to cardiovascular disease may benefit from lifestyle modifications and environmental controls designed to reduce exposure to harmful factors like COEs. Such an integrative approach could significantly improve patient outcomes by addressing both the genetic predispositions and the environmental triggers that often govern the expression of cardiovascular disorders. Moreover, continued research into these interactions is essential to uncovering the multifaceted nature of cardiovascular diseases, which often involve a complex interplay of genetic, environmental, and lifestyle factors in their development and progression.

4.4. Common Cardiovascular Genetic Disorders

The investigation of shared cardiovascular genetic disorders is crucial to comprehending the intricate relationship between genetic predispositions and developmental abnormalities in cardiovascular embryology. One leading example is Tetralogy of Fallot (TOF), a CHD with four distinctive anatomical abnormalities. Recent studies have found rare deleterious genetic variants in the FLT4 gene directly linked with the formation of TOF. These variants, when expressed in primary human endothelial cells, lead to the accumulation of FLT4 protein, interfering with normal cellular function and abnormal heart development. This suggests a specific pathogenic process for FLT4 variants that is different from their function in other disorders, like Milroy disease, and emphasizes the requirement for specific therapeutic interventions addressing these specific genetic mechanisms (Richard et al., 2024). Moreover, dyslipidemia as a genetic disorder also appears to be an important one that is strongly associated with cardiovascular risk, often resulting in atherosclerosis and other associated diseases. Genetic factors determine how lipid metabolism occurs in the body and thus have a key influence on cardiovascular health distinctly in each individual. High levels of low-density lipoprotein (LDL) cholesterol and low levels of high-density lipoprotein (HDL) cholesterol are key contributors to the disorder. The intricacy of lipoprotein interactions and their connection with inflammation only adds to the difficulty in comprehending cardiovascular diseases.

Through a study of the genetic basis for lipid abnormalities, scientists can shed more light on the pathways that lead to conditions like coronary artery disease and myocardial infarction and eventually lead to more effective prevention and treatment (Wazir et al., 2023). Furthermore, the investigation of shared cardiovascular genetic diseases underscores the need for interdisciplinary strategies within cardiology. Genetic screens and cutting-edge imaging technology have become invaluable tools in the identification of high-risk populations and permitting the transition to precision medicine. Such approaches facilitate clinicians to personalize interventions using individual genetic profiles, providing a more tailored method of treatment and prevention. Moreover, lifestyle change and dietetic approaches contribute significantly to controlling the intricacies of genetic susceptibility to cardiovascular disease. Through the promotion of extensive insight into both the genetic foundations and lifestyle components, medical professionals can formulate effective, multi-dimensional strategies against the increasing worldwide trend of cardiovascular disease, thus improving patient outcomes and public health policies (Wazir et al., 2023) (Figure 4.14).

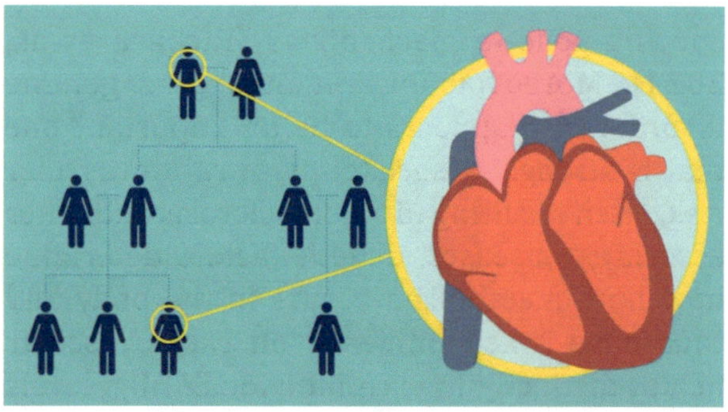

Figure 4.14. Cardiovascular genetic disorders.

Source: https://www.michiganmedicine.org/sites/default/files/styles/article_main_image/public/blog/UMH_C_GENETICHEART.jpg?h=2d703ee9&itok=qSL8LSp0.

4.4.1. Congenital Heart Defects (CHDs)

CHDs are a major group of structural abnormalities of the heart and its related vessels, which can be seen at birth. CHDs result from intricate interplay of genetic and environmental elements during the sensitive stages of cardiac formation during embryology. The pathophysiologic continuum of CHDs varies from simple lesions with no symptoms to severe anomalies that require urgent therapeutic interventions. Studies show that the occurrence of extracardiac anomalies (ECAs) is a strong indicator of co-occurring genetic disorders in infants with CHDs. In a detailed study, it was found that more than 24% of infants with CHDs had recognized genetic conditions, making complete genetic testing important in this group (Benjamin et al., 2024). Recognition of these relationships can result in better management techniques and enhanced prognostic results for involved patients. With advancements in the science of cardiovascular embryology, the hereditary mechanisms of CHDs are being uncovered, and insight is gained into their cause. Mutations involving regulatory genes responsible for controlling cardiac development have been associated with several types of CHDs, reflecting an important relationship between genetics and structural defects. For instance, more recent research has revealed the function of certain proteins, e.g., Pro-rich Coiled-coil Containing Protein 2B (PRRC2B), in modulating cardiac cell proliferation and heart development by mechanisms of alternative splicing.

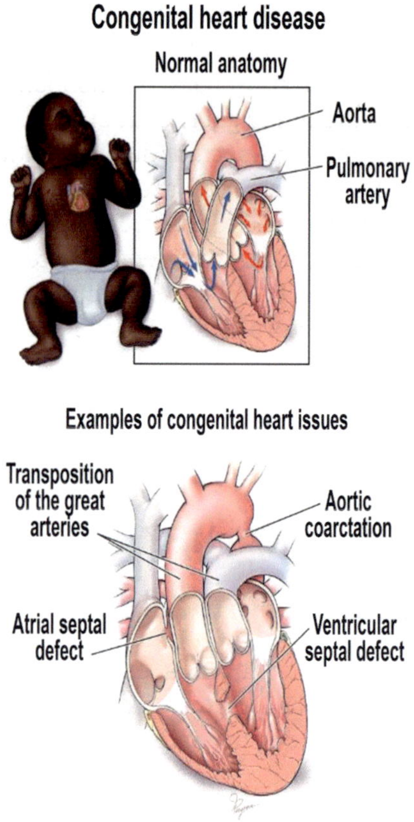

Figure 4.15. Congenital heart defects (CHDs).

Source: https://my.clevelandclinic.org/-/scassets/images/org/health/articles/congenital-heart-disease.jpg.

The perturbation of PRRC2B has been revealed to lead to particular defects such as patent ductus arteriosus (PDA) as well as neonatal lethality, highlighting the functional importance of genetic components in heart development (Das et al., 2024). Such revelations shed light on the multifaceted genetic map that governs CHDs, challenging practitioners and researchers to include genetic testing in the diagnostic workup of all infants with cardiac malformations. The clinical significance of the identification of the complex interplay between CHDs and genetic disease is vast. The delineation of ECAs and target gene mutations necessitates a more individualized approach to screening and management of infants with CHDs. In addition, the knowledge obtained from the study of genes such as PRRC2B can improve diagnostic methods and open up gene-targeted therapy in the future. Since the relatively low predictive capability of using ECA status alone warrants that a complete genetic analysis is not dispensable in neonatal care facilities. The incorporation of genetic screening could not only increase our knowledge of the intricate mechanisms of CHDs but might also reduce the risk of missing crucial, albeit non-phenotypically apparent, genetic disorders within afflicted populations (Benjamin et al., 2024). Furthering cardiovascular embryology and genetics, therefore, holds potential for enhancing health outcomes and guiding therapeutic approaches to congenital heart disease (Figure 4.15).

4.4.2. Genetic Syndromes Associated with Cardiovascular Anomalies

The interaction of genetic syndromes with cardiovascular malformations is an important area of research in the discipline of cardiovascular embryology. A number of genetic diseases, most notably those belonging to the class of RASopathies, have important cardiovascular phenotypes, such as CHDs and hypertrophic cardiomyopathy. Noonan syndrome and other RASopathies are part of an important group of genetic syndromes that require differential diagnosis consideration in persons with congenital cardiovascular malformations. The range of cardiovascular abnormalities seen among RASopathies is not only wide but also is progressive in nature, with certain abnormalities appearing in later years of life. Hence, an in-depth understanding of these syndromes is necessary for correct diagnosis and management. Genetic testing for the established disease genes of RASopathies is becoming increasingly advised because it makes exact prognostic assessments possible and enables the creation of individually tailored treatment plans, which could greatly improve patient outcomes (Zenker et al., 2025). Marfan syndrome and other syndromes related to connective tissue disorders are notable examples of genetic syndromes that cause cardiovascular anomalies. Marfan syndrome, which is also marked by a characteristic marfanoid habitus, ectopia lentis, and aortic dilation, is the paradigm for the crucial interaction between genetics and cardiovascular development. Marfan syndrome patients have high susceptibility to fatal cardiovascular complications such as aortic dissection, and thus early diagnosis becomes essential. Marfan syndrome has overlapping features with other syndromes like Loeys-Dietz syndrome and Beals syndrome, which are also characterized by cardiovascular involvement along with other systemic anomalies. The recognition of these syndromes also helps comprehend the complex network of genes that determine cardiovascular development and highlights monitoring affected individuals for their entire life to prevent risks from possible cardiovascular complications (Anne-Cécile et al., 2025). Beyond the immediate clinical implications of recognizing the genetic syndromes that involve cardiovascular anomalies, they provide clues on the pathogenetic mechanisms governing cardiovascular development. For example, the phenotypes of RASopathy emphasize how disturbances in major developmental pathways can result in substantial cardiovascular malformations. The same applies to the connective tissue disorders of Marfan syndrome and how integrity of connective tissue is essential for maintaining cardiovascular structure and function. The difficulties in diagnosing these conditions, especially in instances of mild or indeterminate symptoms, also emphasize the importance of increased awareness among clinicians. Better awareness and genetic assessment of these syndromes can result in early interventions that not only cover cardiovascular anomalies but also improve the quality of life of individuals suffering from them. With ongoing research, the hope of having targeted therapies that target specific genetic changes is a glimmer of light for many patients with these diseases (Anne-Cécile et al., 2025; Zenker et al., 2025) (Figure 4.16).

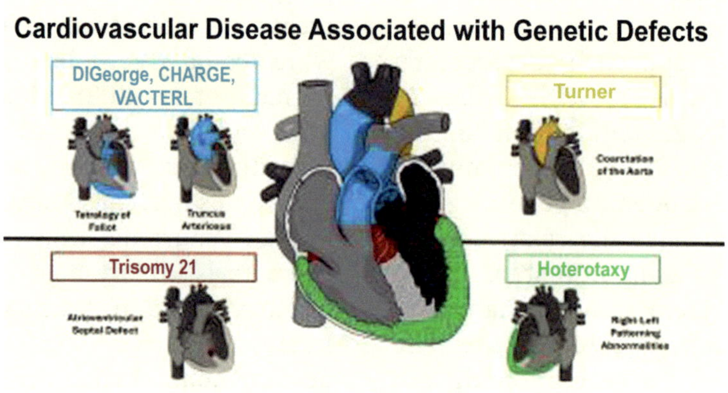

Figure 4.16. Genetic syndromes associated with cardiovascular anomalies.

Source: https://ars.els-cdn.com/content/image/1-s2.0-S1058981324000638-ga1.jpg.

4.4.3. Inherited Arrhythmias and Their Genetic Basis

Inherited arrhythmias are an important and complicated subgroup of genetic conditions with the main feature of abnormal heart rhythms that may have serious implications, such as sudden cardiac death. These disorders, frequently categorized as primary electrical disorders of the heart, generally occur without structural heart defects. Their genetic basis is mainly associated with mutations in ion channel genes of the heart, which are essential for the production and transmission of electrical impulses of the heart. The incidence of these inherited arrhythmias is estimated at under 1 in 2000 people, and they may occur sporadically or within familial distributions, typically by autosomal dominant inheritance. The complex interaction of genetic predisposition with environmental triggers is also a key factor in the clinical phenotype, which varies from asymptomatic carriers to patients presenting with potentially life-threatening arrhythmias, necessitating additional research in this area (Dittmann et al., 2025). The genetic substrate of hereditary arrhythmias is heterogeneous and not yet complete, with existing rates of variant detection varying from 10% to 80%. This knowledge gap underlines the need to keep searching for the underlying genetic causes of these disorders. Dysfunction in ion channels, especially sodium, potassium, and calcium channels, is a frequent pathway via which most inherited arrhythmias are caused. For instance, mutations in the ryanodine receptor 2, a crucial calcium release channel in the cardiac excitation-contraction coupling mechanism, have been known to contribute to diseases like arrhythmogenic right ventricular cardiomyopathy and catecholaminergic polymorphic ventricular tachycardia. These diseases reflect the significance of ion channel biology because the modulation of channel function has a major impact on the initiation and severity of arrhythmias (Marco et al., 2024). In addition, cardiogenetics has brought along the theory of polygenic risk scores but these are still being assessed for their potential clinical application in identifying predisposition to inherited arrhythmias. The phenotypic manifestation of such genetic conditions is varied, both because of genetic modifiers as well as environmental influences adding to the clinical phenotype. This heterogeneity requires individualized management of the patient and also points to the use of genetic counseling and screening in those families with these conditions. Inclusion of genetic testing within the practice of medicine not only increases early diagnosis and disease detection but also facilitates targeted therapeutic approaches that can prevent the risk of serious cardiac events in those with a predisposition for these life-threatening arrhythmias, thereby reinforcing the vital role of genetics in cardiovascular health (Dittmann et al., 2025) (Figure 4.17).

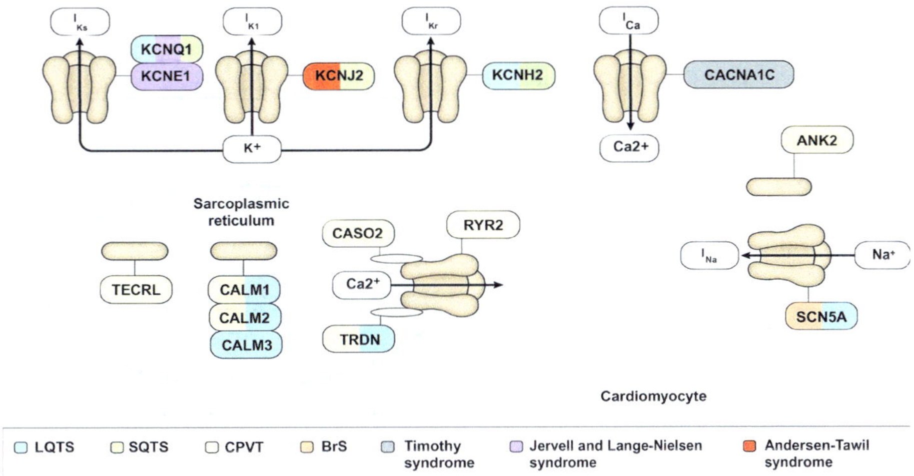

Figure 4.17. Inherited arrhythmias and their genetic basis.

Source: https://media.springernature.com/full/springer-static/image/art%3A10.1038%2Fs41572-020-0188-7/MediaObjects/41572_2020_188_Fig1_HTML.png.

4.5. Diagnostic Approaches

The diagnostic strategies used in detecting cardiovascular embryology-related genetic disorders cover a variety of methods that help in determining the molecular and genetic causes of congenital defects. Genetic analysis has become part of standard diagnostic protocols, especially when family histories indicate hereditary disorders. Novel techniques such as whole-exome sequencing enable extensive screening for genes linked with cardiovascular malformations. In addition, the application of panel genes specifically implicated in cardiac development allows for accelerated diagnosis and potential early intervention. These advances, coupled with conventional imaging modalities such as echocardiography and magnetic resonance imaging (MRI), allow for a multidimensional assessment of these compounded disorders and may greatly enhance prognosis when applied in clinical practice. As the availability of genetic testing continues to progress, the issue is maintaining equal distribution of such resources among diverse groups. Along with molecular diagnostics, the contribution of epigenetics to evaluating cardiovascular embryology cannot be overemphasized. Epigenetic changes affect gene expression without modifying the original DNA sequence, often acting as important markers in developmental stages. Their disruption has been implicated in a number of genetic diseases, mostly of cardiovascular system development. The research of epigenetics in the realm of assisted reproductive technology (ART) raises critical issues about possible long-term consequences in children born after these treatments. The epigenetic signatures set up during gametogenesis are vulnerable to reprogramming that, if poorly controlled, could lead to long-term phenotypic consequences, implying the necessity of strict surveillance throughout assisted reproduction processes. These findings add to a growing appreciation of diagnostic procedures based on sophisticated gene-environmental interactions, allowing new research and clinical applications to emerge (Huntriss et al., 2018). A thorough diagnostic method also requires concerted efforts by healthcare professionals, genetic counselors, and researchers to develop educated guidelines and policies. This collaboration is especially essential in the case of genetic counseling, in which the implications of testing, such as emotional, legal, and ethical considerations, need to be emphasized and translated to patients and their relatives. The heterogeneity of genetic expression and external influences highlight the need for tailored patient care methodologies. For example, heterogeneity of prevalence and expression of disease such as polycystic ovarian syndrome (Wendy et al., 2018) has a direct effect on diagnostic guidelines and patient care strategies. Ultimately, development of standardized diagnostic criteria with flexibility to include variability between populations will improve our overall capacity to understand and treat cardiovascular embryological disorders holistically. This complex diagnostic paradigm is crucial to furthering our understanding and enhancing results in intricate genetic disorders related to cardiovascular development.

4.5.1. Prenatal Screening Techniques

The incorporation of prenatal screening methods in large measure has changed the practice of maternal-fetal medicine, specifically regarding early detection of genetic conditions involving cardiovascular embryology. This major progression of genetic testing has culminated in methods such as non-invasive prenatal testing (NIPT), which have become critical modalities for determining the risk of chromosomal abnormalities, including in heart development. NIPT takes advantage of cell-free fetal DNA present in maternal blood, making it possible to detect potential conditions like CHDs at an early stage. In addition, through the possibility of incorporating these tests into routine care, informed decision-making by expectant parents is promoted, allowing them to seek additional diagnostic tests or treatment options, thus facilitating improved health for the mother and fetus. In this regard, prenatal screening is not only a diagnostic procedure but also a vital component of in-depth prenatal care. Sophisticated genetic testing methods have become the focus in the context of prenatal screening, with profound implications for conditions such as Marfan syndrome, which is linked to cardiovascular complications. Genetic testing helps to quickly diagnose affected individuals by locating specific mutations that predispose individuals to vessel and heart diseases. Such knowledge can prove to be priceless, as it enables prenatal or postnatal diagnosis in future pregnancies, providing families with the opportunity to prepare for possible health issues. Preimplantation genetic diagnosis (PGD) serves as one case of a method that is illustrative of this practice, allowing potential parents to choose embryos without genetic disorders, thereby guaranteeing an unaffected pregnancy. Such treatments are more applicable, especially in cases of families with a history of genetic disorders, since they bring together the practice of reproductive technology and genetics into clinical care, optimizing patient care and results in cardiovascular embryology (Aragon-Martin et al., 2016). The collaboration of geneticists and reproductive health experts has encouraged advances in prenatal screening that balance both ethical concerns and technological innovations. Expert panels, including those organized over recent years by bodies like the European Society of Human Genetics and the European Society for Human Reproduction and Embryology, have reviewed the implications of new genetic findings within clinical settings. These conferences brought to the forefront critical areas like increased carrier screening and the effects of direct-to-consumer genetic testing on reproduction. These convergences, as established by consensus at these conferences, reflect calls to evolve clinical practice based on technological progress, notably through the implementation of massively parallel sequencing in preimplantation genetic testing (PGT). These innovations facilitate future parents to make educated choices about IVF and genetic disorders, an indicator of shifting comprehension concerning epigenetic inheritance and the relevance of prenatal screening in heart irregularities management (Abbott et al., 2017) (Figure 4.18).

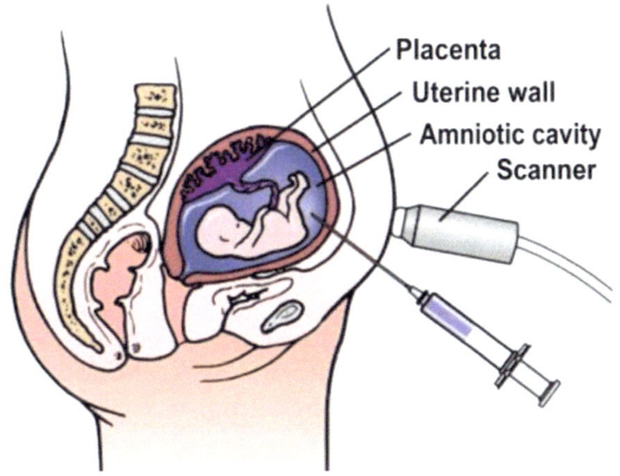

Figure 4.18. Prenatal diagnosis and screening.

Source: https://clinicalsci.info/wp-content/uploads/2022/06/prenatal1.jpg.

4.5.2. Genetic Testing for Cardiovascular Disorders

The integration of genetic testing into the assessment of cardiovascular disorders has transformed our understanding and treatment of these diseases. Genetic testing enables the identification of specific mutations linked to various cardiovascular conditions, such as hypertrophic cardiomyopathy (HCM) and familial hypercholesterolemia. In HCM, it is crucial to initiate appropriate diagnostic procedures, particularly echocardiography or MRI, to assess left ventricular hypertrophy. While genetic testing is often advisable for individuals exhibiting symptoms, emerging evidence suggests its utility may extend to asymptomatic relatives with a family history of sudden cardiac death (SCD). This is particularly true given that pathogenic variants in sarcomeric genes were found to be prevalent among patients diagnosed with HCM, highlighting the importance of a comprehensive family medical history in guiding testing decisions, especially in phenotype-negative relatives as suggested by findings related to genetic testing outcomes (Santos et al., 2025). Furthermore, genetic testing plays a pivotal role in identifying individuals at high risk of atherosclerosis and subsequent cardiovascular events. Elevated LDL cholesterol is recognized as a primary risk factor for myocardial infarction and early mortality, making genetic predisposition to high cholesterol levels a critical focus of cardiovascular genetics. Conditions such as familial hypercholesterolemia demonstrate the need for ongoing monitoring and elucidation of genetic factors contributing to dyslipidemia. By employing genetic testing, clinicians can tailor preventive strategies, such as statin therapy or newer lipid-lowering medications, to manage patients risks effectively. As research shows, the reduction of LDL cholesterol through various pharmacologic interventions significantly decreases the risk of adverse cardiovascular events, thus making genetic testing an essential tool in the arsenal against cardiovascular disease (Wulff et al., 2023). The implications of genetic testing for cardiovascular disorders extend beyond individual patient care to encompass broader public health strategies. By accurately identifying at-risk populations through genetic markers, healthcare providers can implement targeted screening programs to promote early intervention. This preventive approach not only enhances patient outcomes but may also reduce the overall burden of cardiovascular diseases on healthcare systems. Moreover, the evolving landscape of genetic research underlines the necessity for ongoing education and training for healthcare professionals in the interpretation and application of genetic test results. As we advance our understanding of cardiovascular embryology and related genetic disorders, the integration of genetic testing into routine clinical practice stands to optimize both risk stratification and personalized treatment modalities. Thus, the future of cardiovascular health care is increasingly reliant on the insights gained from genetic testing and its subsequent applications (Figure 4.19).

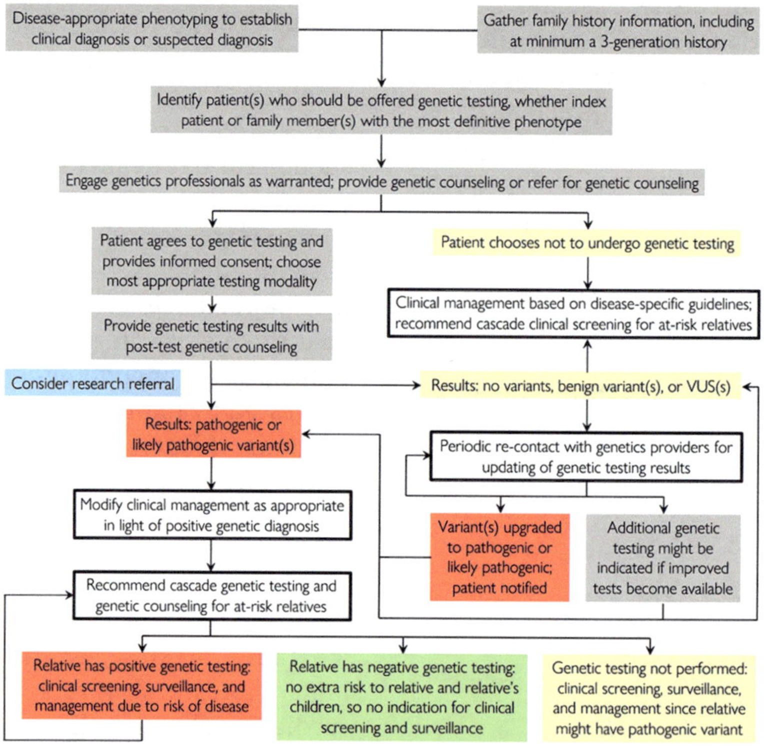

Figure 4.19. Genetic testing for inherited cardiovascular diseases.

Source: https://www.ahajournals.org/cms/10.1161/HCG.0000000000000067/asset/f1f7982a-ba95-4462-b60a-1a412d2deb0f/assets/images/large/hcg.0000000000000067.fig01.jpg.

4.5.3. Imaging Modalities in Assessing Cardiovascular Development

The evaluation of cardiovascular development during embryogenesis is still an intricate task, and advanced imaging modalities need to be integrated into this process. Imaging modalities like ultrasonography, MRI, and computed tomography (CT) are instrumental in the visualization of cardiovascular structures and functions. Ultrasonography, especially fetal echocardiography, has become indispensable for the early diagnosis of CHDs with real-time access to cardiac morphology and blood flow patterns. MRI has become a non-invasive modality that offers precise anatomical and functional information, especially in the evaluation of myocardial development. The advancement in imaging technologies helps elucidate the complex processes of cardiovascular embryology, which is crucial in the detection of genetic disorders and congenital anomalies that can occur during development. In evaluating myocardial perfusion, advanced imaging modalities such as positron emission tomography (PET) and single-photon emission computed tomography (SPECT) offer significant insights into the physiological function of the heart. These modalities allow for the *in vivo* assessment of blood flow and myocardial uptake of tracer molecules, providing a window into the perfusion characteristics of both the trabecular and compact myocardial layers. Current research indicates a discrepancy in perfusion measurements, especially in diseases such as left ventricular noncompaction, where hypoperfusion of the trabeculae can coexist with signs of hyperperfusion in imaging workups. The duality is a result of the malleability of imaging modalities to present diverse images of myocardial health and disease. Therefore, comprehension of the differences between imaging results is imperative for clinicians as they read results and make decisions concerning the treatment of patients with cardiovascular disease, particularly those associated with genetic disorders (Coolen et al., 2022). Eventually, the collaboration of different imaging modalities in the diagnosis of cardiovascular development plays a significant role in developing our comprehension of embryonic heart growth and the possible implications of genetic abnormalities. By using extensive imaging techniques, scientists and medical doctors can evaluate not just anatomical lesions but also functional deficits related to cardiovascular disease. Multimodal imaging will enable a more detailed description of the embryonic heart and help diagnose congenital defects early and guide therapeutic intervention. With evolving technologies, the cardiovascular imaging future is promising to shed light on intricate embryologic processes, improve monitoring for genetic disease, and help achieve better clinical outcomes in affected subjects (The University of Texas Rio Grande Valley, 2018).

4.6. Treatment and Management

The management and treatment of cardiovascular genetic disorders require interdisciplinary interventions that couple advances in genetic studies with clinical intervention. Gene editing technologies, with the recent advent of prime editing (PE), have immense therapeutic potential for cardiac genetic disorders. Not only does this approach enable precise disruptions of the cardiac genetic architecture, but it also poses significant challenges regarding delivery mechanisms and efficacy. The intricate PE tool architecture, size, and immunogenicity are hindrances to *in vivo* use in heart tissues. Future work must overcome these limitations for effective and safe gene editing solutions by maximizing tissue-specific delivery, improving editing components, and refining strategy to reduce off-target effects. By doing this, the face of cardiovascular therapy would change, eventually improving outcomes for patients by addressing genetic origins of many diseases (Hosseini et al., 2024). Besides pharmacological treatment and lifestyle modification, management of cardiovascular disease also entails interventions that are either pharmacological or lifestyle-oriented and directed at the individual needs of the patient. This composite treatment is especially applicable in managing comorbidities common among genetic cardiovascular diseases.

For example, genetic patients with disease predispositions such as psoriasis can develop increased cardiovascular risks that complicate their treatment (Mehta et al., 2024).

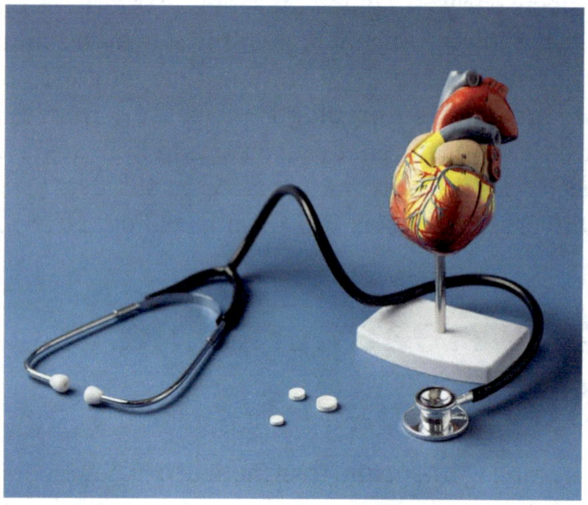

Figure 4.20. The management and treatment of cardiovascular genetic disorders.

Source: https://external-content.duckduckgo.com/iu/?u=https%3A%2F%2Flifecode.life%2Fwp-content%2Fuploads%2F2024%2F09%2FCardiovascular-disease-treatment-mob.webp&f=1&nofb=1&ipt=7cafac3359c0c6439ee89e4c46f83255bffec36bbb1d9d867beb687c4371ff3e.

Effective management includes not just monitoring and controlling these risks through lifestyle adjustments, including diet and exercise, but also pharmacologic therapies that aim to target both cardiovascular and dermatological health. Collaboration between experts, i.e., cardiologists and dermatologists, is crucial in providing integrated care, the efficacy of which can be maximized with ongoing evaluation of treatment impact on cardiovascular risk profiles. Evolving research continues to reinforce therapeutic paradigms for cardiovascular management, especially with investigations into new pharmacologic agents and their efficacy within special populations with genetically associated disorders. Even though conventional treatments such as statins continue to be a mainstay in the treatment of cardiovascular health, newer therapies aimed at targeting certain inflammatory pathways, including IL-17 and IL-23 inhibitors, are under investigation for safety and efficacy in comorbid inflammatory disease patients (Mehta et al., 2024). As more studies focus on the role of Janus kinase inhibitors, there is the potential for a change in treatment practice to bear in mind regarding their cardiovascular implications. With the progress in the field, having specific screening guidelines for cardiovascular risk prediction in patients with such complicated backgrounds becomes critically important. Adopting an integrated strategy will better enhance cardiovascular outcomes, thereby further developing the overall management of genetic cardiovascular diseases (Figure 4.20).

4.6.1. Surgical Interventions for Congenital Heart Defects (CHDs)

Surgical treatments for CHDs have transformed the therapy scenario of patients to provide enhanced survival and quality of life outcomes. Improvements in cardiac surgery, including advancements in minimally invasive technologies, have enabled more advanced and less traumatic methods of treating CHDs. Such surgeries can repair structural abnormalities, allowing for proper blood flow and function. Also, advances in imaging techniques, like echocardiography and MRI, give surgeons high-fidelity images of the anatomy of the hearts. This, in turn, facilitates more accurate surgical planning and better results for patients. In addition, the creation of interventions, such as catheter-based methods, has increased surgical possibilities, enabling less invasive repair of particular defects and emphasizing the requirement for continued research in the new area of precision medicine to make interventions individualized by matching interventions to patient anatomy and genotype as proposed by (Viswanathan et al., 2024). The recognition of the multifaceted relationship between CHDs and genes is essential for the improvement of surgical interventions. Studies show that a high percentage of patients with CHDs can have co-occurring congenital anomalies in other organ systems, for example, in the kidneys, known as congenital anomalies of the kidney and urinary tract (CAKUT) (Amin et al., 2024). This co-occurrence can make the clinical management of CHD challenging, with multi-organ involvement requiring an integrated approach to care. For best surgical results, it is essential to perform careful assessments of possible genetic syndromes behind these defects. These assessments guide surgical planning and postoperative care plans, emphasizing the need for a multidisciplinary team with cardiologists, geneticists, and surgeons. Individualized surgical procedures addressing cardiac defects and concomitant anomalies ultimately favor improved long-term prognoses and improves the quality of life for individuals with such defects. Lifelong monitoring and postoperative care are mandatory aspects of the management plan after surgery for CHDs. In spite of improved surgical methods, patients still contend with problems arising from the long-term implications of their defects and from their respective interventions. For example, patients can develop cardiac dysfunction, arrhythmias, or surgical site-related complications, and for that reason, they must undergo regular follow-up with healthcare providers. In addition, knowledge about the underlying genetic causes of CHDs can guide surveillance during pregnancy and recurrence risk in future gestations for both parents and relatives, as shown by (Viswanathan et al., 2024). Recurring cardiological examination coupled with genetic counseling can give relatives important information regarding the implications of different genetic anomalies. Finally, surgical treatment integrated with genetic information and thorough follow-up care creates a critical paradigm for enhancing immediate and lasting results of patients with CHDs (Figure 4.21).

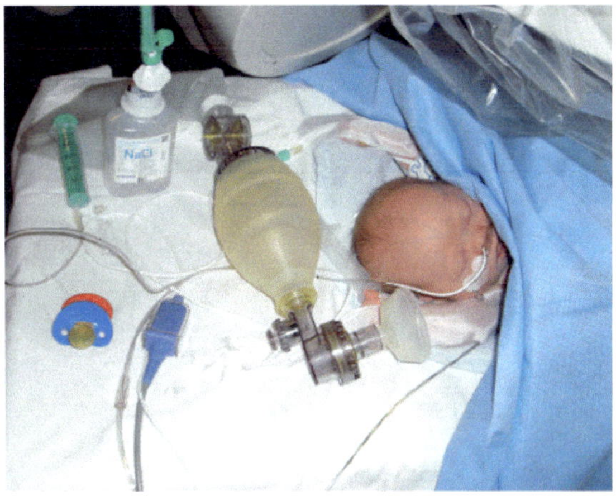

Figure 4.21. Surgical treatments for CHDs.

Source: https://external-content.duckduckgo.com/iu/?u=https%3A%2F%2Fradiologykey.com%2Fwp-content%2Fuploads%2F2020%2F04%2FC2-FF16.gif&f=1&nofb=1&ipt=75ef12176d97481fb7e1ff77fca6e4f8d9c8077bd79a0216a256adc48e77c995.

4.6.2. Pharmacological Treatments for Genetic Cardiovascular Disorders

The pharmacological landscape for treating genetic cardiovascular disorders is characterized by the advent of targeted therapies that address the underlying molecular mechanisms of these conditions. Specific genetic mutations frequently lead to dysregulated pathways that contribute to cardiovascular dysfunction, necessitating innovative treatment modalities. For example, statins have emerged as a cornerstone for managing conditions associated with hyperlipidemia and genetic predispositions to atherosclerosis. These agents not only lower cholesterol levels but also exhibit pleiotropic effects that improve endothelial function and stabilize atherosclerotic plaques. Tailoring pharmacological interventions to the individuals genetic profile enhances the efficacy of treatment, allowing for a more personalized approach that can mitigate severe outcomes associated with genetic cardiovascular disorders, such as sudden cardiac events or heart failure progression. In addition to statins, the use of angiotensin-converting enzyme (ACE) inhibitors and angiotensin receptor blockers (ARBs) extends the pharmacological options available for genetic cardiovascular disorders.

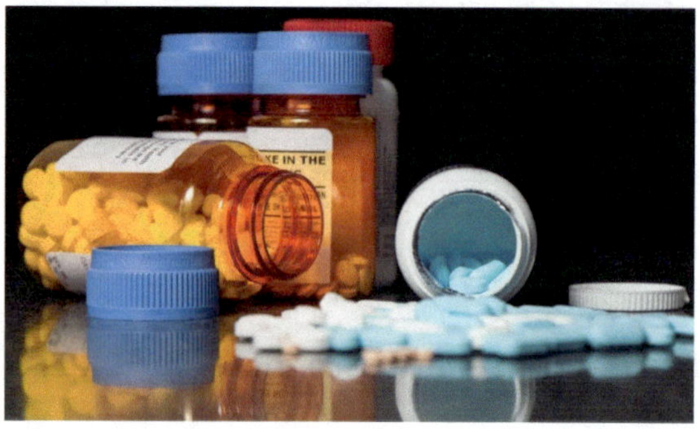

Figure 4.22. Pharmacological Treatments.

Source: https://external-content.duckduckgo.com/iu/?u=https%3A%2F%2Fwww.findatopdoc.com%2Fvar%2Ffatd%2Fstorage%2Fimages%2F_aliases%2Ffb_thumb%2Fhealthy-living%2Fmedical-advancements-new-treatments-and-perspectives-on-fibromyalgia%2Fpharmacological-treatments%2F3584078-1-eng-US%2FP-harmacological-treatments.jpg&f=1&nofb=1&ipt=ffb401be7dc5073731f28995252e3f67fc591f77888b93018f981a6473650777.

These classes of medication are particularly effective in managing conditions such as familial hypercholesterolemia and hypertrophic cardiomyopathy, which are often linked to specific genetic pathways. By inhibiting the renin-angiotensin-aldosterone system, ACE inhibitors and ARBs not only lower blood pressure but also reduce cardiac remodeling and fibrosis, which are critical factors in the progression of heart disease. This pharmacological strategy underscores the importance of early diagnosis and intervention for genetic disorders, emphasizing how timely treatment can improve patient outcomes and potentially halt disease progression. Moreover, advances in pharmacogenomics have begun to illuminate the intricate relationship between genetic variations and drug response in cardiovascular treatments. Identifying specific genetic markers linked to drug metabolism can enhance personalized medicine approaches, allowing healthcare providers to better predict which interventions will yield optimal results for individual patients. For instance, variations in genes such as CYP2C19 can affect the metabolism of antiplatelet agents, which are vital in preventing thrombotic events in individuals with a genetic predisposition to coronary artery disease. The integration of pharmacogenomic testing into clinical practice holds the potential to revolutionize treatment strategies for genetic cardiovascular disorders, as it enables precision medicine tailored to the unique genetic makeup of each patient, thereby improving therapeutic efficacy and safety in managing these complex conditions (Figure 4.22).

4.6.3. Role of Genetic Counseling in Management

The application of genetic counseling to cardiovascular management is especially important, particularly in cases involving diseases such as Marfan syndrome and hypertrophic cardiomyopathy. Genetic counselors act as essential buffers between patients and physicians, facilitating understanding of the issues with genetic testing and family health implications. In disorders like Marfan syndrome, in which symptoms may be highly variable and involve several systems, genetic counseling is critical for proper diagnosis and multi-faceted management plan. By incorporating genetic testing into the patient's care sequence, genetic counselors help families learn about the genetic basis of these disorders, thus facilitating active family planning and screening procedures that can reduce future health hazards. This integrated strategy not only improves clinical results but also enables patients to have the kind of information needed for informed decision-making about their health and that of their family members. Additionally, genetic counseling is important in dealing with the psychological consequences of the results of genetic testing. Patients and families can feel anxious or in doubt when they first hear of their genetic risk, especially in diseases such as hypertrophic cardiomyopathy (HCM), which has severe implications for family members. Genetic counselors are a vital source of support and guidance, explaining the possibility of pathogenic variants and the meaning of such discoveries not just for the patient but also for relatives who might be at risk. They lead families through predictive genetic testing choices, stressing informed consent and comprehension of how these test outcomes might influence family life and medical care. Genetic counseling, therefore, forms a crucial component of ensuring patients are able to manage the emotional and practical consequences of genetic data, helping create an environment of support that promotes active involvement in health care. In addition, integration of genetic counseling as part of cardiovascular genetic disease management comes in the context of the larger objective of personalized medicine. Personalized treatment strategies considering genetic backgrounds will dramatically enhance care for patients. For example, in hypertrophic cardiomyopathy, the identification of known sarcomere mutations by genetic testing permits accurate risk stratification in family members since individuals who are positive for pathogenic variants can be subjected to targeted monitoring and interventions, thereby lowering severe cardiac event risk. Here, genetic counselors' expertise in the interpretation of genetic information makes families aware of inherited risk and the need for repeated assessments. Finally, genetic counseling not only improves clinical management and early intervention measures but also creates a culture of education-driven health choices that appeal to generations, an important element in addressing cardiovascular genetic disorders like those discussed by (Ahluwalia et al., 2020; Akram et al., 2021).

SUMMARY

The interlinking between cardiovascular embryology and genetic disease emphasizes the significance of comprehending developmental processes in both areas. The evidence shows that epigenetic regulation during embryonic development is crucial in the control of gene expression, which can have a profound impact on cardiovascular outcome. As found, disturbances in these processes, more so within assisted reproduction technologies, can increase CHD and other cardiovascular anomaly risks. Thus, a strict scrutiny of epigenetic considerations is crucial to healthcare practitioners engaged in reproductive care so that they can provide insights into possible long-term health issues related to these interventions (Huntriss et al., 2018). Furthermore, the intricate relationship between environmental factors and genetic influences must be appreciated when dealing with the frequency of cardiovascular disease occurring due to embryonic development. For example, disorders like polycystic ovary syndrome illustrate the ways in which endocrine disturbances can influence reproductive outcomes and, in turn, cardiovascular health. The increased prevalence of metabolic disorders like diabetes in these populations serves to illustrate the importance of monitoring and maintaining both reproductive and cardiovascular health in tandem, such that comprehensive patient care is emphasized. Lifestyle changes implemented early, along with screening for comorbidities at an early stage, may reduce risks related to these intertwined disorders (Susan et al., 2013). Lastly, ongoing research is necessary to clarify mechanisms involved in cardiovascular embryology and its resultant genetic disorders. Revealing the epigenetic landscape will not only enhance the predictive ability towards cardiovascular outcomes but also inform the creation of new therapies. Through multidisciplinary interdisciplinarity across developmental biology, genetics, and reproductive medicine, clinicians and researchers can develop integrative models that improve the welfare of patients and advance public health agendas. This collaborative effort will facilitate early identification of populations at risk, enhance preventive measures, and optimize treatment protocols, eventually decreasing the incidence of cardiovascular disease attributed to genetic and developmental causes (Huntriss et al., 2018). The complex domain of cardiovascular embryology forms the basis for comprehending a number of genetic diseases that affect heart development and function. The central focus of this field includes the elaborate interactions among genes and the environment during embryogenesis. Abnormalities resulting from aberrations within the normal mechanisms of heart development may result in CHDs, which are one of the most common of birth defects. By studying critical periods of cardiac development, scientists are able to determine particular genes responsible for cardiogenesis, as well as mechanisms by which these genes communicate with extrinsic factors. This is important in the establishment of therapeutic approaches that can preclude or minimize the impact of such congenital defects. Additionally, an understanding of the genetic basis of these defects enables clinicians to provide more accurate genetic counseling and risk determination for affected families. There has also been recent research emphasizing the role of prenatal environmental exposures that can perpetuate genetic susceptibilities. Studies show that maternal health and lifestyle factors, including diet, stress, and teratogen exposure, are critical in determining embryonic cardiovascular development. For example, insufficient maternal nutrition contributes to defective cardiac morphogenesis, which can possibly interact with inherent genetic predispositions, hence posing a higher risk of CHDs. In addition, examination of epigenetic changes provides evidence of how environmental influences can shape gene expression, complicating further the interplay between genetics and heart health. Further in-depth studies are needed to clarify these complex relationships, which could guide prevention and intervention strategies for safeguarding both maternal and fetal heart development. With the widening scope of cardiovascular embryology, so also does the demand for an interdisciplinary strategy of solving the intricacies associated with related genetic disorders. The management of these conditions is often best left to coordinated effort among geneticists, cardiologists, and obstetricians, ensuring an integrated treatment regimen for affected patients. The outstanding advances in genetic screening have offered the promise of early detection and intervention. Nonetheless, more studies are crucial in creating standard protocols for risk stratification and individualized treatment modalities. Additionally, continuous education among healthcare practitioners regarding the complexities of cardiovascular embryology and associated genetic defects will raise the level of patient care and encourage open discussion of family planning. This intersection of genetics, environmental factors, and clinical practice highlights the need for a multimodal framework to understanding and manage congenital cardiovascular anomalies convincingly.

CLOSER LOOK

HYPERTROPHIC CARDIOMYOPATHY (HCM)

Hypertrophic cardiomyopathy (HCM) is a genetic heart disorder characterized by the abnormal thickening (hypertrophy) of the heart muscle, particularly the interventricular septum — the wall separating the left and right ventricles. This thickening occurs in the absence of another underlying cause, such as high blood pressure or aortic stenosis, and it often interferes with the heart's ability to pump blood effectively.

HCM is the most common genetic cardiovascular disease, affecting approximately 1 in 500 people worldwide. It is typically inherited in an autosomal dominant manner, meaning a child has a 50% chance of inheriting the condition if one parent is affected. The condition is primarily caused by mutations in genes that encode for sarcomeric proteins — the components responsible for muscle contraction in the heart. The most commonly affected genes include *MYH7* and *MYBPC3*.

The hallmark feature of HCM is left ventricular hypertrophy (LVH), which often occurs asymmetrically. In many patients, this results in left ventricular outflow tract obstruction (LVOTO), where the thickened septum blocks the flow of blood from the heart into the aorta. This can lead to a spectrum of symptoms such as chest pain, shortness of breath (dyspnea), fatigue, dizziness, and fainting (syncope). Some individuals remain asymptomatic for years, while others may experience sudden cardiac death (SCD), especially in younger populations and athletes.

Diagnosis of HCM is typically made using echocardiography, which shows the thickened heart muscle and assesses blood flow. Other imaging techniques like cardiac MRI provide more detailed structural information. Electrocardiograms (ECG) and Holter monitors are used to detect arrhythmias or abnormal heart rhythms associated with the condition.

Treatment of HCM depends on the severity of symptoms and the presence of complications. Beta-blockers and calcium channel blockers are commonly prescribed to reduce heart rate and improve symptoms by allowing better filling of the ventricles. In patients with significant LVOTO, septal reduction therapy — such as surgical myectomy or alcohol septal ablation — may be performed to relieve obstruction. Implantable cardioverter-defibrillators (ICDs) are recommended in patients at high risk of sudden cardiac death.

Lifestyle adjustments are also critical. Patients are often advised to avoid intense competitive sports or activities that may trigger arrhythmias or SCD. Genetic counselling and screening of family members are essential, as early identification can significantly impact management and prognosis.

Although HCM can be a life-limiting condition, with proper medical care and monitoring, many individuals live full, active lives. Advances in genetic research and imaging have greatly improved the diagnosis and management of HCM in recent years.

Hypertrophic cardiomyopathy is a prevalent and potentially serious cardiac condition rooted in genetic mutations affecting heart muscle proteins. Early detection, risk stratification, and individualized therapy are essential to improving outcomes and preventing complications, including sudden cardiac death.

REFERENCES

1. Abbott, A., Abulí, A., Amiri-Yekta, A., Bachelot, A., Bustamante-Aragones, A., Coates, A., Diez-Juan, A., et al. (2017). *Recent Developments in Genetics and Medically Assisted Reproduction: From Research to Clinical Applications.* https://core.ac.uk/download/157586216.pdf (accessed on 27 May 2025).
2. Ahluwalia, M., & Ho, C. Y. (2020). Cardiovascular genetics: The role of genetic testing in diagnosis and management of patients with hypertrophic cardiomyopathy. *Heart, 107*, 183–189. https://www.semanticscholar.org/paper/a3d9074a36f699404d1a5f62eb1f30e0114e0310 (accessed on 27 May 2025).
3. Akram, H., Aragon-Martin, J., & Chandra, A. (2021). Marfan syndrome and the eye clinic: From diagnosis to management. *Therapeutic Advances in Rare Disease, 2.* https://www.semanticscholar.org/paper/9906fade9af8e8d63fa87729d330a0b4f652d41e (accessed on 27 May 2025).
4. Alekseev, V., Sharafetdinov, K., & Plotnikova, O. A. (2022). Basic principles of dietary therapy in type 2 diabetes mellitus: Focus on antioxidant protection and endothelial dysfunction. *Voprosy Pitaniia, 91*(4), 6–18. https://www.semanticscholar.org/paper/71499151c0fd442fec4a3d32df7cfba426309a4f (accessed on 27 May 2025).
5. Ambroselli, D., Masciulli, F., Romano, E., Catanzaro, G., Besharat, Z. M., Massari, M. C., Ferretti, E., et al. (2023). New advances in metabolic syndrome, from prevention to treatment: The role of diet and food. *Nutrients, 15.* https://www.semanticscholar.org/paper/37bcd585b4f154648cd815b164c783d57873a057 (accessed on 27 May 2025).
6. Aragon-Martin, J. A., Child, A. H., & Sage, K. (2016). *Genetic Testing in Marfan Syndrome.* https://core.ac.uk/download/287649641.pdf (accessed on 27 May 2025).
7. Baban, A., Calcagni, G., Dallapiccola, B., & De Luca, et al. (2019). *Atrioventricular Canal Defect and Genetic Syndromes: The Unifying Role of Sonic Hedgehog.* https://core.ac.uk/download/188826922.pdf (accessed on 27 May 2025).
8. Barakat, A. J., & Butler, M. (2024). Genetics of anomalies of the kidney and urinary tract with congenital heart disease: A review. *Clinical Genetics.* https://www.semanticscholar.org/paper/3078efe86ce65dcadc0ad8bbf641085b7f7d6397 (accessed on 27 May 2025).
9. Coolen, B. F., Jensen, B., & Petersen, S. E. (2022). *Myocardial Perfusion in Excessively Trabeculated Hearts: Insights from Imaging and Histological Studies.* https://core.ac.uk/download/548783504.pdf (accessed on 27 May 2025).
10. Cowan, S., Lim, S., Alycia, C., Pirotta, S., Thomson, R. L., Gibson-Helm, M., Blackmore, R., et al. (2023). Lifestyle management in polycystic ovary syndrome–Beyond diet and physical activity. *BMC Endocrine Disorders, 23.* https://doi.org/10.1186/s12902-022-01208-y.
11. Das, D., Khor, E. S., Jiang, F., He, J., Kawakami, Y., Wainwright, L., Hollinger, J., et al. (2024). Loss-of-function of RNA-binding protein PRRC2B causes translational defects and congenital cardiovascular malformation. *medRxiv.* https://www.semanticscholar.org/paper/984ef10541bdef624a7e1e96a6685d9367b7cef2 (accessed on 27 May 2025).
12. Debrach, A. C., Ladouceur, M., Trombetti, A., Bouchardy, J., Blondon, M., Robert-Ebadi, H., Ciotu, I. M., et al. (2025). [Marfan syndrome and related disorders]. *Revue Médicale Suisse, 21*(914), 804–808. https://www.semanticscholar.org/paper/7c62dc833874798469bbd4a73897a5a4bd418532 (accessed on 27 May 2025).

13. Dittmann, S., Kerkering, J., & Schulze-Bahr, E. (2025). Cardiac arrhythmias and genetics–Current stage. *Medizinische Genetik*. https://www.semanticscholar.org/paper/72337a2d3ce9416116c19202cd37f9f8fa1f5c76 (accessed on 27 May 2025).
14. Dumesic, D. A., Oberfield, S. E., Stener-Victorin, E., Marshall, J. C., Laven, J. S. E., & Legro, R. S. (2015). Scientific statement on the diagnostic criteria, epidemiology, pathophysiology, and molecular genetics of polycystic ovary syndrome. *Endocrine Reviews, 36*, 487–525. https://doi.org/10.1210/er.2015-1018.
15. Faber, J. E. (2025). Collateral blood vessels in stroke and ischemic disease: Formation, physiology, rarefaction, remodeling. *Journal of Cerebral Blood Flow and Metabolism*. https://www.semanticscholar.org/paper/cbd7a6035eb33a3de891f6bbbc87d17699645c07 (accessed on 27 May 2025).
16. Friedman, C. E. (2020). *Genetic Regulation of Cardiac Differentiation at Single-Cell Resolution.* https://www.semanticscholar.org/paper/68956b14020f4688f83629d4cc86598f789e948a (accessed on 27 May 2025).
17. Giardoglou, P., Deloukas, P., Dedoussis, G., & Beis, D. (2022). Cfdp1 is essential for cardiac development and function. *Cells, 12*. https://www.semanticscholar.org/paper/97c2334c3c3c4a18ad993d890f2b0cdd39bfad4b (accessed on 27 May 2025).
18. Haxel, C. S., Johnson, J. N., Hintz, S., Renno, M., Ruano, R., Zyblewski, S., Glickstein, J., et al. (2022). Care of the fetus with congenital cardiovascular disease: From diagnosis to delivery. *Pediatrics, 150*(Suppl 2). https://www.semanticscholar.org/paper/731950c733a3d3a27f9e4fa935dcc4196bd05739 (accessed on 27 May 2025).
19. Helm, B. M., & Ware, S. M. (2024). Clinical decision analysis of genetic evaluation and testing in 1013 intensive care unit infants with congenital heart defects supports universal genetic testing. *Genes, 15*. https://www.semanticscholar.org/paper/ac887c2cc5096571a6e7ee2d34ff4eb55d84f20b (accessed on 27 May 2025).
20. Hesaraki, M., Bora, U., Pahlavan, S., Salehi, N., Mousavi, S., Barekat, M., Rasouli, S. J., et al. (2022). A novel missense variant in actin binding domain of MYH7 is associated with left ventricular noncompaction. *Frontiers in Cardiovascular Medicine, 9*. https://www.semanticscholar.org/paper/f7f5c756639c2cccfd4b0c14f9fe2b74e59f22d7 (accessed on 27 May 2025).
21. Horne, A. W., & Missmer, S. A. (2022). Pathophysiology, diagnosis, and management of endometriosis. *BMJ*. https://doi.org/10.1136/bmj-2022-070750.
22. Hosseini, S. Y., Mallick, R., Mäkinen, P., & Ylä-Herttuala, S. (2024). Navigating the prime editing strategy to treat cardiovascular genetic disorders in transforming heart health. *Expert Review of Cardiovascular Therapy, 22*, 75–89. https://www.semanticscholar.org/paper/fac06a92652de9a20c79656491dd0a3c23c3b37e (accessed on 27 May 2025).
23. Huntriss, J., Balen, A. H., Sinclair, K. D., Brison, D. R., & Picton, H. M. (2018). Epigenetics and reproductive medicine. *BJOG: An International Journal of Obstetrics & Gynecology, 125*. https://doi.org/10.1111/1471-0528.15240.
24. Jiang, J., Singh, K., Nitin, R., Davis, L. K., Wray, N. R., & Shah, S. (2024). Sex-specific association between genetic risk of psychiatric disorders and cardiovascular diseases. *Circulation: Genomic and Precision Medicine, 17*, e004685. https://www.semanticscholar.org/paper/c9e9aa59b45b7c1b820e209b4017eb23dad26463 (accessed on 27 May 2025).

25. Jin, L., Hwang, B., Rezapourdamanab, S., Sridhar, V., Nandwani, R. K., Amoli, M. S., & Serpooshan, V. (2025). Bioengineering approaches to *in vitro* modeling of genetic and acquired cardiac diseases. *Current Cardiology Reports, 27*. https://www.semanticscholar.org/paper/8b2f27efc9090e9f8d3f5b7f30ea009e446ed01e (accessed on 27 May 2025).

26. Kiełbowski, K., Skórka, P., Plewa, P., Bakinowska, E., & Pawlik, A. (2024). The role of alarmins in the pathogenesis of atherosclerosis and myocardial infarction. *Current Issues in Molecular Biology, 46*, 8995–9015. https://www.semanticscholar.org/paper/040c1d6d57e6b0f459fc1306381925f85d4f1fa1 (accessed on 27 May 2025).

27. Linask, K. K. (2013). The heart-placenta axis in the first month of pregnancy: Induction and prevention of cardiovascular birth defects. https://core.ac.uk/download/208032653.pdf (accessed on 27 May 2025).

28. Maas, A. H. E. M., Rosano, G., Cífková, R., Chieffo, A., van Dijken, D., Hamoda, H., Kunadian, V., et al. (2020). Cardiovascular health after menopause transition, pregnancy disorders, and other gynaecologic conditions: A consensus document from European cardiologists, gynaecologists, and endocrinologists. *European Heart Journal, 42*, 967–984. https://doi.org/10.1093/eurheartj/ehaa1044.

29. Mehta, H., Narang, T., Dogra, S., Handa, S., Hatwal, J., & Batta, A. (2024). Cardiovascular considerations and implications for treatment in psoriasis: An updated review. *Vascular Health and Risk Management, 20*, 215–229. https://www.semanticscholar.org/paper/dcbbad92ad0fdfbb6890a25fb65a29e03adc2cfe (accessed on 27 May 2025).

30. Miotto, M. C., Reiken, S., Wronska, A., Yuan, Q., Dridi, H., Liu, Y., Weninger, G., et al. (2024). Structural basis for ryanodine receptor type 2 leak in heart failure and arrhythmogenic disorders. *Nature Communications, 15*. https://www.semanticscholar.org/paper/09630c570139e424dc2cc58dde1c8a709b5d54dd (accessed on 27 May 2025).

31. Monaghan, R. M., Naylor, R. W., Flatman, D., Kasher, P., Williams, S. G., & Keavney, B. D. (2024). FLT4 causes developmental disorders of the cardiovascular and lymph vascular systems via pleiotropic molecular mechanisms. *Cardiovascular Research*, *120*, 1164–1176. https://www.semanticscholar.org/paper/8d1c0c1fbc14517da5ff2530cb9e4dabf612233d (accessed on 27 May 2025).

32. Paolini, M., Maccario, M., Saredi, V., Verri, A., Calesella, F., Raffaelli, L., Lorenzi, C., et al. (2025). Cardiovascular risk predicts white matter hyperintensities, brain atrophy and treatment resistance in major depressive disorder: Role of genetic liability. *Acta Psychiatric Scandinavica*. https://www.semanticscholar.org/paper/a7f97962e08c25fdf8ceb94ea831759b0445132c (accessed on 27 May 2025).

33. Popov, V. I., Bolotskih, V. I., Makeeva, A. V., Gubin, A. I., & Anufrieva, E. I. (2024). Assessment of the risk of developing cardiovascular pathology in medical university students. *Health Risk Analysis*. https://www.semanticscholar.org/paper/8baefc6c1244d9eb8c57850d316062c67fea57d4 (accessed on 27 May 2025).

34. Rossignol, F., Lamari, F., & Mitchell, G. A. (2025). Phosphoinositide metabolism: Biochemistry, physiology and genetic disorders. *Journal of Inherited Metabolic Disease, 48*. https://www.semanticscholar.org/paper/d82d5681f815e5cbd9fb735b17bcc05ef61b247e (accessed on 27 May 2025).

35. Rzhepakovsky, I., Piskov, S., Avanesyan, S., Shakhbanov, M., Sizonenko, M., Timchenko, L., Nagdalian, A., et al. (2024). Expanding understanding of chick embryo's nervous system development at HH22–HH41 embryonic stages using X-ray microcomputed tomography. *PLOS ONE, 19.* https://www.semanticscholar.org/paper/ed21d1eca9da40528ad6f7de01d00ddf54ab631e (accessed on 27 May 2025).

36. Santos, E. D. S., Research Group in Cardiogenetics of Sergipe, Kuhn, G. D. C., de Almeida, A. G. C., Pimentel, J. V. A., Figueiredo Neto, N. V., Melo, B. C., et al. (2025). Genetic, clinical, and sociodemographic profile in individuals with diagnosis or family history of hypertrophic cardiomyopathy: Insights from a prospective cohort. https://www.semanticscholar.org/paper/970dfb3218e85fdae2866669c68eb28951c989aa (accessed on 27 May 2025).

37. Savirón-Cornudella, R., & Herraiz, I. (2022). Hormones and fetal growth factors. *Gynecological Endocrinology, 38*, 191–192. https://www.semanticscholar.org/paper/6957cb22811823ffac5ef5484f189399c1998351 (accessed on 27 May 2025).

38. Schuermans, A., Truong, B., Ardissino, M., Bhukar, R., Slob, E., Nakao, T., Dron, J. S., et al. (2024). Genetic associations of circulating cardiovascular proteins with gestational hypertension and preeclampsia. *JAMA Cardiology, 9*, 209–220. https://www.semanticscholar.org/paper/d209d380b3e56ace7c13943e102bdb3fb9e8b61c (accessed on 27 May 2025).

39. Shulga, A. (2022). Patterns of development of cardiovascular disorders in patients with COVID-19 (brief review). *Bulletin Physiology and Pathology of Respiration.* https://www.semanticscholar.org/paper/deeb2767f3d94109d892ea646df4a9f1417e9c9e (accessed on 27 May 2025).

40. Sirmans, S. M., & Pate, K. (2013). Epidemiology, diagnosis, and management of polycystic ovary syndrome. *Clinical Epidemiology*. https://doi.org/10.2147/clep.s37559.

41. Sun, J., Chen, Y., Zhao, X., Niu, Z., Gu, Z., Yan, Z., & Wang, W. (2024). Effect and interaction of PINK1 genetic polymorphisms and environmental factors on blood pressure in COEs-exposed workers. *International Journal of Environmental Health Research*. https://www.semanticscholar.org/paper/c9eeb8480d0b6ae867858c979d9c4689b48cc393 (accessed on 27 May 2025).

42. The University of Texas Rio Grande Valley. (2018). *UTRGV School of Medicine Course Catalog 2018–2019*. https://core.ac.uk/download/539651331.pdf (accessed on 27 May 2025).

43. Tyrmi, J., Kaartokallio, T., Lokki, A., Jääskeläinen, T., Kortelainen, E., Ruotsalainen, S., Karjalainen, J., et al. (2023). Genetic risk factors associated with preeclampsia and hypertensive disorders of pregnancy. *JAMA Cardiology, 8*, 674–683. https://www.semanticscholar.org/paper/cddc010ac6ebf0ca3cbfbb469e5b97f5e335cd4e (accessed on 27 May 2025).

44. Vaishnav, V. A. D., & Patel, R. (2025). Genetic factors contributing to hereditary cardiovascular disorders. *Journal of Neonatal Surgery*. https://www.semanticscholar.org/paper/0c6cee211dafebf9155dde31a651f474cad5ad95 (accessed on 27 May 2025).

45. Viswanathan, S., Oza, P. S., Bellad, A., & Uttarilli, A. (2024). Conotruncal heart defects: A narrative review of molecular genetics, genomics research and innovation. *OMICS: A Journal of Integrative Biology, 28*(7), 324–346. https://www.semanticscholar.org/paper/9109fb11f3b047bd9a5bb7d0ef44749d1e8c28a9 (accessed on 27 May 2025).

46. Wazir, M., Olanrewaju, O. A., Yahya, M., Kumari, J., Kumar, N., Singh, J., Abbas Al-itbi, A. Y. A., et al. (2023). Lipid disorders and cardiovascular risk: A comprehensive analysis of current perspectives. *Cureus, 15*. https://www.semanticscholar.org/paper/d59093b6512c59c404002a702420d2824f2ac7a7 (accessed on 27 May 2025).

47. Wolf, W. M., Wattick, R. A., Kinkade, O. N., & Olfert, M. D. (2018). Geographical prevalence of polycystic ovary syndrome as determined by region and race/ethnicity. *International Journal of Environmental Research and Public Health, 15*, 2589. https://doi.org/10.3390/ijerph15112589.

48. Wulff, A., Mortensen, M., & Nordestgaard, B. (2023). Low-density lipoprotein cholesterol cannot be too low after a myocardial infarction. *Journal of Internal Medicine, 294*. https://www.semanticscholar.org/paper/733e246d0014cf53113f81bc428fe41ef68afc7c (accessed on 27 May 2025).

49. Yang, Z., Macdonald-Dunlop, E., Chen, J., Zhai, R., Li, T., Richmond, A., Klarić, L., et al. (2022). Genetic landscape of the ACE2 coronavirus receptor. *Circulation, 145*, 1398–1411. https://www.semanticscholar.org/paper/5ef0eec4fd490b3471e3f7762e1856c685d6c9e4 (accessed on 27 May 2025).

50. Yap, C., Henders, A., Alvares, G., Giles, C., Huynh, K., Nguyen, A., Wallace, L., et al. (2023). Interactions between the lipidome and genetic and environmental factors in autism. *Nature Medicine, 29*, 936–949. https://www.semanticscholar.org/paper/3d2fae88030d1009ccca22328170d344819e4ad0 (accessed on 27 May 2025).

51. Yehuda, R., & Lehrner, A. (2018). Intergenerational transmission of trauma effects: Putative role of epigenetic mechanisms. *World Psychiatry, 17*, 243–257. https://doi.org/10.1002/wps.20568.

52. Zenker, M., & Wolf, C. (2025). Cardiovascular aspects of Noonan syndrome and related disorders. *Medizinische Genetik, 37*, 113–124. https://www.semanticscholar.org/paper/9b2769480b12a465c7824d349ad00ce4e4e919b3 (accessed on 27 May 2025).

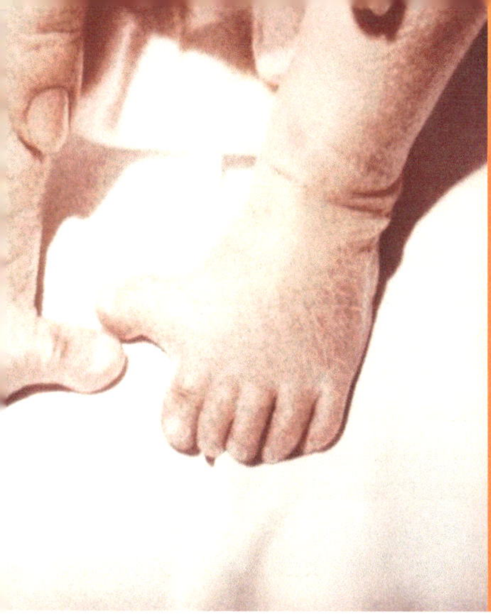

Chapter 5

LIMB AND SKELETAL DEVELOPMENT

Contents

Introduction

The complex processes regulating limb and skeletal development form the basis for comprehending human physiology and anatomy. Limb development is a highly complex interaction between genetic and environmental factors that coordinate the differentiation of progenitor cells into functional osteoprogenitor lineages. New developments in multi-omic profiling have enabled a greater understanding of the regulatory networks underlying embryonic bone and joint development. For example, studies that use transcriptional and epigenetic profiling of embryonic tissues have revealed several cell states and their epigenetic landscapes and described the differentiated pathways that are involved in the formation of skeletal structure. This is particularly clear in the analysis of limb and cranial osteoprogenitor trajectories that elucidates the pivotal role of intrinsic and extrinsic signals in cell fate decision in forming the developing skeleton (To et al., 2024). Equally important in the development of limbs is maternal health, more specifically maternal obesity, which can negatively influence myogenic cell migration that is required to produce skeletal muscles. Myogenic progenitor cell migration to limb areas is essential for muscle development and is regulated by several pathways that influence it. Current studies have shown that maternal obesity leads to the down-regulation of crucial genes involved in the process of myogenic migration, thereby impairing the formation of normal skeletal muscle in the embryo. Pathways such as hepatocyte growth factor signaling and fibroblast growth factor (FGF) signaling have been associated with the process of migration, with the findings of research showing that their inhibition results in impaired ability of myogenic cells for migration in limb development (Gao et al., 2024). These interactions not just shed light on the nature of limb development but also bring a question regarding physical fitness in children and the role of mothers' health. Overall, it is the interaction between genetic, epigenetic, and environmental factors that controls the complex process of limb and skeleton formation in the human. Novel multi-omic paradigms offer researchers a solid basis to explore regulatory mechanisms intrinsic to bone formation and skeletal maturity. This goes hand-in-hand with an understanding of how maternal influences, e.g., obesity, impact these pathways to development and illuminates the importance of a comprehensive grasp of intrinsic and extrinsic factors on fetal development. These findings offer avenues for future investigation to treat developmental musculoskeletal disorders and their etiologies in embryonic and maternal environments and, ultimately, to expand our understanding of human health and disease (Figure 5.1).

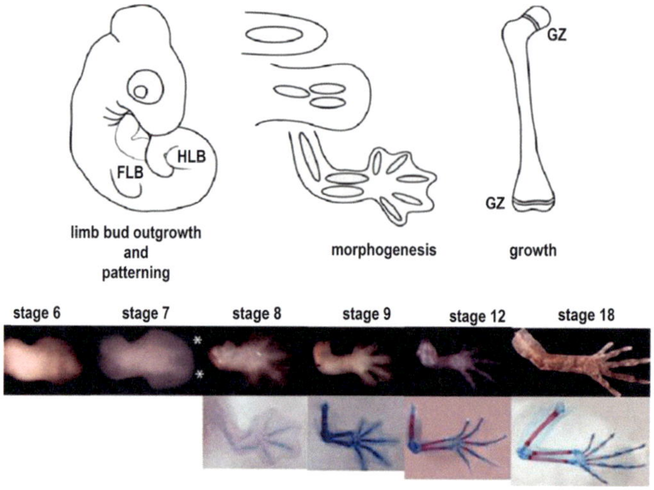

Figure 5.1. Limb development.

Source: https://www.researchgate.net/profile/Jonathan-Losos/publication/51578615/figure/fig1/AS:393904479326221@1470925554871/a-Summary-of-limb-and-long-bone-development-Limb-development-proceeds-through-several.png.

Definition of Limb and Skeletal Development

Limb and skeletal development involve a very complex interplay of anatomical and physiological changes during the embryogenesis phase and subsequently. It begins with the formation of the limb bud, which consists of ectodermal and mesodermal tissues that give origin to muscles, bones, tendons, and skin. After additional growth, the proximal-distal axis is established, which acts as a basis for further anatomical differentiation. This specificity is regulated by genetic and environmental factors, e.g., signal pathways that guide tissue interaction. These are significant because abnormal limb and skeletal development can lead to congenital malformations or functional deficiencies that can have a profound impact on a human's mobility and overall health. The intricacy of arm and bone development does not respite in the independent growth of bones and muscles, but in an intricate network of body modules whose coordination is critical for operational proficiency. Recent studies using Anatomical Network Analysis (AnNA) have lent better insight into how these anatomical components develop into integrated shapes without compromise in functionality. For instance, research has contrasted patterns of development of forelimbs and hindlimbs in humans and chimpanzees and found that even though the two limbs have different functions, they possess some degree of modularity and sophistication that defies earlier assumptions regarding their evolutionary trajectory. This analytical strategy highlights the importance of considering both hard and soft tissues in evaluating anatomical integration and modularity during development, providing an overall picture of limb and skeletal evolution (Esteve-Altava et al., 2018). Of importance for understanding limb and skeletal development is the contribution of evolutionary adaptations that form anatomical structures between species. By using sophisticated quantitative methods like AnNA, scientists are able to reasonably determine variations in limb design between species and gain insights into their evolutionary histories as well as functional diversity. Importantly, studying pathology also brings to light anatomical integration because such conditions tend to interfere with normal developmental processes, giving rise to limb configuration variations. The discoveries of these studies have significant implications, not just for developmental biology and orthopedics but also for paleontology, because they spark controversies on vertebrate evolutionary relationships. Therefore, the complex interaction between anatomy, development, and evolution is the key to understanding limb and skeletal development (Goswami et al., 2015).

Importance of Studying Limb and Skeletal Development

The underlying theme of limb and skeletal development lies in understanding normal physiology, as well as most pathological conditions. All these processes are highly intricate and have complex interactions among genes, cells, and the environment. Science has made important pathways such as those controlled by fibroblast growth factors (FGFs) and bone morphogenetic proteins (BMPs) that control limb and bone formation. Knowledge of these pathways offers insight into congenital disease, allowing scientists to uncover the genetic basis that contributes to abnormalities such as polydactyly or limb reduction disorders. In addition, this information lies at the core of implementing individualized therapeutic approaches that can cure or manage these conditions. With advancing fields, the incorporation of more sophisticated molecular methods will increasingly improve our understanding of the multiplex signals that coordinate limb development and enable more successful intervention in skeletal dysplasia and other related conditions. Beyond congenital disease, the conclusions of research on limb and skeletal development also have widespread consequences for regenerative medicine and tissue engineering. By describing the mechanisms of limb regeneration in certain animals, scientists are motivated to explore potential regenerative medicine applications in human beings. As an illustration, studies on model organisms such as zebrafish and salamanders have yielded information about cellular plasticity and limb regeneration following loss. This may be followed by new approaches in the management of traumatic injury as well as musculoskeletal degenerative diseases. Furthermore, advances in 3D bioprinting and biomaterial science rely on our understanding of the formation of the skeleton, enabling the creation of scaffolds that can be employed to regenerate and repair tissue, eventually translating into better patient care. Thus, the integration of limb development research into regenerative therapy strategies holds the promise of transforming medical practice. The connection between skeletal development and health in general cannot be overemphasized, as skeletal development affects other physiological systems and disease states throughout life. Diseases like osteoporosis and arthritis are associated with the basic mechanisms of bone formation and homeostasis. Understanding these processes allows scientists to recognize possible biomarkers for early diagnosis and disease risk assessment. In addition, new studies are investigating the microbiota-gut-brain axis in relation to skeletal health, highlighting the interconnection of body systems in achieving homeostasis. The make-up of the microbiome can influence bone density and healing by different pathways, such as immune response and metabolic cross-talk. As we gain more information regarding these interactions, the future for interdisciplinarity develops with a true understanding of how limb and skeletal formation influences health throughout life. Hence, in order to approach these systems fully, both for preventative and therapeutic applications in medicine, an integrated approach is necessary (Figure 5.2).

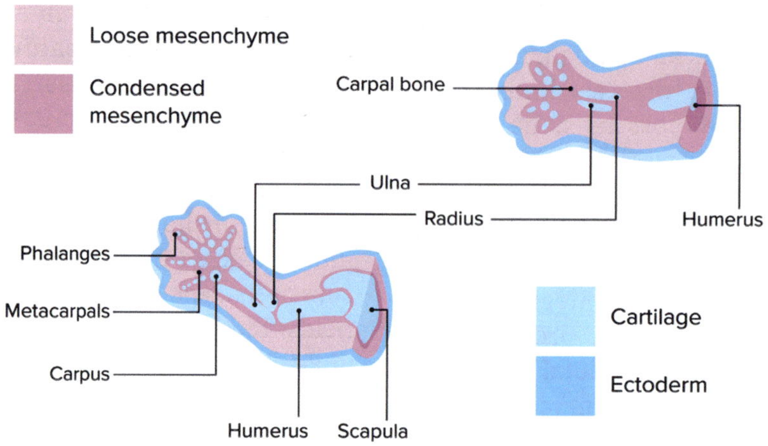

Figure 5.2. Limb and skeletal development.

Source: https://cdn.lecturio.com/assets/Cartilage-development.png.

5.1. Embryonic Development of Limbs

Embryonic limb development in the study of organism development shows a key understanding of how organisms pattern and shape their limbs early in their development. In amphibians, development can be vastly different from that occurring in direct-developing species compared to those species that go through metamorphosis. For example, the direct-developing salamander *Plethodon cinereus* has a fascinating limb patterning involving early digit formation, specifically digit II, which forms in continuity with the ulnar/fibular arch. This association replicates the amniote anatomical features, indicating an evolutionary adaptation of limb formation in direct-developing species. The fact that preaxial zeugopodial cartilage differentiation takes place without acceleration compared to postaxial cartilages further explains the distinctive development pattern of this salamander, implying a necessity for extensive studies in evolutionary biology to comprehend limb morphology variation among species (Blackburn et al., 2018). Knowledge of the molecular basis of limb development provides invaluable information on developmental biology. The expression patterns of the regulatory genes sox9 and col2a1 have critical roles in the skeletal patterning in embryonic limb development. Conservation of these gene expression patterns in direct-developing salamanders gives evidence of a common developmental program among different species. But then again, the normal models of digit identity in amphibians might not be universal. The fact that *P. cinereus* lacks vestigial digits highlights the need to reconsider current explanations of digit formation and identity within the confines of direct development. Through the comparison of gene expression patterns in this salamander with other amphibians, scientists can reveal important evolutionary trends and changes in limb development that distinguish the direct-developers from their more metamorphic relatives (Blackburn et al., 2018). In addition, the consequences of interfering with normal vascular mechanisms during embryonic development should not be underestimated. Vascular integrity is essential for maintaining the required blood supply to limbs undergoing development, and any disruption may result in serious limb abnormalities. Studies emphasize the complex interactions between limb formation and blood flow, wherein arterial dysgenesis is a frequent condition that may occur. Expert consultations show a treasure trove of information regarding vascular disruption and its effects on the development of bones. Knowing the correlation between vascular anomalies and malformations of the limbs helps generate preventive measures and therapeutic approaches for congenital limb malformations. Even though this field needs to be further investigated, most importantly in terms of models utilized, the interrelated development of vascular and skeletal tissues is a vital area of focus for continued research and developmental work (Figure 5.3).

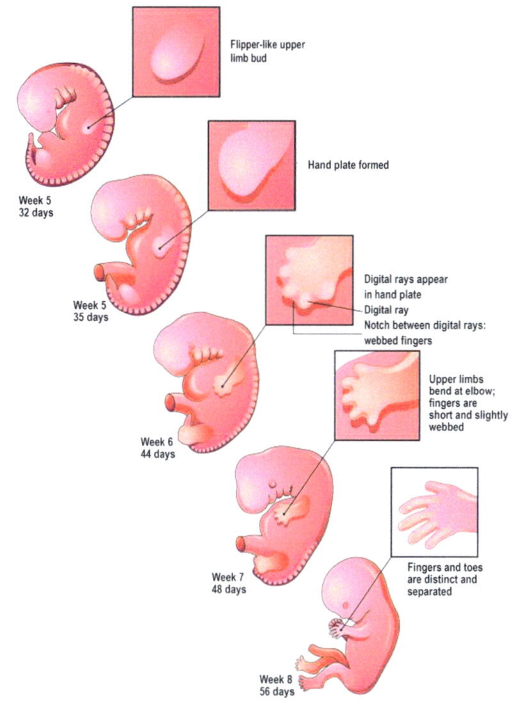

Figure 5.3. Development of limbs.

Source: https://i0.wp.com/obgynkey.com/wp-content/uploads/2020/03/f016-003-9780323611541.jpg?w=960.

5.1.1. Stages of Limb Formation in Embryonic Development

The mechanisms of limb development during embryogenesis are characterized by highly interactive processes of genetic and cellular mechanisms that govern limb formation. Limb buds originate from the somatic mesoderm, after interaction with many signaling molecules like FGFs and BMPs. These embryonic structures serve as a precursor to limbs and provide the scaffolding for future skeletal development. With continued development, the zone of polarizing activity (ZPA) and apical ectodermal ridge (AER) determine the anterior-posterior and proximal-distal axes, respectively. The spatial arrangement is essential in determining limb structure and function, illustrating the significance of embryonic signaling in directing the exact anatomy of limbs throughout development. Later stages include immense cellular differentiation and patterning, especially by apoptosis, which is essential for correct joint and digit development.

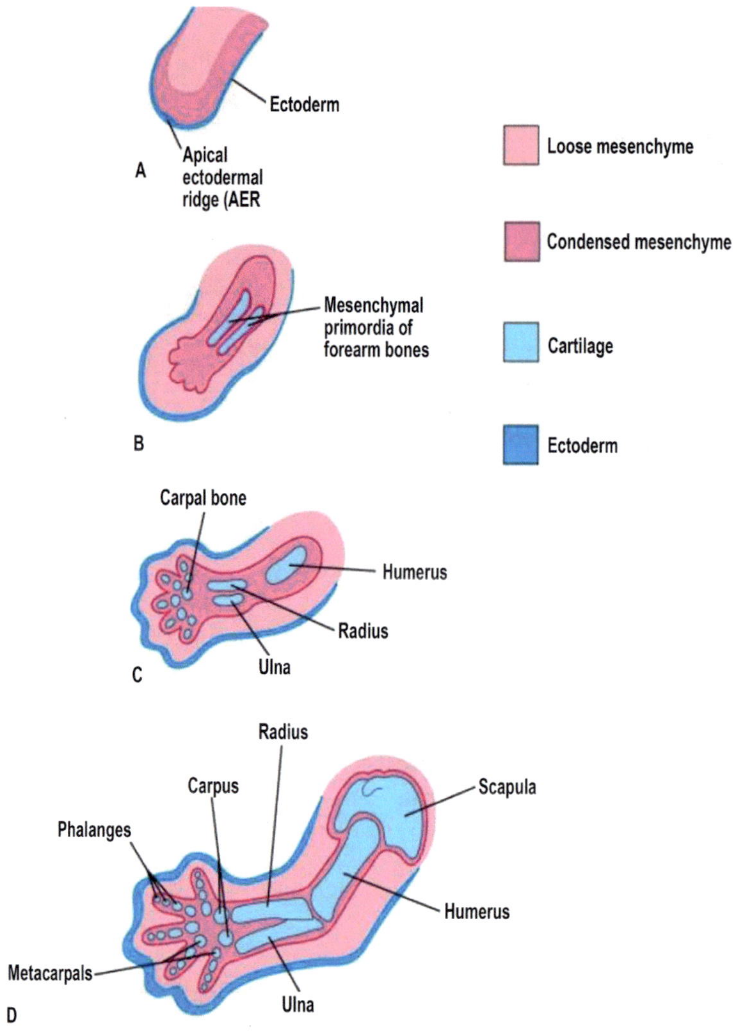

Figure 5.4. Stages of limb formation in embryonic development.

Source: https://i0.wp.com/obgynkey.com/wp-content/uploads/2020/03/f016-007-9780323611541.jpg?w=960.

As the limb matures, patterns of cell death help in the digit separation and the establishment of articulated joints. The embryonic remodeling process is best illustrated by the degradation of interdigital tissues to enable the development of discretely formed digits. A study documents the function of epigenetic regulators Uhrf1 and Uhrf2, which are expressed temporally and spatially in apoptotic tissues (Cristina Sánchez–Fernández et al., 2019). Their control of chromatin structure and differentiation factors plays a critical role in balancing cell proliferation and apoptosis in the transition phase, highlighting the complex management of cellular events leading to limb development. Genetic mutations also play a significant role in limb development, as evident in disorders like fibrodysplasia ossificans progressiva (FOP), where skeletal malformations arise due to aberrant differentiation. The ACVR1/ALK2 gene mutation for FOP demonstrates the manner in which alterations of signal transduction pathways can lead to profound developmental abnormalities, such as deformed digits and the development of heterotopic bone (Salin et al., 2012). During embryonic development, the effects of such mutations can be dramatic, highlighting the sensitivity of regulatory networks controlling limb morphogenesis. Recognition of these stages and related genetic influences not only illuminates normal limb formation but also gives insights into congenital limb deformities and targets of future therapeutic interventions (Figure 5.4).

5.1.2. Role of Mesoderm in Limb Development

The mesoderm is primarily responsible for limb development as it acts as a precursor to several structures of the limbs, such as bones, muscles, and connective tissues. With the progression of embryonic development, the mesoderm differentiates in a manner that is essential for the development of the limb buds. The limb buds are the early stages of limb formation and are mainly formed from the lateral plate mesoderm and paraxial mesoderm. The cell signal pathways that control this differentiation are intricate and consist of many interactions among cells within the mesoderm and with their local environment. Elucidating the regulatory processes in mesodermal tissue is crucial to understanding how alterations in these mechanisms might result in limb malformations, making this tissue of key importance in both normal development as well as possible pathological processes. Recent studies have shown that certain gene families in the mesoderm play key roles in proper limb development. For example, the TET family of DNA demethylases shows a critical function in mesodermal cells, specifically in mesenchymal stem cells (MSC) that give rise to bone. In research involving Tet gene deficiency, loss of TET function in mesodermal cells was found to cause profound skeletal defects, highlighting the significance of TET proteins in ensuring genomic flexibility during limb development. Additionally, TET proteins also interact with central transcription factors, including RUNX2, to enable bone development by chromatin remodeling and regulating genes. The interaction between mesoderm-originated stem cells and such regulatory proteins reinforces the mesoderms role in limb and skeletal development, demonstrating elaborate dependencies which, if interrupted, can result in severe congenital abnormalities (Wang et al., 2022). Apart from gene regulation, signaling pathways arising from the mesoderm play a crucial role in cartilaginous and bony limb elements. The IL-6/STAT3 signaling pathway is a prime example of how mesodermal interactions are responsible for limb skeletal integrity. Conditional loss of STAT3 in the limb mesenchyme has been found to give rise to a range of limb deformities, such as irregular growth plate development and fracture susceptibility. This result highlights the wider function of mesoderm in not just controlling the growth of limb tissues but also their repair process following injury. A discovery of how these signaling pathways operate at various stages of cartilage and bone development could reveal new therapeutic targets for the management of musculoskeletal diseases. Thus, the role of mesoderms in limb development goes beyond structural functions to include intricate signaling and regulatory processes that assure ideal limb function and durability (Rigueur et al., 2021) (Figure 5.5).

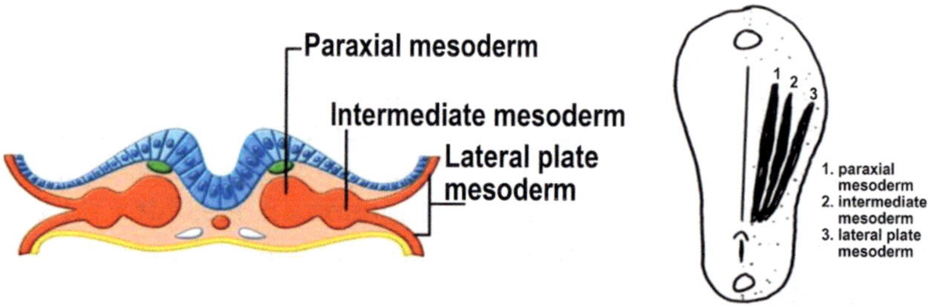

Figure 5.5. Role of mesoderm in limb development.

Source: https://wisc.pb.unizin.org/app/uploads/sites/58/2017/01/Figure-1.jpg.

5.1.3. Genetic Factors Influencing Limb Growth

The delicate involvement of limb development with genetics is highlighted by the function of multiple genes that control the development and differentiation of skeletal elements of the limbs. These genes have an important function during periods of significant development, and not only influence growth patterns but also the shape of the limbs. Mutations or polymorphisms in genes such as the FGF and Wingless Integration Site (Wnt) signaling pathway are known to impact limb shape and size. The mutations in the genes can lead to gross issues, one of which includes growth disorders. Environmental variables, although strong, are largely modulated by genetic predisposition in their turn, showing that inheritable characteristics play a basic role in limb and skeletal development. Further, genetic syndrome studies demonstrate how inherited illnesses contribute to changing limb growth. Conditions such as achondroplasia, or dwarfism, are good examples of how changing one area of the genome can lead to unequal limb growth, and the exceedingly connected relationship between genotype and phenotype. Research has indicated that changes in genes like FGFR3 can lead to defective chondrocyte, which affects bone growth longitudinally. Similarly, genetic factors may regulate limb's capacity to adapt and respond to mechanical forces, again indicating that genetics actively contributes to defining not only physical characteristics but also functional abilities. As researchers move into understanding these genetic processes, a clearer image emerges on the possibility of therapeutic interventions that will be able to reverse certain growth abnormalities. In addition to these direct effects on limb development, genetics also intersect with more general physiological processes that influence overall skeletal health. For instance, genetic predispositions toward chronic conditions like osteoporosis can influence bone density and, consequently, limb structure integrity as a person ages. It has been noted in studies on chronic venous disease that genetic considerations also encompass the vascular networks in limbs, which is critical in the maintenance of healthy blood flow needed for proper growth and healing. This is an inter-disciplinary note whereby the genetic background affects not just the structure of the limbs but also the functional usability of the limbs in the long term. As such, understanding these relationships is crucial in the development of effective strategies for enhancing limb and bone health across human development stages, especially considering the aging population that is progressively struggling with degenerative diseases linked to genetic factors (Feng et al., 2025; Gwozdzinski et al., 2024).

5.2. Skeletal System Overview

The skeletal system allows for a complex architecture that supports and allows the body to move in conjunction with performing essential physiological functions. The bone, cartilage, ligaments, and tendons that make up this system are unique in that they are not just a structure of solidity but also a dynamic organism that continues to develop, adapt, and renew itself. Skeletal system development begins in utero, as mesenchymal cells transform into chondrocytes and osteoblasts. This process determines the fundamental outline of the skeleton, such as the development of both the axial and appendicular portions. Each developmental stage is important since it establishes the overall morphology and helps to determine the functional potential of the limbs. Further, knowledge of skeletal developmental mechanisms serves to reveal some of the pathological conditions that can occur due to abnormal development or environmental factors affecting growth. Recent advances in single-cell transcriptomics have significantly improved our understanding of the cellular diversity of skeletal systems during development.

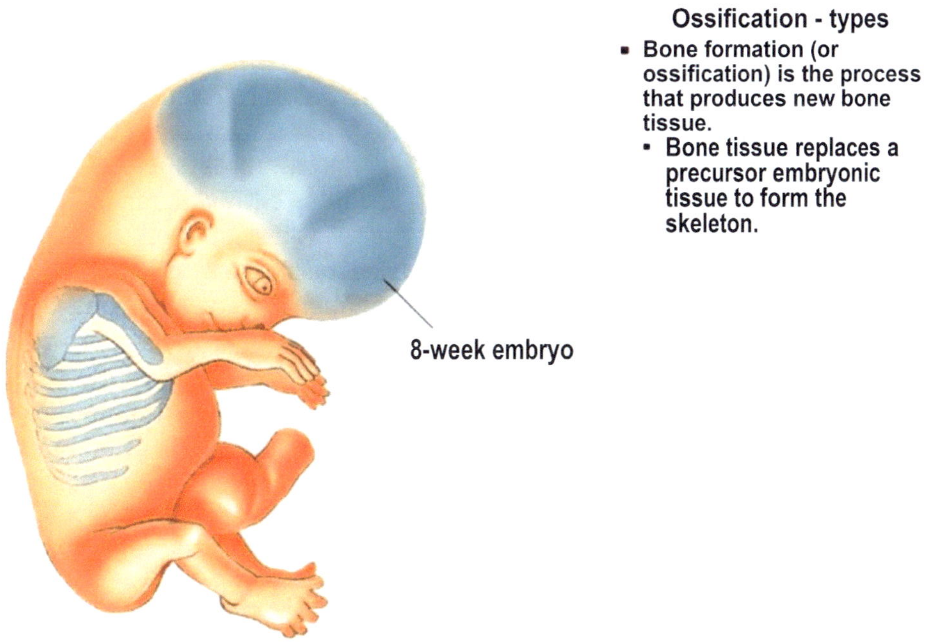

Figure 5.6. Skeletal system.

Source: https://i.ytimg.com/vi/p-3PuLXp9Wg/maxresdefault.jpg.

With scRNA-seq technologies, scientists have started building comprehensive atlases of limb skeletal cells, from their early precursors to mature bone. For example, one of the most detailed atlas created from 10 individual scRNA-seq datasets identified 133,332 cells across 39 cell states and thus shed light on the intricate lineage dynamics and interactions of the limb skeleton. This information not only accentuates how interlinked the skeletal system is with the hematopoietic niches and metabolic functions but also reveals the essential gaps in current organism-wide reference atlases. As future studies build upon these datasets, the findings that will emerge are expected to shed light on new avenues for developmental biology, regenerative medicine, and the treatment of skeletal disease, further justifying ongoing investigation in this area (Herpelinck et al., 2024). In addition, new therapeutic approaches are becoming available to treat conditions of skeletal muscle, illustrating the overlap between the research on skeletal development and clinical application. One of these approaches is the delivery of genetic material into skeletal muscles, which could provide cures for crippling disorders such as Duchenne muscular dystrophy (DMD). Current advances using lipid-based nanobubbles have the potential to increase the permeability of muscle tissue for intravascular delivery of nucleic acids. In experimental systems, these nanobubbles, in addition to ultrasound exposure, enabled effective delivery of plasmid DNA and antisense morpholino oligomers to destination limb muscles with a marked increase in dystrophin expression in DMD model mice. This strategy is not just an interesting application of limb and skeletal development research, but also an exciting path to creating targeted neuromuscular disease therapies, highlighting the immediate clinical relevance of knowing about limb and skeletal development (Sekine et al., 2023) (Figure 5.6).

5.2.1. Composition of the Skeletal System

The skeletal system is an intricate framework made up of different types of tissues which collectively supply the body with structure and allow for movement. The components of this system are bones, cartilage, and ligaments, which contribute to the system distinct properties for function as a whole. Bones, being rigid, are made up of a mineralized matrix with high calcium phosphate content that supplies strength as well as elasticity. Cartilage, however, is elastic tissue that supports joints and provides for smooth movement. Ligaments, fibrous connective tissues, hold bones to one another and stabilize the skeletal system. Knowledge of the makeup and interplay of these structures is vital in understanding how limb and skeletal development takes place, especially during growth periods and when subjected to physical stresses and traumas. Additionally, the organization of the skeletal system is also influenced by genetic and environmental factors and results in variation in skeletal function and health. A sensitive balance between bone formation by osteoblasts and bone resorption by osteoclasts is responsible for skeletal integrity. A shift in this balance can lead to bone diseases like osteoporosis, which is marked by loss of bone and greater susceptibility to fractures. Current research centers on the role of extracellular matrix (ECM) molecules in transmitting biological signals that are relative to bone development and regeneration. Tissue-derived materials, such as acellular extracellular matrix-based hydrogels, have demonstrated potential in enhancing skeletal health by promoting tissue regeneration, enhancing perfusion, and bringing in muscle progenitor cells in response to ischemic damage, as evidenced in current studies (Braden et al., 2016). In addition, muscle-skeleton interaction is also a key factor in determining the composition of the skeletal system, particularly locomotor muscle functionality and performance. Muscle distribution and type could affect overall movement ability and effectiveness. For instance, studies have observed that piglets of lower birth weight have differences in force generating capacity but not necessarily differences in muscle fiber composition but a reduction in total force generated overall. These considerations suggest that while the skeleton provides the framework for movement, the functional characteristics of locomotory muscle contribute a significant amount to defining the efficacy with which the framework is utilized (Aerts et al., 2019). Usually, the intricate interaction between muscle and skeletal composition is central to analyzing limb and skeletal development because both components must cooperate in unity for efficient motor function and structural support (Figure 5.7).

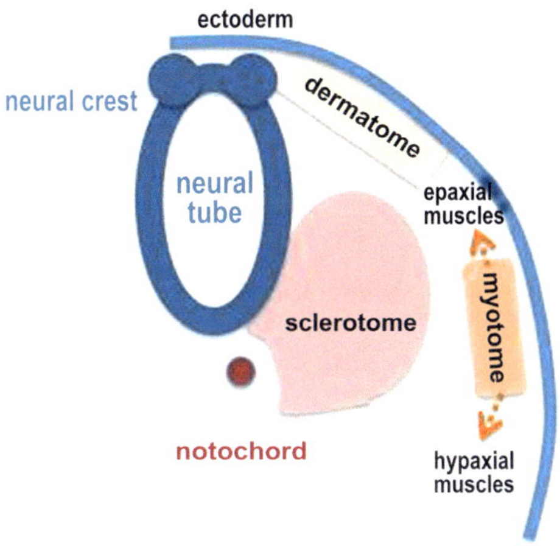

Figure 5.7. Composition of the skeletal system in embryology.

Source: https://embryology.med.unsw.edu.au/embryology/images/b/b9/Somite_cartoon5.png.

5.2.2. Functions of the Skeletal System

The skeletal system performs several essential functions that are integral to overall health and mobility, especially in the context of limb and bone development. First and foremost, it gives structural support, creating a framework that allows the body to keep its shape and stand erect. This is not only important for posture but also for allowing movement since the skeleton serves as a site of attachment for muscles. The interaction of the bones with different muscle groups enables human beings and animals to perform complex movements, from running and walking to subtle gestures. The significance of this interaction is highlighted through research in biomechanics focusing on the mechanical benefits offered by skeletal structure, determining how movements are carried out efficiently and effectively, especially during physical exercises that require agility and strength (Seth et al., 2018). Another basic role of the skeletal system is protection of important organs. For example, the rib cage protects the heart and lungs, and the skull protects the brain by housing it in a hard protective coat against which the outside world cannot easily act. This protective aspect is vital during the formation of limbs because the skeletal framework allows the bones to be able to withstand stresses and impacts repeatedly encountered in movement. In addition, the skeletal system supports mineral homeostasis—specifically calcium and phosphorus—stored in bone tissue.

This storage of minerals is critical for physiological stability during growth phases, when demand for these nutrients is greater because of accelerated limb and skeleton growth. Such multi-functionality is evidence of the integrated nature of the skeletal system in total body health and locomotion (Bogin et al., 2018). Lastly, the skeletal system also has a central function in hematopoiesis, the creation of new blood cells. Red bone marrow, located within specific bones, is where red blood cells, white blood cells, and platelets are created, which again shows the skeletal systems contribution in addition to structure and support. This process is especially pertinent during growth and development, like during adolescence, when blood cell formation is important in maintaining augmented metabolic needs and facilitating proper oxygen transport to the body. Furthermore, interaction between bone and the immune system has also been investigated by recent studies showing how bone status is linked to immune function in general. The complex functions of the skeletal system thus cut across developmental processes, influencing both the function of the limbs and systemic health (Seth et al., 2018) (Figure 5.8).

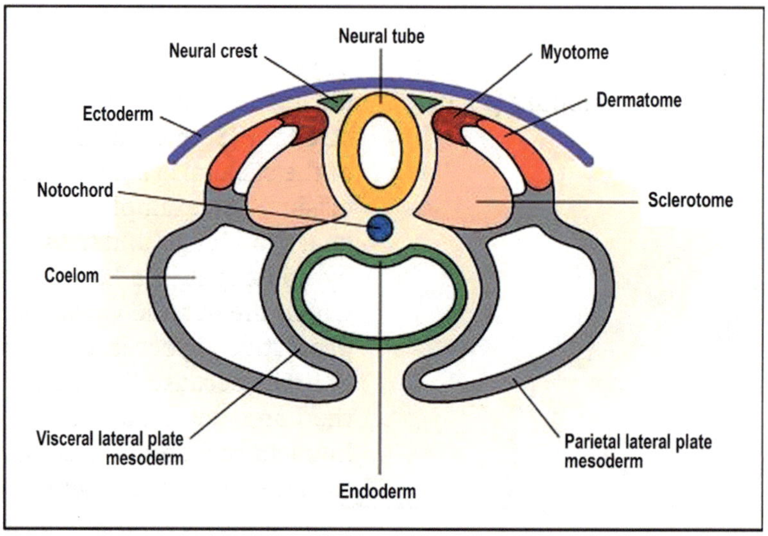

Figure 5.8. Functions of the skeletal system in embryology.

Source: https://radiologykey.com/wp-content/uploads/2019/10/C14-FF1.gif.

5.2.3. Types of Bones and Their Roles in the Body

Knowledge of the different kinds of bones found in the human body is central to the understanding of their functions in both skeletal and limb development. Bones can be categorized primarily into four groups: long bones, short bones, flat bones, and irregular bones. Long bones like the femur and humerus play crucial roles in support and movement and are levers for movement. In contrast, short bones like those of the wrists and ankles help in stability and offer little motion, whereas flat bones like the skull and ribs protect important organs and function in hematopoiesis, or blood cell production. Irregular bones, such as vertebrae and facial bones, have specialized functions, such as support and protection, but also play a role in the overall design of the skeleton, illustrating the ordered complexity required for an effective musculoskeletal system. The bone's structural and functional characteristics go beyond their categorization to involve complex development patterns based on genetic and environmental influences. Early in limb development, signaling pathways like Sonic hedgehog (Shh) and FGF coordinate the differentiation of mesenchyme to cartilaginous precursors, allowing them to ossify into bone later on. The process points to the central role that primary cilia play in conveying these signals since they function as sensory organelles that sense and transduce signaling information critical for embryonic patterning and organogenesis. The significance of these structures becomes apparent; disruptions in ciliary function have the potential to cause a range of skeletal abnormalities, highlighting the fine line between genetic regulation and environmental influence required for normal bone development and growth (Kim et al., 2023). Also, genetic mutation of bone developmental pathways has the potential to cause conditions such as split hand/foot malformation (SHFM), which highlights the clinical relevance of underlying bone biology. SHFM involves abnormal skeletal development, such as aplasia or hypoplasia of the digits, which may be caused by mutations in the DLX5 gene, a transcription factor involved in limb development (Ullah et al., 2016). This illustration highlights the way complexities in bone forms and developmental processes may lead to congenital malformations. A grasp of these genetic factors provides insight into possible therapeutic interventions against improving malformations in the skeleton. With ongoing research aimed at elucidating the molecular pathways of bone formation, it becomes more apparent that an intricate grasp of bone categories is essential not merely for developmental biology but also for improving clinical approaches in treating skeletal diseases (Figure 5.9).

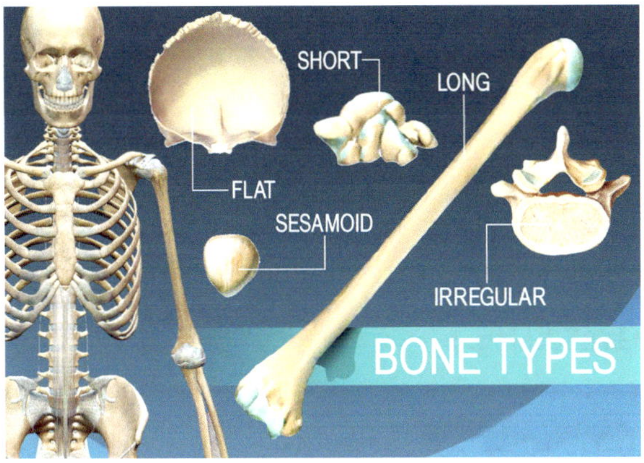

Figure 5.9. Types of bones and their roles in the body.

Source: https://www.visiblebody.com/hs-fs/hub/189659/file-2122072719-

jpg/Learn_Articles/Skeleton_System/Set_1_Bone_Types/1-Five-Types-Of-Bones-1232W.jpg.

5.3. Growth and Maturation of Bones

Bony growth and development are essential steps in the formation of vertebrate limb and skeletal structures. The development of bones begins with bones being developed by the process of endochondral ossification, wherein cartilage models are sequentially substituted with bone tissue. This is initiated by condensation of mesenchymal cells to cartilage, which acts as a scaffold for bone formation. Bone maturation entails a sequence of highly organized activities, namely the proliferation and differentiation of chondrocytes, mineralization of the matrix of cartilage, and recruitment of osteoblasts subsequently, which deposit new bone. The complex regulation of this activity is critical to normal growth of the skeleton, determining the general architecture as well as function of the limbs. An understanding of these dynamics is key to clarifying mechanisms of congenital skeletal malformations and growth abnormalities in human and other animal forms. The involvement of transcription factors, including the Forkhead box proteins FOXC1 and FOXC2, has been suggested in chondrocyte maturation in limb development. The proteins are found in the mesenchymal cells condensing at the initiation of endochondral ossification and are thus crucial during the stage of skeletal progenitor cells. Experimental models, including the Prx1-cre mouse, have shown that loss of Foxc1 and Foxc2 in limb progenitor cells leads to severe skeletal abnormalities, including reduced limb length and impaired cartilage formation. As mentioned, loss of these factors induces chondrocyte maturation delay and a decreased hypertrophic chondrocyte zone, thereby affecting the development of the primary ossification center. This evidence highlights the important functions of FOXC1 and FOXC2 in coordinating the processes that direct the maturation and remodeling of chondrocytes necessary for normal bone development and limb growth, as supported by the results in applicable research (Almubarak et al., 2024). Furthermore, the role of RNA-binding proteins like Elavl1 (HuR) further reveals the intricate regulatory network involved in bone maturation. Loss of Elavl1 has been shown to be lethal, mainly because it is crucial for progenitor cell maintenance in different tissues. Interestingly, deletion of Elavl1 in limb bud mesenchyme showed no visible abnormalities in the embryonic limb skeleton, implying that its roles could be different at different stages of development and in different cell types. While Elavl1 may be non-essential for limb formation, its function in other precursor cells challenges the differential dependencies that occur during bone development. This emphasizes the need to know how such regulatory proteins are involved in the complex balance of proliferation, differentiation, and maturation in the skeletogenesis system, hence affecting overall limb and skeletal development as part of growth processes (Parsha et al., 2024) (Figure 5.10).

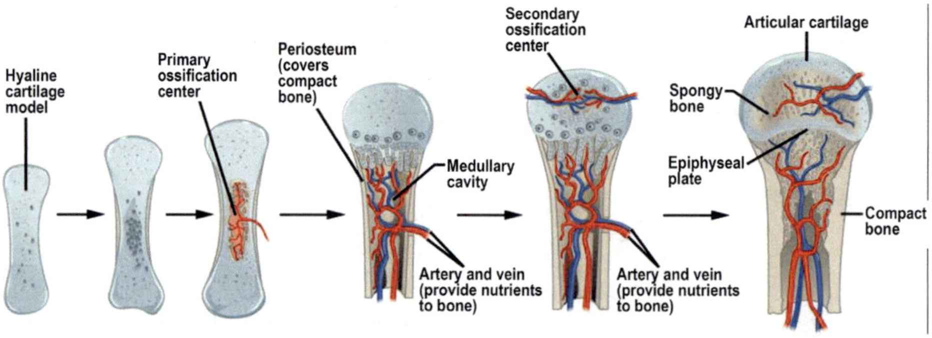

Figure 5.10. Growth and maturation of bones.

Source: https://s3-us-west-2.amazonaws.com/courses-images/wp-content/uploads/sites/1223/2017/02/08000442/Figure_38_02_06-1024x378.jpg.

5.3.1. Processes of Bone Growth: Ossification and Remodeling

The mechanisms of bone growth, that is, ossification and remodeling, are crucial to the formation and sustenance of the skeletal system. There are two basic modes of ossification: intramembranous and endochondral ossification. Intramembranous ossification is the direct transformation of mesenchymal cells into bone to constitute flat bones like the skull and clavicles. In contrast, endochondral ossification is initiated by a cartilaginous model of the bone that becomes increasingly substituted by osseous tissue. This process is especially important for long bone formation in extremities and spine, where a complex chain of cellular and molecular processes govern the conversion from cartilage to bone, providing the basis for the mature skeletal design. Unraveling regulatory mechanisms of ossification reveals the biological complexity that must occur for correct limb and skeleton formation, highlighting the dynamic nature of bone as living tissue (Blumer, 2021). Bone remodeling, a continuous life-long process, is necessary to preserve skeletal integrity and function. This sophisticated mechanism allows bone structure to adapt to different physiological requirements, including mechanical loading and trauma. Remodeling is an orderly process that involves the juxtaposed functions of osteoclasts, bone-resorbing cells, and osteoblasts, bone-building cells. A key feature of this process is the equilibrium between formation and resorption; imbalances can lead to bone pathologies. Recent research has shed light on the role of Hox genes, particularly expressions of the Hox11 gene, in the regulation of bone remodeling, especially after fractures caused by injury. Loss of Hox11 function has been shown to cause severe defects in endochondral ossification and irregular bone matrix arrangement during the remodeling process, which points out to the genetic elements that regulate skeletal regeneration (Rux et al., 2017). Additionally, the dynamic interactions among the different cells in the bone microenvironment are responsible for the overall health of the skeletal system. Osteocytes, the most common bone cells, are in charge of perceiving mechanical stresses and organizing the remodeling process. They communicate with osteoclasts and osteoblasts and thus act as a regulatory center of the bone. Moreover, remodeling is regulated by several factors like hormones, nutrition, and mechanical stress, which altogether instruct bone to react to interior and exterior changes. This fine balance illustrates the flexibility of the skeletal system in that it is continuously undergoing ossification and remodeling to meet the functional demands imposed on it throughout life. A full understanding of these processes not only sheds light on the physiology of the bone but also potential therapeutic interventions utilized in treating skeletal pathology (Blumer, 2021) (Figure 5.11).

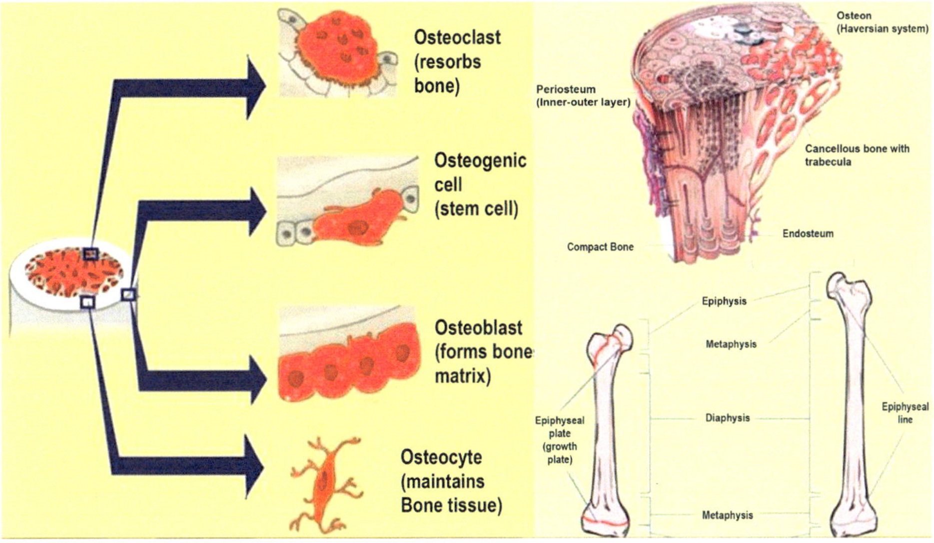

Figure 5.11. Ossification (bone growth and development).

Source: https://biologynotesonline.com/wp-content/uploads/2023/06/Ossification-Bone-Growth-and-Development-Definition-Steps-Importance.jpg.

5.3.2. Hormonal Influences on Bone Growth

Hormones are key regulators of the bone development and skeletal growth process, especially for the critical stages in life like puberty and menopause. Estrogens, a class of hormones that contain 17β-estradiol, are well recognized for their reproductive and sexual development roles but have strong nonreproductive actions on the bone. Estrogen encourages the maturation of osteoblasts, the bone-forming cells, and at the same time suppresses the activity of the bone-resorbing osteoclasts. This equilibrium between bone resorption and bone formation is critical to the preservation of bone density and skeletal integrity. Grasping the mechanisms of these hormonal effects can shed light on the fundamental mechanisms concerning bone health, particularly in women, who go through changing estrogen levels during their menstrual cycle that can influence bone and calcium metabolism, musculoskeletal well-being, and function (Sarah et al., 2024). Together with estrogens, thyroid hormones play a noteworthy role in bone development. They induce osteoblast differentiation and increase their activity and so allow for long bone growth and maintenance of skeletal integrity. Thyroid hormones interact with other hormonal systems and may influence muscle function and energy metabolism, additionally affecting limb and skeletal development. Hematopoietic progenitor cells, specifically myogenic progenitor cells, have variable responses to thyroid hormones that determine the functional properties of muscle fibers. The interaction between thyroid hormones and muscle physiology is crucial because it is responsible for the strength and condition of muscles needed for dynamic activities like jumping or running. This plasticity in physiology consequently underscores the necessity of hormonal control for maximum skeletal development, especially under changing environmental and dietary demands (Hoh, 2023). The interplay between hormonal forces and bone development is of particular relevance to health, notably in relation to physical activity and the prevention of injury. Studies demonstrate that both the menstrual cycle and the consumption of hormonal contraceptives can affect calcium metabolism and hence the strength of bones in physically active females. The myosin heavy chain differentiation, which is driven by neural signals and thyroid hormones, is critical in muscle adaptation that has direct implications for the function and load-carrying capacity of the skeletal system. Those fine changes can guide the planning for the optimization of musculoskeletal health among athletes and other physically demanding groups. Finally, understanding the many functions of hormones during bone development not only improves our understanding of limb and skeletal development but also offers a model for addressing health concerns associated with bone density and muscle function among different populations (Hoh, 2023; Sarah et al., 2024) (Figure 5.12).

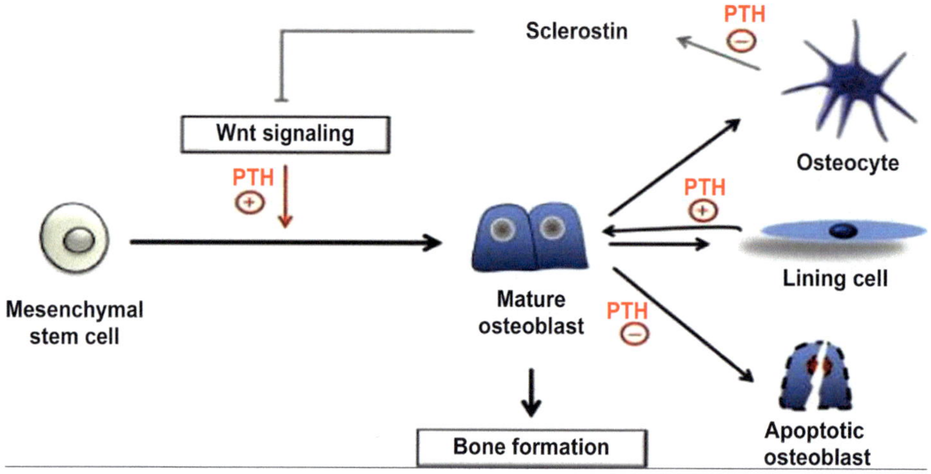

Figure 5.12. Hormonal influences on bone growth.

Source: https://ars.els-cdn.com/content/image/3-s2.0-B9780124160156000150-f15-01-9780124160156.jpg.

5.3.3. Factors Affecting Bone Density and Strength

Bone density and bone strength are supported by a variety of interacting factors, a complex web that changes over the course of an individual's lifetime. Diet is essential, with nutrients such as calcium and vitamin D at the forefront of health bone physiology. A lack of calcium can lead to lower bone mineral density, a predisposing factor for osteoporosis, particularly in the elderly where bone turnover is already compromised. Also, normal vitamin D levels are necessary as they facilitate the absorption of calcium in the intestine and enable bones to be dense and strong. Precisely, a study suggests that patients with Parkinsons disease diagnosis may experience more osteoporosis due to inadequate nutritional status and consequent malnourishment, which further reduces bone mineral content and causes adverse health effects (Fucheng et al., 2023). Apart from nutrition, exercise is an essential aspect in maintaining healthy and dense bones. Weight-bearing exercises performed consistently strengthen bones by promoting the growth of bones and reducing bone resorption, a factor that is very vital during developing years and beyond into adulthood. The gradual loss of physical activity witnessed predominantly in elderly people accelerates skeletal muscle wasting and bone mineral density loss, a condition typically termed as sarcopenia. Such a decline has extensive implications for health since muscle mass and strength are essential in preventing falls and fractures among elderly populations (Littner, 2011). Additionally, studies reveal that physical activity levels are affected by cognitive and emotional health; for example, those suffering from depression or having cognitive deficits might take part in physical exercises less, which in turn results in the deterioration of both muscle and bone health (Fucheng et al., 2023). Hormonal influences also have a significant role to play in measuring bone density and strength, especially at crucial times like puberty, menopause, and old age. Both estrogen and testosterone are hormones that are vital in maintaining bone density, and their reduction will be linked with a higher risk of osteoporosis. Women after menopause have a marked reduction in their estrogen levels, which leads to rapid bone loss and thus more fractures. On the other hand, male androgens decline gradually and can also impact bone density in the long run. This decline with age highlights the need to track changes in hormones and their impact on skeletal health during old age. Additionally, chronic illnesses and medications influencing hormone levels further make the situation complicated, requiring overall management techniques to reduce risks imposed by lower bone density (Littner, 2011).

5.4. Limb Proportions and Variability

Limb proportions are vital in the understanding of skeletal growth among species and differences in individuals within a population. Limb proportions are defined as the relative lengths and breadths of the different segments in the limbs, and they can have a significant impact on locomotion and functionality. For example, species living in particular environments tend to show specific limb proportions that are favorable to their survival. These adaptations point to the strength of understanding both the morphological features and what they mean for survival. Limb proportions can be used by researchers to establish correlations between form and function, giving us information about the mechanics of motion and the evolution of skeletal configurations. This investigation of proportion not only adds to our understanding of biomechanics but also adds to our appreciation of the evolutionary routes followed by different taxa. Proportional variation among limbs is contingent upon a multiplicity of factors, such as genetic, environmental, and nutritional factors. Such differences can lead to the great range of limb types within a species and can cause such things as sexual dimorphism, in which the male and female members of a species have different limb sizes and shapes. Also, environmental stresses, including the presence of resources or climatic conditions, can affect the development of the limbs, demonstrating the adaptability of skeletal growth. Research has noted that factors beyond the organism itself, such as diet at key periods of growth, contribute importantly to the determination of limb structure. Knowledge of such factors offers much insight into how organisms may morphologically fit into their environments, an issue that remains a fundamental area of inquiry in evolutionary biology and functional morphology. The applications of knowing limb proportions and variability go beyond scholarly interest; they have real-world implications in agriculture and medicine. In cattle, for instance, the correct limb proportions can mean market readiness in terms of meat quality and health of the animal, as deviations can point to certain heritable factors influencing production. Also in human medicine, knowledge of limb variability is significant in treating conditions like sarcopenia, where with age, there is the loss of muscle mass and function accompanied by changes in limb proportions and efficiency (citing points discussed in (Larsson et al., 2018)). As scientists delve further into the genetic and environmental foundations of limb proportions, the prospect of using the findings to enhance healthcare outcomes and farming practices becomes more important. The interaction of limb proportions, variability, and health consequences is an expression of a general understanding of limb and skeletal development that is crucial to both evolutionary biology and applied use (Figure 5.13).

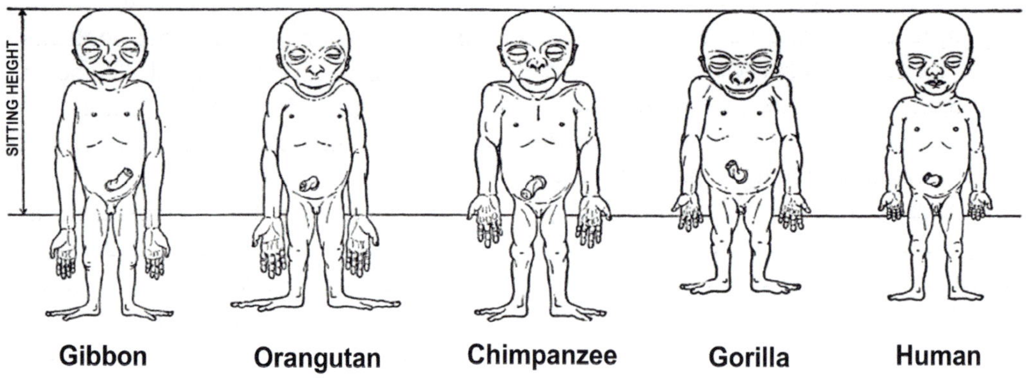

Figure 5.13. Limb proportions and variability.

Source: https://www.mdpi.com/ijerph/ijerph-07-01047/article_deploy/html/images/ijerph-07-01047f7-1024.png.

5.4.1. Genetic Factors Influencing Limb Proportions

Amongst the numerous factors that affect limb proportions, genetic factors play a key role in determining how individuals develop their skeletal frameworks during growth. Genetic inheritance determines the patterning of long bones, which in turn affects the proportion of limbs. Each person's genetic template comes together to form the potential maximum length, width, and density of their bones, leading to naturally occurring differences in limb proportions. Studies have shown that various populations have different average proportions of the limbs, which can be explained by genetic selection compared to environmental adjustment over generations. The genetic variation between populations points towards a greater understanding of how certain alleles can determine growth patterns, which could shed light on normal development as well as on conditions that have skeletal abnormalities, thus pointing towards the importance of genetics in limb and skeletal development. The interaction between environmental influences and genetic predisposition is highly demonstrated by the investigation of limb proportions. Genetic tendencies do not explain the variations seen in measurements of limbs; rather, they interact with the external stimuli received during developmental stages. Food supply, mechanical loading due to exercise, and disease states are among the external influences that may affect bone growth and remodeling. For example, how limb bones respond to mechanical loading could be influenced by genetic sensitivity, which would result in differences in bone density and structure across people of differing genetic makeup. These interactions are central to the explanation of population-scale trends in limb proportions because they demonstrate how pressures exerted by an environment might guide the expression of genes over the course of time to impact limb morphology within different contexts and populations. Further investigations have highlighted the role of specific genetic markers in determining limb proportions and their functional outcomes. Genetic studies have identified qtls (quantitative trait loci) associated with skeletal traits, underscoring the complexity of genetic influences on limb development. Consequently, understanding these genetic factors can significantly enhance our knowledge of not only average population limb characteristics but also the variances observed in individual cases. For instance, the covariation of cortical bone and dentine volume among various skeletal elements highlights the extent to which genetic determinants of bone density may influence limb proportions as a whole. This is further complicated by evidence that particular genetic features could respond differently to environmental stressors, finally determining limb proportions in people with varied backgrounds. Studying such genetic effects is critical for formulating targeted solutions to correct skeletal growth disorders, highlighting the significance of genetics in limb and skeletal development (Figure 5.14).

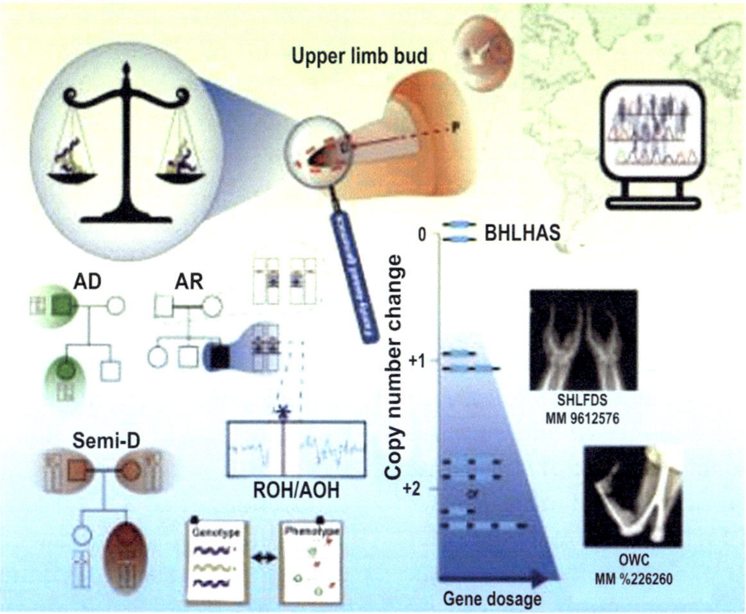

Figure 5.14. Developmental genomics of limb malformations.

Source: https://ars.els-cdn.com/content/image/1-s2.0-S2666247722000483-fx1.jpg.

5.4.2. Environmental Influences on Limb Development

The interaction between environmental influences and limb development is a subject of vital research in the overall study of limb and skeletal development. Different external factors, such as nutrition, exercise, and weather, have a direct impact on limb growth patterns in humans as well as in other animals. For example, proper nutrient intake during childhood is critical for optimal bone accretion, with such factors as peak bone mass and skeletal health later in life being affected. Inadequate essential nutrients can lead to abnormal bone modeling and potential risks for diseases like osteoporosis later in life. In addition, the environment in terms of geographic location and elevation can change the biomechanical load on the musculoskeletal system, resulting in adaptations that maximize limb function across life, illustrating the significant effect of environmental factors on limb growth (Signe et al., 2021). Studies on gorilla skeletal growth illustrate how the environment, such as locomotion, climate, and diet, dictates limb morphology variation. An overall comparison of gorilla skeletons illustrates that limb proportions greatly differ between species inhabiting various environments. For example, it is noted that high-altitude gorillas have longer thoracic vertebrae as adaptations for reduced oxygen levels. Likewise, the general limb lengths and proportions are determined by the gorillas' requirement to move about their habitats efficiently, with differences being an expression of locomotor adaptations required for survival. These morphological differences highlight the importance of both genetic and environmental factors at developmental stages, depicting a dynamic interplay wherein environmental pressures can modify aspects of the skeleton to patterns important for adaptation and survival (Ruff et al., 2021). The implications of such work go far beyond sheer anatomical differences; they highlight the importance of environmental factors in the context of developmental health. Conditions like childhood malnutrition or lack of physical activity can inhibit maximum limb development, with long-term impacts in adulthood such as compromised bone quality or general lower height. These detrimental impacts underscore the need for public health programs directed towards enhancing nutritional intake during childhood and encouraging exercise to facilitate good skeletal development. Grasping the critical periods when environmental effects are most significant can assist in developing strategies to counteract related health hazards and offer insights into the control of skeletal disorders associated with growth impairment. Therefore, incorporating understanding of both environmental and genetic factors is fundamental to a holistic method of promoting limb and skeletal health across the life cycle (Signe et al., 2021).

5.4.3. Variability in Limb Development Across Populations

Population variation in limb development is an essential component of understanding human biology. Both genetic, environmental, and lifestyle components contribute to variation observed in limb morphology among groups. Research indicates that growth of the skeleton has intrinsic plasticity and can allow for populations to adapt to their specific ecological niches. For instance, populations in colder climates are more likely to have shorter, stronger limb proportions as an adaptation to preserve heat, while warmer climate populations have longer limbs for enhanced loss of heat and movement. Furthermore, activity levels and cultural practices dictate the development of muscles, which also gets expressed in the structure of the limbs, showing the intricate nature of factors involved in shaping human anatomy in different populations. Studies of muscle development have also yielded striking inter-population differences that underscore the complexity of limb adaptability. Advanced methods, such as the use of ultrasound technology in conjunction with artificial intelligence (AI), allow for accurate determinations of muscle quality and volume. Studies employing such measures have demonstrated repeatability of measurements across populations, which implies that geography and clinical environments may influence the characteristics of muscle. For example, the use of the MyoVision-US instrument has provided evidence that change in limb muscle structures is not just a product of genetic variation but also of earlier lifestyle impact and health disparity within populations. The intricate framework highlights the capability of technological advances to value variety in limb and muscle growth, proposing a need for further examination of these associations across human populations (Rivera et al., 2025). Besides, the role of skeletal stem cells (SSCs) remains a core focus in examining limb developmental diversity. Research indicates that m6A modification in SSCs plays a significant role in their differentiation and overall limb development. Genetic regulation by m6A modification appears to be population-specific, with implications for how SSCs maintain their role and, accordingly, skeletal integrity. For instance, mutations in genes related to m6A methyltransferase activity may disrupt regular bone formation, leading to complex clinical presentations such as dwarfism or low bone density (Wang et al., 2025). These findings highlight the importance of epitranscriptomic control in limb variability and propose further investigations into cellular processes behind limb growth variability across populations. By uniting genetic research with analysis sensitive to populations, researchers are better able to unveil the intricate patterns of limb formation that define human variability (Figure 5.15).

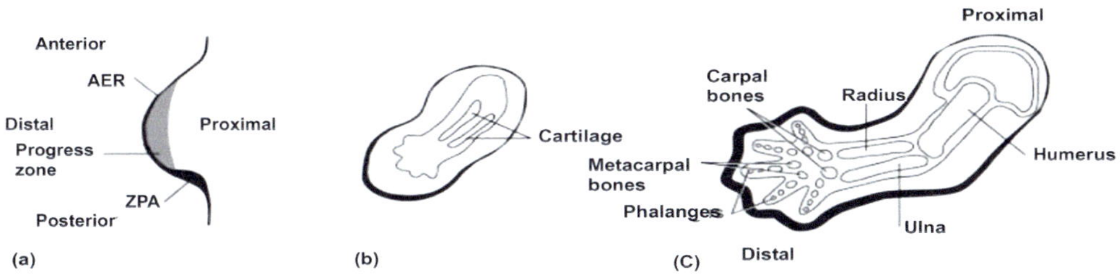

Figure 5.15. Variability in limb development.

Source: https://ars.els-cdn.com/content/image/3-s2.0-B9780123708779000232-gr11.jpg.

5.5. Common Limb and Skeletal Disorders

When one looks at the prevalent limb and skeletal disorders, it is important to reflect on the numerous factors that lead to their occurrence. These disorders, such as osteoarthritis, rheumatoid arthritis, and osteoporosis, have a serious effect on the musculoskeletal system, causing pain, reduced mobility, and compromised quality of life. Osteoarthritis, commonly linked to ageing, is caused by the deterioration of cartilage and characteristically occurs in weight-bearing joints like the knees and hips. In contrast, rheumatoid arthritis is an autoimmune disease characterized mainly by joint inflammation, which results in severe disability if not properly treated. Both diseases demonstrate the manner in which underlying biological processes and environmental determinants may converge, testing the mettle of both individuals and healthcare systems in coming up with effective management and rehabilitation plans. Early treatment of these disorders in their course can help maintain joint function and improve patients' overall health. Aside from arthritis, skeletal conditions like scoliosis and limb malformations pose special difficulty in limb and skeletal growth. Scoliosis, which is a lateral deviation from the normal curve of the spine, may cause physical pain and respiratory dysfunction complications. Limb malformations, like clubfoot or developmental dysplasia of the hip, may compromise normal movement and must be addressed early for best results. The therapy for such disorders usually includes multidisciplinary treatment, including orthopedic experts, physiotherapists, and, where required, surgical treatments. The role of environmental factors and genetics is highly significant in the expression of such conditions, highlighting the multifaceted nature of skeletal and limb disorders from a developmental perspective. Ongoing research into the disorders is essential to further enhance diagnostic techniques and therapeutic interventions.

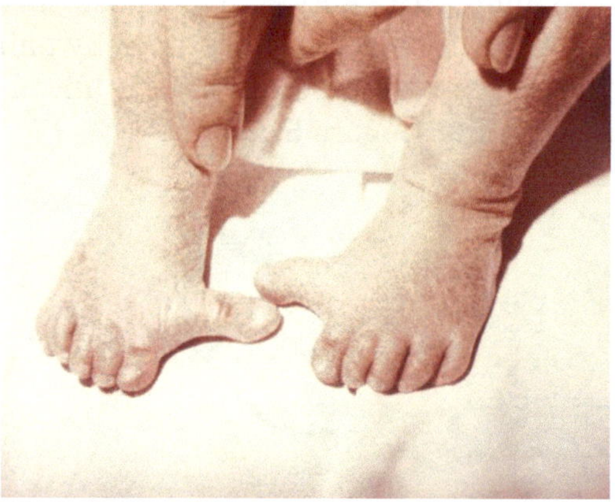

Figure 5.16. Limb and Skeletal Disorders.

Source: https://embryology.med.unsw.edu.au/embryology/images/b/bf/Polydactylia.jpg.

Knowledge of the epidemiology of these prevalent limb and skeletal disorders is essential for guiding public health programs and healthcare policy. The Global Burden of Diseases, Injuries, and Risk Factors Study offers useful information on the prevalence and burden of these disorders, noting the increasing non-fatal disease burden documented in aging populations (Spencer et al., 2018). In addition, the World Health Organizations guidelines support routine physical activity as a preventive measure for musculoskeletal disorders, highlighting not only the need for exercise but also the necessity of customized programs for vulnerable groups (Bull et al., 2020). By combining recommendations for exercise and increased awareness of the disorders, public health programs can encourage healthy living, thereby leading to enhanced quality of life. Increased awareness of risk factors and preventive care can significantly reduce the occurrence of common limb and skeletal disorders, with benefits to the individual and to society (Figure 5.16).

5.5.1. Congenital Disorders Affecting Limb Development

Development of the limbs is a highly intricate process that can be extremely disturbed by congenital conditions, which occur due to genetic, environmental, or both factors during embryogenesis. They have the capability of producing a vast number of malformations such as syndactyly, polydactyly, and reduction limb defects. These conditions usually result from malfunction in the signals controlling limb outgrowth and skeletal patterning, which are important for the determination of normal anatomy and function of limbs. The complex interplay between these developmental processes and genetic factors makes research imperative. Knowing how disruption of such early signals leads to certain limb malformations is essential for designing useful interventions and enhancing patient outcomes in patients with such congenital malformations. Another important aspect of congenital limb disorders is their relation to minor physical anomalies (MPAs), which may reflect more extensive developmental disruption. For instance, 22q11.2 deletion syndrome (22q11DS) shows how a general genetic condition can express through particular limb and craniofacial dysmorphologies, which in turn results in both limb-based and psychological problems. Studies show that those with 22q11DS tend to have distinctive physical characteristics, like unusual finger or ear shape, that can be seen at birth and develop over the course of their lives. These characteristic dysmorphic features serve as a glimpse into early embryologic development and underscore the significance of recognizing such markers since they could be associated with subsequent health status. As illustrated through research with high-tech imaging modalities, precise identification of these anomalies will play an important role in facilitating earlier diagnosis and intervention plans and, by extension, improving the quality of life of individuals so afflicted. Advances in multi-omic profiling in the recent past have further shed light on the intricacies of limb and skeletal development, including the regulatory pathways governing congenital disease. Transcriptional and epigenetic data integration in a study brought forth important information on the fate of osteoprogenitor cells during joint and limb morphogenesis, proposing that aberrations within these processes could be the underlying cause for several congenital limb malformations. These results suggest the possibility of using genetic knowledge to shape therapies for limb development disorders. Furthermore, forecasts of cellular origins of chondrocytes from non-canonical sources highlight the dynamic nature of developmental biology and its implications for congenital disease. By investigating the regulatory processes underlying normal and pathological development, researchers have the ability to reveal new targets for intervention, ultimately working to limit the effects of these congenital disorders on the patient and family (Roalf et al., 2024; To et al., 2024) (Figure 5.17).

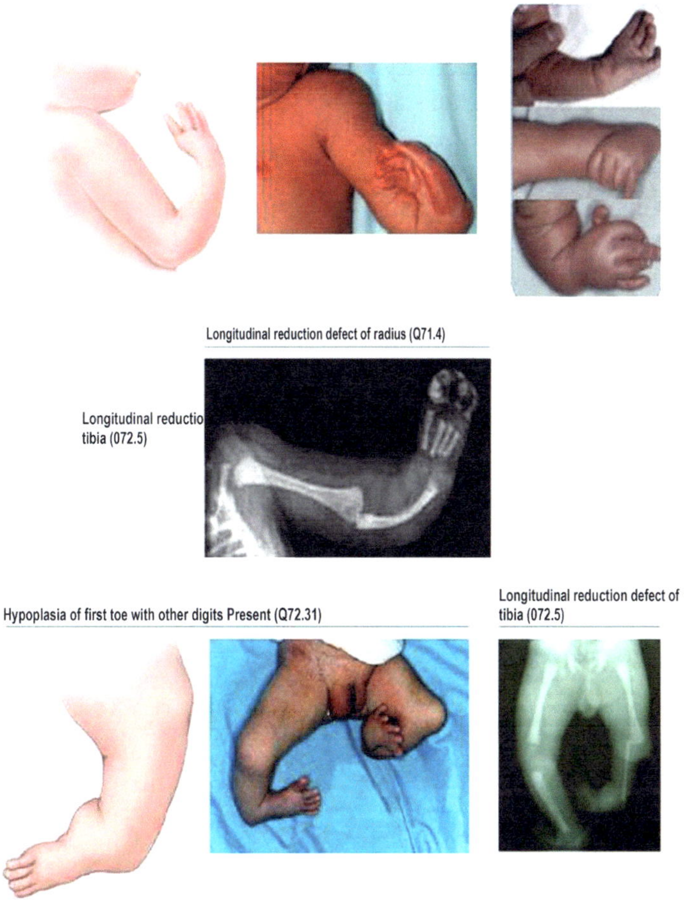

Figure 5.17. Congenital disorders affecting limb development.

Source: https://archive.cdc.gov/www_cdc_gov/ncbddd/birthdefects/surveillancemanual/chapters/chapter-4/chapter4_9f_html_files/Fig.-4.39.-Longitudinal-preaxial.jpg.

5.5.2. Acquired Skeletal Disorders and Their Impact

Acquired skeletal disorders pose immense challenges in the realm of limb and skeletal development, emphasizing the intricate relationship between bone health and mechanical stress. Immobilization of some form due to illness or injury can cause negative skeletal effects like osteopenia, which is a state of diminished bone density. This mechanical unloading reduces the physiological stimuli required to preserve bone integrity, evidenced by the correlation between levels of physical activity and skeletal health. Although certain disorders may be caused by genetic predispositions, the acquired status of these conditions is given emphasis by highlighting the input of environmental factors, such as inactivity and immobilization, in perpetuating skeletal deficiencies. Appreciating this dynamic is important in formulating effective interventions that not only treat prevailing disorders but also ensure optimal skeletal growth. The effects of decreased physical activity on the skeleton are most detectable in populations with limb fractures. Physical activity has been measured to decrease substantially by adolescents in immobilization related to limb fracture, with declines ranging from 30.1% to 84.4% based on fracture type. This lack of activity causes significant reductions in bone loading that elicit a physiological response leading to disuse-related bone mineral loss and eventually osteopenia. Such observations provide further emphasis on the necessity of providing sufficient movement and mechanical loading to young skeletons, especially during these essential developmental stages. Since healthcare professionals are dealing with the injured population, it is essential that there is prioritization of techniques that reduce immobilization time and promote safe rehabilitation exercises, thus lessening the effect of such acquired skeletal disorders on bone integrity. Besides the physical effects of acquired skeletal disorders, there are also general implications for mobility and overall quality of life. The social and psychological aspects of skeletal conditions can have a tremendous impact on individuals affected by them, causing them to feel isolated or lowered self-efficacy. In addition, the effect of missing physical activity is not limited to the immediate skeletal problems and can extend to other body systems, causing cascades of health outcomes. As recent studies demonstrate, the function of long non-coding RNAs (lncRNAs) in the adaptation and metabolism of skeletal muscle is increasingly evident, and they may prove to be of therapeutic significance in preventing muscle atrophy caused by extended immobilization. Knowledge of the pathways through which muscular responses to immobility not only benefits the management of improved outcomes for patients with acquired disorders but also highlights the complex relationships underlying limb and skeletal development in diverse contexts (Alessio et al., 2019; Heinonen et al., 2011).

5.5.3. Treatment and Management of Limb and Skeletal Disorders

The effective treatment and management of limb and skeletal disorders often necessitate a multifaceted approach that addresses not only the physical symptoms but also the broader impact on the patient's quality of life. This includes both pharmacological and non-pharmacological interventions tailored to individual patient needs. Pharmacological treatments may involve the use of analgesics to manage pain, nonsteroidal anti-inflammatory drugs (NSAIDs) to reduce inflammation, and, in more severe cases, corticosteroids or disease-modifying antirheumatic drugs (DMARDs) for conditions like rheumatoid arthritis. Moreover, physical therapy plays a crucial role, enhancing mobility while strengthening muscles surrounding afflicted joints. Such therapies can improve functionality and reduce disability, thus alleviating the social and psychological burdens often experienced by individuals suffering from limb and skeletal disorders. A comprehensive treatment strategy is vital to maximize patient well-being and long-term health outcomes, particularly as these disorders evolve and necessitate ongoing care (Vos et al., 2017). In addition to conventional treatments, advanced methodologies such as regenerative medicine and surgical interventions are garnering interest in the management of limb and skeletal disorders. Regenerative techniques, including stem cell therapy and tissue engineering, have the potential to repair damaged tissues and restore function in cases where traditional treatments fall short. For instance, the application of stem cells can promote healing and regeneration in patients with osteoarthritis, significantly improving their quality of life. On the surgical front, orthopedic procedures, including joint replacements and corrective surgeries for skeletal deformities, can provide significant relief and restore function. Nevertheless, these interventions often require substantial rehabilitation efforts to achieve optimal outcomes. Thus, integrating innovative approaches with established practices forms a cornerstone of contemporary management strategies for limb and skeletal disorders, ultimately leading to better patient satisfaction and improved clinical results (Margaret et al., 2017). The importance of early diagnosis in the treatment and management of limb and skeletal disorders cannot be overstated. Timely intervention correlates with better prognoses and enhances the efficacy of treatment regimens. For conditions like osteogenesis imperfecta or disorders stemming from enzyme deficiencies, early identification allows for prompt initiation of supportive therapies, potentially mitigating long-term complications. Furthermore, advancements in genetic testing are enhancing our ability to diagnose hereditary disorders earlier, enabling tailored therapeutic approaches that address the specific needs of patients. Establishing a collaborative care model that involves physicians, therapists, and support networks can significantly enrich management strategies by fostering proactive monitoring and adjusting treatments as needed. Collectively, these elements underscore the necessity of a comprehensive, interdisciplinary approach to effectively manage limb and skeletal disorders, enhancing both physical and psychosocial outcomes (Vos et al., 2017) (Figure 5.18).

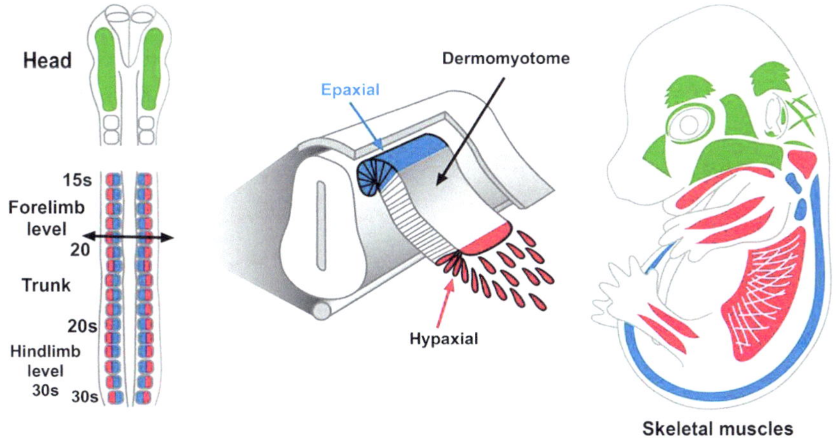

Figure 5.18. Treatment and management of limb and skeletal disorders.

Source: https://www.researchgate.net/publication/315526863/figure/fig3/AS:11431281246825003@1716470517161/Embryonic-origins-of-skeletal-muscles-Myogenic-cells-of-skeletal-muscles-have-two.tif.

5.6. Advances in Research and Technology

Recent advancements in research and technology have significantly enhanced our understanding of limb and skeletal development, paving the way for innovative therapeutic approaches. The integration of high-throughput genomic technologies has allowed researchers to identify key genetic regulators involved in osteogenesis and chondrogenesis. For example, the development of CRISPR-Cas9 gene editing tools has made it possible to make targeted changes in genes that are involved in skeletal diseases, allowing for more in-depth exploration into the pathophysiology of diseases like osteogenesis imperfecta. Furthermore, improved imaging modalities, such as 3D computed tomography (CT) and magnetic resonance imaging (MRI), have enabled unparalleled observations of morphological and structural alterations during limb and skeletal development. These technologies improve not only our knowledge of normal developmental processes but also hasten the diagnosis and treatment of congenital limb malformations and degenerative skeletal diseases, ultimately enhancing patient outcomes through targeted interventional approaches. Additionally, the integration of tissue engineering and regenerative medicine methodology has revolutionized the landscape of limb and skeletal treatment approaches. By using biomaterials in conjunction with stem cell technology, scientists are leading the way in regenerating missing or injured bones. Advances in scaffold design for the engineering of bone tissue have shown potential to imitate the extracellular matrix of the body, supporting cell growth and differentiation. Improvements in bioprinting technology also offer the capability of printing complex 3D structures that can be implanted to enable limb regeneration. These technologies, in conjunction with advanced drug delivery systems, provide for the release of therapeutic agents in a controlled fashion to maximize regeneration processes. As these technologies advance, they promise to revolutionize treatment regimens for patients with traumatic injury or degenerative disease, extending the limits of what is achievable in limb and skeletal repair. The study of the microbiota's impact on skeletal and limb growth has become a crucial field of research in the current field. The microbiota-gut-brain axis, a complex network of communication between gut microbiota and the central nervous system (CNS), was found to be involved in multiple physiological processes, such as skeletal health. Current evidence indicates that microbial metabolites may have an impact on bone homeostasis via the regulation of immune responses and regulation of osteoclast and osteoblast differentiation. Exploring how early-life factors, including mode of delivery and dietary patterns, form the microbiota structure and thus influence limb and skeletal development can produce new avenues for prevention. As our knowledge of this axis increases, it creates new avenues for therapeutic interventions to enhance skeletal outcomes through diet modification or probiotic supplementations, demonstrating the deep interrelationship of our microbiome and skeletal well-being, ultimately enriching limb and skeletal development research.

5.6.1. Role of Stem Cells in Limb Regeneration

The stem cells' function in limb regeneration is vital, especially considering their differentiating ability and what controls it. In the context of skeletal growth, stem cells, mainly MSCs, have demonstrated high ability to differentiate into different cell types such as chondrocytes and osteoblasts, which play fundamental roles in the development and regeneration of limb structures. Research has identified that these stem cells have the ability to dynamically respond to their microenvironment, regulating their lineage commitment in accordance with intrinsic and extrinsic cues. In addition, myogenesis research reveals that muscle stem cells or satellite cells are key to skeletal muscle regeneration through the reactivation of myogenic programs, further supporting that the regenerative potential of limbs is directly related to the efficacy and control of stem cell functions in development and repair (De-Shi et al., 2021). Of equal importance when considering limb regeneration is the complex interaction between stem cells and the nervous system. The peripheral nervous system, including sympathetic and sensory innervation, is directly implicated in the regulation of the functions of many cell types utilized in bone metabolism and regeneration. Neurotransmitters secreted by these nerve fibers have been demonstrated to regulate the activity of osteoblasts, osteoclasts, and MSC during endochondral ossification, which is very important for limb growth. This intersection of neural and stem cell interactions implies that regenerative potential of limb tissues may not be solely a function of intrinsic stem cell properties but is also contingent on extrinsic signals propagated by the nervous system, thus pointing towards a multidimensional regulatory paradigm (Sässel, 2014). Additionally, elucidating the molecular and cellular processes that drive stem cell-mediated limb regeneration also raises compelling issues related to therapeutic utility in regenerative medicine. Understanding how stem cells react to certain signaling pathways may lead to the creation of novel mechanisms to promote limb repair after injury or degenerative disease. Analysis of the post-transcriptional regulation of gene expression and the functions of RNA-binding proteins during stem cell differentiation and tissue regeneration is a promising area of research in this field. Increasing our understanding of these regulatory mechanisms may result in better practices in the treatment of musculoskeletal diseases and the creation of successful limb regeneration therapies. These improvements would not only advance skeletal development science but can also be applied across many regenerative medicine fields, highlighting the central position of stem cells during recovery and reconstruction (De-Shi et al., 2021) (Figure 5.19).

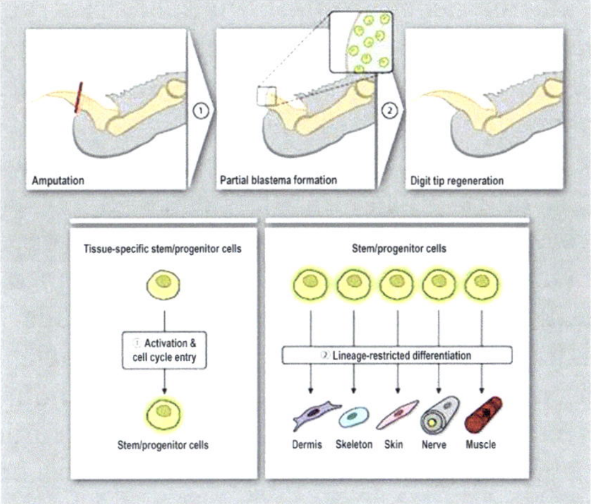

Figure 5.19. The role of stem cells in limb regeneration.

Source: https://www.tandfonline.com/cms/asset/07db8a58-349d-4f0c-9ae9-dda6cc88ee6c/kogg_a_1163463_f0003_oc.gif.

5.6.2. Innovations in Orthopedic Treatments

The orthopedic treatment landscape has come a long way, especially through novel pharmaceutical strategies that seek to treat skeletal dysplasia disorders like achondroplasia. Achondroplasia, which is expressed by limb length and growth abnormalities, has classically been resistant to patient management, causing numerous orthopedic complications. Advanced pharmacological therapies have, in recent times, offered prospective alternatives to surgery. Vosoritide, an analog of the C-type natriuretic peptide, was approved by the FDA in 2021, a landmark advance in the treatment of this disorder. Its availability not only provides promise for enhanced linear growth for involved children but also signifies the value of biochemical knowledge in the design of specific therapies for disorders of skeletal growth. The continuous research of other prospective candidate drugs such as TransCON CNP and recifercept also shows the dedication to broadening therapy options, in the end, improving the quality of life for achondroplasia patients (Patrycja, 2025). Minimally invasive techniques (MIT) are another important breakthrough revolutionizing orthopedic therapies, particularly for complicated lower limb fractures. The new surgical methods focus more on minimizing tissue injury and recovery time while preserving effectiveness. Conventional orthopedic operations typically entail large incisions and long periods of rehabilitation, which can be an obstacle to patient recovery. The advent of MIT, though, permits fractures to be stabilized with accuracy and precision using minimally invasive incisions. External fixation and locked intramedullary rods are examples of the trend towards less invasive methods. Intraoperative imaging and surgical navigation systems have further improved the accuracy of procedures, reducing the risk of complications. While difficulties like the initial learning curve for new technology remain, the promise of quicker recovery and reduced post-operative complication incidence makes these technologies essential to developing orthopedic practice (Ant Mônia Fiorott et al., 2024). The incorporation of cutting-edge technologies in orthopedic therapies is not limited to surgical procedures and drugs but includes biomechanical innovations in prosthetics and orthopedic appliances. Modern prosthetic designs aim not only to replace lost function but also to enhance the quality of limb and skeletal development. With the advent of smart technologies, prosthetics can now respond dynamically to user movements, providing a more natural experience. For instance, myoelectric prosthetics use electrical signals from residual muscle activity to control movement, offering users improved control and comfort. In addition, 3D printing technology has transformed the process of customizing orthopedic devices to fit unique anatomical differences. These advancements reflect a larger movement toward personalized medicine in orthopedics, with treatments being designed and optimized to suit the unique requirements of each individual patient, resulting in better functional results and quality of life (Ant Mônia Fiorott et al., 2024; Patrycja, 2025).

5.6.3. Future Directions in Limb and Skeletal Research

As the field of limb and skeletal research continues to evolve, future directions are increasingly focused on integrating advanced imaging modalities and molecular biology to enhance our understanding of musculoskeletal disorders. Non-invasive techniques like CT and MRI have already revolutionized the capacity to assess vascular-related conditions such as peripheral artery disease (PAD). Researchers are now advocating for a multi-modality imaging approach combined with molecular markers, which include those associated with inflammation and oxidative stress. This convergence is expected to provide a comprehensive view of limb and skeletal pathology and could uncover previously unrecognized mechanisms underlying limb diseases. Addressing the technical challenges inherent in these imaging modalities, as noted in (Chan et al., 2023), is crucial for the successful implementation of these future directions, as they may significantly improve patient outcomes and therapeutic strategies. Moreover, the investigation of skeletal muscle atrophy presents a compelling avenue for research within limb and skeletal development. Understanding the molecular mechanisms driving muscle wasting could lead to innovative therapeutic interventions for various conditions that lead to limb disabilities. The identification of specific E3 ubiquitin ligases, such as MuRF1, has demonstrated their significance in the atrophy cascade. Future studies investigating the role of MuRF1 in regulating genes like Dusp4, as discussed in

(Haddock et al., 2016), will be essential for delineating these pathways. By dissecting the transcriptional networks influenced by these factors during muscle atrophy, researchers may be able to identify novel targets for intervention, ultimately contributing to advancements in treatments for age-related and disease-induced muscular degeneration, thereby enhancing the quality of life for affected individuals. Finally, embracing interdisciplinary collaboration among researchers specializing in biomechanics, genetic engineering, and regenerative medicine will be critical in shaping the future of limb and skeletal research. By fostering dialogue and cooperation across these diverse fields, innovative strategies could emerge that synergize anatomical insights with cutting-edge technologies. For instance, applications of CRISPR-Cas9 gene editing have the potential to correct genetic defects associated with skeletal disorders, while advancements in 3D bioprinting could lead to more effective tissue engineering solutions for limb regeneration. The combination of genetics and biomechanics is especially pertinent for understanding not just the structural but also the functional implications of mutations or injuries in the skeletal system. As such, the trajectory of future research should embrace an integrative approach, ensuring that progress in limb and skeletal development is holistically achieved.

SUMMARY

The complex processes involved in limb and skeletal formation expose the depth of the relationship between genetic inputs and phenotypic results. Recent advances, for example, in the study of acromesomelic dysplasia associated with the BMPR1B gene, demonstrate how certain genetic mutations can lead to marked skeletal deformities, such as brachydactyly and postaxial polydactyly. This case illustrates the diversity of skeletal phenotypes and indicates the necessity for ongoing genetic research in the study of the complete range of osteochondrodysplasias. The capability to connect genetic results with clinical presentations not only increases our understanding of limb development but also provides opportunities for potential therapeutic treatments aimed at these genetic diseases, the way forward for better patient care and outcomes in individuals suffering from such disorders (Ibrahim et al., 2024). In addition, the significance of early orthodontic treatment at the most critical phases of skeletal growth, as observed in children with mixed dentition, cannot be overemphasized. Interceptive orthodontics provides a preventive strategy through which meaningful improvements in dental position and general skeletal relationship can be achieved. Research shows that prompt orthodontic treatment can result in a notable decrease in overjet and improvement in occlusion, promoting better dental growth. This not only illustrates the importance of intervention during formative years but also reinforces the notion that the timing of treatment can significantly influence long-term skeletal and dental health (Sandhu et al., 2024). By addressing these developmental issues proactively, clinicians can mitigate more severe complications that could arise from untreated malocclusions, emphasizing the critical role of timely interventions in skeletal development. Finally, the integration of genetic studies and clinical practice offers a holistic approach towards understanding limb and skeletal development. Inasmuch as the interaction between genetics and environmental factors is further unraveled, specialists in the field need to continue in their guard against a one-dimension approach to diagnosis and treatment. The implications of the findings on BMPR1B-related conditions and the advantages of interceptive orthodontics ought to form the cornerstones of future research and clinical practice guidelines. Through the implementation of genetic knowledge along with evidence-based orthodontics, healthcare practitioners can more effectively address the issues raised by skeletal anomalies and ensure optimal development results. This integrative approach will not only improve outcomes for individual patients but could also lead to a more comprehensive understanding of skeletal development, ultimately refining the quality of care provided within this specialist discipline (Ibrahim et al., 2024; Sandhu et al., 2024).

The formation of limbs and skeletal features is regulated by a myriad of biological processes and environmental stresses. Central discussions suggest the complex interaction between genetics and environmental stresses in influencing skeletal morphology. Studies show that during early life, the microbiota is very critical in determining developmental pathways, affecting aspects of health and neurological functions. Disturbances at this point, due to influences such as infection or poor diet, can have permanent effects on skeletal growth and function, highlighting the necessity for a multidisciplinary approach in understanding the development of the skeleton. Data indicate that microbial metabolites affect bone growth and density patterns, an idea that opens the door to further investigation of the gut-microbiota-skeletal axis as a regulatory process in skeletal biology (John et al., 2019). Furthermore, the bioarcheological past reveals how human remains become critical data in the understanding of the tempo and mode of skeletal development across thousands of years. The contribution of skeletal work in archaeology has changed over time, with greater emphasis on the contextual influences of diet, culture, and mobility on anatomical differences. Preferably, developments in the subject have moved away from typological divisions towards an integrative framework that explores the aggregated record of a person's life history as expressed in their bones. This view discloses valuable observations on how environmental and social influences impact skeletal adaptation, robustness, and diversity between populations. The use of multidisciplinary techniques in bioarcheology, such as genetic and isotopic analysis, has enriched our knowledge on the intricate relationship between biological principles and life choices in terms of skeletal formation (Larsen, 2018). Additionally, the continued investigation of limb and skeletal formation has far-reaching implications for current anthropology and medical research. The dynamic quality of bone, as confirmed by new research, suggests that morphology of bone is not a static condition but a result of ongoing adaptation to mechanical and environmental forces. It has implications for understanding mechanisms that can translate into clinical practice for the management of bone health, osteoporosis, and other skeletal conditions. As we continue to refine our understanding of the interactions between behavior and biology in the growth of skeletons, subsequent research will continue to aim towards converging knowledge from multiple fields to clarify the complex processes that shape the growth of limbs and bones. The possibility of identifying microbial connections and other biocultural contributors holds the potential to inform further understanding of the development of the skeletal systems and its implications for human health and evolution more generally (John et al., 2019).

CLOSER LOOK

SARCOPENIA

Sarcopenia is a generalized and progressive skeletal muscle disease with loss of muscle mass, strength, and function, which is mainly related to aging. It is a key element of frailty syndrome in older people and markedly increases the risk of falls, fractures, physical disability, and loss of autonomy. While long considered a natural consequence of aging, sarcopenia is now understood to be an intricate condition determined by numerous factors, such as physical inactivity, poor nutrition (particularly protein and vitamin D deficiencies), chronic illness, inflammation, hormonal alterations, and neural degeneration. The loss of muscle mass usually starts in the fourth decade of life and becomes more pronounced after 60 years of age. Sarcopenia may be primary, age-related, or secondary if it occurs due to other reasons like chronic disease, malnutrition, or physical inactivity.

Sarcopenia pathophysiology entails muscle protein synthesis versus degradation imbalance. With aging, anabolic resistance occurs, which reflects muscles' decreased sensitivity to growth stimuli like exercise and dietary protein. Additionally, mitochondrial impairment, oxidative stress, chronic low-grade inflammation (inflammaging), and hormonal losses (such as testosterone, estrogen, and growth hormone) also lead to muscle catabolism. Neuro-muscular junction deterioration and motor neuron loss further compromise muscle regeneration and coordination. Clinical diagnosis of sarcopenia usually depends on criteria given by organizations such as the European Working Group on Sarcopenia in Older People (EWGSOP), consisting of quantitative measures of muscle strength (e.g., handgrip strength), muscle quantity or quality (e.g., through DXA or MRI), and functional performance (e.g., gait speed or chair stand test).

Prevention and treatment of sarcopenia are multi-faceted. Resistance training is the foundation of therapy since it has been demonstrated to induce significant gains in muscle strength and mass in older individuals. Exercise combined with sufficient protein intake—particularly leucine-dense sources—augments anabolic response. Recommendations are frequently that for older individuals' protein intake should be 1.0–1.2 grams per kilogram of body weight daily, more than the usual recommendation. Vitamin D supplementation might also aid in the maintenance of muscle function, especially in those who are deficient. Pharmacologic treatments, including hormone replacement therapy and myostatin inhibitors, are under investigation but are not currently in standard use because of a lack of good evidence and associated side effects.

As populations globally age, sarcopenia is increasingly posing a public health problem. Not only does it impact individuals' quality of life but also burdens health systems with greater hospitalization, rehabilitation requirements, and long-term care. Early detection and preventive management are essential. Regular screening of sarcopenia among older adults, particularly at risk due to chronic diseases, immobility, or malnutrition, may facilitate early intervention. With proper lifestyle changes, most importantly in the form of physical activity and nutritional status, development of sarcopenia can be delayed, and functional independence can be maintained. Further research is needed to unravel the pathogenesis of sarcopenia and evolve specific therapies to effectively address this disabling condition.

REFERENCES

1. Abdelrazek, I. M., Knaus, A., Javanmardi, B., Krawitz, P., Horn, D., Abdalla, E. M., & Kumar, S. (2024). Acromesomelic dysplasia with homozygosity for a likely pathogenic BMPR1B variant: Postaxial polydactyly as a novel clinical finding. *Molecular Genetics & Genomic Medicine, 12*. https://www.semanticscholar.org/paper/9f0748577d1cc5f01f4ddf24bae061ead0b6e00d (accessed on 27 May 2025).

2. Aerts, P., Ayuso, M., Prims, S., Van Cruchten, K., et al. (2019). Does intrauterine crowding affect the force generating capacity and muscle composition of the piglet front limb? https://core.ac.uk/download/287940318.pdf (accessed on 27 May 2025).

3. Alessio, E., Bertoli, A., Buson, L., Cagnin, A., et al. (2019). Single cell analysis reveals the involvement of the long non-coding RNA Pvt1 in the modulation of muscle atrophy and mitochondrial network. https://core.ac.uk/download/185556788.pdf (accessed on 27 May 2025).

4. Almubarak, A., Zhang, Q., Zhang, C. H., Abdelwahab, N., Kume, T., Lassar, A. B., & Berry, F. B. (2024). FOXC1 and FOXC2 regulate growth plate chondrocyte maturation towards hypertrophy in the embryonic mouse limb skeleton. *Development (Cambridge, England), 151*. https://www.semanticscholar.org/paper/65a1a035953b06011c48871a487aa5389601d8a5 (accessed on 27 May 2025).

5. Augoyard, M., Zanolli, C., Profico, A., Thibeault, A., Cazenave, M., Oettlé, A., Abbé, E. N. L., et al. (2025). Exploration of the covariation signal between cortical bone and dentine volumes across the upper limb bones and anterior teeth in modern humans and relevance to evolutionary anthropology. *Journal of Anatomy*. https://www.semanticscholar.org/paper/ea00fd7f282bfe527d84b9fb8bf7ada2620d7d47 (accessed on 27 May 2025).

6. Beck-Nielsen, S., Greggio, N. A., & Hagenäs, L. (2021). Defining a growing and maturing skeleton and its relevance in diseases that affect skeletal growth, such as X-linked hypophosphatemia (XLH). *International Journal of Rare Diseases & Disorders*. https://www.semanticscholar.org/paper/7173c8fff329379ccf7a7cf143b834093e2033cc (accessed on 27 May 2025).

7. Beermann, J., Piccoli, M. T., Viereck, J., & Thum, T. (2016). Non-coding RNAs in development and disease: Background, mechanisms, and therapeutic approaches. *Physiological Reviews, 96*, 1297–1325. https://doi.org/10.1152/physrev.00041.2015.

8. Blackburn, D. C., Hanken, J., & Kerney, R. R. (2018). Early limb patterning in the direct-developing salamander *Plethodon cinereus* revealed by *Sox9* and *Col2a1*. https://core.ac.uk/download/214067168.pdf (accessed on 27 May 2025).

9. Blumer, M. (2021). Bone tissue and histological and molecular events during development of the long bones. *Annals of Anatomy–Anatomischer Anzeiger, 235*, 151704. https://doi.org/10.1016/j.aanat.2021.151704.

10. Bogin, B., Varea, C., Hermanussen, M., & Scheffler, C. (2018). Human life course biology: A centennial perspective of scholarship on the human pattern of physical growth and its place in human biocultural evolution. *American Journal of Physical Anthropology, 165*, 834–854. https://doi.org/10.1002/ajpa.23357.

11. Braden, R. L., Christman, K. L., Dzieciatkowska, M., Elhag, A., et al. (2016). Extracellular matrix hydrogel promotes tissue remodeling, astrogenesis, and perfusion in a rat hindlimb

ischemia model. https://core.ac.uk/download/323065138.pdf (accessed on 27 May 2025).

12. Bull, F., Al-Ansari, S. S., Biddle, S., Borodulin, K., Buman, M. P., Cardon, G., Carty, C., et al. (2020). World Health Organization 2020 guidelines on physical activity and sedentary behavior. *British Journal of Sports Medicine, 54*, 1451–1462. https://doi.org/10.1136/bjsports-2020-102955.
13. Chakkalakal, S. A., Zhang, D., Culbert, A. L., Convente, M. R., Caron, R., Wright, A. C., Maidment, A. D. A., et al. (2012). An *Acvr1* R206H knock-in mouse has fibrodysplasia ossificans progressive. *Journal of Bone and Mineral Research, 27*, 1746–1756. https://doi.org/10.1002/jbmr.1637.
14. Chan, D. Y. S., Chong, T. T., Gan, J., & Hausenloy, D., et al. (2023). Multi-modality imaging of atheromatous plaques in peripheral arterial disease: Integrating molecular and imaging markers. https://core.ac.uk/download/573841607.pdf (accessed on 27 May 2025).
15. Cryan, J. F., O'Riordan, K. J., Cowan, C. S. M., Sandhu, K. V., Bastiaanssen, T. F. S., Boehme, M., Codagnone, M. G., et al. (2019). The microbiota-gut-brain axis. *Physiological Reviews, 99*, 1877–2013. https://doi.org/10.1152/physrev.00018.2018.
16. Esteve-Altava, B., Villmoare, B., Rolian, C., et al. (2018). First anatomical network analysis of fore- and hindlimb musculoskeletal modularity in bonobos, common chimpanzees, and humans. https://core.ac.uk/download/157769144.pdf (accessed on 27 May 2025).
17. Feng, B., & Zhao, Y. (2025). Development of techniques for measuring lower limb flexibility in the elderly. *AHFE International*. https://www.semanticscholar.org/paper/238b9d82bab5f95d082958957fc78e2011789a0e (accessed on 27 May 2025).
18. Fiorott, M. A. R., Neto, J. S., Eller, L. M., Coelho, I. B., Scarpat, E. D., Pinheiro, A. S., Silva, I. A. P., et al. (2024). Advances in orthopedic surgery. *Health and Society*. https://www.semanticscholar.org/paper/257316dea03869232d4ef346d6947492d96eb328 (accessed on 27 May 2025).
19. Gao, Y., Hossain, M. N., Zhao, L., deAvila, J., Law, N. C., Zhu, M. J., Murdoch, G. K., et al. (2024). Spatial transcriptomics analysis: Maternal obesity impairs myogenic cell migration and differentiation during embryonic limb development. *International Journal of Molecular Sciences, 25*. https://www.semanticscholar.org/paper/6b594a7c22610afb85c9c94ca05ba39091fe1452 (accessed on 27 May 2025).
20. Goswami, A., Porto, A., Leroi, A. M., Esteve-Altava, B., et al. (2015). Anatomical network comparison of human upper and lower, newborn and adult, and normal and abnormal limbs, with notes on development, pathology and limb serial homology vs. homoplasy. https://core.ac.uk/download/36779022.pdf (accessed on 27 May 2025).
21. Grässel, S. (2014). The role of peripheral nerve fibers and their neurotransmitters in cartilage and bone physiology and pathophysiology. *Arthritis Research & Therapy, 16*. https://doi.org/10.1186/s13075-014-0485-1.
22. Gwozdzinski, L., Pieniazek, A., & Gwozdzinski, K. (2024). Factors influencing venous remodeling in the development of varicose veins of the lower limbs. *International Journal of Molecular Sciences, 25*. https://www.semanticscholar.org/paper/b4776f733408906846e1c3be8e517253c226947c (accessed on 27 May 2025).
23. Haddock, A. N. (2016). Transcriptional regulation of dual-specificity phosphatase 4 (Dusp4) by muscle RING finger 1 (MuRF1) and myogenic regulatory factors. https://core.ac.uk/download/71998703.pdf (accessed on 27 May 2025).

24. Heinonen, A., Leblanc, A. D., Nilsson, A. E. U., Cassell, C., Riddoch, C. J., Craig, C. L., Slemenda, C. W., et al. (2011). Decrease of physical activity level in adolescents with limb fractures: An accelerometry-based activity monitor study. https://core.ac.uk/download/pdf/8567398.pdf (accessed on 27 May 2025).

25. Herpelinck, T., Ory, L., Verbraeken, T., Nasello, G., Barzegari, M., Bolander, J., Luyten, F., et al. (2024). An integrated single-cell atlas of the limb skeleton from development through adulthood. *bioRxiv*. https://www.semanticscholar.org/paper/ac8bcd1ebf17912c6cfbd7ec07cefada0212c7b5 (accessed on 27 May 2025).

26. Hoh, J. (2023). Developmental, physiologic and phylogenetic perspectives on the expression and regulation of myosin heavy chains in mammalian skeletal muscles. *Journal of Comparative Physiology B, 193*, 355–382. https://www.semanticscholar.org/paper/9d1a53041a05c01fcba22369fe9d34a61df52d7b (accessed on 27 May 2025).

27. Hootnick, D. R., & Vargesson, N. (2017). Arterial dysgenesis and limb defects: Clinical and experimental examples. https://core.ac.uk/download/131024852.pdf (accessed on 27 May 2025).

28. James, S. L., Abate, D., Abate, K. H., Abay, S. M., Abbafati, C., Abbasi, N., Abbastabar, H., et al. (2018). Global, regional, and national incidence, prevalence, and years lived with disability for 354 diseases and injuries for 195 countries and territories, 1990–2017: A systematic analysis for the Global Burden of Disease Study 2017. *The Lancet, 392*, 1789–1858. https://doi.org/10.1016/s0140-6736(18)32279-7.

29. Jędrzejewska-Rzezak, P. (2025). Advances in the treatment of achondroplasia. *Journal of Education, Health and Sport*. https://www.semanticscholar.org/paper/da18823513a82e8c53cbca5a6917668183c77234 (accessed on 27 May 2025).

30. Kim, S. E., Nechipurenko, I., & Christensen, S. (2023). Editorial: Signaling by primary cilia in development and disease. *Frontiers in Cell and Developmental Biology, 11*. https://www.semanticscholar.org/paper/a50cb3d67f5970d4c43a5dd6b10f7b1a2c6d324c (accessed on 27 May 2025).

31. Kokoba, E. G. (2024). Temporal dynamics of the morphological characteristics of the Abkhazian children and adolescents in changing living conditions of the population. *Moscow University Anthropology Bulletin*. https://www.semanticscholar.org/paper/644cd7889abbda51a16531a06982124051c31999 (accessed on 27 May 2025).

32. Larsen, C. S. (2018). Bioarcheology in perspective: From classifications of the dead to conditions of the living. *American Journal of Physical Anthropology, 165*, 865–878. https://doi.org/10.1002/ajpa.23322.

33. Larsson, L., Degens, H., Li, M., Salviati, L., Lee, Y. I., Thompson, W. J., Kirkland, J. L., et al. (2018). Sarcopenia: Aging-related loss of muscle mass and function. *Physiological Reviews, 99*, 427–511. https://doi.org/10.1152/physrev.00061.2017.

34. Littner, M. (2011). Chronic obstructive pulmonary disease. *Annals of Internal Medicine, 154*(ITC4-1). https://www.semanticscholar.org/paper/5aa67d7bb2e620d8dbd73f653546d96999c1d93e (accessed on 27 May 2025).

35. McGovern, M. M., Avetisyan, R., Sanson, B.-J., & Lidove, O. (2017). Disease manifestations and burden of illness in patients with acid sphingomyelinase deficiency (ASMD). *Orphanet Journal of Rare Diseases, 12*, Article 57. https://doi.org/10.1186/s13023-017-0572-x.

36. Myers, S. J., Knight, R. L., Wardle, S., Waldock, K. A., O'Leary, T. J., Jones, R., Muckelt, P. E., et al. (2024). Effect of menstrual cycle and hormonal contraception on musculoskeletal health and performance: Protocol for a prospective cohort design and cross-sectional comparison. *JMIR Research Protocols, 13*. https://www.semanticscholar.org/paper/2a1c3f27083680d9535b4ed44a9e2ae2358d92f8 (accessed on 27 May 2025).

37. Parsha, R., & Kota, S. (2024). Elavl1 is dispensable for appendicular skeletal development. *bioRxiv*. https://www.semanticscholar.org/paper/45ad25c557949836c20b64c6010092d1f59dfa98 (accessed on 27 May 2025).

38. Picard, B., & Gagaoua, M. (2020). Muscle fiber properties in cattle and their relationships with meat qualities: An overview. *Journal of Agricultural and Food Chemistry, 68*, 6021–6039. https://doi.org/10.1021/acs.jafc.0c02086 (accessed on 27 May 2025).

39. Qiu, F., & Kong, X. (2023). Analysis of related factors in patients with Parkinson's disease and osteoporosis. *International Journal of Science and Engineering Applications*. https://www.semanticscholar.org/paper/52ef83ee1d0f2e16399f8102c22dc5db945947e2 (accessed on 27 May 2025).

40. Rigueur, D., Lopez, N., & Lyons, K. (2021). A requirement for STAT3 in limb development. *The FASEB Journal, 35*. https://www.semanticscholar.org/paper/fe3aa2f5532ae349e4000cff319c3292a5e12228 (accessed on 27 May 2025).

41. Rivera, Z. C., González-Seguel, F., Horikawa-Strakovsky, A., Granger, C., Sarwal, A., Dhar, S., Ntoumenopoulos, G., et al. (2025). Development of an artificial intelligence powered software for automated analysis of skeletal muscle ultrasonography. *Scientific Reports, 15*(1), 14936. https://www.semanticscholar.org/paper/0a649b6a05de858dc2e026c8115a74a2767ef913 (accessed on 27 May 2025).

42. Roalf, D., McDonald-McGinn, D. M., Jee, J., Krall, M., Crowley, T., Moberg, P., Kohler, C., et al. (2024). Computer-vision analysis of craniofacial dysmorphology in 22q11.2 deletion syndrome and psychosis spectrum disorders. *Journal of Neurodevelopmental Disorders, 16*. https://www.semanticscholar.org/paper/b8d248a58d114d4451242d7a13d0ce5420c1ad26 (accessed on 27 May 2025).

43. Ruff, C., Junno, J. A., Burgess, M., Canington, S. L., Harper, C. M., Mudakikwa, A. B., & McFarlin, S. (2021). Body proportions and environmental adaptation in gorillas. *American Journal of Biological Anthropology, 177*(3), 501–529. https://www.semanticscholar.org/paper/47a1c93009c3a1d9f3aa7ea3361daae501446b1a (accessed on 27 May 2025).

44. Rux, D., Song, J. Y., Pineault, K. M., Mandair, G. S., Swinehart, I. T., Schlientz, A. J., Garthus, K. N., et al. (2017). *Hox11* function is required for region-specific fracture repair. *Journal of Bone and Mineral Research, 32*, 1750–1760. https://doi.org/10.1002/jbmr.3166.

45. Sánchez–Fernández, C., Lorda-Diez, C. I., García-Porrero, J. A., Montero, J. A., & Hurlé, J. M. (2019). UHRF genes regulate programmed interdigital tissue regression and chondrogenesis in the embryonic limb. *Cell Death and Disease, 10*. https://doi.org/10.1038/s41419-019-1575-4.

46. Sandhu, A., Sakaria, B. A., Patel, S. D., Ahuja, G., Jadeja, N., Mehta, A., & Kakkad, D. (2024). The impact of early orthodontic intervention on dental and skeletal development in children with mixed dentition. *Journal of Pharmacy & Bioallied Sciences, 16*, S818–S820. https://www.semanticscholar.org/paper/6046fed693706c40ff78db60c269ba0c63b90c8d (accessed on 27 May 2025).

47. Sekine, S., Mayama, S., Nishijima, N., Kojima, T., Endo-Takahashi, Y., Ishii, Y., Shiono, H., et al. (2023). Development of a gene and nucleic acid delivery system for skeletal muscle administration via limb perfusion using nanobubbles and ultrasound. *Pharmaceutics, 15*. https://www.semanticscholar.org/paper/e915c7add0d773cdf7ba47bf871cb60b4ed946f1 (accessed on 27 May 2025).

48. Seth, A., Hicks, J. L., Uchida, T. K., Habib, A., Dembia, C. L., Dunne, J. J., Ong, C., et al. (2018). OpenSim: Simulating musculoskeletal dynamics and neuromuscular control to study human and animal movement. *PLoS Computational Biology, 14*, e1006223. https://doi.org/10.1371/journal.pcbi.1006223.

49. Shi, D. L., & Grifone, R. (2021). RNA-binding proteins in the post-transcriptional control of skeletal muscle development, regeneration and disease. *Frontiers in Cell and Developmental Biology, 9*. https://doi.org/10.3389/fcell.2021.738978.

50. To, K., Fei, L., Pett, J. P., Roberts, K., Blain, R., Polański, K., Li, T., et al. (2024). A multi-omic atlas of human embryonic skeletal development. *Nature, 635*, 657–667. https://www.semanticscholar.org/paper/e68c462466814d53da020a0c80374b22aefcca30 (accessed on 27 May 2025).

51. Ullah, A., Ullah, M. F., Khalid, Z. M., & Ahmad, W. (2016). Novel heterozygous frameshift mutation in distal-less homeobox 5 underlies isolated split hand/foot malformation type 1. *Pediatrics International, 58*. https://www.semanticscholar.org/paper/1c7b351c60e4bb3053859f09c07a5c43038acf0c (accessed on 27 May 2025).

52. Vos, T., Abajobir, A. A., Abate, K. H., Abbafati, C., Abbas, K., Abd-Allah, F., Abdulkader, R. S., et al. (2017). Global, regional, and national incidence, prevalence, and years lived with disability for 328 diseases and injuries for 195 countries, 1990–2016: A systematic analysis for the Global Burden of Disease Study 2016. *The Lancet, 390*, 1211–1259. https://doi.org/10.1016/s0140-6736(17)32154-2.

53. Wang, J., Liu, W., Zhang, T., Cui, M., Gao, K. K., Lu, P., Yao, S. Q., et al. (2025). An epitranscriptomic program maintains skeletal stem cell quiescence via a METTL3-FEM1B-GLI1 axis. *The EMBO Journal, 44*, 2263–2278. https://www.semanticscholar.org/paper/9ad157ff632336623a6d98347c8ddeb2b6b5d231 (accessed on 27 May 2025).

54. Wang, L., You, X., Ruan, D., Shao, R., Dai, H. Q., Shen, W., Xu, G. L., et al. (2022). TET enzymes regulate skeletal development through increasing chromatin accessibility of RUNX2 target genes. *Nature Communications, 13*. https://www.semanticscholar.org/paper/47262d9458a6fc365808e0a901f855d13c4382af (accessed on 27 May 2025).

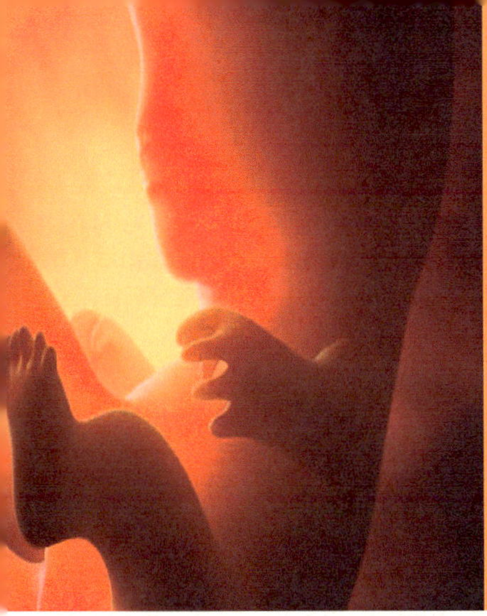

Chapter 6

GENITAL AND URINARY SYSTEM DEVELOPMENT

Contents

Introduction

Development of the genital and urinary systems is a complex and multifaceted process that is at the core of human health and involves intricate interactions among genetic, hormonal, and environmental factors. Understanding these pathways of development is not only necessary for an appreciation of normal physiology but also for the recognition of the abnormalities that result in clinical conditions. Critical stages of system development occur during embryogenesis, where the formation of the mesodermal tissues gives rise to the kidneys, ureters, and reproductive system. Management of these processes enhances insight into congenital anomalies that are capable of having a significant effect on an individual's lifestyle. Furthermore, it is important that these systems interact with each other; the function of the urinary system in homeostasis and excretion is really linked with reproduction health, as imbalances within one area affect the performance of the other, thereby emphasizing the importance of studying these fields together. The significance of understanding genital and urinary system development extends far beyond that of simple anatomical knowledge because it is of utmost significance to fetal and maternal health. Throughout pregnancy, changes in both systems not only occur normally but are essential to the successful outcome of gestation. For instance, the system of the urinary adapts to increased blood volume and metabolic needs, while the genital system must adapt to fetal growth and development.

Complications arising from such dysfunction, as evidenced in the literature for postpartum purulent-septic complications, illustrate the risk factors potentially compromising maternal mortality and shaping neonatal outcomes (Feyta et al., 2018). A preventive strategy in the foreseeing of risks and management of health implications for pregnancy relies on an overall understanding of such systems, hence the importance of research and study of this kind. In studying growth of the genital and urinary system, it is essential to consider the implications of healthcare and social factors that necessitate further inquiry. Problems like availability of prenatal care, reproductive health education, and pre-existing condition control have significant effects on the course of maternal and fetal well-being. Studies of the initiation of septic complications in the postpartum period illustrate the way that the coming together of gynecological history, extragenital pathosis, and obstetric complication can create high-risk categories that need to be addressed through targeted prevention (Feyta et al., 2018). Moreover, the contemporary evidence base for maternal health calls for an approach that integrates these biological phenomena with social determinants in order to substantially decrease morbidity and mortality. Continuing education and research efforts are essential, as they provide the foundation for creative interventions and enhanced health literacy regarding reproductive and urinary health concerns (Figure 6.1).

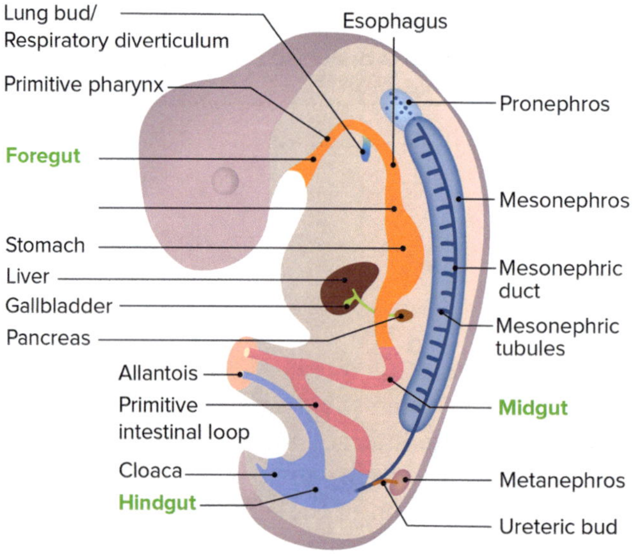

Figure 6.1. Development of the urogenital system.

Source: https://cdn.lecturio.com/assets/Developmental-location-of-the-pronephros-mesonephros-and-metanephros-in-the-developing-embryo_NEW.png.

Definition of the Genital and Urinary Systems

The urinary and genital systems, while separate in their functions, are fundamentally intertwined in the human body and commonly learned about as a unit. The genital system is tasked with reproduction and sexual differentiation, including the structures of the ovaries, testes, external genitalia, and other internal channels that guide the reproductive processes. By contrast, the urinary system is important for the elimination of waste and homeostasis, which consists mainly of the kidneys, ureters, bladder, and urethra. With their interconnected functions, any examination of human development that investigates these systems is not only necessary to examine their own properties but also how they interact and coordinate with each other during development. This mutual dependence places strong emphasis on an understanding of each system by both medicine and biology as well as by biomedical informatics, in which correct anatomical definitions are necessary for clear communication as well as adequate therapeutic procedures. Among the most important factors of determining the genital and urinary systems is to comprehend their functional and anatomical correlations. Adherence to terminological precision in anatomical and medical language is crucial because it ensures healthcare professionals are able to venture into the complexities of human anatomy successfully. For example, the *Terminologia Anatomica* is a hierarchical textbook that delimits anatomical terminology, but inconsistency in representation may lead to confusion and complexity in practice. The repercussions of such structures are more profound than simply anatomical designation; they determine our medical education strategy and affect controlled medical terminologies applied in electronic health records. The interplay between class inclusion and part-whole relationships in anatomical terms, which has been subject to analysis in research in Terminologia, emphasizes the importance of precision in designating the genital and urinary systems (Rosse et al., 2000). This level of precision is crucial in the advancement of biomedical informatics and has a direct influence on the way anatomical knowledge is structured and utilized. Other than issues regarding terminologies, spatial interrelationships between genital and urinary system anatomical structures are important in developing comprehensive biomedical ontologies. As shown by the Basic Inclusion Theory (BIT), understanding parthood and spatial relations among anatomical classes is essential to developing correct ontologies that enable automatic reasoning (Bittner et al., 2006). Formal spatial theories integrated in anatomy provide a more coherent description of anatomical knowledge and facilitate better integration of the urinary and genital systems into biomedical paradigms. By rectifying ambiguity in existing ontologies, researchers are able to standardize anatomical information more and make it interoperable, thereby augmenting its utility in clinical as well as research settings. Finally, a clear comprehension of the definitions and semantics of the genital and urinary systems is needed for informed advances in medicine that facilitate successful disease diagnosis and treatment within these critical anatomical locations (Figure 6.2).

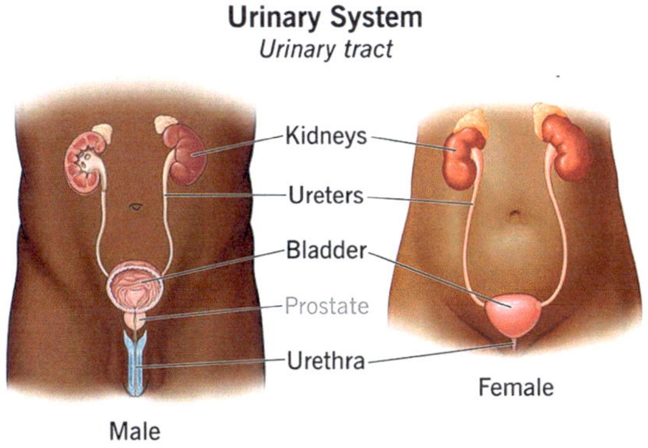

Figure 6.2. Genital and urinary systems.

Source: https://my.clevelandclinic.org/-/scassets/images/org/health/articles/21197-urinary-systems.

Importance of Studying System Development

To understand system development is valuable for many reasons, particularly in the case of urinary and genital system development. An essential reason is the ability to detect developmental defects that can be caused by environmental or hereditary factors. It aids in the detection of many disorders, which can lead to early intervention. For example, the Global Burden of Diseases, Injuries, and Risk Factors Study (GBD) illustrates how specific conditions associated with failures of systems make tremendous contributions to the rates of mortality in the entire globe (Gregory et al., 2018). This calls for immediate research on developmental processes because early detection and management of such conditions make contributions towards the enhancement of quality of life and survival rates. Therefore, the research into system development not only adds to our understanding of normal physiology but also provides healthcare professionals with the means to conduct effective diagnosis and treatment. Furthermore, a clear understanding of development of the genital and urinary system has far-reaching implications for clinical practice and public health programs. With increasing knowledge, we begin to understand the complex interplay of hormonal signaling and body shape to foster an enhanced appreciation of reproductive health and urological disease. One of the best examples of how changing knowledge is more directly translated into enhanced clinical management is the revised clinical practice guidelines for congenital adrenal hyperplasia (Speiser et al., 2018). This highlights the importance of integrating newer evidence into health systems to facilitate best patient outcomes and utilization of resources. In addition, by placing emphasis on the quest for learning during system development, future healthcare professionals will better be able to navigate the complexity of such systems, yielding a resilient healthcare setup that is responsive to emerging health challenges. Finally, system development study is significant not only for one's health but also in order to understand the overall impact on society. Abnormalities of genital and urinary system development can have some grave implications, not only for the patient diagnosed with them but also for their communities and families. An extremely exhaustive exploration of such systems will lead to the determination of environmental or social risk factors for their formation, leading to public health intervention in the manner of prevention and education. Furthermore, with the redirection of global health programs towards more individualized medicine, it is all the more important to appreciate variation in system development as a function of genetic background. This information can be utilized to support optimization of intervention in a way that interventions can be optimized among the target population. Finally, learning system development in the context of genital and urinary systems cannot be overemphasized because it forms the foundation upon which medical knowledge can be built and improved health outcomes are enhanced worldwide.

Overview of Key Developmental Stages

Genital and urinary system formation begins early on during the embryonic phase, specifically during week four of pregnancy. The formation begins with the formation of urogenital ridges, which are essential organs that form the two systems. These three sets of excretory organs form from the ridges: the pronephros, the mesonephros, and the metanephros. These phases are progressive evolutionary adaptation, with the metanephros being the adult kidney. The highly precise regulation of gene expression within these structures is necessary to allow proper development. For example, displacement from the process can lead to malformations such as renal agenesis or congenital urinary tract malformations and illustrates the delicate balance that has to be achieved during these early, critical stages of development. As pregnancy progresses into the weeks to come, differentiation by hormone becomes the key. The role of sex steroids, particularly the androgens and estrogens, becomes significant in determining the primary and secondary sexual characteristics of the developing fetus. In embryonic males, testosterone evokes the differentiation of the Wolffian ducts to other male reproductive system structures, including the epididymis and vas deferens. In contrast, female development is contingent on the lack of these androgens, in which case the Wolffian ducts degenerate and the Müllerian ducts develop into the fallopian tubes, uterus, and upper portion of the vagina.

This critical effect of hormones speaks to the intricate interplay of environment and genetics during sexual differentiation. The complexity of genital and urinary tract formation highlights the importance of learning human and animal models, above all the mouse, in this field. Investigations have established that while mouse models yield valuable insights owing to their genetic homology and developmental processes, anatomical and hormonal divergence require a careful interpretation of results. For example, although mice show a similar phenotype for some human genetic diseases, significant differences in organogenesis and hormone function must be respected to prevent false conclusions. Thus, studies should highlight those features of mouse models that can be clearly seen as having relevance to human reproductive tract development with an understanding of the limitations involved in cross-species extrapolation. Identifying these subtleties is crucial for moving forward our knowledge of normal and abnormal development of the genital and urinary systems (Baskin et al., 2019; Foster et al., 2010).

6.1. Embryonic Development of the Genital System

The complex embryonic development of the genital system is controlled by a sophisticated interaction of genetic, hormonal, and environmental influences. The genital ridges in the initial stages develop from mesodermal tissues, which serve as the platform for the development of the gonads. Testosterone and anti-Müllerian hormone, markers of the male phenotype, guide the formation of the male reproductive organs, including the epididymis and seminal vesicles, whereas their absence permits the formation of female reproductive organs. Recent progress in techniques such as light sheet fluorescence microscopy (LSFM) has shed new light on previously unappreciated details of this process, enabling investigators to witness the formation of both external and internal genitalia with clarity unrivaled by earlier approaches. This novel strategy underscores the significance of knowing the morphological transformations that take place during embryogenesis and calls for further investigation of the gene regulatory networks (GRNs) operating in the development of the genitalia. The study of model organisms consolidates the knowledge on human embryonic genital development via comparative analysis. Mice have been especially useful in this context, acting as a model for human development based on the substantial molecular and anatomical conservation between the two species. There are significant differences as well that need to be weighed with caution when taking conclusions from mouse models to human conditions. It has been found through studies that although developmental processes are conserved, the actual timing and hormonal controls can vary significantly. This disparity requires a complete examination of the confluence as well as divergence in organogenesis in the male and female reproductive tracts. It is important to comprehend these differences in order to extrapolate knowledge from animal models to human disease and create useful treatments for congenital diseases of the genitalia, according to research on the importance of both mouse and human reproductive tract development (Baskin et al., 2019). Recent research in LSFM has also added depth to the knowledge of formation in the human fetal genital system, giving insights into tissue dynamics and protein localization. The method makes imaging at high resolution of previously inaccessible developmental stages possible, thus building high-resolution three-dimensional models of the embryonic urogenital system. The technique employed in these studies includes meticulous preparation, clearance, immunostaining, and imaging of human fetal material, which may reveal crucial interactions between forming tissues. As a result, researchers have begun to reconstruct the complex story of how external and internal genitalia form during embryogenesis. This data not only furthers scientific understanding but also informs clinical practices in reproductive health and birth defects (Baskin et al., 2020). By applying frontier imaging technologies to developmental biology, the field stands to develop an even richer, more nuanced appreciation of the development of human genital and urinary tracts (Figure 6.3).

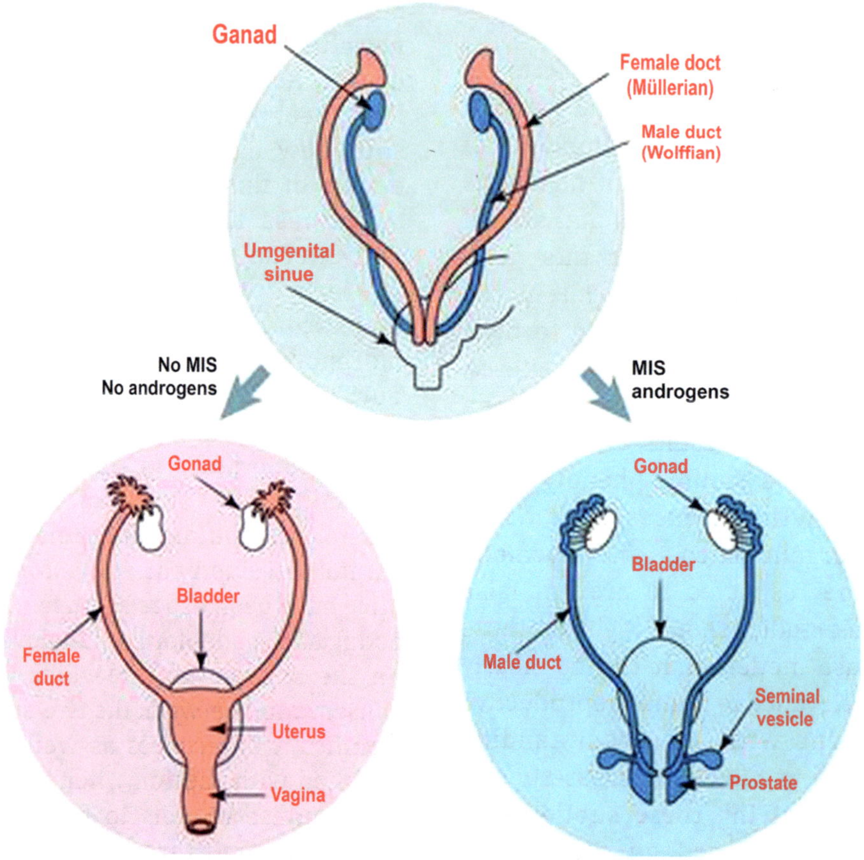

Figure 6.3. Development of reproductive systems at the embryo stage.

Source: https://static.cambridge.org/binary/version/id/urn:cambridge.org:id:binary-alt:20210224074621-20686-mediumThumb-74438fig1_1.jpg?pub-status=live.

6.1.1. Formation of the Gonads

Formation of the gonads is a very important part of genital and urinary system development, which requires complex genetic and hormonal interactions during stages of embryonic growth. The bipotential gonads form first from the intermediate mesoderm of the early embryo and provide sexual differentiation. A presence of the SRY gene on the Y chromosome is necessary for the development of the male gonads. This gene leads to the development of indifferent gonads into testes, which then produce hormones required for male phenotypic traits. However, the lack of this gene leads to the formation of ovaries, and it directs the process towards female sexual differentiation. Therefore, the SRY gene is a master switch in sex determination of the embryo, with a well-defined biochemical pathway underlying the development of the gonads. In addition, the hormonal milieu is also a strong force in gonadal development. During male embryos, testosterone secretion by the embryonic testes is essential for masculinizing external genitalia and forming internal sex organs. This involves the conversion of testosterone into dihydrotestosterone (DHT), which helps in the differentiation of male tissues. In contrast, during female development, the lack of these male hormones results in the development of female reproductive structures in a process that is fairly passive.

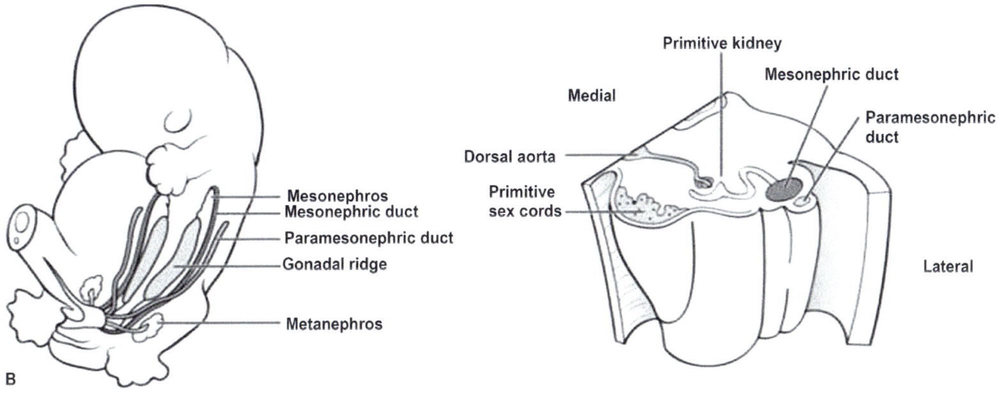

Figure 6.4. Genetic basis of gonadal and genital development.

Source: https://oncohemakey.com/wp-content/uploads/2017/01/B9781416055839001180_f1b.jpg.

Recent developments in the understanding of ovarian development have shown that estradiol and other related hormones, whilst being produced to a lesser degree during this period, are just as critical in determining the female phenotype. This illustrates that although the pathways branch, both hormonal impacts are equally crucial for successful gonadal development. In more intricate organisms, like mammals, intricacies in gonadal development can complicate our comprehension further. Investigations have revealed alternate routes of androgen manufacture, specifically in species like marsupials, which indicate more than one pathway to affecting sexual differentiation and gonadal evolution. The identification of novel androgens in the different hyperandrogenic disorders suggests that the interruption of these processes can result in rather substantial sexual development abnormalities. For example, research across a number of species, including the shortnose green eye, has investigated gonadal anatomy and reproductive tactics, demonstrating that taxa may engage in disparate developmental paths. These studies reinforce the importance of learning about both the hormonal and genetic control systems of gonad development, since these are important not just for general biological knowledge but also for regulating species populations and solving reproductive disease in human and veterinary medicine (Figure 6.4).

6.1.2. Differentiation of Male and Female Reproductive Systems

Male and female reproductive system differentiation is an extremely intricate process beginning in embryonic life and influenced by genetic, hormonal, and environmental factors. Both sexes have a shared set of structures initially, such as indifferent gonads, which can differentiate into testes or ovaries based on signals provided by genes. The SRY gene's presence on the Y chromosome triggers testis formation, leading to the production of testosterone and anti-Müllerian hormone (AMH). Male hormones stimulate male reproductive organs to develop while simultaneously stimulating the regression of the Müllerian ducts, which would otherwise develop female reproductive organs. This intricate balance of the diagram shows how chromosomal diversity leads to various anatomical implications, predisposing the ultimate morphogenetic differentiation of the male and female reproductive system by a series of developmental events critical for subsequent reproductive functions.

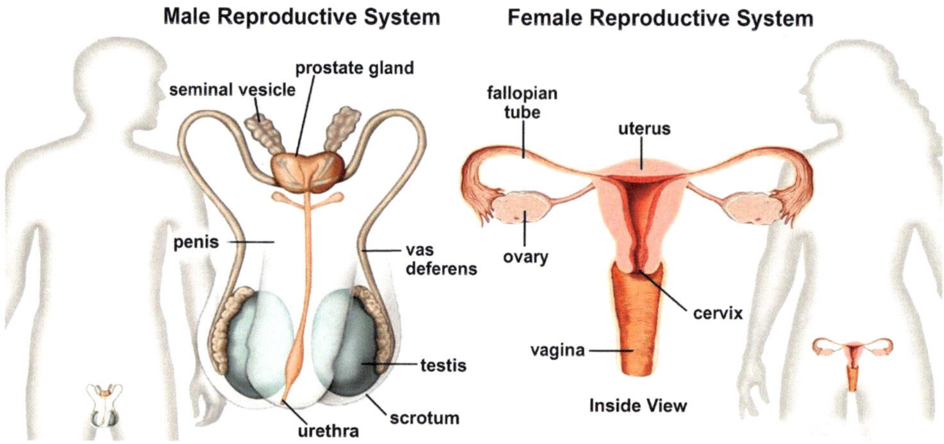

Figure 6.5. Differentiation of male and female reproductive systems.

Source: https://cdn.britannica.com/31/94931-050-41A3B5F4/females-puberty-organs-hormones-males-reproduction-egg.jpg.

As growth unfolds, the differentiating processes become more distinct, with substantial anatomical transformation in both male and female embryos. The differentiation of Wolffian ducts to epididymis, vas deferens, and seminal vesicles in males happens due to testosterone, establishing their role in the male reproductive system. On the other hand, the absence of testosterone in females allows for the continuance of Müllerian ducts to form major structures like the fallopian tubes, the uterus, and the upper two-thirds of the vagina. This disparity underscores the role of hormones in the development of reproductive anatomy, pointing out the impact of steroids in determining the internal structures that are involved in reproduction. This developmental specificity not only points to evolutionary concessions but also to pivotal information regarding congenital defects developing when these processes are impaired. Advances in imaging technologies, especially LSFM, in recent times have transformed the exploration of human genital development to enable scientists to directly visualize the anatomical changes during pivotal embryonic stages. The cutting-edge method achieves high-resolution observations of the spatial and temporal dynamics of the urogenital systems, including the developing external and internal genitalia, as well as the kidneys. Through the clarification of the interactions between differentiation signals and tissue morphogenesis, LSFM has enabled pioneering research into protein localization and structural organization in such systems. Additionally, comprehension of such processes gives a basis for tackling developmental disorders since aberrations in the normal differentiation pathways may lead to developmental abnormalities like hypospadias or ambiguous genitalia. The continuous convergence of high-end imaging techniques into developmental biology represents the possibility for greater understanding of reproductive system differentiation and its relevance to disease and health (Acien et al., 2017; Baskin et al., 2020) (Figure 6.5).

6.1.3. Role of Sex Chromosomes in Development

The sex chromosomes' role in development is also pivotal in determining how the genital and urinary systems develop. For mammals, the presence of the Y chromosome is generally responsible for starting male sexual differentiation through the action of the SRY gene. This gene initiates testes formation, which further leads to the production of male hormones such as testosterone. Testosterone is required for masculinization of the external genitalia and formation of male internal structures, including the vas deferens and seminal vesicles. The lack of the Y chromosome tends to result in the formation of female characteristics, where the default pathway provides for the development of female anatomical structures. Therefore, the interaction between genetic information on sex chromosomes and hormonal effect deeply influences reproductive system formation. Additional intricacies stem from findings of sexual differentiation alternative pathways, as underscored by recent studies. Although traditional wisdom suggests that male genitalia need direct contact with androgenic substances, recent evidence reveals a backdoor androgen formation pathway, especially common in marsupials. In humans, abnormalities of this pathway may cause conditions of sexual development, including congenital adrenal hyperplasia (CAH) and disorders of sex development (DSD). Backdoor steroids, such as androsterone, are mainly of placental progesterone metabolism in non-testicular tissues, as do recent studies. These results indicate that biochemical pathway variations contribute importantly to establishing sexual phenotypes, consonant with the dynamic interactions among genetic profile and hormonal cues in genital development. Shaughnessy and co-researchers delineated this complex interplay, giving impetus to understanding the etiology of sexual development disorders. The implications of sex chromosome function modification pertain to diseases linked to DSD, which includes a variety of intersex variations. These disorders usually arise due to unusual chromosomal pairings, gene mutations, or endocrine imbalances at critical periods of fetal growth. Knowledge of the role of sex chromosomes is most important here, as it determines clinical strategies for diagnosis and possible therapeutic measures. Genetic and hormonal analysis, for example, may determine treatment, which might reduce the psychosocial consequence of the condition. Second, the intricacy of DSD suggests that educating practitioners and the general public about the biological complexity of sex development is a pressing need. Such realization goes beyond simple biological categorizations, where individuals with differences in sex development need to be treated with a holistic care approach that values the person's identity (Davies et al., 2023). With ongoing research, it is still important to have an integrative concept of how genetics, hormones, and their interplay affect development of the genital and urinary systems (Figure 6.6).

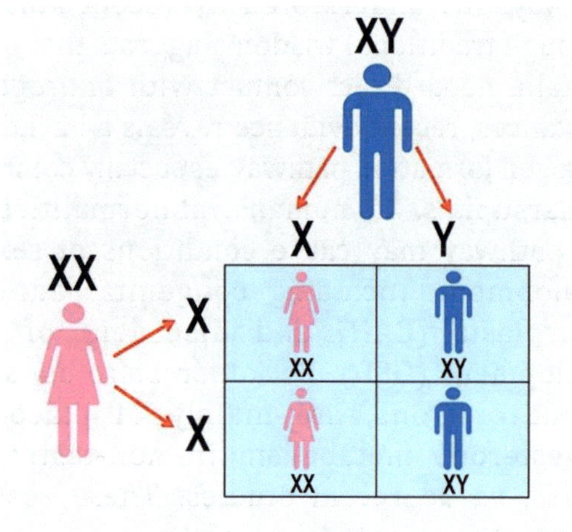

Figure 6.6. Role of sex chromosomes in development.

Source: https://cdn.storymd.com/optimized/Nq4yKbmS7A/thumbnail.webp.

6.2. Embryonic Development of the Urinary System

The embryonic growth of the urinary system is a sophisticated process that requires synergistic coordination of genetic and environmental cues. It starts in the third week of pregnancy with the development of the mesonephric kidney, or Wolffian body, which is a temporary excretory organ. As growth continues, the definitive kidney, or metanephros, becomes functional by the fifth week. The metanephros arises from the metanephric mesenchyme and the ureteric bud and interacts with each other through mutual signaling pathways. These interactions are essential for the normal branching and development of the ureteric bud, which subsequently gives rise to the renal collecting system. Appreciation of these initial developmental milestones underscores the complexities of the formation of the urinary system, and shows how interruptions can result in congenital anomalies, like renal agenesis or ectopic kidneys, which are important clinical problems in pediatric urology. Besides genetic factors, the contribution of hormonal factors to urinary system development cannot be overemphasized. In particular, the interaction of sex hormones with the developing urinary and genital organs is critical. Murine model research demonstrates how androgens can impact urinary tract anatomy and function, on both kidney development and ureter development. Although the mouse model is useful, researchers caution that proper knowledge of mouse vs. human embryonic development must be understood to avoid invalid extrapolations. In particular, significant anatomical and developmental differences require extreme care when employing rodent models to make inferences about human urinary system development (Baskin et al., 2019). Awareness of these differences is essential to further our knowledge and therapy of urinary system disorders that can occur during embryogenesis. New technology, especially in imaging methods, has greatly improved our insight into urinary system development. Three-dimensional (3D) reconstruction methods, including LSFM, enable high-resolution visualization of forming human fetal structures, including the urinary tract and kidneys, at previously unachievable resolutions. This approach provides researchers with the ability to examine the dynamic organ development processes in a manner not possible before. The use of LSFM to fetal specimens offers great insights into the detail of organogenesis and changes in the shape of organs during critical stages of development (Baskin et al., 2020). In addition, this technology is not only useful for identifying normal development but also supports the investigation of pathological states that may arise during this critical phase. As such, improved imaging techniques are central to expanding our understanding of normal and abnormal urinary system formation (Figure 6.7).

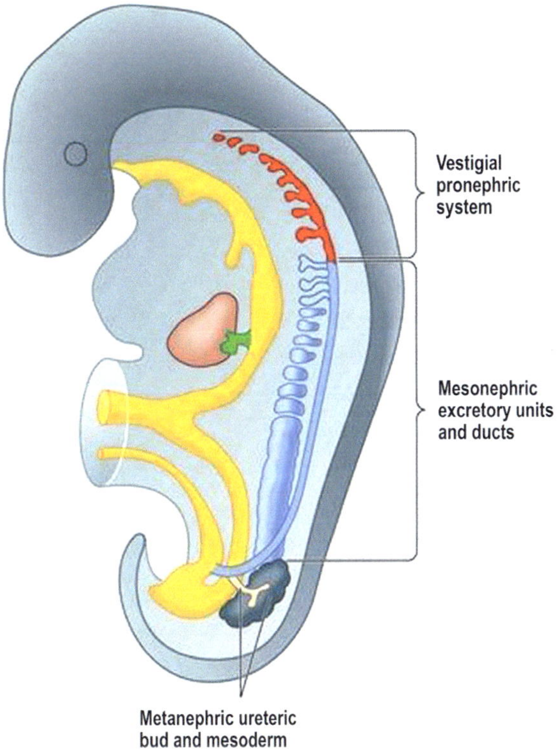

Figure 6.7. Embryonic development of the urinary system.

Source: https://static.cambridge.org/binary/version/id/urn:cambridge.org:id:binary-alt:20180930192054-94155-mediumThumb-66713fig12_2.jpg?pub-status=live.

6.2.1. Formation of the Kidneys

Kidney development is an essential process of the genital and urinary system formation comprising a series of complex embryological processes. Early on, the nephric structures derive from the mesoderm in the first couple of weeks of pregnancy. The development begins with the emergence of the pronephros, a temporary and primitive structure developing into the mesonephros. This second phase, the mesonephros, is a temporary function of filtration and is central to the origin of the permanent kidneys called the metanephros. The metanephros starts developing by the fifth week of pregnancy, eventually giving rise to the working kidneys that develop by the end of the first trimester. The passage through these stages depicts the intricate coordination of embryonic development that establishes the foundation for the renal apparatus, which takes a key role in homeostasis once functional. As the kidneys form from the metanephric blastema, key interactions between the ureteric bud and underlying mesenchyme direct the morphologic and functional differentiation of the kidneys. The ureteric bud arises from the Wolffian duct and grows out into the metanephric mesenchyme, and it goes on to cause a cascade of branching processes that form the renal collecting system. These mesenchymal-epithelial interactions are regulated through significant signaling pathways, some of which include fibroblast growth factors (FGF), bone morphogenetic proteins (BMP), and transforming growth factor-beta (TGF-β). These signaling molecules play a pivotal role in facilitating structural arrangement and differentiation in the developing kidneys. Moreover, disturbances in these signal processes can lead to congenital malformations or defects in the kidney development function, and this emphasizes the importance of the precise regulation of such interactions in embryogenesis. The use of novel imaging methods, including LSFM, has dramatically changed our views of the developmental morphology of kidneys during embryonic life. This approach enables researchers to see the complex dynamics of kidney development in three-dimensional space and gain insights into protein localization and tissue architecture. With the application of LSFM to study human fetal tissues, researchers have been able to trace the developmental path of the renal system with an unprecedented level of precision. Such a study not only advances our knowledge of the normal development of the kidney but also has implications in identifying aberrations that lead to developmental abnormalities. With our investigative methods for examining human urogenital development evolving with increasing precision through time, the capacity to anatomically dissect complicated interactions in real time has the potential to advance knowledge of mechanisms of congenital renal disease, ultimately to improved clinical outcomes (Baskin et al., 2018; Baskin et al., 2020) (Figure 6.8).

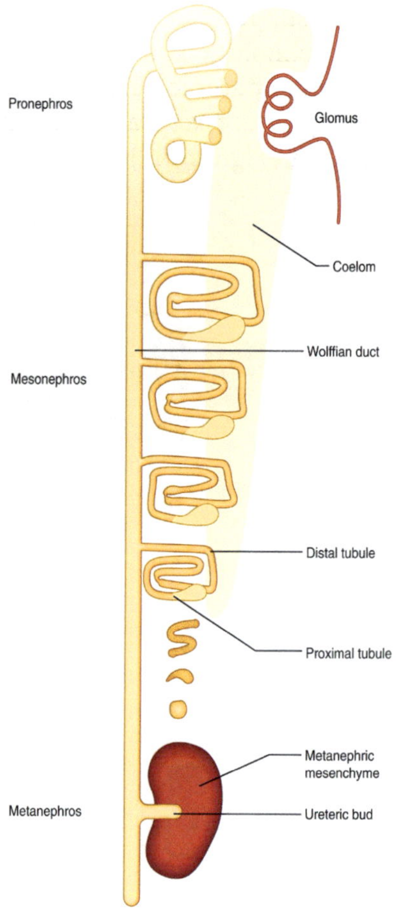

Figure 6.8. Embryonic development of the kidney.

Source: https://media.springernature.com/lw685/springer-static/image/chp%3A10.1007%2F978-3-642-27843-3_1-1/MediaObjects/149891_0_En_1-1_Fig2_HTML.gif.

6.2.2. Development of the Urinary Tract

The process of developing the urinary system is a multifactorial process that starts during embryonic life and encompasses many complicated interactions among genetic, environmental, and hormonal influences. The urinary system arises mostly from the intermediate mesoderm, in which particular structures differentiate to give rise to the kidneys, ureters, bladder, and urethra. Formation of these organs occurs in a sequential manner, initially the pronephros, which is transient, followed by the mesonephros, and subsequently the metanephros, which develops into the working kidneys. All stages of this development are critical as any break would lead to severe congenital defects. An understanding of the development biology of such structures allows researchers and clinicians to identify potential complications and act early when complications arise, thereby demonstrating the relevance of this research both in clinical and basic settings. The interaction between various signaling pathways, especially the transcription factors and the hormones, is very important in urinary tract development. For instance, studies have proven that the coordinated regulation of Pax2 and Gdnf genes is required during nephron development, a critical process that defines kidney development. In addition, the function and differentiation of urinary organs are regulated by hormones, particularly those of the endocrine system. This biochemical choreography must be read with respect to animal models that, although not entirely equivalent to human development, provide information on potential genetic abnormalities of the urinary tract. Scientists' warning about species differences points to careful extrapolation of data from animal models to human patients and thereby bridging the gap between developmental biology and therapeutic application (Baskin et al., 2019). The applicability of urinary tract development is not just in embryogenesis, but is also closely related with the well-being of adult human beings. Problems like urinary tract infection, kidney stones, and chronic renal disease often have their origin in developmental abnormalities. Also, the mother's condition during pregnancy may have an effect on the fetus's development of the urinary tracts, so it is important to learn about the factors at risk. Studies have indicated that extragenital pathologies may lead to pregnancy complications in the fetal and maternal urinary systems (Feyta et al., 2018). As such, the importance of urinary tract development extends beyond the immediate outcomes of organogenesis to long-term well-being. Such aspects demand intensive comprehension by medical practitioners who endeavor to mitigate risks associated with urinary dysfunctions throughout a person's life cycle (Figure 6.9).

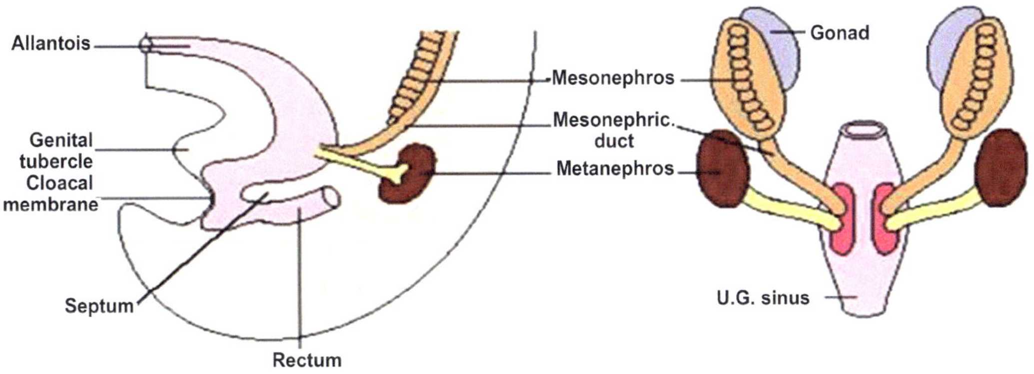

Figure 6.9. Development of the urinary tract.

Source: https://media.springernature.com/lw685/springer-static/image/chp%3A10.1007%2F978-3-642-38482-0_163-1/MediaObjects/272888_0_En_163-1_Fig4_HTML.png.

6.2.3. Interaction Between Urinary and Reproductive Systems

The interaction between the urinary and reproductive systems is an important aspect of human anatomy, particularly in developmental biology. The two systems are functionally distinct but anatomically and developmentally identical, an indicator of the tight interrelationship of the two. For instance, both systems arise from the intermediate mesoderm during embryonic development, and development in one system affects another significantly. The urogenital sinus is an extremely significant junction as a site where the two systems converge, indicating the combined function of the two systems. During fetal growth, where the spatial relationships of associated organs, such as the bladder and reproductive organs, establish their position and organization, the interpretation thereof determines their location and thus demand explicit understanding of these interactions to ensure medical science and anatomy education (Bittner et al., 2006). Furthermore, the urinary and reproductive systems are also functionally interdependent, with implications for disease and health. For example, the periurethral anatomic location of the female urethra in relation to the vaginal canal produces an increased risk for urinary tract infection, particularly for women. Endocrine variation throughout the menstrual cycle, peri- and post-pregnancy, also underscore the dynamic interaction between the systems, which affects urinary function as well as reproductive health. The male prostate gland, which surrounds the male urethra, is also employed for both reproductive fluid secretion and regulation of the urinary stream, further indicating the coordination between these systems. An understanding of these intricacies not only teaches us about normal physiology but also teaches clinicians about complications that can occur, illustrating their relevance to biomedical science and clinical practice (Campo et al., 2006). Along with anatomical and functional relations, the evolutionary perspective also provides valuable information regarding the evolution of urinary and reproductive systems. The common origins of the two systems imply that adaptations would have presumably occurred under evolutionary pressures to maximize functions involved in reproduction and excretion. Morphological and physiological homologies can be found in other organisms that imply common ancestry and adaptive mechanisms that have endured over time. Comparative anatomy is therefore a means of gaining knowledge of the mechanisms responsible for functional integration of urinary and reproductive systems in man. The evolutionary context necessitates questions about congenital defects and the effect of such defects on health, necessitating increased research into the field. Increased precision in terms of such matters is likely to enhance treatment of genital and urinary system conditions (Bittner et al., 2006).

6.3. Hormonal Influences on Development

Hormones are key to genital and urinary system development, and they direct not only the physiological organization but also functional potential of these systems. Sex hormones, specifically androgens and estrogens, lead the differentiation of reproductive and urinary organs from common precursor structures during embryonic and fetal development at key times. The action of testosterone, for example, is necessary for male genital development, and the lack of substantial androgen exposure leads to female structure formation. Such hormonal control of sexual differentiation highlights its complexity, with excess or insufficiency of hormone levels potentially causing sexual development disorders, reflecting the fine balance required for organ development and function. In addition, puberty is the period when hormonal changes reprogram already determined systems to bring about functional maturation and reproductive ability. Addition of androgens in male development not only defines genital structures but also affects the urinary system profoundly. Sex hormones' influence is not limited to embryogenesis, but it reaches into manipulative and adaptive life periods, where their application can bring about significant physiological changes. For instance, the abuse of androgenic anabolic steroids (AAS) has been associated with a multitude of complications involving the genital and urinary tracts. As noted, the drugs may cause elevated levels of lipids and hormonal imbalances that could predispose the body to cardiovascular complications, thus reflecting on the fine balance between hormones in ensuring homeostasis. The possible consequences of AAS abuse underscore the necessity of more awareness about the hormonal context that influences genital and urinary well-being. Therein lies an imperative reminder about the subtleties involved in hormonal effects, since derangements have the potential to cascade into serious developmental and health concerns (Abrão et al., 2020). Additionally, newer research highlights the probiotic functions of the microbiota in supporting hormonal equilibrium and, in turn, the optimal development and operation of the genital and urinary tracts. The studies have increasingly focused on how the microbiome influences the host hormone systems, with respect to the potential that a healthy microbiome could contribute to controlling hormones like estrogen and testosterone, important for sustaining reproductive well-being. Dysbiosis or microbiota imbalances may have negative consequences on hormonal homeostasis, causing illnesses that affect not just sexual development but also the health of the urinary tract. The direct correlation between microbiota and the regulation of hormones thus calls for a thorough understanding of both the hormonal control as well as the microbial community that plays a role in genital and urinary system development. Such insights propel further inquiry, potentially revealing novel therapeutic avenues for addressing developmental disorders and enhancing overall health (Hou et al., 2022) (Figure 6.10).

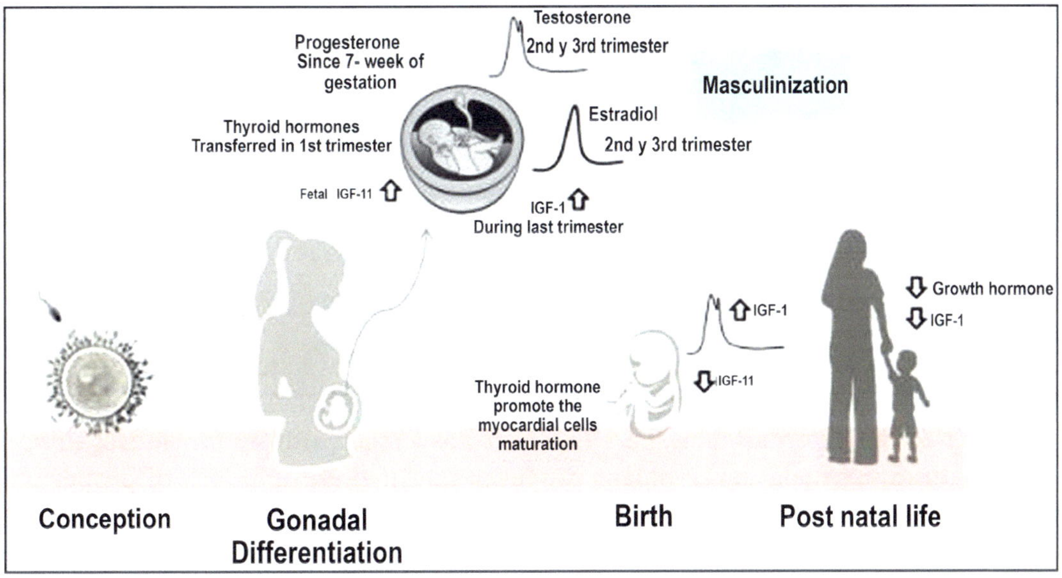

Figure 6.10. Hormonal influences on development.

Source: https://media.springernature.com/lw685/springer-static/image/chp%3A10.1007%2F978-3-031-32554-0_2/MediaObjects/480145_1_En_2_Fig3_HTML.png.

6.3.1. Role of Androgens in Male Development

Androgens, and notably testosterone, play a vital part in the development of males, particularly the development of genitalia and the urinary system. Through the presence of the Y chromosome, during embryogenesis, testes are induced to develop, which subsequently secrete testosterone. Testosterone is involved in the differentiation of the internal male reproductive organs, i.e., seminal vesicles and prostate, and external genitalia, i.e., penis and scrotum. As Baskin et al. (2019) explains, the evolution of these processes through research provides key insights into how anatomical differentiation in males is guided by hormonal cues. Additionally, testosterone functions in a multi-level process, affecting gene expression and cellular differentiation, key to upholding male-specific attributes of the reproductive tract.

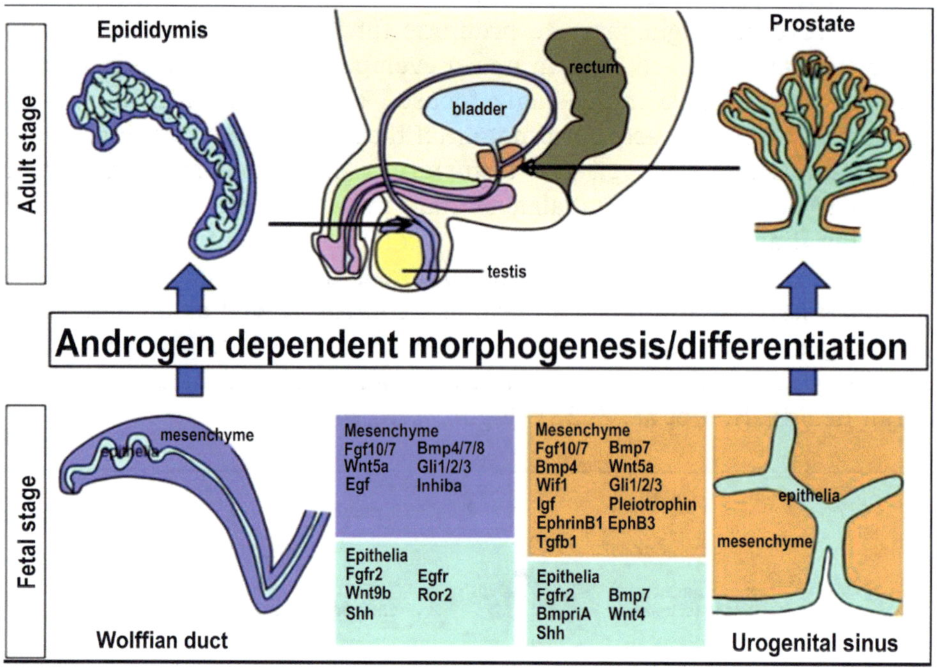

Figure 6.11. Role of androgens in male development.

Source: https://ars.els-cdn.com/content/image/1-s2.0-S1874939914001266-gr1.jpg.

The androgenic action on male genitalia involves not only testosterone but other androgenic drugs like DHT. While testosterone initiates the development of male structures, DHT ensures the final completion of the external genitalia because it has higher affinity for androgen receptors. The classical pathway of male development proposes that if there is a lack of proper androgen levels, then sexual development disorders are possible, with which people possess ambivalent or underdeveloped male genitalia. Recent research, as mentioned by Auchus et al. (2019), has suggested an alternative backdoor pathway of androgen synthesis that can also contribute to these processes. Understanding these pathways reaffirms the importance of androgens in regulating male reproductive structure and function. Furthermore, the effects of androgen signaling are not only about physical development; they also inform us about the types and etiology of numerous genetic disorders and how they present themselves phenotypically in terms of male development. Genetic changes in androgen synthesis or receptor activity could generate a spectrum of disorders, including androgen insensitivity syndrome or 5-alpha reductase deficiency. These disorders document the essentiality of androgens to masculine sexual differentiation and emphasize the complexity of hormone regulation in developmental biology. As elucidated in studies, such as comparative model organism observations, researchers emphasize the need for physical exercise to prevent overgeneralization of conclusions from animal models to human conditions, due to differences in hormonal pathways and processes of development, which Baskin et al. (2019) correctly outlines. This nuanced examination of androgen studies in male development then sharpens our understanding of both normal and abnormal development of the genital and urinary system (Figure 6.11).

6.3.2. Influence of Estrogens in Female Development

The function of estrogens in feminization is central, especially during the development of the genital and urinary tracts. These steroid hormones, mainly estradiol, play a crucial role during essential stages of development like pregnancy and puberty. In addition to their function in the control of secondary sex characteristics, estrogens enable the growth and differentiation of reproductive tissues, impacting structures like the ovaries, uterus, and vagina. In addition, estrogens are of profound importance in the onset of gametogenesis and the menstrual cycle. Current research emphasizes the role of ideal estrogen levels during such developmental stages, as this can result in disorders like polycystic ovary syndrome and other gynecological problems, indicating the complex interrelation between hormonal balance and women's reproductive health, as quoted in detailed guidelines for treating hormonal disorders among women (Speiser et al., 2018). The effects of estrogens are not localized to the reproductive organs and have profound effects on the urinary system. Estrogen receptors have been found in several tissues, such as bladder and urethral tissues, indicating that estrogens play a role in the development and functioning of these organs. At puberty, estrogen levels are responsible for the development of the urinary tract, influencing tissue elasticity and sensitivity to other hormonal stimuli. This hormonal effect is crucial for the preservation of urinary tract health and averts disorders like urinary incontinence, which tend to arise from functional deficits in the supportive tissues regulated by hormonal mechanisms. As women grow older and estrogen levels change, especially at menopause, the incidence of urinary system disease rises, highlighting the necessity for continued research into therapeutic intervention addressing estrogen pathways for the preservation of urinary health (Matthew et al., 2017). Besides, as the development of estrogens role in the female continues to grow, so do the implications for therapies. Hormone replacement therapy (HRT) is one such case where estrogens impact is put to critical use, particularly among postmenopausal women. HRT is designed to reduce the symptoms of estrogen deficiency, which can range from alterations in urinary function. The dosing and timing of HRT are critical parameters of which professionals need to take note since inappropriate application will worsen health hazards instead of alleviating them. Knowledge of the pharmacokinetics and dynamics of estrogens further enhances effective therapies so that female health can be managed on a more individualized basis. By incorporating an understanding of estrogens multidimensional functions in the urinary and genital systems, healthcare professionals can improve the quality of care for women at all stages of life, meeting both reproductive as well as urinary health needs efficiently (Speiser et al., 2018) (Figure 6.12).

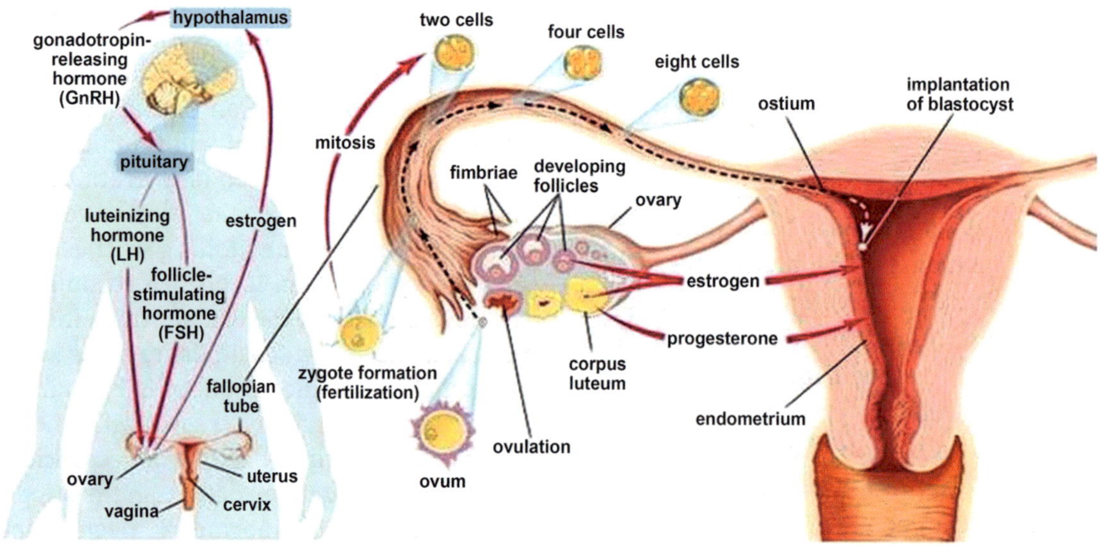

Figure 6.12. Estrogens in female development.

Source: https://www.creative-diagnostics.com/blog/wp-content/uploads/2018/03/Estrogen-and-Progesterone.jpg.

6.3.3. Impact of Hormonal Imbalances on System Development

The formation of the urinary and genital systems is closely associated with hormonal signaling, underlining the extreme influence that hormonal imbalances have upon these systems. Testosterone, estrogen, and progesterone are among the hormones that are important for reproductive differentiation and organ formation. For example, differences in testosterone levels can cause hypospadias or cryptorchidism in males, respectively, which include malformations or undescended positions of the penis. These disorders represent the extent to which deviations from normal hormonal profiles can derail the normal developmental pathways of the genital system and result in long-term health issues. Beyond that, hormonal imbalance also has the potential to impinge upon the urinary tract, potentially contributing to urinary incontinence or bladder dysfunction, demonstrating the extent to which the health of the hormones plays a role in proper formation of both the genital and urinary tracts. Aside from direct developmental effects, hormonal imbalances can trigger a series of additional physiological problems that may occur during adulthood and puberty. For instance, dysregulations in the estrogen-progesterone balance may result in profound alterations in the menstrual cycle, influencing feminine reproductive health and resulting in disorders like PCOS. PCOS is defined by irregular menstrual periods and hyperandrogenism, and this can also disturb the development and integrity of the urinary system. This speaks to the interconnectedness between hormonal instability and systemic development. Dysbiosis, or a lack of balance within the microbiota, could be a contributory factor, impacting endocrine signaling and further complicating irregulation of these hormones. Therefore, it is important to comprehend the pathogenic mechanisms of hormonal imbalance in developing treatment strategies for affected individuals. In addition, the significance of hormonal imbalance goes beyond reproductive and physical aspects. Hormonal changes can cause a disturbance in microbiota of different body systems, which, in turn, affect general health. Human microbiota, such as that found in the genitourinary tract, has important functions in metabolic processes, immune function, and hormonal metabolism. Dysbiosis within the microbiota can be involved in the regulation of hormone production and response, establishing a feed-forward loop that perpetuates hormonal imbalance. The relationship between urinary tract microbiota and hormonal status is an area that has become more recognized, with the potential for a two-way relationship where changes in one system have the capacity to meaningfully affect the other. This interrelatedness highlights the significance of holistic consideration when examining the health and development of the genital and urinary systems, implying that balance in the hormones is essential for systemic health and preventing disease (Amicuzi et al., 2024; Barajas Vélez et al., 2021).

6.4. Congenital Anomalies of the Genital System

The formation of the genital system is a multifaceted process controlled in part by genetic and environmental conditions. Abnormalities in this developmental stage may lead to a number of disorders like hypospadias, cryptorchidism, and genital agenesis. The physical health is not affected alone, but these conditions have significant psychological consequences on the afflicted individuals. For instance, hypospadias, a condition in which the urethral opening is on the penis's underside, is among the most prevalent congenital urethral disorders of the male genitalia. The condition can manifest as problems with urination, sexual function, and self-esteem, making it compulsory to treat it with full medical and psychological care. Such problems need to be dealt with at an early development stage because anomalies left untreated tend to result in more serious complications down the line, again accentuating the need to grasp normal genital system development and congenital anomalies' probable effects. Etiology of congenital anomalies in the genital system tends to involve a complex interplay between teratogenic causes and genetic predisposition. For example, pregnancy exposure to some medications, infections, or toxins in the environment may interfere with normal fetal development of the genitalia, leading to conditions such as vaginal agenesis or DSD. In addition, genetic syndromes such as Turner syndrome and Klinefelter syndrome present with congenital abnormalities of the genitals and other systemic manifestations, highlighting the importance of interdisciplinary assessment and management in affected individuals. The implications of these anomalies are more than immediate physical impairment, as they also have effects on reproductive health and the psychosocial state of the individual. Thus, continuous research into a better understanding of the effects is imperative for enhancing diagnostic, preventive, and therapeutic approaches related to congenital anomalies of the genital system. Standards for managing and treating congenital genital anomalies are updated with ongoing research evidence and clinical practice issues. In this regard, the revised best practice guidelines for the management of conditions such as congenital adrenal hyperplasia endorse the need to integrate patient safety, quality of life, and cost considerations into treatment strategies (Speiser et al., 2018). This ensures that patients have access to comprehensive care, from diagnosis to ongoing management, tailored to their unique needs. Additionally, the analysis of global health data reveals disparities in the prevalence and outcomes of these conditions across different populations, highlighting the necessity for localized health strategies and awareness initiatives (Gregory et al., 2018). These newer views of congenital genital system anomalies bring a more refined understanding that emphasizes both clinical effectiveness and the greater general welfare of affected patients, ultimately enhancing health outcomes (Figure 6.13).

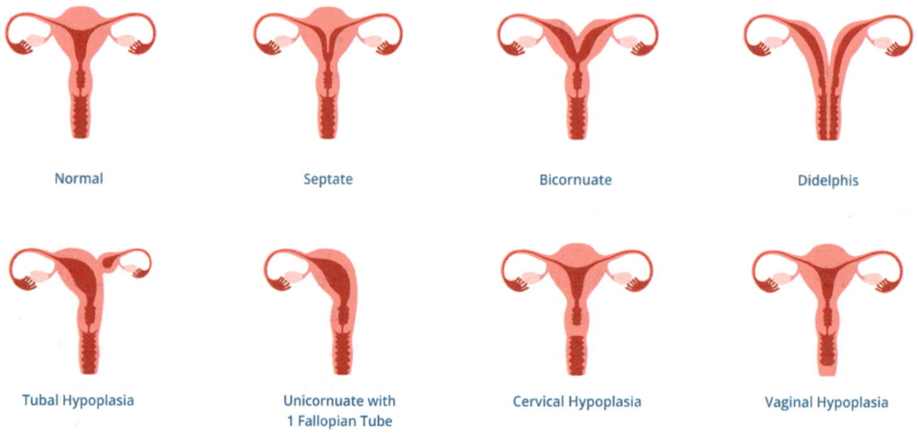

Figure 6.13. Congenital anomalies of the female genital tract.

Source: https://womenandchildren.avisena.com.my/wp-content/uploads/2024/10/CART-article-diagram.jpg.

6.4.1. Common Congenital Disorders

Congenital abnormalities of the genital and urinary systems are numerous and have a profound impact on an individual's health and well-being. Of these, hypospadias is a widespread urogenital defect in which the opening of the urethra is found on the underside of the penis rather than at the tip. This condition occurs in about 1 in 200 to 300 live births and can introduce future complications such as issues with urination, sexual function, or fertility. Hypospadias tends to occur concomitantly with other congenital defects, so patients must be carefully assessed for the overall urogenital health. Surgical procedures are usually needed to repair the positioning of the urethra, improving both function and cosmetic appearance, eventually affecting the psychosocial status of affected patients as they become adults. Another common congenital anomaly is cryptorchidism, defined by the non-descent of one or both testes into the scrotum during fetal life. It is exceedingly common, occurring in approximately 3% of term infants and roughly 30% of preterm infants. The importance of treating cryptorchidism is not just its possible effect on fertility but also because it occurs with higher risks for testicular cancer in the future. Treatment is most often surgical, with the operation called orchidopexy, to bring the undescended testicle to the scrotum and fix it there. Early detection and corrective surgery are essential since intervention in the first year of life is advised to maximize the possibility of normal testicular growth and function, thus minimizing long-term health risk for the individual. Finally, congenital anomalies like bladder exstrophy and epispadias also highlight the intricacies of genital and urinary tract development. Bladder exstrophy is an uncommon condition in which the bladder develops outside the body, occurring in about 1 in 50,000 births. This is a challenging condition to manage, with the need for extensive surgical repair within a short time of birth. Epispadias, which is usually associated with bladder exstrophy, is a malformation in which the opening of the urethra is on the upper surface of the penis, which may complicate urinary and sexual function. These conditions require multidisciplinary management, including pediatric urologists, surgeons, and counseling, to treat both the physical and emotional consequences for individuals and families involved. Placing these conditions in the context of genital and urinary system development highlights the need for early diagnosis and intervention measures to enhance prognosis in those affected (Figure 6.14).

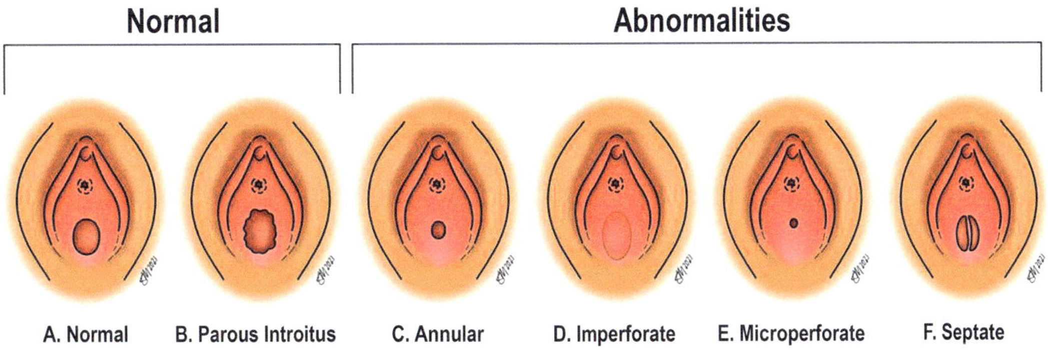

Figure 6.14. Congenital disorders affecting the genital and urinary systems.

Source: https://urogynecology.nm.org/uploads/1/3/2/8/132816529/fig-6-rev2-hymenalabnormalities_orig.jpg.

6.4.2. Causes and Risk Factors

Embryogenesis of the genitourinary systems is regulated by a heterogeneous set of intrinsic and extrinsic factors that have the potential to very significantly influence both function and anatomy. Inherited dispositions, particularly those which arise from chromosomal aberrations or mutations, are similarly of paramount importance as regulators of susceptibility to developmental abnormalities. For instance, conditions like Turner syndrome or Androgen Insensitivity Syndrome result from sex chromosome arrangement abnormalities in genetics, leading to abnormal genital and urinary system development. Other maternal factors for concern, including pre-existing conditions such as diabetes or hypertension, can also render pregnancy risky, ultimately impacting fetal development. The intricate interaction of these genetic and maternal factors illustrates the importance of appropriate prenatal care for minimizing risks of urinary and genital system abnormality. Environmental factors other than maternal also contribute to heightening the risk for congenital abnormality of the urinary and genital system. Teratogenic environmental exposure during sensitive periods of fetal development is accountable for other developmental defects. For example, exposure to certain pharmaceuticals, alcohol, or environmental toxins can disrupt typical embryonic development and cause defects such as hypospadias or renal agenesis. Dosing and timing of exposure are critical in that certain stages of organogenesis are particularly vulnerable to such injury. In addition, pregnancy infections and nutritional deficiencies are of significant concern. In particular, hyperglycemia or gestational diabetes has been linked with an increased incidence of urinary tract abnormalities. It is significant to recognize these environmental factors so that prevention methods can be formulated and healthier pregnancy outcomes ensured to preserve the developmental integrity of the urinary and genital systems. Psychosocial factors can indirectly affect the risk of having complications in the genital and urinary systems as well. Maternal mental health, stress, and levels of anxiety can have a tangible effect on fetal growth and pregnancy outcomes. Higher levels of maternal stress have been associated with adverse birth outcomes, which, although less anatomically connected, may complicate pre-existing conditions or introduce complications in the birthing process. Such programs of maternal care need to address the psychosocial factors along with the traditional medical monitoring to minimize these risks appropriately. Moreover, access to health resources and education regarding prenatal care varies widely between diverse socioeconomic groups, which develops disparities in risk factors for genital and urinary system formation. Without intervention on these social determinants of health, risk groups are vulnerable to increased degrees of developmental abnormalities in these systems, with long-standing health impacts to those individuals (Carter et al., 2014; Feyta et al., 2018).

6.4.3. Implications for Health and Treatment Options

Genital and urinary system embryogenesis is important in understanding various health implications and therapies which can be applied in related disorders. System abnormalities could lead to chronic diseases, which make an impressive impact on patients' quality of life. Chronic primary pain (CPP) is such a disease, where patients experience constant pain with no easily detectable cause. This diagnosis challenges caregivers to adopt a biopsychosocial approach that addresses biological, psychological, and social determinants of the patients pain experience. Individualized treatment plans should be employed in the management of such multicausative disorders with the guarantee that treatment not only addresses physiological needs but also emotional and social requirements. Through the understanding of the multilateral interaction of these dimensions, medical practitioners are able to develop more effective treatment strategies, as highlighted by current research in managing and classifying pain in patients suffering from genital and urinary system diseases (Michael et al., 2018). Additionally, some conditions of the genital and urinary system, such as congenital adrenal hyperplasia (CAH), underscore the importance of tailored treatments. CAH is typically caused by enzyme 21-hydroxylase deficiency, which leads to hormonal imbalances seen in several clinical presentations. The updated clinical practice guidelines of the Endocrine Society highlight the importance of the integration of best practices in accordance with the latest evidence and expert opinion.

The guidelines address not only clinical management of CAH but also patient safety and overall quality of life. These treatment interventions must be responsive to the overall needs of patients, both biological and psychosocial, positioning providers to enhance outcomes by way of communication and education (Speiser et al., 2018). Together with individualized treatments, continued research into the implications of genital and urinary system development guides future practice and intervention. Ongoing developments underpin increased awareness of genetic and environmental determinants affecting these systems, which in turn inform preventive interventions and early treatment. Practitioners are urged to keep up with developments in this area to facilitate proactive health management. Increased awareness of pitfalls and patient participation in collaborative decision-making can create more rewarding treatment experiences. Finally, awareness of the varied ramifications involved with genital and urinary system disorders guarantees that healthcare providers are able to modify treatment decisions to enhance both physiological function and psychological resilience so that the quality of care in this vital area of health is enhanced (Michael et al., 2018).

6.5. Congenital Anomalies of the Urinary System

Congenital urinary tract anomalies are an important field of developmental biology, in which organogenesis is highlighted as a complex set of processes. Congenital urinary tract anomalies can be caused by a number of genetic and environmental mechanisms during embryonic development, leading to severe structural and functional urinary tract abnormalities. Detailed genetic studies have now started to untangle the intricate underlying causes of these disorders and identified certain genes crucial in the development and differentiation of renal structures. To cite an example, the mutation of the SHROOM4 gene has been implicated in a variety of congenital abnormalities affecting the urinary system as well as the anorectal and cardiovascular systems. This association highlights the multifactorial origin of developmental malformations, as attested by reports wherein mutations in this gene were associated with extreme developmental abnormalities in many organ systems, which indicates a more general function of SHROOM4 during embryogenesis (Adamczyk et al., 2022). A critical element towards congenital anomalies of the urinary tract is the function of signaling pathways, specifically the glial cell-line derived neurotrophic factor (Gdnf) signaling pathway. This pathway is essential for kidney development and differentiation, affecting essential processes like kidney branching and ureter differentiation. Mutations in the essential elements of this signaling pathway, like Gfra1 and Ret, have been associated with a range of congenital disorders, including solitary congenital anomalies of the kidney or urinary tract (CAKUT) and disorders like Hirschsprung disease. The lethality seen in knockout models with deficiencies in these genes highlights their non-redundant function in embryonic development. As more is learned about the molecular mechanism of Ret signaling, the phenotypic diversity arising from its dysfunction yields salient information about the etiology of these congenital disorders, ultimately refining our understanding of normal urinary system development (Jain et al., 2009).

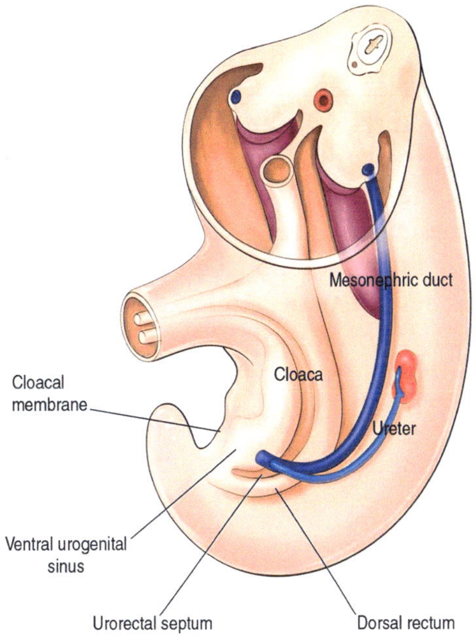

Figure 6.15. Embryology and congenital anomalies of the urinary tract, rectum, and female genital system.

Source: https://i0.wp.com/obgynkey.com/wp-content/uploads/2021/11/f02-01-9780323697835.jpg?w=960.

The effect of congenital anomalies extends beyond the direct physical health of individuals into psychological and social aspects as well. Several of these anomalies are complex to repair surgically and must be managed medically throughout life, resulting in higher healthcare expenses and burdens for affected families. Early detection with the help of advanced imaging modalities and genetic testing is essential in managing these conditions to permit timely treatment and enhanced quality of life for patients. In addition, the continuing studies on the genetic origin of congenital urinary malformations emphasize the need for a multidisciplinary strategy involving urology, genetics, and developmental biology. As our knowledge from the scientific community improves our understanding of the genetic, environmental, and mechanistic factors underlying these malformations, public health policy can be improved to better offer preventive care and support services to affected individuals and families (Figure 6.15).

6.5.1. Overview of Urinary Tract Anomalies

Urinary tract anomalies encompass a range of congenital malformations that can significantly impact renal and bladder function, as well as overall individuality. These anomalies can be classified broadly into structural and functional defects, with structural abnormalities frequently arising during the embryonic development of the urogenital system. During this critical period, the mesoderm gives rise to the kidneys and associated structures, and any disruption in this development can lead to issues such as renal agenesis, ectopic kidneys, and more complex formations like horseshoe kidneys. Such anatomical distinctions often manifest in varying degrees of severity, necessitating a comprehensive understanding of normal embryogenesis to differentiate between benign variations and clinically significant anomalies.

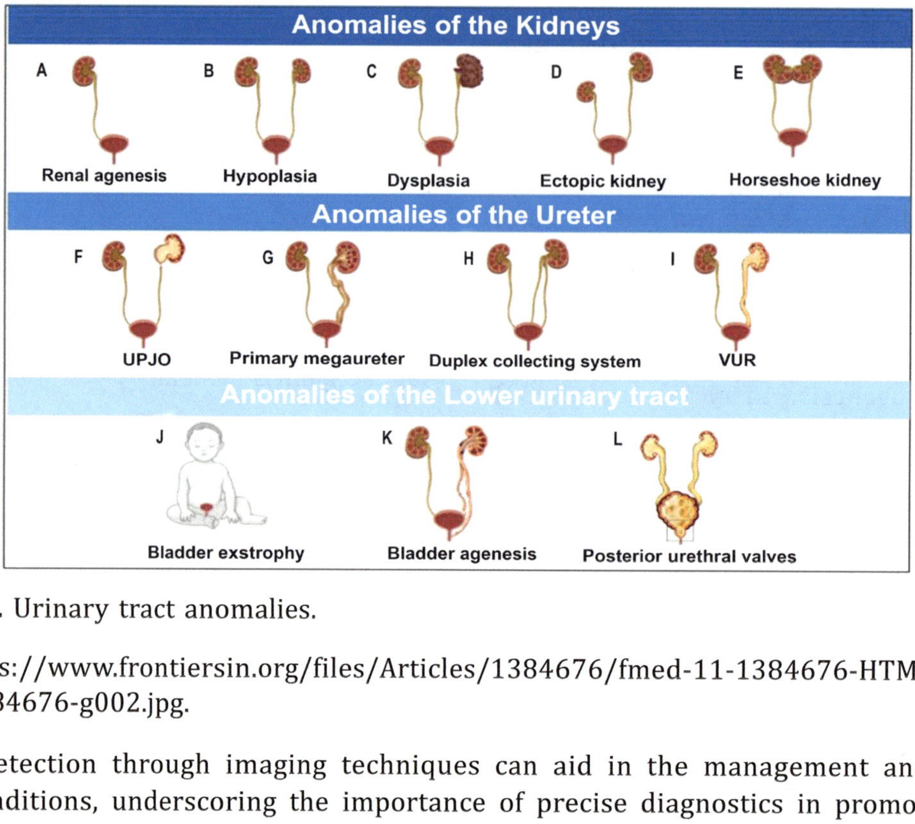

Figure 6.16. Urinary tract anomalies.

Source: https://www.frontiersin.org/files/Articles/1384676/fmed-11-1384676-HTML/image_m/fmed-11-1384676-g002.jpg.

Early detection through imaging techniques can aid in the management and treatment of these conditions, underscoring the importance of precise diagnostics in promoting healthy outcomes in affected individuals. The interrelationship between urinary tract anomalies and genetic disorders has been the focus of increasing attention in recent research. For instance, conditions such as Turner syndrome and disorders of sex development also bear significant correlations with urinary tract malformations, suggesting a multifactorial origin for many anomalies.

Key steroidogenic pathways, often implicated in developmental abnormalities, highlight the necessity of examining hormonal influences alongside genetic factors. In a clinical setting, as evidenced by recent studies, patients with complex presentations, such as hydronephrosis accompanied by severe polyhydramnios, have shown elevated levels of steroidogenic enzymes, suggesting a hormonal component in certain congenital cases (Foster et al., 2010).

Understanding these connections is essential for clinicians, as it can lead to more targeted approaches in both diagnosis and management, particularly in cases where multiple organ systems are involved. The variability seen in urinary tract anomalies demands a comprehensive approach to both management and treatment. Innovations in prenatal imaging have facilitated earlier detection of these anomalies, allowing for more effective intervention strategies soon after birth. However, the complexity of conditions like congenital hydronephrosis or renal dysplasia often necessitates a multidisciplinary approach, involving nephrologists, urologists, and genetic counselors. Moreover, understanding the developmental biology of urogenital structures, particularly the similarities and differences between human and murine models, can provide critical insights into the underlying mechanisms of these anomalies (Baskin et al., 2019). Comprehensive care for affected individuals extends beyond immediate surgical interventions, encompassing long-term monitoring and supportive therapies to address potential complications such as urinary tract infections or hypertension. This holistic consideration of urinary tract anomalies exemplifies the importance of integrating developmental biology, clinical expertise, and patient-centered care in managing complex congenital conditions (Figure 6.16).

6.5.2. Diagnosis and Management of Conditions

The diagnosis and management of conditions related to the genital and urinary systems are vital in ensuring proper reproductive and renal health. A comprehensive approach must be employed, integrating clinical history, physical examination, and diagnostic procedures. For instance, myofascial pelvic pain (MFPP) often complicates chronic pelvic pain syndromes but may go unrecognized. Effective management necessitates awareness of myofascial trigger points within the pelvic floor, which can radiate pain to adjacent anatomical regions. Treatments such as trigger point release, biofeedback, and electrical stimulation have proven beneficial. The involvement of an interdisciplinary team is crucial for identifying MFPP early and administering effective therapies. This multi-faceted approach emphasizes the need for holistic evaluations that consider both physiological and psychosocial factors influencing the patient's condition. Advancements in prenatal diagnosis have significantly enhanced the management of conditions affecting the genital and urinary systems, particularly regarding congenital anomalies. In pregnant women, routine genetic counseling has become paramount, allowing for early identification of potential defects in the fetus, such as congenital heart defects (CHDs), which can be closely linked to urinary system abnormalities. Studies reveal that various factors, like maternal somatic health and biochemical markers, offer critical insights into fetal development risks. For example, genetic counseling evaluated mothers with chronic conditions, noting the prevalence of cardiovascular issues as risk factors for congenital anomalies (Helner et al., 2019). Early detection through non-invasive prenatal testing (NIPT) and other diagnostic tools can inform clinical interventions, potentially leading to improved outcomes for both mothers and infants while guiding clinical decisions throughout pregnancy. Postnatal management remains crucial to address identified conditions within the genital and urinary systems. Following birth, healthcare practitioners often employ a variety of diagnostic imaging techniques, such as ultrasound or MRI, to assess for congenital anomalies or developmental issues. For instance, management strategies may include personalized monitoring and treatment plans designed to minimize complications associated with conditions like urinary tract infections or structural abnormalities. Regular follow-up and assessment are necessary to identify any changes in the child's health status that may require intervention. Furthermore, education for families about the signs and symptoms of potential issues enhances early detection and promotes a proactive approach to care. Through ongoing research and clinical practice, the integration of diagnostic and management strategies continues to evolve, ensuring better health outcomes for affected children and families in the long term.

6.5.3. Long-Term Effects on Health

The long-term impact of health complications of the genital and urinary systems can pose serious implications for women's overall well-being and quality of life, especially after childbearing. Maternal sepsis is also a very serious issue in the area of postpartum complications, which may result in major health problems or even death in women. Studies have proven that postpartum purulent-septic complications (PPSC) significantly account for maternal death rates, with about one-tenth of those deaths worldwide. Further, the risk posed by several obstetric and gynecologic disorders, such as preeclampsia, chronic inflammatory conditions, and labor complications, highlights the importance of early detection and specialist prevention measures. Successful management of such risk factors may lead to a considerable decrease in the incidence of PPSC, further improving women's long-term health and well-being after delivery (Feyta et al., 2018). Apart from the short-term risks during the postpartum period, the long-term health complications arising from untreated or poorly managed conditions in the urinary and genital systems may extend to men also, especially to those surviving genitourinary cancer. Development of patient self-report instruments, like the Lymphoedema Genito-Urinary Cancer Questionnaire (LGUCQ), is a preventive action for identifying and managing long-standing symptoms that occur after treatment. These devices not only enable enhanced detection of symptoms but also promote enhanced interaction between patients and health professionals about alterations in health. The continued involvement in monitoring such conditions indicates the possibility of sustained effects on survivors' physical health, emotional welfare, and general quality of life, and the need for individualized assessments and interventions (Fitzpatrick et al., 2014).

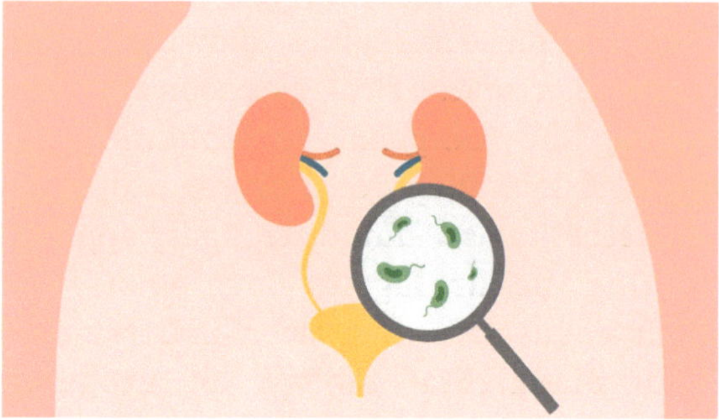

Figure 6.17. The long-term effects of health complications in the genital and urinary systems.

Source: https://images.everydayhealth.com/images/urinary-conditions/urinary-tract-infection/uti-causes-and-risk-factors-alt-1440x810.jpg?sfvrsn=8ee2c4b5_3.

Additionally, the complex interdependence between early detection, risk factor management, and long-term health outcomes represents a critical paradigm within obstetric and urological care. Recognizing the complex nature of complications originating from inadequate genital and urinary health benefits not only in the prevention of immediate emergencies but also highlights the need for integrated healthcare practices that can treat these matters along an individual's lifetime. More importantly, the occurrence of extragenital pathologies complicates this further by associating poor health results with a variety of other chronic illnesses. Therefore, the development of preventive strategies and inter-disciplinary management plans incorporating individuals' special needs will ultimately be key to optimizing strong long-term health in this population (Feyta et al., 2018) (Figure 6.17).

6.6. Comparative Development Across Species

The study of genital and urinary system evolution across species has been seen to display an interesting interplay between evolution, genetics, and environmental pressures. Different species have unique adaptations in their reproductive and excretory systems that mirror their ecological niches and biological demands. For example, most mammals exhibit clear gonadal development controlled by intricate Android signals, whereas the avian organisms depict a lesser level of complexity in their reproductive apparatus, focusing on the evolutionary shortcuts in favor of efficiency over redundancy. Such discrepancies not only show the variety of reproductive strategies but also point out the adaptive value of these systems in securing reproduction and species survival. At the cellular level, the metabolic profiles of varying species also play an important role in determining the morphogenesis of the urinary and genital systems. The latest research points out that changes in metabolic processes are associated with the general health of the reproductive systems. For instance, dysbiotic vaginal microbiota have been recognized as major players in cervical carcinogenesis and genital inflammation among women. In other species like mice, the same metabolic derangements can affect fertility and pregnancy. Comparison of these pathways between species gives valuable information about the host-microbe interactions and systemic dysfunctions that may occur in preserving reproductive health, as shown by the results that metabolic signatures are modulated by the onset of cancer, genital inflammation, and microbiota dynamics (Ilhan et al., 2019). In addition, developments in medical technology have also influenced our knowledge of genital and urinary tract development throughout species. Procedures like the application of lasers to correct a number of gynecological pathologies reflect notable evolutionary adaptations to handle human reproductive problems. The results indicate that energy therapies efficiently facilitate healing and restoration of vaginal integrity following pathologies, highlighting the significance of regenerative processes in evolutionary biology. Studies have shown how therapeutic procedures with thermal energy exposure may result in increased collagen production and better lubrication, evidence of humanity's adaptability in sexual and urinary health. These findings support a greater understanding of developmental processes not as singular events but as holistic components influenced by both evolutionary factors and contemporary clinical interventions (Tadir et al., 2017).

6.6.1. Similarities in Genital System Development

The formation of both the male and female genitalia share basic similarities that are critical to understanding sexual differentiation and reproductive biology. During early embryonic development, bipotential gonads develop and become testes or ovaries upon stimulation by certain genetic and hormonal influences. This common embryonic origin emphasizes the core processes in genital development, pointing to the work of genes like SRY in males, which triggers testicular differentiation, while the absence of this gene triggers ovarian development in females. Also, the Müllerian and Wolffian ducts, which are precursors to female and male reproductive tracts respectively, also show the complex developmental processes that arise from a shared structure, ending up in distinct reproductive anatomies. In examining the yolk sac and coelomic mesoderm contributions to developing genital systems, there are additional similarities. Both the systems make use of undifferentiated mesenchymal tissues which get differentiated into important structures like the genital ridges that are involved in the formation of gonads. The development of the ridges is affected by the same signaling pathways and growth factors, proposing a conserved evolutionary mechanism to develop the reproductive organs. In addition, the mutual dependence upon the same vascular and nerve supply during early development proves that despite differing endpoints—testes vs. ovaries—much of the developmental foundation is surprisingly similar. This highlights an important evolutionary factor where reproductive development most effectively adapts comparable embryonic tissues to serve divergent functional needs. Additionally, both systems depend on similar endocrine and paracrine factors for their formation. Hormones like androgens are responsible for crucial roles in the development of male genitalia while, conversely, estrogen and other ovarian hormones coordinate female genital development. This duality stresses the cooperation between genetic, hormonal, and environmental determinants that all together guide the processes. Recent mouse model studies have indicated that even though anatomical and physiological variations exist, the basic pathways that control reproductive tract development are very similar, and such findings have implications in providing potential therapeutic interventions for reproductive disease. These observations underscore the need to define male and female developmental pathways in order to have a comprehensive concept of human sexuality and reproductive health, especially considering the possibility of overlapping pathophysiological conditions that may occur in these systems (Baskin et al., 2019; Venuti et al., 2008) (Figure 6.18).

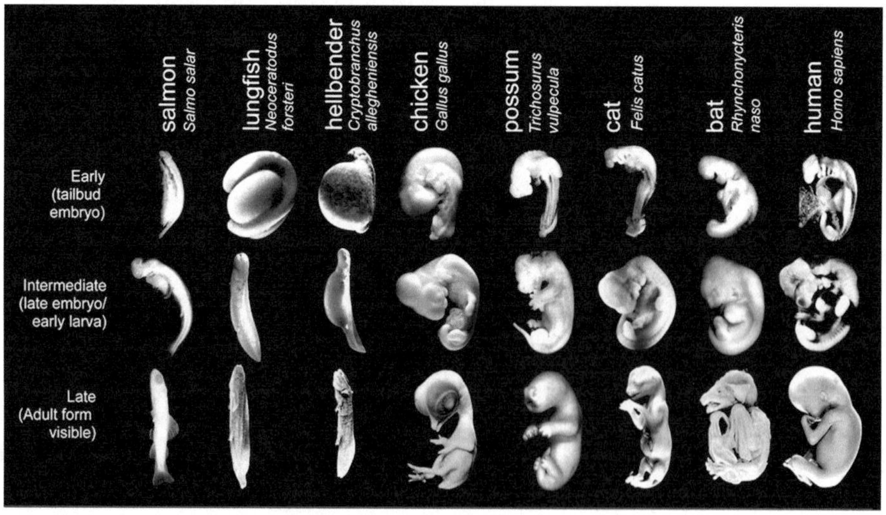

Figure 6.18. Similarities in genital system development across species.

Source: https://external-content.duckduckgo.com/iu/?u=http%3A%2F%2Ffarm2.staticflickr.com%2F1214%2F1139590175_f033109a49_z.jpg&f=1&nofb=1&ipt=8855b6d5f844ea5a6c82eaa70afa1e5f3d5fe797ca8c59d64bcd6b76015a3e34.

6.6.2. Differences in Urinary System Development

Urinary system development's complexity demonstrates extremes in differences during embryonic phases, especially between the sexes. Early development starts with the creation of the pronephros, mesonephros, and metanephros, which are key processes in developing functional kidneys. Incidentally, though both males and females follow identical developmental processes during these initial periods, the following processes of differentiation drastically split based on the action of sex-specific hormones. When the metanephros develops, the action of androgens in males causes retention of some of the mesonephric structures, which eventually form part of male reproductive anatomy. Females, on the other hand, have regression of these structures, thereby providing for the formation of the female urinary system. This divergence points to the complex interplay of urinary and reproductive system development, which requires a sophisticated comprehension of organogenesis and hormonal control within this context. An accurate analysis of urinary system development must also consider anatomical and functional diversities evolving out of genetic and environmental determinants. The mouse model has been generally used in developmental biology to make comparisons and contrasts between murine and human urogenital development. Yet, although this model has been informative, there are substantial anatomical and developmental disparities, especially regarding hormonal activity and organogenesis. For example, renal structure differentiation and the capabilities of function can provide some understanding of how human urinary systems develop in varying states. An awareness of these differences is paramount in ensuring that results from murine research are correctly put into perspective when translated to human development, given that several aspects may not be directly translatable. It is important to comprehend these differences, particularly because they influence overall health and pathology in the human organism. Clinically, an appreciation of the differences in the development of the urinary system can shape patient evaluation and treatment modalities, especially in those populations plagued by genitourinary disease. As an example, in the design and use of patient self-report instruments for identifying symptoms concerning the urinary and genital health, the implications of dissimilarities in development increase the validity and applicability of the instruments. There has been a recent study that brought the importance of including the views of several patients and experts in the formulation of the assessment tools, like the LGUCQ. These instruments are essential in managing under-reported conditions and securing total care for patients. Through an understanding of the individualized developmental pathways and diversities of the urinary system, healthcare professionals can enhance their knowledge and treatment methodology, ultimately driving higher quality of life for patients suffering from genitourinary disease (Fitzpatrick et al., 2014).

6.6.3. Insights from Animal Models for Human Health

In looking into evidence from animal models about human health, especially when it comes to the development of the genital and urinary systems, one sees that the models are priceless when it comes to appreciating chronic ailments and how they progress. Animal models allow for the exploration of intricate biological and genetic mechanisms that underlie human issues. For example, diseases like Long COVID have shown that there is a need for root scientific research to decipher underlying mechanisms involving numerous organ systems, including the urinary and genital systems. Studying animal models, which include genetically altered mice and nonhuman primates, enables researchers to view symptoms and mechanisms similar to those in human conditions, hence enabling the formulation of effective preventative and therapeutic modalities that might reduce these health problems (Zhang et al., 2025). Therefore, this emphasizes the likely effectiveness of using animal models to mimic different features of human health problems. Animal models are also vital to the development of organ-on-a-chip technology, which mimics physiological structures related to the urinary and genital systems. The level of sophistication in biological interactions within these systems is difficult to reproduce in the more conventional two-dimensional cell cultures. Rather, new technologies such as microfluidic devices enable scientists to develop three-dimensional models more akin to *in vivo* environments. These technological advances improve the research of individual organ functions, including renal filtration and reproductive endocrine regulation, critical in determining how diseases may develop or advance in humans. Merging of these systems with sensor technologies can provide real-time monitoring, tremendously fast-tracking the research. Ongoing improvement and use of such models can offer a true reflection of human health, filling gaps in our existing knowledge on associated diseases (Hu et al., 2025). Finally, the information obtained from animal models is vital not just for basic research but also for informing targeted interventions within clinical contexts. By precisely mimicking disease states and treatment responses, investigators are able to evaluate the effectiveness of novel therapeutic strategies for enhancing human health outcomes associated with the genital and urinary tracts. The flexibility and expandability of animal models guarantee that they will continue to lead the way in medical research, especially as they continue to incorporate the latest technologies. Finally, capitalizing on these findings will enable a deeper understanding of how problems in the genital and urinary systems affect overall health and will enable the development of creative solutions to critical public health issues (Hu et al., 2025; Zhang et al., 2025).

SUMMARY

The complex mechanisms of the genital and urinary system development are important in the understanding of human physiology and pathology. During embryonic development, several signaling pathways and genes coordinate the development of these systems to ensure they develop appropriately for their reproductive and excretory functions. The interaction of hormones and genetic determinants, particularly at times of critical development, has been demonstrated to play a role not only in the physical structures of the genitalia and urinary tract but also in their long-term functioning. With new information arising, it is increasingly clear that disturbances during this developmental period can result in a variety of disorders, highlighting the significance of knowing about these processes both in clinical and developmental contexts. In addition, the intersection of information from genetics, molecular biology, and clinical experience points to the promise of novel therapeutic strategies that target abnormalities in the genital and urinary tract. For example, examination of the functions of dominant proteins and signaling molecules can offer insights into disease such as congenital defects, hypospadias, or urinary tract infections. Therapeutic interventions can encompass the use of pharmacological agents acting on select pathways or genetic counseling in hereditary disorder-affected families. Further, insight into the impact of disorders in these systems helps develop prevention and serves as a foundation for better patient care. Enhancing our knowledge in this regard will assist in better clinical outcomes for the subjects confronted by such issues. The growth of the urinary and genital systems is marked by intricate biological mechanisms that not only form the foundation of human health but also serve to explain the underlying pathogenesis of a range of disorders. The recent progress in investigations, specifically with regard to the efficacy and safety of treatments targeting associated conditions, like those targeting SGLT-2 inhibitors, signifies the imperative of continued research in this area (Carter et al., 2014). The implications are significant, as such abnormalities can have a direct influence on quality of life and health outcomes. With researchers illuminating the intricacies of genital and urinary tract formation, there is potential to convert the knowledge into real-world solutions, thereby improving preventive and therapeutic measures for impacted individuals (Ahmed-Sarwar et al., 2016). The way ahead lies in the development of interdisciplinarity and innovation to improve our understanding of these vital systems.

Genital and urinary system development is a sophisticated process that is intricately coordinated with genetic, environmental, and biochemical elements. The basic blueprint of these systems is formed early in embryogenesis based on the interaction between the mesoderm and the genital ridges. This interaction leads to differentiation into either a male or female structure based on the presence of certain sex-determining genes. Some of the key milestones are the indifferent stage formation, in which both the Mullerian and Wolffian ducts form. This indifferent stage is crucial as it provides the foundation on which further differentiation shall take place, leading to the formation of ovaries or testes, and finally having an impact on external genital development, thereby creating all-important points of sexual differentiation. The action of hormones secreted by developing gonads is also very significant at the phase of differentiation. In males, testosterone and anti-Mullerian hormone (AMH) cause the regression of the Mullerian ducts while inducing differentiation of the Wolffian ducts. In females, lacking these hormones, the Mullerian ducts develop into the uterus and fallopian tubes. Hormonal signal timing and balance are also important because interruptions can cause congenital abnormalities, including hypospadias or cryptorchidism in males and sexual development disorders in women. Knowledge of the hormonal pathways not only explains normal genital and urinary system development but also shows the risk for pathological development from disruptions. Making this developmental terrain even more complex are conditions such as endometriosis, which manifests as an especially vexing condition within the urinary and genital tracts. It is defined by the existence of endometrial-type tissue outside the uterus, and it is marked by debilitating pain and infertility, as well as significant economic costs to healthcare systems. Recent guidelines highlight early detection and treatment, demonstrating the complex nature of diseases affecting the genital and urinary systems. In spite of advancements in knowledge regarding determinants of endometriosis, such as congenital and environmental factors, as well as processes like retrograde menstruation, the disease remains mysterious and heterogeneous across individuals, with the need for continued research and enhanced clinical practices in women's health (Christian et al., 2022; Smolarz et al., 2021).

CLOSER LOOK

THE WOLFFIAN DUCT

The Wolffian duct, or the mesonephric duct, is a key structure in embryonic development of the urogenital system, specifically in the development of male reproductive organs and the early kidney apparatus. Developing from the intermediate mesoderm, the Wolffian duct is initially seen in the fourth week of human embryonic development as a caudally extended longitudinal epithelial tube originating from the mesonephric tubules towards the cloaca. Its initial role in early development is to serve as a drainage system for the mesonephros, the second of three consecutive kidney systems (pronephros, mesonephros, metanephros) that emerge in embryogenesis. While in humans the mesonephros and its duct are transient structures, they play an important role in normal renal and reproductive organ development. In males, through the action of testosterone produced by the fetal testes, the Wolffian duct develops into several important structures of the male urogenital system, such as the epididymis, vas deferens, seminal vesicles, and ejaculatory ducts. This is regulated tightly by androgens and the presence of functional Sertoli and Leydig cells. In women, lack of these androgens causes regression of the Wolffian duct, which is mediated by AMH produced by Sertoli cells, which at the same time causes regression of the paramesonephric (Müllerian) ducts in males. Though in women, the Wolffian duct mostly regresses, some parts may be left behind as vestigial structures like Gartner's ducts or epoophoron. Notably, the distal end of the Wolffian duct is also an essential inductor of metanephric blastema formation, the embryonic origin of the mature kidney, the metanephros. As the ureteric bud, derived from the caudal Wolffian duct, invades the metanephric mesenchyme at approximately the fifth week, it triggers a two-way interaction that is pivotal to the development of nephrons and the collecting system. This exchange induces the branching morphogenesis of the ureteric bud into renal pelvis, calyces, and collecting ducts, as well as causing the surrounding mesenchyme to differentiate into nephron structures such as the glomeruli and renal tubules. The Wolffian duct itself, therefore, does not form kidney tissue directly, but its structural and inductive functions are crucial in the initiation of definitive kidney formation. In addition, abnormalities of the development of function of the Wolffian duct or its derivatives may cause congenital anomalies including renal agenesis, ureters that are ectopic, or reproductive tract abnormalities in the male. In short, the Wolffian duct is a critical embryonic structure that aids in both urinary and reproductive system formation via direct differentiation and inductive signaling, whose final fate is sexually dimorphic and under strong control of hormonal signaling pathways during early embryogenesis.

REFERENCES

1. Abrão, J. M., Araújo, A. C., Figueiredo, F., & Figueiredo, D. L. A. (2020). Acute myocardial infarction in a young bodybuilder: A case report and review of the literature. *American Journal of Case Reports, 21*, e924796. https://doi.org/10.12659/ajcr.924796.
2. Acién, P., Acién, M., Agic, A., Annabi, B., Annunziata, G., Laganà, A. S., et al. (2017). *Unas Pro Omnibus, Omnes Pro Uno: A Novel, Evidence-Based, Unifying Theory for The Pathogenesis of Endometriosis.* https://core.ac.uk/download/84600731.pdf (accessed on 27 May 2025).
3. Adamczyk, P., Bartik, L., Bayat, A., Dworschak, G., et al. (2022). X-linked variations in SHROOM4 are implicated in congenital anomalies of the urinary tract and the anorectal, cardiovascular and central nervous systems. https://core.ac.uk/download/618187399.pdf (accessed on 27 May 2025).
4. Ahmed-Sarwar, N., Nathan, K. T., & Werner, P. M. (2016). SGLT-2 inhibitors: A novel mechanism in targeting glycemic control in type 2 diabetes mellitus. https://www.ingentaconnect.com/content/ascp/tcp/2016/00000031/00000005/art00003.
5. Amicuzi, U., Balsamo, R., Barone, B., Coppola, M., et al. (2024). Exploring the multifactorial landscape of penile cancer: A comprehensive analysis of risk factors. https://core.ac.uk/download/636827512.pdf (accessed on 27 May 2025).
6. Auchus, R. J., & Miller, W. L. (2019). The "backdoor pathway" of androgen synthesis in human male sexual development. https://pmc.ncbi.nlm.nih.gov/articles/PMC6464227/.
7. Barajas Vélez, M. Á., Cabello Olmo, M., Encío Martínez, I., Martínez, M., et al. (2021). Human microbiota network: Unveiling potential crosstalk between the different microbiota ecosystems and their role in health and disease. https://core.ac.uk/download/491328734.pdf (accessed on 27 May 2025).
8. Baskin, L. S., Cao, M., Cunha, G. R., Ricke, W. A., et al. (2019). Reproductive tract biology: Of mice and men. https://pmc.ncbi.nlm.nih.gov/articles/PMC7339118/.
9. Baskin, L., Calvert, M., Cao, M., Cunha, G. R., et al. (2020). Imaging the developing human external and internal urogenital organs with light sheet fluorescence microscopy. https://www.sciencedirect.com/science/article/abs/pii/S0301468119300799?via%3Dihub.
10. Baskin, L., Cao, M., Cunha, G. R., Liaw, A., et al. (2018). Development of the human bladder and ureterovesical junction. https://www.sciencedirect.com/science/article/abs/pii/S0301468118301038?via%3Dihub.
11. Becker, C. M., Bokor, A., Heikinheimo, O., Horne, A. W., Jansen, F., Kiesel, L., King, K., et al. (2022). ESHRE guideline: Endometriosis. *Human Reproduction Open, 2022*(1), hoac009. https://doi.org/10.1093/hropen/hoac009.
12. Beeson, M. S., Ankel, F., Bhat, R., Broder, J., Paradise, S., Gorgas, D. L., Jones, J. S., et al. (2020). The 2019 model of the clinical practice of emergency medicine. *Journal of Emergency Medicine, 59*(1), 96–120. https://doi.org/10.1016/j.jemermed.2020.03.018.
13. Bittner, T., Donnelly, M., & Rosse, C. (2006). A formal theory for spatial representation and reasoning in biomedical ontologies. https://core.ac.uk/download/pdf/9412351.pdf (accessed on 27 May 2025).

14. Cabiddu, S., Cau, A., Follesa, M. C., & Porcu, C. (2010). Gonad development and reproduction in the monoecious species *Chlorophthalmus agassizi* (Actinopterygii: Aulopiformes: Chlorophthalmidae) from the Sardinian Waters (Central-Western Mediterranean). https://core.ac.uk/download/pdf/54567398.pdf (accessed on 27 May 2025).

15. Campo, M. S. (2006). Bovine papillomavirus: Old system, new lessons? https://core.ac.uk/download/1393674.pdf (accessed on 27 May 2025).

16. Carter, C. A., Pittet, D., Mavalankar, D., Yealy, D. M., Karunajeewa, H. A., et al. (2014). The effect of surveillance and appreciative inquiry on puerperal infections: A longitudinal cohort study in India. https://core.ac.uk/download/19506505.pdf (accessed on 27 May 2025).

17. Davies, K. (2023). An introduction to differences in sex development (DSD). https://core.ac.uk/download/613862253.pdf (accessed on 27 May 2025).

18. Feyta, Y. (Yuliya), & Pyrohova, V. (Vira). (2018). Assessment of risk factors of septic complications of the puerperium. https://core.ac.uk/download/301580699.pdf (accessed on 27 May 2025).

19. Fitzpatrick, B., Hendry, D. S., Leung, H. Y., et al. (2014). Development of the lymphoedema genito-urinary cancer questionnaire. https://core.ac.uk/download/42355541.pdf (accessed on 27 May 2025).

20. Foster, H., Goumenou, A., Karamouti, M., Karteris, E., et al. (2010). Congenital imperforate hymen with hydrocolpos and hydronephrosis associated with severe hydramnios and increase of maternal ovarian steroidogenic enzymes. https://core.ac.uk/download/336910.pdf (accessed on 27 May 2025).

21. Helner, N. (Nadiya), Makukh, H. (Halyna), Prokopchuk, N. (Natalia), & Sharhorodska, M. (2019). Medical genetic counseling of women with congenital heart diseases of fetus. https://core.ac.uk/download/301580705.pdf (accessed on 27 May 2025).

22. Hou, K., Wu, Z. X., Chen, X. Y., Wang, J. Q., Zhang, D., Xiao, C., Zhu, D., et al. (2022). Microbiota in health and diseases. *Signal Transduction and Targeted Therapy, 7*, Article 135. https://doi.org/10.1038/s41392-022-00974-4.

23. Hu, W., Wang, Y., Han, J., Zhang, W., Chen, J., Li, X., & Wang, L. (2025). Microfluidic organ-on-a-chip models for the gut-liver axis: From structural mimicry to functional insights. *Biomaterials Science*. https://www.semanticscholar.org/paper/58198f7b5fe724fbfc481025992a9aefd2ccc249 (accessed on 27 May 2025).

24. Ilhan, Z. E., Łaniewski, P., Thomas, N., Roe, D. J., Chase, D. M., & Herbst-Kralovetz, M. M. (2019). Deciphering the complex interplay between microbiota, HPV, inflammation, and cancer through cervicovaginal metabolic profiling. *EBioMedicine, 44*, 675–690. https://doi.org/10.1016/j.ebiom.2019.04.028.

25. Jain, S. (2009). *The Many Faces of RET Dysfunction in Kidney*. https://core.ac.uk/download/70378095.pdf (accessed on 27 May 2025).

26. Katzman, W. B., & Pastore, E. A. (2012). Recognizing myofascial pelvic pain in the female patient with chronic pelvic pain. https://pmc.ncbi.nlm.nih.gov/articles/PMC3492521/.

27. Nicholas, M. K., Vlaeyen, J. W. S., Rief, W., Barke, A., Aziz, Q., Benoliel, R., Cohen, M., et al. (2018). The IASP classification of chronic pain for ICD-11: Chronic primary pain. *Pain, 160*(1), 28–37. https://doi.org/10.1097/j.pain.0000000000001390.

28. Rizk, M. L., Zou, L., Savic, R. M., & Dooley, K. E. (2017). Importance of drug pharmacokinetics at the site of action. *Clinical and Translational Science, 10*(3), 133–142. https://doi.org/10.1111/cts.12448.

29. Rosse, C. (2000). *Terminologia Anatomica: Considered from the Perspective of Next-Generation Knowledge Sources.* https://core.ac.uk/download/pdf/9412243.pdf (accessed on 27 May 2025).

30. Roth, G. A., Abate, D., Abate, K. H., Abay, S. M., Abbafati, C., Abbasi, N., Abbastabar, H., et al. (2018). Global, regional, and national age-sex-specific mortality for 282 causes of death in 195 countries and territories, 1980–2017: A systematic analysis for the Global Burden of Disease Study 2017. *The Lancet, 392*(10159), 1736–1788. https://doi.org/10.1016/S0140-6736(18)32203-7.

31. Smolarz, B., Szyłło, K., & Romanowicz, H. (2021). Endometriosis: Epidemiology, classification, pathogenesis, treatment and genetics (Review of literature). *International Journal of Molecular Sciences, 22*(19), 10554. https://doi.org/10.3390/ijms221910554.

32. Speiser, P., Arlt, W., Auchus, R. J., Baskin, L. S., Conway, G. S., Merke, D. P., Meyer-Bahlburg, H. F. L., et al. (2018). Congenital adrenal hyperplasia due to steroid 21-hydroxylase deficiency: An Endocrine Society clinical practice guideline. *The Journal of Clinical Endocrinology & Metabolism, 103*(11), 4043–4088. https://doi.org/10.1210/jc.2018-01865.

33. Tadir, Y., Gaspar, A., Lev-Sagie, A., Alexiades, M., Alinsod, R., Bader, A., Calligaro, A., et al. (2017). Light and energy-based therapeutics for genitourinary syndrome of menopause: Consensus and controversies. *Lasers in Surgery and Medicine, 49*(2), 137–159. https://doi.org/10.1002/lsm.22637.

34. Venuti, A., Borzacchiello, G., Raso, C., Rizzo, C., Urraro, C., Paolini, F., et al. (2008). Detection of bovine papillomavirus type 2 in the peripheral blood of cattle with urinary bladder tumors: Possible biological role. https://core.ac.uk/download/55012241.pdf (accessed on 27 May 2025).

35. Zhang, Y., Chen, H., Li, Y., Luo, C., Zhu, Y., Zhou, X., Wang, R., et al. (2025). Animal models for long COVID: Current advances, limitations, and future directions. *Journal of Medical Virology, 97*(2), e70237. https://www.semanticscholar.org/paper/28f78db4cbc02faf35e7455df1b7c670fc4abdf6 (accessed on 27 May 2025).

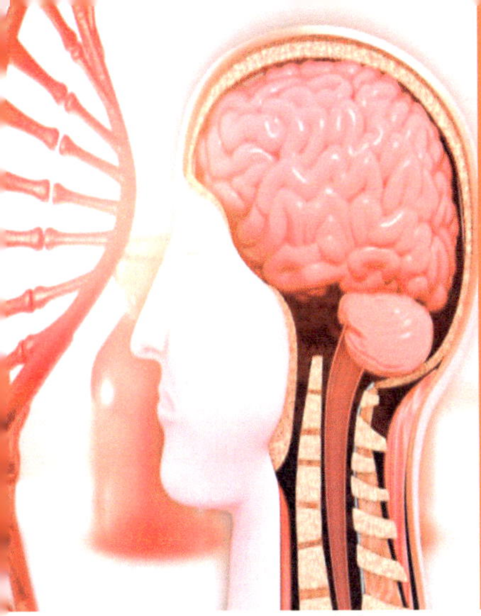

Chapter 7

CRANIOFACIAL DEVELOPMENT AND GENETICS

Contents

Introduction

During pregnancy, craniofacial development happens under the influence of many genetic and environmental factors. It is very important to understand this process, because abnormalities can result in different craniofacial issues such as craniosynostosis, where the skull sutures fuse too early. It can change the way a person looks and may also have major effects on mental development and general health. Genetics has recently helped us understand the routes and genes that are necessary for proper formation of the face and head, showing how important genetic studies are for finding risk factors of these conditions. The role of the Human Phenotype Ontology (HPO) in providing a standardized framework for describing phenotypic abnormalities underlines the necessity for comprehensive data in both clinical and research contexts (Sebastian Köhler et al., 2020). Genetic factors are extremely important in how the face and skull develop. Normal growth can be disrupted and developmental disorders may occur when genetic mutations, either inherited or not, occur. As an illustration, changes in the genes that control cranial sutures can result in abnormal joining which changes the shape and structure of the skull. Also, the way genes and the environment interact plays a role in causing the variety of symptoms seen in craniofacial conditions. With the integration of genomic studies and advancements in genetic testing, clinicians can now better predict the likelihood of craniofacial anomalies (CFAs) and implement early intervention strategies. A strong foundation in genetics is essential for both understanding these developmental processes and for informing clinical guidelines to optimize patient outcomes, as emphasized in recent expert recommendations (Mathijssen, 2020). Because craniofacial genetics is advancing, it is very important for experts from different fields to collaborate. Using genetic information in clinical practice helps doctors give a more complete diagnosis and treatment. For example, a recent review of the literature on craniosynostosis guidelines found that early referral and correct diagnosis are very important for effective treatment. Also, when new phenotypes and mutations are discovered, the guidelines and care plans must be updated to keep up with the new information. Working on detailed guidelines points out that doctors and healthcare workers must always learn and adapt. It is crucial to harness this knowledge to improve treatment approaches, prevent complications, and enhance the quality of life for individuals affected by CFAs (Figure 7.1).

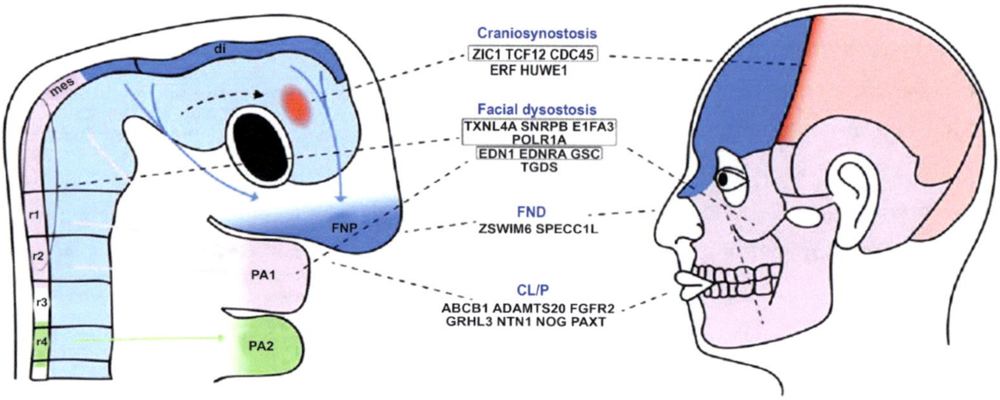

Figure 7.1. Development of the head and face and recently identified craniofacial.

Source: https://www.researchgate.net/profile/Steve-Twigg/publication/278731343/figure/fig2/AS:667176394571791@1536078656784/Development-of-the-head-and-face-and-recently-identified-craniofacial-genes-An-embryo-is.png.

Definition of Craniofacial Development

Craniofacial development refers to the complex biological processes that occur in the formation and differentiation of the skull and facial structures during embryogenesis. It is concerned with the interplay between the genetic, molecular, and environmental factors responsible for directing the growth and morphology of the structures. When the ectodermal and mesodermal tissues migrate, proliferate, and differentiate during early development, they contribute to the formation of the cranial neural crest cells necessary for facial feature development. The neural crest cells give rise to bones, cartilage, and connective tissues in the craniofacial complex. Characterization of the complexities within these pathways is significant, as dysmorphologies in craniofacial development can contribute to a myriad of conditions such as cleft lip and palate (CLP), which are functionally and esthetically relevant. The genetic underpinning of craniofacial development is extremely complicated, reflecting the multifactorial complexity of these phenotypes. Studies have identified particular genetic loci responsible for a range of craniofacial characteristics, with allelic variation having an impact on morphology outcomes. More recent studies have indicated the presence of quantitative trait loci (QTL) that have variable expression depending on environmental factors, demonstrating a clear relationship between genotype and phenotype in this context of development (Albertson et al., 2016). These findings highlight the importance of considering not only genetic predispositions but also environmental pressures during craniofacial development since they can offer hints towards adaptive evolution via morphological diversity. This intersection of environment and genetics is central to understanding craniofacial phenotypes since it suggests a dynamic system that encompasses inherited characteristics as well as functional adaptations over the lifespan of an individual. Besides genetic forces, modularity of craniofacial features also plays a powerful role in developmental processes, mapping the manner in which some structures develop irrespective of other structures. Variational modularity is a concept that posits that some features covary and vary together because of gene and environmental interactions. Studies on craniofacial modularity have found that quite minor genetic changes are able to induce radical changes in trait covariance without enormous changes to overall morphology (Albertson et al., 2018). This is a sign that the craniofacial structure may possess intrinsic tendencies towards certain phenotypic outcomes, enabling rapid evolution. Understanding these module-specific dynamics not only enriches evolutionary biology but also sheds light on clinical maneuvers in the correction of craniofacial abnormalities, reinforcing the necessity to integrate genetic and developmental factors in this field.

Importance of Genetics in Craniofacial Formation

The relationship between genetics and craniofacial development is a complex process with wide-ranging effects on developmental processes. Craniofacial growth and morphogenesis are controlled by numerous genetic elements, and several genes coordinate the development of each skeletal element. Information on such genetic underpinnings is not only important in the comprehension of normal craniofacial development, but also in the management of congenital malformations such as craniosynostosis and CLP. The genetic material determines the cellular processes responsible for craniofacial tissue differentiation, including bone and cartilage, to achieve facial feature development appropriately. The intricate relationship between the genetic components and the consequent phenotypic influences underscores the significance of genetics in CFA prediction and treatment. The function of cartilage in craniofacial morphogenesis has been elucidated by recent research, delineating its bimodal role during morphogenesis. Cartilage also serves as a precursor template for endochondral bones within the chondrocranium and is thus significant in the determination of skull shape. As suggested in recent research, some of the predominant characteristics of hyaline cartilage facilitate directional growth, allowing for the development of facial structures that are adjacent. Nevertheless, cumulative evidence also indicates the potential for other roles of cartilage beyond being mere templates. The interactions between osteogenic and chondrogenic cells in development show that cartilage influences the position of the adjacent facial bones, which implies its involvement in direct and indirect craniofacial morphogenesis pathways (Smith et al., 2025). All of these findings indicate the sophisticated way by which craniofacial development is influenced by genetic factors mediated through cartilage. Furthermore, the role of individual genes and epigenetic processes in craniofacial abnormalities is ever more trendy in the literature. For instance, methytransferase-like gene 3 (Mettl3) was implicated in craniofacial development through its m6A RNA modification role. Zebrafish studies revealed that knockdown of mettl3 causes extreme CFAs, suggesting the gene's critical role in regulating stem cell differentiation and tissue development, among other important biological processes. These findings suggest that dysregulation of methylated m6A pathways can have dramatic impacts on craniofacial morphology (Ma et al., 2024). Clarification of the genetic regulation of craniofacial development not only informs medical management of congenital anomalies but also calls for critical consideration of the broader relevance of genetic research to public health and precision medicine (Figure 7.2).

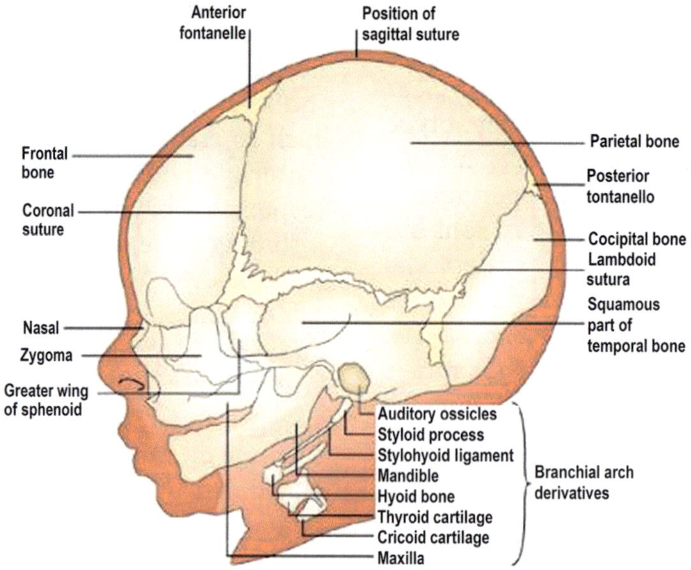

Figure 7.2. Genetics of craniofacial development.

Source: https://media.springernature.com/full/springer-static/image/art%3A10.1038%2F35076601/MediaObjects/41576_2001_Article_BF35076601_Fig1_HTML.gif.

7.1. Overview of Craniofacial Anatomy

Craniofacial anatomy is a very basic foundation for understanding the structural intricacy and developmental dynamics of the human face and skull. Composed of hundreds of bones, soft tissues, nerves, and vascular components, craniofacial anatomy holds paramount importance in a wide range of sciences, including medicine, dentistry, and plastic surgery. The human skull is made up of numerous bones, including the frontal, maxillary, and zygomatic bones, each with a particular role in the formation of facial features and bearing the sensory apparatus. Most importantly, cranial sutures, the fibrous joints between the skull's bones, are dynamic actors in skull development themselves. Their interaction strongly influences the ultimate head and facial form, offering strong underpinnings for understanding how genetic mechanisms give rise to specific craniofacial disorders and variations, a testament to the intricate interdependence of anatomical form and gene expression. Engagement of craniofacial anatomy and genetics is also improved by an investigation of developmental processes governing facial architecture. They are defined by a complex interaction of signaling molecules and transcription factors regulating cell proliferation, migration, and differentiation during embryogenesis. The neural crest cells, which migrate to give rise to parts of the facial skeleton, are especially important to normal craniofacial development. Mutations in the genes of these pathways may cause a range of congenital anomalies that are known as craniofacial syndromes. For instance, genetic mutations that regulate face structural growth, such as in craniosynostosis syndromes, are found to be responsible for premature closure of the sutures of the cranial bones, resulting in abnormal facial anatomy and potential functional hindrances. This convergence of anatomy and genes determines that craniofacial development research needs to be interdisciplinary. On top of that, improvements in technological methods such as virtual reality (VR) and computer modeling have opened new windows of opportunity for craniofacial anatomy acquisition and cognition. Current research has highlighted the advantages of the use of VR to optimize the acquisition of knowledge from accessing and seeing craniofacial structures three dimensionally. Interactive software such as this allows increased understanding of anatomical relationships and the impact of genetic factors on craniofacial malformations. The worth of such technology also augments the rising emphasis on personalized medicine, whereby information about an individual's craniofacial anatomy (coupled with genetic data) can provide access to tailored therapeutic strategies. The more the integration between genetics and anatomy advances, the more tools like the Mouse Genome Informatics (MGI) database are a necessity. MGI supports continuous research by providing required genetic data to explain biological processes of craniofacial development and its associated pathologies, thereby bridging gaps between theory and practice in craniofacial genetics (Janan, 2017; Jiang et al., 2021) (Figure 7.3).

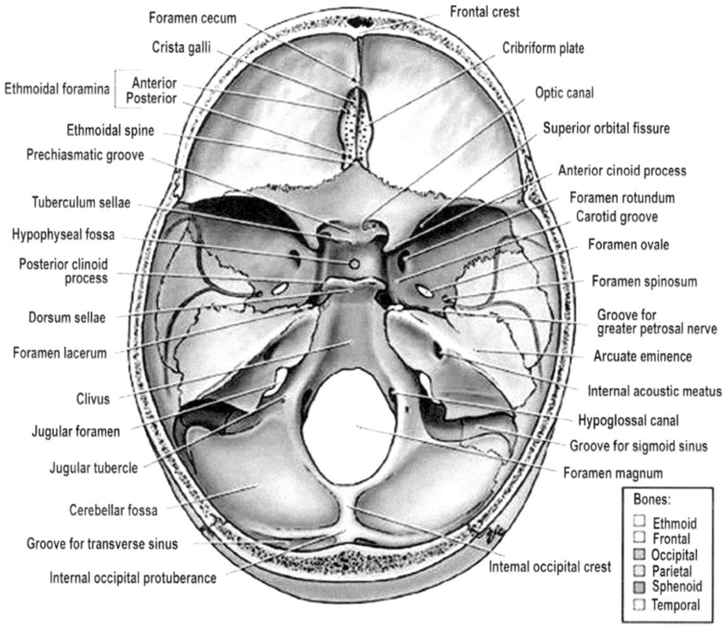

Figure 7.3. Craniofacial anatomy in embryology.

Source: https://pocketdentistry.com/wp-content/uploads/1008/image003723.jpeg.

7.1.1. Key Structures of the Craniofacial Region

The craniofacial complex is a very complex structure composed of numerous bones, muscles, and tissues that are involved in functions such as respiration, mastication, and speech. The maxilla and mandible are the focal points within this complex, representing the upper and lower jaw, respectively. Both structures need to have proper alignment and growth for oral function and facial appearance. Deformities in the development of these bones can lead to congenital conditions such as CLP. Understanding the genetic and developmental pathways that regulate the formation of these important structures allows for better treatment and management of CFAs. Interplay of environmental forces and genetic input during embryonic development is critical to the proper patterning of the craniofacial skeleton, for any disturbance may result in severe functional deficits and health issues of the patient. While the maxilla and mandible play essential roles, the nasal cavity and associated structures also contribute significantly to craniofacial functionality. The cartilaginous nasal framework and nasal bones support the stability of structures while preventing respiration and olfaction. It is that subtle interplay between these osseous and soft tissues that is most critical, as any defect will cause compromised airway performance and nasal contour. Importantly, advances in genetic research have provided insights into conditions affecting the nasal region, such as choanal atresia, which obstructs the nasal passage in newborns. Through research of the genetic foundation and developmental biology of these structures, scientists anticipate the identification of therapeutic targets through which congenital disorders of the craniofacial region can be intervened, thereby gaining deeper understanding of its complexity and clinical importance. One of the most significant characteristics of the craniofacial region is the involvement of several musculature that governs movement and function.

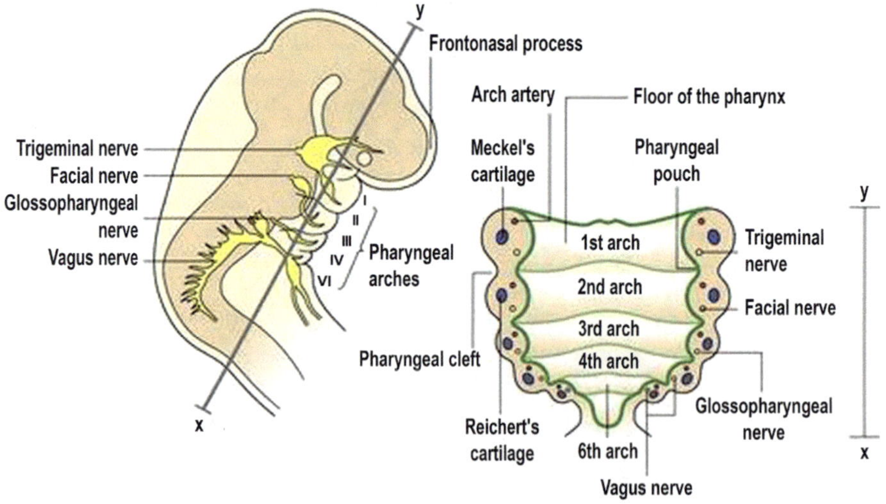

Figure 7.4. Key structures of the craniofacial region in embryology.

Source: https://pocketdentistry.com/wp-content/uploads/285/B9780723434504000055_f7.jpg.

Mastication muscles, including the temporalis, masseter, and pterygoid muscles, are accountable for the mechanical processes of mastication and speech. These muscles also have intricate relationships with the skeletal elements, relying heavily on the precise spatial location of the craniofacial bones for their normal functioning. Changes either in the musculature or in the development of the skeletal structures can result in temporomandibular joint disorders or malocclusion, affecting the quality of life in humans. Genetic breakthroughs have also identified some gene variants that are associated with such muscular and skeletal interactions, which have contributed to the knowledge of the mechanisms of such CFAs. Insights gained from studies focusing on craniofacial structure and muscle interaction propel forward the fields of genetic counseling and therapeutic practices aimed at ameliorating craniofacial dysfunctions, ultimately fostering interdisciplinary collaboration in patient care and treatment planning (Figure 7.4).

7.1.2. Developmental Stages of Craniofacial Anatomy

The craniofacial region undergoes a complex series of developmental stages that are vitally important to normal form and function. Beginning in the embryo stage, craniofacial formation is predominantly regulated by the interaction of various populations of cells, including neural crest cells and mesodermal tissues. They migrate and differentiate to give rise to specialized structures that make up the face and skull. The first critical event is the formation of pharyngeal arches, which serve as the building blocks for subsequent development. As further development proceeds, formation of the frontonasal prominence, maxillary processes, and mandibular processes must occur for construction of the basic framework of the face. Disruption at any one of these stages can lead to severe congenital anomalies, thus reflecting the significance of these developmental events in craniofacial anatomy. Genetic inputs to craniofacial development are significant too, leading to an organizational template through which physical structure arises. Transcription factors, such as Pbx family members, have key roles in modulating the morphogenetic process of the midface. These proteins are involved in the regulation of cell proliferation and apoptosis at sites of fusion of facial processes. In loss-of-function mutation experiments, researchers have found that disruptions in Pbx1, Pbx2, or Pbx3 are able to cause characteristic CLP malformations.

These findings illustrate the interconnectedness of genetic regulation and developmental outcome and therefore present a framework on which to base explanations for the genetic etiology of orofacial clefting and other malformations. The complexity of such relationships underlines the necessity for further study in ascertaining the genetic mechanisms of craniofacial malformations (Berkes et al., 2018). One of the revolutionary resources to enhance our understanding of craniofacial development is the Fish Face Atlas, an Internet-based resource designed to provide insight into the cellular events that underlie craniofacial skeletal development.

The atlas takes the form of three-dimensional imaging data from zebrafish embryos to determine particular anatomical structures and how these develop over time. With the assistance of advanced techniques such as fluorescent optical projection tomography, researchers can visualize the intricate process of cartilage and bone formation, critical in understanding variation in craniofacial anatomy between species. The information compiled in the atlas not only advances our understanding of developmental dynamics but also serves as a standard for comparative analysis and mutational research. Therefore, the Fish Face Atlas is a giant leap forward toward craniofacial biology progress, marrying analytic insight and clear visual presentation toward our further enrichment of craniofacial intricacy (DeLaurier et al., 2013) (Figure 7.5).

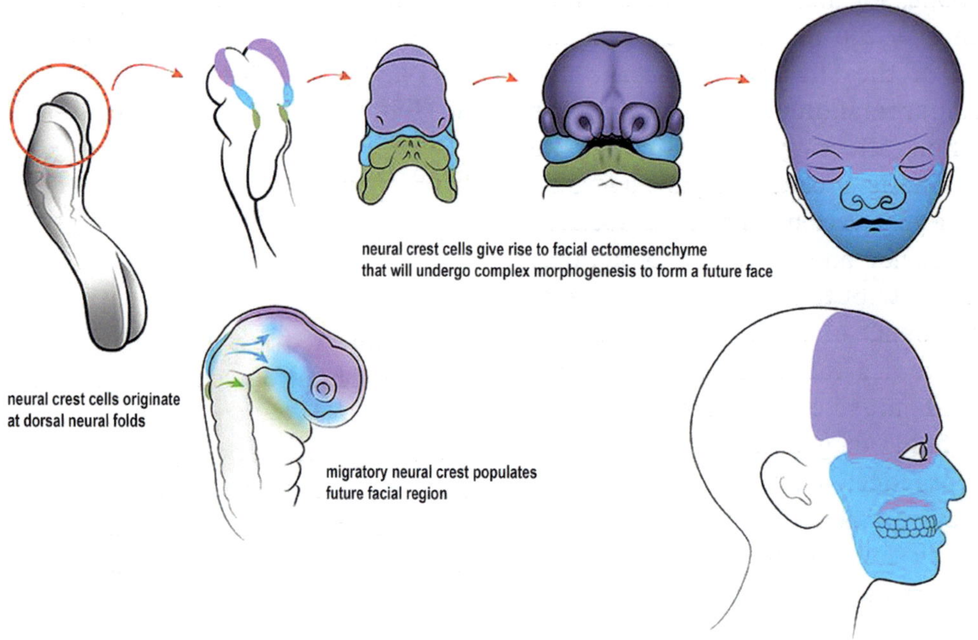

Figure 7.5. Developmental stages of craniofacial anatomy.

Source: https://images-provider.frontiersin.org/api/ipx/w=1200&f=png/https://www.frontiersin.org/files/Articles/185323/fphys-07-00049-HTML/image_m/fphys-07-00049-g001.jpg.

7.1.3. Functional Significance of Craniofacial Structures

The craniofacial region plays an integral part in functional as well as esthetic aspects of human anatomy. The intricate design of craniofacial structures provides for vital functions such as respiration, mastication, and phonation. For instance, the maxilla and mandible form the dental arch to facilitate proper chewing and grinding of food, which aids in digestion. On top of that, the nasal passage, supported by facial bones, is essential for air filtration and smell. Their arrangement in space also gives the resonance essential for speech production. Due to the complex interaction of genes present in craniofacial development, any variance will create malformation not only inhibiting functionality but even with social and psychological impact as well. The functional significance of such structures directs surgical and medical therapy to reconstruct quality of life in these patients. Craniofacial morphology is controlled by genetic mechanisms that predominantly determine their functional dynamics. A variety of gene families, such as the TGF-β family, are implicated to be essential for craniofacial development by being involved in cellular proliferation, differentiation, and tissue repair. TGF-β, for instance, is defined by the broad set of functions that it performs in regulating these processes, highlighting why TGF-β is one of the best-studied factors in craniofacial genetics (Morikawa et al., 2016). Dysregulation of genetic signaling can lead to developmental abnormalities such as CLP, which detrimentally affects the mechanics of chewing, speaking, and breathing. Hence, the genetics of craniofacial structures not only unravels the biological intricacy of these structures but also unlocks new avenues to specific therapies aimed at restoring function in subjects suffering from developmental disorders. Moreover, functional significance of craniofacial structures extends to their influence on overall health and well-being. Proper alignment and operation of the craniofacial skeleton are vital for the maintenance of oral health and prevention of associated complications such as temporomandibular joint disease or obstructive sleep apnea. Additionally, elements of the craniofacial complex belong to appearance identity; variations in their shape can have a significant impact on self-esteem and social interactions. Clinical guidelines demand that healthcare professionals must comprehensively investigate these factors while making a diagnosis and drawing up plans for intervention in CFAs (Members et al., 2014). Through the treatment of both craniofacial functional and psychosocial aspects of aesthetics, the medical community can implement a more integrated strategy, wherein not only do patients restore physiological function but also attain quality of life improvement.

7.2. Genetic Factors Influencing Craniofacial Development

The intricate relationship between the genetic factor and the development of craniofacial structures has captivated researchers who have tried to unlock the hidden biological processes that govern facial form. The high heritability of craniofacial dimensions in one of the initial studies to contrast monozygotic and dizygotic twins has been demonstrated. More recently, the study documented that monozygotic twins had significantly greater genetic contribution for vertical craniofacial dimensions than corresponding dizygotic twins. This finding emphasizes the importance of genetics in craniofacial morphology, suggesting that the same genetic qualities of monozygotic twins are the central elements in the development of their craniofacial morphology. Moreover, stability of dermatoglyphic characteristics in zygosity verification reiterates the research protocol for genetic research in this regard, emphasizing the importance of genetic heritage in craniofacial growth (KVV et al., 2025). Apart from genetic explanations identified using twin studies, multiple signal pathways take part in craniofacial morphogenesis. Of those, the Hedgehog (Hh) pathway, namely Indian Hedgehog (Ihh) and Gli zinc finger transcription factor 1 (Gli1), is a central controller of cranial bone and cartilage development. Ihh plays a role in the proliferation and differentiation of chondrocytes, necessary for the formation of cranial structures like the temporomandibular joint (TMJ). Malformation of the cranium and defective ossification are caused by aberration in Ihh signaling, illustrating the effect of interaction between genes on physical growth. The identification of Gli1 as a master regulator during bone development highlights the reciprocal dependence between genetic determinants and signaling pathways in shaping the craniofacial complex (Sun et al., 2024). Moreover, the relationship between Gli1 and Ihh illustrates the complex regulatory networks responsible for directing craniofacial development. Evidence indicates that Gli1+ cells act as master mesenchymal stem cells (MSCs) of craniofacial bones, and this highlights their differentiation and morphogenesis function. The cooperative control of Ihh and Gli1 not only ensures effective function of the Hh signaling pathway but also illustrates the intricacy of genetic regulation in craniofacial development. Understanding of such interactions is vital since it enlightens us regarding prospective therapeutic methods for craniofacial malformations and highlights the significance of research with accuracy towards tissue regeneration. These genetic components are addressed by treating them for novel clinical uses of orthodontics and craniofacial reconstruction with inheritable properties required for typical craniofacial morphology (Sun et al., 2024) (Figure 7.6).

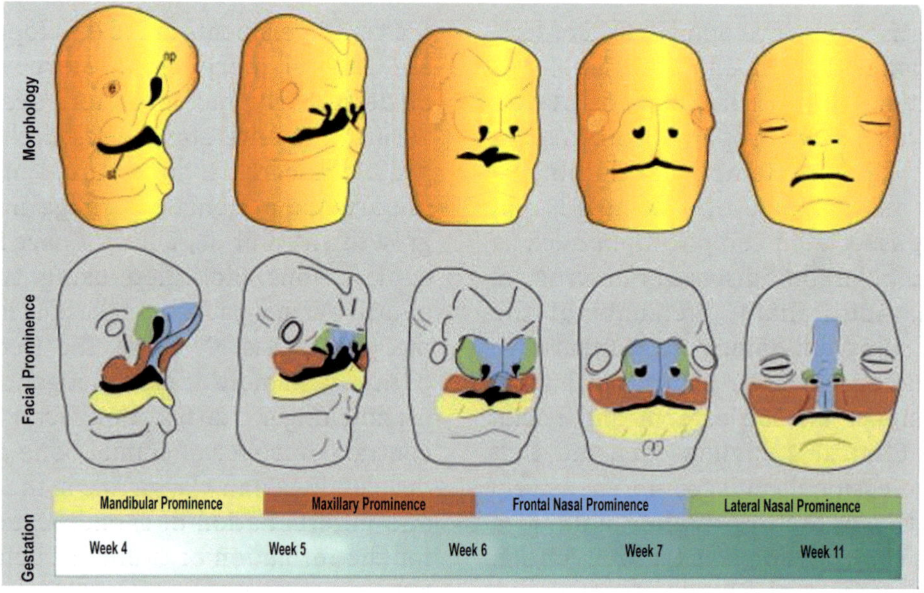

Figure 7.6. Genetic factors influencing craniofacial development.

Source: https://ars.els-cdn.com/content/image/3-s2.0-B9780124059450000351-f35-01-9780124059450.jpg.

7.2.1. Role of Specific Genes in Craniofacial Formation

The craniofacial region is a complex anatomical entity that is influenced by a vast array of genetic factors. Some genes are in charge of coordinating the complex process of craniofacial formation. For example, genes such as MSX1, PAX9, and AXIN2 are accountable for most CFAs such as agenesis of teeth and jaw deformities. Identification of such markers has come a long way in de-mystifying malocclusions. This genetic data allows more tailored treatment modalities in the orthodontics department, where methods can be tailored to the individuals' genetic tendencies. With ongoing progress in genetic research, the possibility of enhancing diagnoses and treatment planning for craniofacial deformities increasingly becomes a valid consideration, revolutionizing traditional practice within the field of orthodontic therapy and enhancing patient outcomes in general (Farran et al., 2024). Other than the genes identified above, Six1 has also been implicated in playing an essential function in craniofacial morphogenesis, specifically in mandibular development. The involvement of Six1 in such morphogenesis illustrates the function of transcription factors in controlling cranial neural crest-derived structures. Research into Six1 knockout mouse models suggests that removal of the gene leads to severe craniofacial malformations, including microsomia and high-arched palates. Besides, Six1 expression in ectomesenchyme is critical in the development of the mandible as its knockout affects the osteogenic gene expression vital for optimal craniofacial architecture. Such evidence reveals not only the pivotal role of Six1 but also the complex regulatory networks that guide craniofacial development, connecting genetic expression with phenotypic consequences in the craniofacial field (Luo et al., 2023). The collective action of these genetic elements accounts for a wider picture of craniofacial growth and associated disorders. Demystifying the genetic etiology of CFAs would allow researchers to make an important contribution to the development of diagnostics, treatment strategies, and even prophylactic interventions. Bringing genetic testing into clinical practice allows for early identification of susceptibilities to CFAs and optimal effectiveness of therapeutic interventions. It also opens up windows for new paradigms, such as gene therapy, which may be able to correct or modulate defects at the genomic level. In the course of developing research, the integration of genomic data into orthodontic and craniofacial therapy will not only refine treatment schedules but also illuminate a better understanding of human craniofacial biology, with a focus on genetics interactions with phenotypic expressions (Farran et al., 2024) (Figure 7.7).

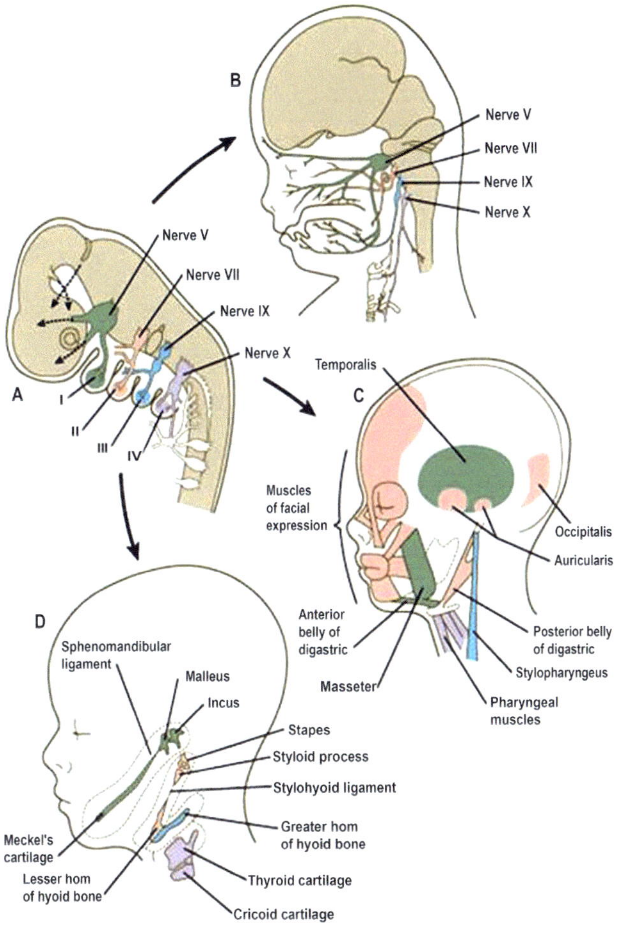

Figure 7.7. Role of specific genes in craniofacial formation.

Source: https://external-content.duckduckgo.com/iu/?u=https%3A%2F%2Fembryology.oit.duke.edu%2Fcraniofacial%2FheadEmbryoImage6.jpg&f=1&nofb=1&ipt=477b3eb52c310796028b0a96c075f130d97e64cb1defac093eec28bebc73f87e.

7.2.2. Genetic Mutations and Their Impact on Development

Genetic mutations play a vital role in craniofacial development since they influence facial structure morphology and function. Genetic mutations, such as in the EPHRIN-B1 gene, are responsible for craniofrontonasal syndrome (CFNS), a disorder characterized by typical CFAs. Interactions between EPHRIN-B1 and receptors, such as EPHB1, EPHB2, and EPHB3, play a crucial role in normal facial morphogenesis. Research has indicated that their loss results in drastic facial morphological alterations, implying that there has to be precise genetic control for ideal craniofacial growth. A study examined the facial morphologies of various mouse mutants devoid of these receptors, revealing particular patterns such as wider orbits and altered nasal placements in triple homozygous nulls, underscoring the additive and unique impacts of individual genetic components on overall facial structure (Mincer et al., 2021). Further consideration of genetic mutations demonstrates intricate interactions between CFAs and developmental pathways. As evident from the example of the EPHB receptor genes, individual mutations have non-linear impacts on facial morphology, demonstrating the intricacy of craniofacial development. This is also complicated by potential additional genetic influences, which may interact with the EPHRIN-B1 signaling pathways. For example, mutations in additional growth and regulatory genes can exacerbate or mitigate the phenotypic expression of craniofacial syndromes, resulting in heterogeneous clinical findings. Clarification of these genetic interactions is important for a comprehensive insight into craniofacial development and the pathogenesis of related syndromes, with the aim of informing therapeutic strategies in patients with genetic mutations (Mincer et al., 2021). Additionally, broader implications of genetic mutations extend beyond structural anomalies to functional impairments and syndromic outcomes. Genetic risk factors such as those associated with apolipoprotein E (APOE) illustrate the connection between craniofacial development and broader systemic health conditions. For example, certain alleles of APOE have been implicated in neurodegenerative diseases, suggesting that genetic impacts can cascade through multiple systems including craniofacial structure and function. The complexity of these interactions underscores the necessity of an integrated approach to studying craniofacial genetics, in which susceptibility genes are combined with environmental factors during growth. Investigating these interactions provides greater insight into how CFAs are not discrete entities, but rather part of a web of interrelated genes that guide individual health trajectories (Figure 7.8).

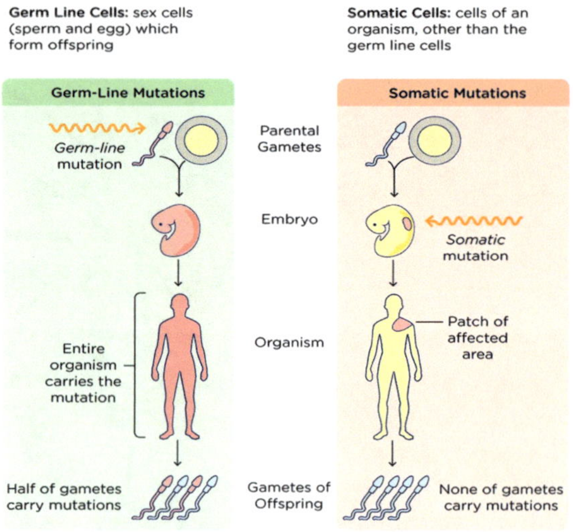

Figure 7.8. Genetic mutations and their impact on development.

Source: https://external-content.duckduckgo.com/iu/?u=https%3A%2F%2Falevelbiology.co.uk%2Fwp-content%2Fuploads%2F2019%2F03%2FMutations_1.jpg&f=1&nofb=1&ipt=b5de0fff5c4ef7a64c5e5106cb40b6a41393e9390039daeceb43aa585f992c5e.

7.2.3. Hereditary Patterns Observed in Craniofacial Anomalies (CFAs)

Studies on CFAs reveal that genetic patterns play a critical role in their development. The majority of CFAs are always linked to specific genetic mutations that affect craniofacial shape and performance. Syndromic CFAs, for instance, typically occur due to one gene alteration or intricate interactions between groups of genes inherited from parents. Evidence is suggestive of the fact that the majority of these syndromic conditions have patterns that are primarily autosomal dominant, with others being encountered as sporadic or de novo in nature. One of the retrospective reviews has indicated that the disease-causing genes implicated like FGFR2 and IRF6 have a crucial role to play in explaining the genetic basis of various craniofacial disorders, and thus increasing the possibility of targeted intervention and genetic counseling (Aaron et al., 2024). In clinical practice, the identification of hereditary patterns in CFAs is critical in the development of useful genetic testing algorithms. These algorithms enable practitioners to assess risk factors and facilitate the early diagnosis of such conditions, thus contributing to better patient outcomes. Through collaboration between genetics and pediatrics providers, there have been consensus-driven algorithms for orofacial clefts and craniosynostosis. These algorithms are crucial instruments in guiding best practice genetic assessment. By streamlining the testing protocol, clinicians are well-positioned to render patients timely and accurate diagnosis, which in turn benefits maximal medical management strategies as well as surgical interventions (Emily et al., 2024). Moreover, the intricate interaction between genetic factors and CFAs demands further research be carried out to unravel the secrets surrounding their hereditary models. Identification of new variants, for instance, those associated with Van der Woude syndrome and Crouzon's syndrome, sheds light on the varied genetic landscape of CFAs. With our appreciation of these hereditary characteristics growing, implications for future clinical practices become ever more important. Genetic counseling informed by full genetic analysis has the capacity to empower families with information, facilitating comprehension of recurrence risks and guiding reproductive decisions. Current studies that explore common and rare craniofacial syndromes will facilitate further insight into the mechanisms involved, leading eventually to the advancement of the science of craniofacial development and genetics (Figure 7.9).

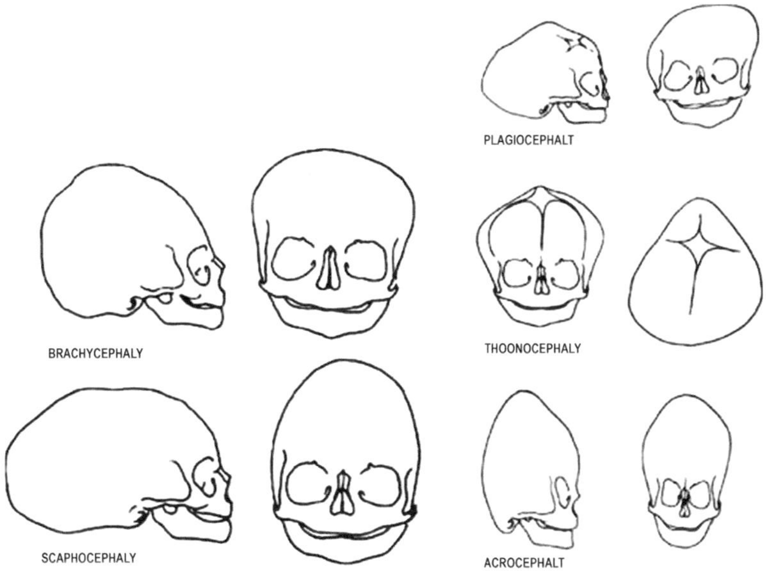

Figure 7.9. Hereditary patterns observed in craniofacial anomalies.

Source: https://external-content.duckduckgo.com/iu/?u=https%3A%2F%2Fentokey.com%2Fwp-content%2Fuploads%2F2016%2F07%2FDA2-DB1-DC1-C41-FF10.gif&f=1&nofb=1&ipt=0c5d8784ff524c5bcd4ad127a4961fca12f9d2b73d79761c5b5d2efe41b597ac.

7.3. Environmental Influences on Craniofacial Development

The intricate interplay of environmental and genetic determinants truly dictates craniofacial development, along with the intricacy of biological growth. Maternal nutrition and health during pregnancy are some of the principal environmental determinants. Lack of particular nutrients, including folic acid, is related to a myriad of CFAs, including CLP. They may be the result of both prenatal predispositions and noxious conditions, and thus a full understanding of developmental forces is necessary. For instance, the timing and nature of nutrient intake during critical embryonic intervals can shape not just short-term health status but also craniofacial form in the long run. These findings necessitate further exploration of the role of environmental factors, supporting the premise that CFAs are not merely a reflection of genetic susceptibility but also a reflection of developmental external factors. Moreover, environmental exposure to noxious agents has the potential to disrupt normal craniofacial growth, and being responsive to exogenous insult at susceptible periods of development is therefore imperative. This has been demonstrated by research that indicates that exposure to chemicals such as tobacco smoke, alcohol, and some chemicals can result in extensive malformations and developmental abnormalities. Teratogenic factors can interact with genetic susceptibility to increase the risk of CFAs among susceptible populations. Researchers are now examining how gene-environment interaction works, particularly among children with genetic predisposition that renders them more vulnerable to environmental causes. By identifying these associations, clinicians are able to craft efficient interventions with regard to both environmental exposure and genetic predisposition, thus improving preventive strategies against craniofacial disorders. Finally, the intersection of modern technology with craniofacial research has illuminated novel pathways through which environmental factors contribute to craniofacial development. Advanced methodologies such as high-resolution imaging and genetic analysis, as discussed in contemporary studies, allow researchers to visualize and understand craniofacial morphology profoundly. These methods enhance the knowledge regarding how environmental factors, in concert with genetic ones, determine craniofacial outcomes. Additionally, this interdisciplinary approach promotes the development of individualized medicine endeavors, as clinicians are able to tailor treatment and prevention protocols based on both genetic and environmental histories. Ultimately, understanding craniofacial development through the lens of environmental influences reveals a compelling narrative about growth that necessitates both genetic and external considerations, as highlighted in current research challenges and future directions (Juhi, 2023; Wang et al., 2025).

7.3.1. Maternal Factors Affecting Craniofacial Growth

Maternal factors play an important role in craniofacial growth and development by influencing genetic expression and environmental interactions that shape cranial structures. Nutrition in utero is an important factor, as insufficient intake of required nutrients, most notably folic acid, has been associated with numerous CFAs, including CLP. Evidence indicates that adequate folate enables DNA synthesis and repair, which are fundamental necessities for cell division in the development of developing organs and tissues, including the craniofacial complex. Moreover, maternal lifestyle choices, such as alcohol and tobacco consumption, negatively impact fetal craniofacial development. Both drugs disrupt normal growth and can cause a variety of congenital defects, once more indicating the contribution of maternal health to the prevention of craniofacial defects in pregnancy. The maternal environment will influence the genetic predisposition to CFAs through epigenetic processes. Exposure to environmental toxins, such as heavy metals or endocrine-disrupting chemicals, during critical periods of fetal development has been linked to altered gene expression that impacts craniofacial morphology. For instance, maternal exposure to high levels of lead has been associated with increased rates of cranial malformations, emphasizing the need for protective measures in expecting mothers. The intricate relationship between genetic and environmental exposures highlights the mechanism through which maternal factors significantly shape craniofacial development, necessitating a harmonized method of prenatal care that considers biological and environmental health determinants. In addition to dietary and environmental conditions, maternal disease conditions, such as obesity or diabetes, are critical maternal factors impacting craniofacial development. These diseases have the capability of inducing developmental disparities due to alterations of the metabolic environments during pregnancy. For example, gestational diabetes may lead to macrosomia, posing risks not only during birth but also for subsequent craniofacial growth patterns. Surprisingly, such maternal conditions are also correlated with syndromic forms of craniosynostosis, as maternal diabetes can disrupt the complex signaling pathways required for normal sutural closure and cranial shape formation. Innovations in prenatal diagnostics, as reflected in recent guidelines (Pierpont et al., 2018) and research initiatives (Mathijssen, 2015), are essential for identifying at-risk pregnancies and ensuring timely interventions that promote optimal craniofacial outcomes in offspring, underscoring the pivotal role of maternal health in craniofacial genetics (Figure 7.10).

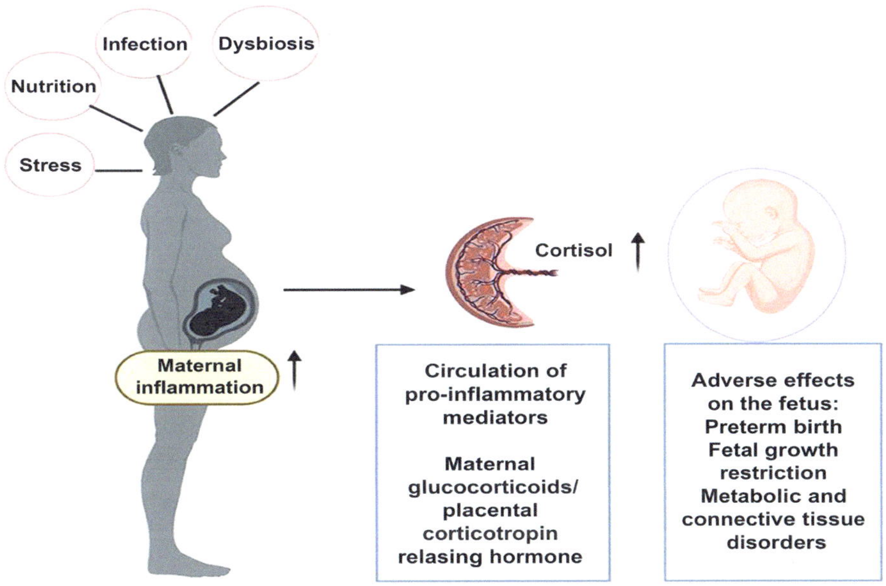

Figure 7.10. Maternal factors affecting craniofacial growth.

Source: https://www.frontiersin.org/files/Articles/735634/froh-02-735634-HTML/image_m/froh-02-735634-g002.jpg.

7.3.2. Teratogens and Their Effects on Craniofacial Structures

The disruption of teratogens in craniofacial development is one of the most serious concerns in the etiology of most CFAs. Teratogens may either be environmental factors such as some drugs, alcohol, and infections that may disrupt normal developmental activities during critical stages of gestation. Evidence suggests that teratogenic exposure during embryonic stages can lead to abnormal craniofacial morphogenesis, resulting in conditions such as CLP, craniosynostosis, and other dysmorphologies. This association is strongest in syndromic craniosynostosis, with the exposure to teratogens reinforcing underlying genetic predispositions, illustrating the dynamic interaction of environmental and genetic factors in CFAs. Not only is the timing but also the dosage of teratogenic exposure critical, as both determine the kind and degree of subsequent anomalies. These findings are pivotal in the development of preventive strategies and clinical management aimed at protecting fetal craniofacial development. Current research has also highlighted the importance of genetic susceptibility to teratogenic action during craniofacial development. For instance, individuals belonging to specific genetic backgrounds may be more susceptible to teratogens, and this might lead to a greater incidence of craniofacial anomalies.

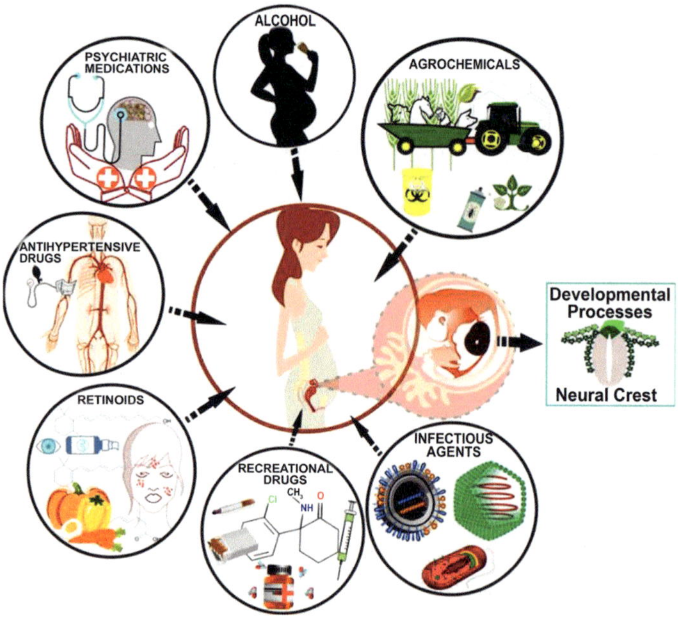

Figure 7.11. Teratogens and their effects on craniofacial structures.

Source: https://www.researchgate.net/profile/Manuel-Aybar/publication/338536974/figure/fig2/AS:905303281381376@1592852530035/Graphical-Abstract-Teratogenic-factors-disrupt-the-normal-morphogenesis-of-the-neural.png.

Clarifying the genetic mechanisms for such susceptibility can give hints for individualized prenatal care. By integrating knowledge of genetic predispositions with data on teratogenic exposure, healthcare providers can better assess risks and implement targeted prevention strategies. In addition, advances in genomic technology enable scientists to be capable of determining the complex interactions between various teratogens and gene influences, giving the platform for improved surveillance and intervention of vulnerable groups. Continued research to specify and categorize these interactions is important in decreasing the incidence of teratogen-induced CFAs. The impact of teratogens on craniofacial development also extends beyond individual structural defects, with extensions to functional and psychosocial implications for those affected. Patients born with CFAs typically face communication difficulty in speech, hearing, and socialization that leads to long-term psychosocial implications. The effects of teratogen exposure are not only observed physically but also reverberate through various processes of life, influencing cognitive development and emotional status. The diagnosis and treatment of these broader effects require a multi-disciplinary intervention in the form of genetic counseling, surgical intervention, and psychological treatment. The establishment of comprehensive care pathways for children with teratogen-related CFAs can enhance their quality of life and ensure that they receive holistic support. Consequently, this underscores the importance of proactive prenatal education and awareness regarding teratogens, bridging the gap between genetics, environmental factors, and their cascading effects on craniofacial health across the lifespan (Figure 7.11).

7.3.3. Interaction Between Genetics and Environmental Factors

Understanding of the intricate relationship between genetics and environmental factors is at the heart of deciphering the complexity of craniofacial development. Genetic mutations cause the formation of numerous CFAs, and certain mutations directly contribute to disorders such as orofacial clefts and prognathism. Such genetic predispositions, however, often interact with environmental influences such as maternal smoking, nutritional insults, or teratogenic exposures. This exchange not only confounds the etiology of craniofacial disorders but also demands a multifaceted approach in the research and clinical settings to unravel how such exogenous factors may exacerbate genetic susceptibilities. As noted, many of the genetic risk factors associated with CFAs can manifest differently when exposed to environmental triggers, leading to a diverse range of phenotypes and developmental outcomes (Jaruga et al., 2022). A significant issue in studying craniofacial development lies in the under-researched area of how environmental exposures impact genetically predisposed individuals. Extensive research is necessary for the determination of the entire spectrum of interactions present; e.g., CFM is a prime example where genetic factors, e.g., specific genomic loci, are involved in the condition but where environmental conditions during strategic stages of embryonic life are not very well understood to contribute to the condition. Current research has just begun to unveil these relationships, demonstrating that certain environmental risk factors, including paternal behaviors, raise the risk of CFM development when combined with a polygenic risk score (Xu et al., 2021). Thus, the continuation of this research can improve diagnoses and inform prenatal screening, which will ultimately result in reduced incidence and improved patient outcomes. The incorporation of a detailed appreciation of gene-environment interactions into clinical practice can facilitate more suitable management and preventive measures in CFAs. The advance in our appreciation of genetic susceptibilities, particularly through the identification of significant loci and their risk associations, facilitates better risk stratification and focused interventions. Further, the appreciation of the role of environmental factors, such as lifestyle and socio-economic determinants, provides an integrated picture of craniofacial development. From this consciousness, healthcare professionals can develop personalized counseling for risk populations to augment information and proactive actions to mitigate environmental factors that could exacerbate the vulnerabilities offered by their genes. The convergence of genetics and environment in CFAs indicates the need for inter-disciplinary integration to spearhead future research, clinical care, and patient education (Jaruga et al., 2022).

7.4. Common Craniofacial Disorders

Craniofacial anomalies are a heterogenous collection of congenital deformities that arise during facial and head development. They can present as structural abnormalities, from CLP to more complex syndromes such as 22q11.2 deletion syndrome. The latter is particularly noteworthy due to its association with characteristic facial dysmorphology and a heightened risk of psychotic illnesses, including schizophrenia. Current studies using 3D laser surface imaging and geometric morphometrics reveal striking similarities in facial morphology between 22q11.2DS patients and schizophrenia patients, highlighting the importance of facial dysmorphology in diagnosis and clinical handling of these allied disorders. This confluence of craniofacial and psychological phenomena underscores the multifaceted implications of craniofacial disorders and the need for interdisciplinary genetic and clinical studies (Aggarwal et al., 2015). The genetic basis of craniofacial disorders is key to understanding their etiology, which is multifactorial in nature. For instance, the CFDP1 gene on chromosome 16q22.2-q22.3 is linked to a variety of craniofacial malformations and plays a critical role in the chromatin remodeling process. Aberrant expression or dysfunction of CFDP1 not only disrupts normal craniofacial development but also can directly cause developmental disorders resulting in infant morbidity and mortality. By examining cellular processes of the CFDP1 protein, researchers have found its role in chromosome organization and cell cycle regulation, uncovering the intricate molecular mechanisms controlling craniofacial development. This research therefore offers insight into how genetic and epigenetic disruptions can manifest as CFAs, with a need to more carefully consider their developmental etiology (Atterrato et al., 2017). As we enhance our understanding of common craniofacial disorders, it becomes clear that early diagnosis and treatment are the most critical factors. Clinicians are now able to use sophisticated imaging modalities and genetic assessments that allow for the diagnosis of such disorders at a young age. Therapies such as surgical corrections in CLP have been found to be effective in improving both aesthetic and functional outcomes, significantly impacting the quality of life of patients. Furthermore, ongoing genetic research promises to refine our understanding of CFAs, identifying new biomarkers and therapeutic targets that could alter the disease trajectory.

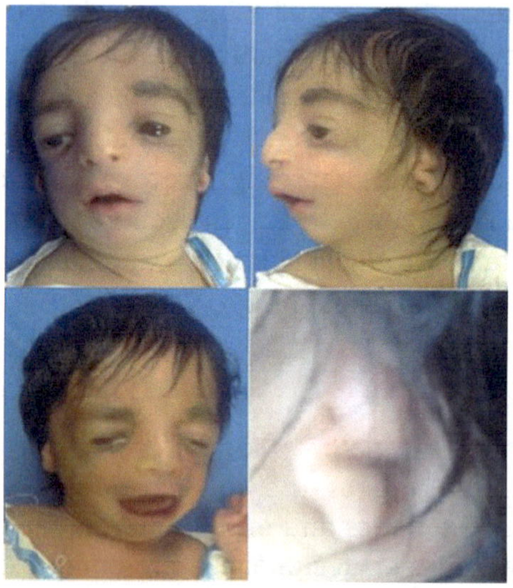

Figure 7.12. Craniofacial disorders.

Source: https://cdnintech.com/media/chapter/73154/1512345123/media/F4.png.

By integrating genetic insights with clinical practices, healthcare providers can better tailor their approaches to individual patients, ultimately leading to enhanced outcomes and an overall improved quality of care for those affected by craniofacial disorders (Figure 7.12).

7.4.1. Overview of Cleft Lip and Palate (CLP)

The development of CLP occurs during embryogenesis at an early period and is one of the most common congenital malformations that are encountered in clinical practice. The embryological development of the face and the palate occurs by the fusion of the various facial processes that happen between the 4th and 10th weeks of gestation. Disruptions in this process are also accountable for the incomplete fusion of the lip and palatine structures that result in the varied presentations of CLP. Understanding the critical timeline and mechanisms of craniofacial development is relevant for healthcare professionals, particularly ultrasonographers who are involved in prenatal screening. In-depth knowledge of these embryological processes can enhance diagnostic accuracy, with the overall goal of enhancing outcomes for affected infants and their families.

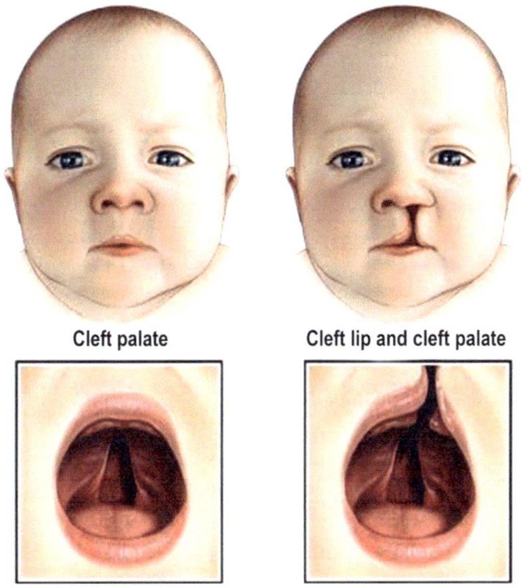

Figure 7.13. Overview of cleft lip and palate (CLP).

Source: https://www.mayoclinic.org/-/media/kcms/gbs/patient-consumer/images/2013/08/26/10/45/ds00738_ds00998_im02607_fl7_cleft_palatethu_jpg.png.

Moreover, knowledge of the significance of these developmental stages highlights the requirement for targeted ultrasound screening that can identify these conditions early, enabling early intervention and management (Smarius et al., 2017). Postnatally, CLP are classified into various types based on the anatomy involved and the severity of the defect. This classification system is also helpful to healthcare providers as they coordinate care within multidisciplinary teams that may include surgeons, orthodontists, speech therapists, and genetic counselors. Classification also assists in the development of treatment plans that respond to the individual needs of each patient. A consistent approach to the management of CLP cannot be understated; each patient's experience varies, and the repair and rehabilitation must also be individualized. Furthermore, handling associated issues such as feeding difficulties and potential speech disability is significant for the child's development. Given the complexities of the cases of CLP, efficient communication among healthcare teams is crucial in order to supply general care, meaning the role of a highly developed classification system in improved patient outcomes (Smarius et al., 2017). CLP may occur with other disorders such as Robin sequence (RS), making diagnosis and management even more complicated. Robin sequence is characterized by micrognathia, glossoptosis, and upper airway obstruction that may appear as isolated anomalies or as part of more involved syndromic presentations. The subjective nature of the diagnosis of micrognathia can be challenging in the clinical evaluation, necessitating consensus-derived best practices to ensure standardized examinations. Effective management of RS is closely related to an understanding of how airway compromise can exacerbate feeding difficulties, particularly in infants with cleft palates. A uniform approach to the clinical evaluation of such disorders serves to empower health professionals to introduce evidence-based remedies for managing the unique issues presented by each case. Lastly, extensive knowledge pertaining to craniofacial development and associated syndromes, such as RS, is necessary to optimize care for affected infants and to facilitate their long-term growth and development (Figure 7.13).

7.4.2. Syndromic Craniofacial Disorders

Syndromic craniofacial disorders are a group of disorders characterized by the abnormal formation of craniofacial structures and often linked with genetic predispositions. Syndromic craniofacial disorders are presented in association with the concomitance of well-defined facial features and systemic illness, a peculiarity among presentation complexities and treatment needs. Clinical presentation variability is a reflection of syndromic craniofacial complexity because of the diversity of genetic mutations that can result in similar phenotypic expressions. The interaction of genetic influences with environmental determinants, such as teratogen exposures during pregnancy, also makes the etiology and course of development of these conditions more complicated. Critical studies indicate that an epigenetic framework can offer insight into how environmental factors affect gene expression, potentially elucidating the mechanisms that underlie disorders like microtia, known for its significant craniofacial implications (Chen et al., 2024). CFM serves as a prominent example of syndromic craniofacial disorders that arise from disruptions in embryonic development affecting the first and second branchial arches. CFM is typified by a spectrum of deformities, which can include underdevelopment of the jaw and ear anomalies, and it poses both aesthetic and functional challenges for affected individuals. Research reveals that CFM and related syndromes have garnered considerable attention within the clinical community, accomplished through a comprehensive bibliometric analysis that illustrates the growing interest in this field over the last three decades (Liu et al., 2023). The analysis of published literature suggests that research in this area is increasingly focused on clinical characteristics, classification systems, and advanced surgical techniques, such as mandibular distraction osteogenesis, which aimed to improve the quality of life for affected patients. The implications of syndromic craniofacial disorders extend beyond physical presentation, highlighting the need for interdisciplinary approaches in their management. Genetic counseling plays a crucial role in addressing familial risks and informing prospective parents about potential outcomes associated with known syndromic conditions. Additionally, advancements in genetic testing and sequencing technologies have facilitated the identification of specific mutations linked to various syndromes, enabling more tailored treatment options. An increased understanding of the genetic underpinnings also encourages proactive measures in prenatal care and early intervention, essential for optimizing health outcomes in affected individuals. As research continues to evolve, it is imperative to maintain focus on the genetic and epigenetic factors influencing craniofacial development, allowing for improved diagnostics and therapeutic strategies in managing syndromic craniofacial disorders (Figure 7.14).

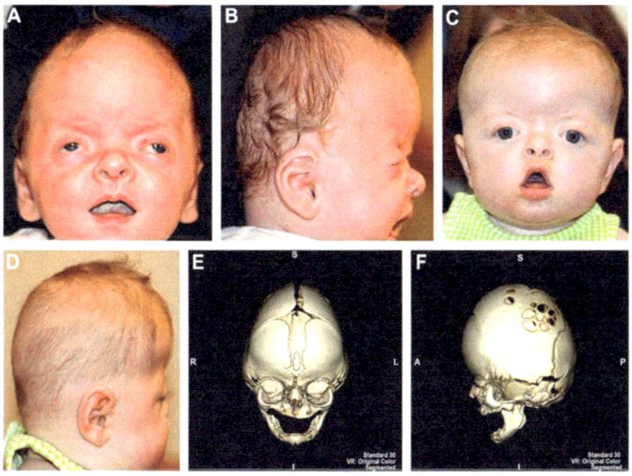

Figure 7.14. Syndromic craniofacial disorders.

Source: https://www.facialplastic.theclinics.com/cms/10.1016/j.fsc.2023.07.002/asset/e7cc5fd7-bae5-400a-8a0a-ae9134afb8a3/main.assets/gr1_lrg.jpg.

7.4.3. Non-Syndromic Craniofacial Anomalies (CFAs)

Non-syndromic craniofacial malformations, particularly orofacial clefts, are a major area of study in the realm of craniofacial development and genetics. Such malformations occur in isolation without being influenced by syndromic diseases and commonly in the general population, one of the most prevalent being orofacial clefts. Their multifactorial origin is due to synergistic interaction between genetic as well as environmental predispositions, which renders them extremely challenging to study as well as prevent. In recent years, extensive research has been conducted on the genetic etiology of such conditions, and several gene polymorphisms have been identified as having a potential to cause the presence of non-syndromic cleft lip with or without cleft palate (nsCL/P). By studying the inheritance patterns and associated risk factors, investigators aim to uncover the molecular driving forces underlying such malformations, which can lead to improved prevention and treatment. One of the most important aspects of the nature of non-syndromic CFAs is the way in which epigenetic processes, that is, DNA methylation, are involved. Various studies have detailed the manner in which variations in levels of DNA methylation can influence gene expression, which then proceeds to form orofacial clefts. For instance, research on patients with nsCL/P has noted variable patterns of hypermethylation and hypomethylation of specific genes and chromosome regions, underscoring the complexity of epigenetic regulation of craniofacial development. These methylation changes could be a consequence of varying exposures to the environment and genetic susceptibilities, underscoring the need for an integrative model that incorporates both genetic and environmental data. Elucidation of these mechanisms may pave the way for early detection and new interventions that may counteract the impacts of non-syndromic CFAs in humans. Apart from genetic and epigenetic effects, the impact of clinical guidelines and health policies in controlling non-syndromic CFAs should not be exaggerated. The ESC guidelines, while primarily cardiovascular in nature, illustrate the importance of overall care strategies in clinical practice, which also apply in CFAs. Medical practitioners are obligated to use clinical judgment based on the latest scientific evidence and to focus on sensitivity to the social and psychological impacts for individuals with craniofacial disorders. This accommodating outlook assures medical treatments become patient-specific, with ethical considerations incorporated, which is pivotal in treating patients with such conditions. Upon the incorporation of clinical practice guidelines and genetic research, there is space for more effective management strategies that not only address physical conditions of such anomalies but also enhance overall patient well-being (Figure 7.15).

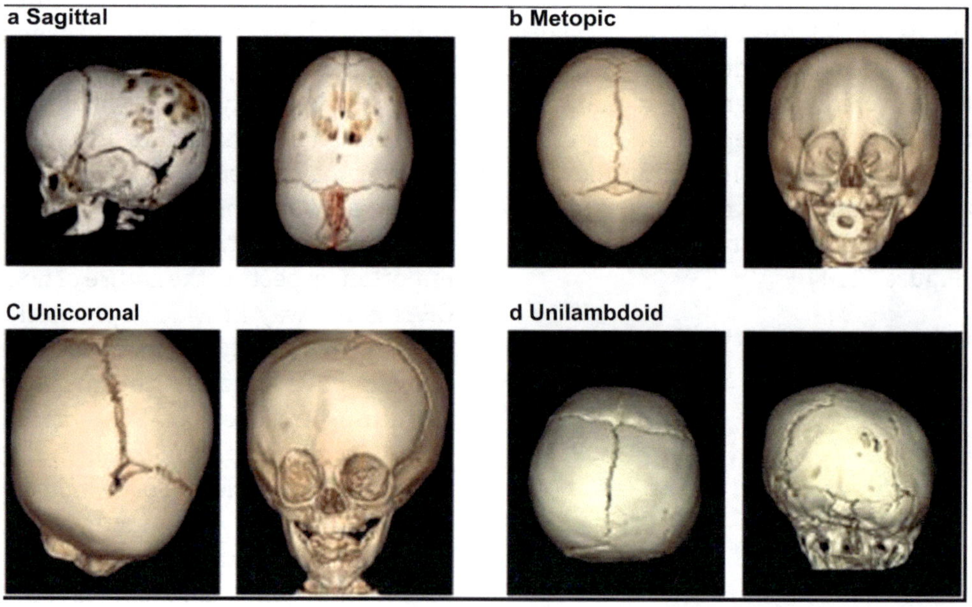

Figure 7.15. Non-syndromic craniosynostosis.

Source: https://media.springernature.com/lw685/springer-static/image/art%3A10.1038%2Fs41572-025-00607-4/MediaObjects/41572_2025_607_Fig3_HTML.png.

7.5. Advances in Genetic Research

Recent results of genetic research have significantly enhanced understanding of craniofacial development with inherent interactions between genetic determinants and morphological consequences being intricate. Modularity of craniofacial features is crucial as it involves developmental and evolutionary biology. From research, morphological variability was found to be indicative of developmental processes controlled by genetic variability. For example, research with zebrafish has shown that quite subtle alterations of genes may have profound effects on craniofacial covariance without severely deforming general shape. This suggests that specific genetic mutations will selectively induce just some latent modularity patterns, thus allowing the skull to be structurally coherent while facilitating rapid evolutionary adaptation. As a result, this well-balanced view of the genetic determinants can unveil new avenues to more effective approaches in the therapy of CFAs through targeted genetic manipulation (Albertson et al., 2018). Particularly, genetic dissection has demonstrated the richness of syndromes such as 22q11.2 deletion syndrome, which forms a pivotal example in craniofacial genetics. Patients with the syndrome are frequently distinguished by distinctive facial dysmorphologies, which have been well delineated using advanced imaging techniques like 3D laser surface imaging. A recent study identified that, while the facial contours of subjects with 22q11.2DS resemble those of subjects with schizophrenia, there are also distinct differences that become evident, especially facial length and prominence in some areas. These anatomic variations underscore the subtle interaction between genetics, craniofacial morphology, and developmental pathways. These findings not only make possible the comprehension of the phenotypic expressions of genetic disease but also highlight the therapeutic value of specialized clinical studies that can follow the developmental etiology of most CFAs and, by doing so, highlight the value of genetic investigation (Aggarwal et al., 2015). Further, the comprehension that is made possible by progress in genetic research finds relevance in broader implications for evolutionary biology and therapeutic intervention in craniofacial development. By unraveling the genetic etiology of craniofacial morphology and evolutionary forces, researchers can have a better idea about how specific traits predispose specific populations to specific phenotypic expression. Understanding how modularity patterns influence adaptive evolution is important to found successful interventions in craniofacial syndromes and anomalies. Ongoing debate on genetic influences and implications for development not only enriches academic discourse but also unfolds new perspectives for personalized medicine. As the genetic context surrounding craniofacial development is increasingly well understood, there is an increased opportunity to take these findings and apply them in practical terms within clinical settings that will further enhance patient care and treatment protocol, ultimately addressing the inherent significance of genetic research within the field (Aggarwal et al., 2015; Albertson et al., 2018).

7.5.1. Techniques Used in Craniofacial Genetic Studies

In craniofacial genetics, a range of advanced techniques are employed to describe the intricate interaction between genetics and craniofacial development. Among the most prominent techniques employed is genome-wide association studies (GWAS), where genetic differences between groups of individuals are compared to find specific loci associated with craniofacial morphology. This approach employs a massive number of single nucleotide polymorphisms (SNPs) to detect genetic susceptibility to such diseases as cleft palate and craniosynostosis. In addition, the next-generation sequencing (NGS) platforms allow for comprehensive examination of the genetic mutations influencing craniofacial morphology. The sequence technologies, through giving a wider view of the genome, make identification of rare variants that contribute to complex facial anomalies (CFAs) more feasible. Therefore, as a whole, the methods reveal the doors of individualization of treatment methods along with the creation of craniofacial disorder-specific therapies through enhanced clinical outcomes. In addition, advancements in bioinformatics have completely transformed the process of handling genetic information in craniofacial research. Extremely sophisticated computer programs enable researchers to decipher and analyze vast amounts of data sets obtained from genomic research in an effortless manner. With machine learning algorithms, researchers can detect faint patterns as well as interactions between genes that control craniofacial development. For instance, bioinformatics pipelines align gene expression profiles of healthy and affected craniofacial tissues to produce data on dysregulated pathways that can lead to malformations. Furthermore, the incorporation of comparative genomics allows researchers to evaluate the evolution of craniofacial genes in different species and contextualize human craniofacial genetics. Integration of these bioinformatics tools enhances the potential for identifying new genetic determinants of craniofacial phenotypes and clarification of underlying biological processes. Finally, in silico simulation and trans-regulatory analysis are also staples of craniofacial genetics investigation. Computer modeling enables researchers to examine GRNs with specific emphasis on craniofacial development transcription factors. Genetic interaction simulation software enables researchers to simulate phenotypic effects from specific genetic alterations. Above all, studies have also highlighted the involvement of transcription factors SOX2, KLF4, and MITF that are of significant importance in craniofacial morphogenesis and brain formation. The simulations not only elucidate genetic interactions but also indicate likely therapeutic targets for craniofacial diseases. Above all, the incorporation of these approaches ensures a comprehensive understanding of craniofacial genetics, ultimately impacting treatment methodology research. By combining these many different strategies, scientists are continually broadening our understanding of craniofacial development and its genetic underpinnings (Figure 7.16).

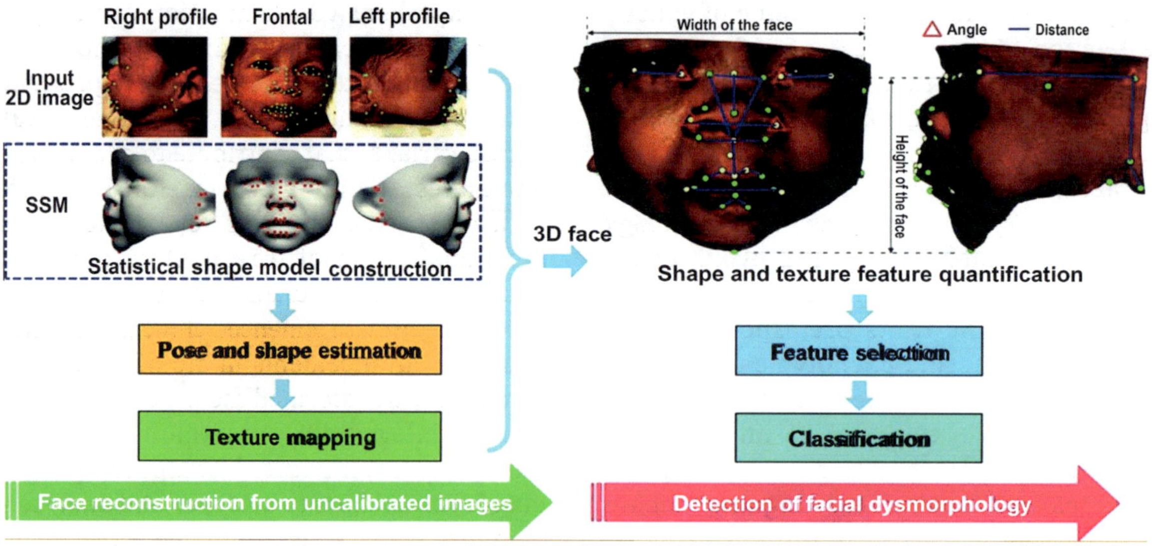

Figure 7.16. Techniques used in craniofacial genetic.

Source: https://scx2.b-cdn.net/gfx/news/hires/2019/anewfacialan.jpg.

7.5.2. Recent Findings in Craniofacial Genetics

More recent developments in craniofacial genetics have stressed the contribution of environmental factors to the development of facial form. The use of Danio rerio, or zebrafish, has emerged as a valuable model for elucidating the impact of environmental toxins on craniofacial form. Recent studies have offered a systematic review of the impact of various chemical pollutants, including herbicides and pesticides, on zebrafish embryonic craniofacial development. Analysis of a number of articles revealed that these toxicants have the capacity to negatively impact facial morphology and jaw formation in these organisms, suggesting parallels to the potential for impacts in mammalian and human systems. These results highlight the need to also consider environmental aspects alongside genetic predispositions in investigating CFAs, offering a broader context for environmental and genetic interplay in craniofacial development (Firdaus, 2018). In addition to environmental factors, genetic mutations are at the core of craniofacial abnormalities such as craniosynostosis. Molecular genetic progress in recent years has allowed for the identification of close to 57 genes associated with the condition, pointing to the complexity of its etiology. As next-generation DNA sequencing techniques continue to improve, the discovery of new genetic markers and mutations has been significantly sped up, offering the promise of improving understanding of craniosynostosis. While research has established that craniofacial disorders have environmental and genetic underpinnings, gaps persist in linking clinical presentations to specific genetic markers and the involved signaling pathways. Such investigations are worth pursuing, as they would potentially elucidate mechanotransduction events in the development of craniofacial abnormalities and ultimately guide better therapeutic strategies (Al Rekabi et al., 2016). In addition, the intersection of developmental biology and craniofacial genetics highlights the importance of animal models in advancing research. Through the integration of genetic research and cell mechanics research, scientists are obtaining useful insights into how craniofacial structures are developed and the pathways that control the process. Understanding the contributions of both biomechanical forces and genetic expression allows for a more nuanced view of craniofacial development, one that reveals how specific gene variants can modulate cell responses to mechanical stress. Such a coming together of disciplines not only enhances our knowledge of craniofacial development but also serves to underscore the need for additional research to fill gaps between genotype and phenotype. In so doing, we can better appreciate the craniofacial multifactorial genetics and how it pertains to human disease and health (Al Rekabi et al., 2016).

7.5.3. Implications of Genetic Research for Treatment

The clinical implications of genetic research in craniofacial development are vast, most fundamentally in patient outcome and clinical practice improvement. Genetic insight into craniosynostosis, for instance, has led to the creation of individualized treatment plans to consider the specific genetic mutations responsible for causing an individual's condition. Genetic markers for craniosynostosis enable clinicians to risk stratify patients and tailor surgical intervention and postoperative care accordingly. Notably, these genetic investigations have encouraged the development of a multidisciplinary model incorporating genetic assessment and counseling, with the recommendation to be aware of the genetic background of a patient prior to treatment. This renewed interest places emphasis on clinicians staying current regarding new genetic advancements in the field of craniofacial disorders because they form an essential component of simplifying treatment protocols for these patients (Mathijssen, 2020). Moreover, the application of genetic diagnostics within clinical models has very profound implications for early detection as well as intervention strategies. By employing prenatal genetic screening, medical practitioners are currently in a position to identify CFAs such as craniosynostosis prenatally, thus allowing them to commence early discussions with their specialist care teams. An early diagnosis ensures that families are provided with extensive counseling on both potential treatment options and anticipated outcomes before the child is born. This preventive approach not only optimizes the management of craniosynostosis but also addresses the potential comorbidities of CFAs. Genetics not only informs treatment protocols but also offers parents information and counseling to help them make a choice. This shift towards a preventive model of care reflects the increased applicability of genetic research in delivering a better quality of overall care in craniofacial development (Lyons et al., 2020). The effect of genetic studies is also being felt in the long-term management of craniofacial anomalies. With the increasing knowledge of genetics, clinicians are now better able to anticipate treatment outcome as well as complications given a patient's genetic background. Such information augments a more finesse approach to postoperative care, for instance, individualized follow-up routines that are sensitive to the specific needs of different genetic subtypes of craniosynostosis. In addition, there is developing evidence of the potential of gene therapy for the therapeutic correction of individual genetic defects, possibly resulting in new therapies that will limit the need for long-term, invasive surgical treatment. This sort of radical possibility of genetics implies not simply an expansion of existing treatments but also the hope for entirely new treatments in the future. Lastly, the active incorporation of genomic data in the disease management of CFAs will bring about improved outcomes and quality of life for the affected (Mathijssen, 2020).

7.6. Clinical Applications and Interventions

Knowledge of craniofacial growth and genetics is imperative in the development of clinical interventions and applications for the treatment of CFAs. Recent advances in genomic science have unraveled the genetic pathogenesis of diseases, and it is now achievable to utilize targeted therapy with enhanced patient outcomes. For instance, conditions such as Treacher Collins syndrome presenting with unilateral facial appearance and hearing impairment have been confirmed through multidisciplinary therapies that include surgical management together with genetic guidance. As earlier discussed in recent SCGDB meetings, collaboration among clinicians and researchers promotes the innovation of surgical techniques and regenerative medicine, thereby improving management of craniofacial differences. Such a collaborative culture is important in translating laboratory discoveries into useful clinical applications that resonate with both the form and function of craniofacial disease. Translational research is instrumental in closing laboratory breakthrough and clinical utility in craniofacial genetics. Emerging technologies such as spatial transcriptomics are being explored to shed light on gene expression profiles in the development of craniofacial structures. Such frontier technologies were referenced in SCGDB meetings to have immense potential towards deconvoluting intricate signaling pathways as well as the molecular etiology of CFAs. Through elucidating these genetic mechanisms, clinicians are able to create personalized treatment regimes, surgery and adjunct therapy that are tailored to address the individualized requirements of the patient. The emphasis on novel solutions at professional meetings not only strengthens the knowledge base of the research community but keeps clinical procedures evidence-based and patient-centered. Furthermore, the importance of mentoring and collaboration between craniofacial scientists cannot be overemphasized. The SCGDB discussions offer venues whereby junior researchers engage with veteran scientists, promoting the ethos of collaborative innovation and learning. Hands-on training workshops in manuscript writing and preparation train such professionals even more for contribution-making. Such courses make the craniofacial genetics community as a whole stronger so that future researchers are able to handle the challenges of CFAs more efficiently through clinical applications and interventions. Since each new discovery is established and the degree of genetic influence on craniofacial development intensifies, the commitment to developing ability and cooperation will remain key to achieving successful clinical outcomes.

7.6.1. Genetic Counseling for Affected Families

Genetic counseling is an important intervention in craniofacial anomaly-affected families, and it provides essential information and emotional support at a time of stress. The understanding of the genetic etiology of craniofacial conditions allows families to become active partners in taking care of the health of their child. Genetic counselors provide explanation regarding inheritance patterns of disorders like frontonasal dysplasia, particularly those that involve mutations in genes like ALX1. Such genetic data empowers families so that they can make reproductive choices and adjust interventions that can optimize the developmental trajectory of the child. Furthermore, successful counseling addresses the emotional impact of having a child with craniofacial deformities, enhancing resilience and adaptive coping mechanisms in families who feel overwhelmed with the uncertainty they face (Pini et al., 2020). In addition to the relay of information regarding genetic predispositions, counseling is a fundamental means of introducing families to broader resources. By granting access to multidisciplinary interventions, genetic counselors help families grasp medical, surgical, and therapeutic options that have the potential to profoundly influence craniofacial development. In addition to health issues of a direct nature, counselors will often relay information about ongoing research in genomics as well as future clinical trials that may be useful to the afflicted child. This integration of knowledge keeps families informed with developments in treatment and postnatal care modalities. With more genetic advancements breaking down the complexities of craniofacial disorders, the role of genetic counseling in bridging gaps between families and the health system becomes increasingly important (Pierpont et al., 2018). Last but not least, genetic counseling is extremely important for improving psychosocial well-being among families. Growth of craniofacial disorders generally provokes a combination of feelings, for instance, guilt, fear, and anxiety concerning the future. The counselors are proficient in providing coping strategies, improving communication in the family, and facilitating the adoption of a positive attitude. Their function is to bridge support groups, where families provide experiences and coping strategies to one another, thus legitimizing their experience. In addition, counseling sessions also entail a regular discussion of the consequences for members of extended families of genetic findings, through which the latter develops a sense of belonging and common consciousness. Therefore, the assistance of genetic counselors extends not only to the biological conditions of craniofacial disorders but also encompasses their emotional and relationship-based conditions influencing family dynamics and coping (Pini et al., 2020) (Figure 7.17).

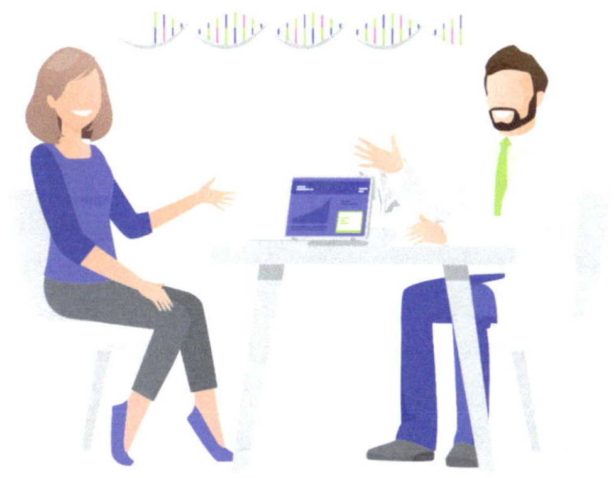

Figure 7.17. Genetic counseling.

Source: https://external-content.duckduckgo.com/iu/?u=https%3A%2F%2Fwww.genomemedical.com%2Fwp-content%2Fuploads%2F2019%2F09%2F1-e1567546844132.png&f=1&nofb=1&ipt=76fda5693a8a9297ab74c97e6a49d07ae5976c5bf9c0ac1773bd64a469355ec9.

7.6.2. Surgical Interventions for Craniofacial Disorders

Surgical corrections of craniofacial anomalies are instrumental in the repair of congenital deformities that compromise the structural and functional integrity of the face and cranium. Surgical operations for these conditions tend to be reliant on well-established classifications, including Tessiers system, which serves as a foundation for diagnosing and treating various craniofacial clefts and associated deformities. For instance, techniques like spectacle osteotomy and facial bipartition osteotomy are specially tailored to meet the demands of defects like orbital hypertelorism, which is an abnormally increased distance between eyes. Besides trying to remedy cosmetic problems, these techniques try to restore functional potential too, underlining the twofold goals of reconstruction in patients with such birth defects. Thorough preoperative evaluation lies at the heart of determining the best surgical approach, emphasizing the multidisciplinary nature of effective craniofacial care (As'adi et al., 2025). Postoperative outcomes are an important parameter in assessing the success of craniofacial surgeries for disorders. According to recent studies, postoperative infection and cerebrospinal fluid (CSF) leakage are possible complications that can happen, for which careful monitoring and management are crucial. Within the group of craniofacial cleft syndromes and orbital hypertelorism patients, a reported 9% infection rate and 22.7% leakage of CSF illustrate some of the challenges that surgeons of this type of specialty might face. Not only do these complications influence clinical outcomes but they also form the basis of the need for individualized surgical planning to the unique anatomical challenges posed by each patient's condition. Thus, meticulous postoperative management and follow-up are crucial in ensuring that patients realize significant aesthetic and functional improvements, which in return provide their quality of life (As'adi et al., 2025). The interplay between surgery and genetics ensures the importance of accurate genetic assessments in treating craniofacial disorders. Collaborative efforts by pediatricians and geneticists have made it possible to develop algorithms based on consensus for genetic testing among people with typical craniofacial malformations, such as orofacial clefts. The algorithms are beneficial in directing practice, particularly in institutions that lack direct access to genetics specialties. Early identification of genetic defects can determine medical management plans, thus maximizing surgical interventions. By integrating genetic information into the therapy process, practitioners can optimize both the preoperative planning process and long-term outcomes in patients with craniofacial abnormalities. This integration of genetic and clinical information ultimately emphasizes the role of genetics in informing surgical techniques and optimizing patient treatment (Figure 7.18).

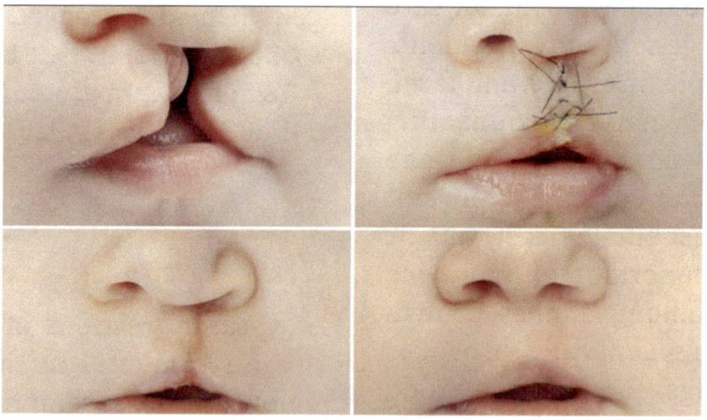

Figure 7.18. Surgical interventions for craniofacial disorders.

Source: https://149727273.v2.pressablecdn.com/wp-content/uploads/2023/06/craniofacial-plastic-surgery.jpg.

7.6.3. Future Directions in Craniofacial Treatment

Looking ahead in craniofacial therapy, advances in tissue engineering have enormous potential for craniofacial repair and regeneration. Researchers are increasingly integrating cross-disciplinary perspectives such as material science, mechanical engineering, and genetics to construct innovative approaches that have the ability to simulate the local biological environment. Of special interest is the creation of scaffolds wherein tissue regeneration can be facilitated through the creation of optimal conditions for cell growth and differentiation. Such scaffolds may employ a combination of cells and matrices from various materials and seek to deliver more efficacy to oral regenerative therapies that are on par with established practices in bone tissue engineering. By creating the materials and manufacturing technologies for scaffolds, the objectives are not only to restore function but also to achieve better overall aesthetic outcomes in craniofacial operations, a sign of a more interdisciplinary treatment method (Chocholata et al., 2019). Further, by addressing the role of genetic factors in CFAs, insights are gained into future paths for individually tailored treatment methods. Genetic syndromes such as Noonan syndrome and related RASopathies have characteristic facial appearance and corresponding health conditions. Enhanced recent diagnostics in the diagnosis of the genetic basis of these diseases cast lights on potential therapeutic targets and allow more targeted intervention strategies. Understandings of the pathophysiologic and functional consequences of RASopathy-causing mutations can inform the design of specific therapies that can overcome complicating situations inherent in these syndromes. Personalized medicine is more essential now than ever before in craniofacial medicine due to its ability to greatly enhance therapeutic outcomes and quality of life in patients with these conditions (Mylène Tajan et al., 2018). Moreover, the integration of computational modeling and digital technologies in craniofacial therapy is just the start of a new era of revolutionary surgical planning and delivery. Sophisticated imaging modalities have the capacity to create precise digital models of an individual patient's craniofacial anatomy, enabling personalized treatment planning. Using computer-aided design software, these technologies can lead to the production of patient-specific implants and guides that are specifically tailored to fit each patient's unique anatomical needs. Besides, augmented and virtual reality devices will be employed to make pre-operative simulation more realistic so that surgeons can rehearse complex operations on a simulation before undergoing real surgeries. With future developments in progress, these technologies will ensure greater precision in surgery, reduced recovery time, and enhanced patient satisfaction, hence innovation will become vital for the future of craniofacial therapy (Chocholata et al., 2019).

SUMMARY

The study of craniofacial development and genetics, it is necessary to understand the intricate interaction between embryonic and genetic processes regulating craniofacial structure formation. The findings of numerous distinct studies demonstrate that specific genes exhibit conserved patterns of expression in a variety of vertebrate species. This conservation renders the discovery that information obtained using model organisms like mice and zebrafish can be highly relevant to the understanding of human craniofacial disorders.

The identification of shared molecular mechanisms not only improves the understanding of the etiology of orofacial clefts and other disorders but also highlights the potential of such models for therapeutic development (Liu et al., 2024). Additionally, the past of craniofacial development research illustrates the trajectory of methods development and interdisciplinarity. From the early studies that took into account only morphological considerations, the field has evolved through the use of molecular genetics and cutting-edge imaging. Studies, such as those from the recent conference on craniosynostosis, demonstrate the usefulness of such collaborative efforts in expanding our knowledge of complex biological processes (Morriss-Kay, 2024). As we expand our understanding of CFAs through rigorous experimental methods, the background data from previous researchers remain vital. Lastly, the future of craniofacial genetics research is in its commitment to new approaches and the search for understanding bridging basic research and clinical practice. By continuing to clarify the genetic underpinnings of craniofacial development, researchers can lay the groundwork for targeted interventions that can prevent congenital defects. The integration of data from both empirical findings and genetic studies will ultimately lead to better diagnosis and treatment and decrease the burdens of craniofacial defects. While research is ongoing, the translational potential of these advances must be kept in mind, so that evolved knowledge is used to enhance both patient treatment and scientific understanding.

The area of craniofacial genetics and development encompasses numerous essential themes that reflect the complexity and the intricate aspects involved in facial structure establishment. Transcriptional dynamics and cell type-specific aspects that participate in craniofacial morphogenesis are one of the main issues. Interestingly, the newer study employing single-nucleus RNA sequencing has provided details regarding seven significant cell types in human embryonic development, highlighting the important interaction between CNCCs and muscle progenitors (Khouri-Farah et al., 2025). These investigations highlight the gene expression heterogeneity in accordance with these cell populations and outline the core role of CNCCs, which are highly evolutionarily variable, thus influencing facial shape and carrying major implications for understanding congenital malformations. In addition to resolution of cellular dynamics, the genetic origins of craniofacial structures have emerged as an essential area of study.

The association of face shape and genetic difference has been well established by comparative analyses that demonstrate common and rare variants associated with craniofacial development (Khouri-Farah et al., 2025). Surprisingly, the identification of Neanderthal-introgressed sequences near key genes further strengthens this narrative by suggesting an explanation of the evolutionary origins of the genetic blueprints shaping modern human facial structure. This dynamic dialogue addresses complex genetic interactions in favor of explanation of craniofacial development not only biologically but also through an evolutionary approach, hence further elucidating normal and abnormal facial morphogenesis. Moreover, developmental diseases affecting craniofacial structures, such as orofacial clefts, emphasize the vital implications of deciphering genetic effects on craniofacial anatomy. The continuing study of how some mutations of the genes are linked to quantifiable morphological changes puts this research squarely at the top of relevance for clinical utility. By examining both retained and distinctly human characteristics in craniofacial development, researchers aim to set the stage for new therapeutic strategies that may reverse the actions of genetic disease upon facial development. Thus, a comprehensive study of craniofacial growth and genetics not only enables academic research into human evolution but also promises limitless hope for developing therapeutic intervention in CFAs.

CLOSER LOOK

CRANIOFACIAL MICROSOMIA (CFM)

CFM is a birth defect in which there is undergrowth of the bones of the face, typically on one side of the face (unilateral), but occasionally on both sides (bilateral). It is the second most common facial birth defect, after CLP, and has been reported to occur in 1 in 3500 to 1 in 5600 live births. CFM encompasses a variety of anomalies of the ear, mandible (jawbone), mouth, and sometimes the eye and soft facial tissues. The severity of CFM can be extremely variable, from mild asymmetry to severe underdevelopment that affects function and appearance. One of the typical features of CFM is microtia, a small deformed external ear, which may be accompanied by hearing loss due to hypoplastic middle or inner ear structures. The involved side of the mandible is typically smaller (mandibular hypoplasia), resulting in facial asymmetry, dental malocclusion, and difficulties with chewing and speech. There can also be a lack of soft tissue of the cheek and surrounding areas, whereas others clefts occur in the mouth or facial clefts extending towards the eye.

The exact cause of CFM is not fully understood but is believed to result from interference with the development of the first and second branchial arches early in fetal development, either due to vascular problems or environmental and genetic factors. Most cases are sporadic, but familial cases and atypical genetic mutations have been reported. Diagnosis is typically established clinically based on physical exam at birth, and CT or MRI imaging is used to determine the extent of bony and soft tissue involvement. A classification system, the OMENS system (Orbit, Mandible, Ear, Nerve, Soft tissue), is commonly used to classify the severity and extent of anomalies in affected individuals. Early intervention is required for management of functional issues such as breathing, feeding, and hearing. Optimal care requires a team approach involving specialists in pediatrics, craniofacial surgery, otolaryngology, audiology, dentistry, speech therapy, and psychology.

Treatment of CFM is highly customized and often staged over time, beginning in infancy and continuing through adolescence. Hearing loss is often treated early with bone conduction hearing aids or other assistive devices. Surgery may include ear reconstruction, mandibular distraction osteogenesis to lengthen the jaw, and orthognathic surgery to realign the jaws. Soft tissue reconstruction and orthodontics are also common components of care. Psychosocial support is also important, as facial difference can significantly impact self-esteem and social development. Most individuals with CFM can anticipate good functional and aesthetic outcomes with adequate treatment and support. Research continues to improve the understanding of the genetic and developmental basis of CFM as well as to optimize treatment strategies. In conclusion, while CFM presents with phenomenal challenges, advancements in medical and surgical care have drastically enhanced the quality of life for affected individuals and their families.

REFERENCES

1. Aaron, R., Chellappa, R. K., & Danda, S. (2024). Analysis of phenotypic characteristics and mutation patterns in syndromic craniofacial anomalies: Insights from a tertiary care medical genetics unit in South India. *Journal of Cleft Lip Palate and Craniofacial Anomalies*. https://www.semanticscholar.org/paper/bfcc9739e189a1a0b2023d13d1a75872d8d9d1d7 (accessed on 27 May 2025).

2. Aggarwal, A., Allanson, J., Antshel, K., Armando, M., Bassett, A., Bayer, M., et al. (2015). Craniofacial dysmorphology in 22q11.2 deletion syndrome by 3D laser surface imaging and geometric morphometrics: Illuminating the developmental relationship to risk for psychosis. https://core.ac.uk/download/42358302.pdf (accessed on 27 May 2025).

3. Albertson, R. C., Campbell, C., Concannon, M., Ea, I., et al. (2016). Foraging environment determines the genetic architecture and evolutionary potential of trophic morphology in cichlid fishes. https://core.ac.uk/download/46558799.pdf (accessed on 27 May 2025).

4. Albertson, R. C., Crespel, A., Harris, M. P., Killen, S. S., et al. (2018). Conserved but flexible modularity in the zebrafish skull: Implications for craniofacial evolvability. https://core.ac.uk/download/157582972.pdf (accessed on 27 May 2025).

5. Al-Rekabi, Z., Cunningham, M. L., & Sniadecki, N. J. (2016). Cell mechanics of craniosynostosis. *ACS Biomaterials Science & Engineering, 3*, 2733–2743. https://doi.org/10.1021/acsbiomaterials.6b00557.

6. As'adi, K., Ahmadi, S., & Mirsalehi, M. (2025). Surgical treatment of craniofacial cleft and orbital hypertelorism: A single-center cohort study. *Neurosurgical Focus, 58*(1), E4. https://www.semanticscholar.org/paper/587e554b321cb2303c34714a613c3f7b75decc30 (accessed on 27 May 2025).

7. Atterrato, M. T., Dimitri, P., Losada, A., Messina, G., et al. (2017). The human Cranio Facial Development Protein 1 (Cfdp1) gene encodes a protein required for the maintenance of higher-order chromatin organization. https://core.ac.uk/download/98337830.pdf (accessed on 27 May 2025).

8. Benítez-Burraco, A., Uriagereka, J., & Nataf, S. (2023). The genomic landscape of mammal domestication might be orchestrated by selected transcription factors regulating brain and craniofacial development. *Development Genes and Evolution, 233*, 123–135. https://www.semanticscholar.org/paper/0c96f85f6c2f6688d2bda21857fdb024f4022327 (accessed on 27 May 2025).

9. Berkes, C., Blaschke, R. J., Brendolan, A., Britanova, O., Buck, A., Bush, J. O., Capellini, T. D., et al. (2018). Pbx loss in cranial neural crest, unlike in epithelium, results in cleft palate only and a broader midface. https://pmc.ncbi.nlm.nih.gov/articles/PMC6036936/.

10. Breugem, C. C., Evans, K. N., Poets, C. F., Suri, S., Picard, A., Filip, C., Paes, E. C., et al. (2016). Best practices for the diagnosis and evaluation of infants with Robin sequence. *JAMA Pediatrics, 170*, 894. https://doi.org/10.1001/jamapediatrics.2016.0796.

11. Brugmann, S. A., Clouthier, D., Fantauzzo, K. A., Harris, M. P., Jeong, J., Saint-Jeannet, J., Stottmann, R., et al. (2024). The Society for Craniofacial Genetics and Developmental Biology 46th Annual Meeting. *American Journal of Medical Genetics Part A, 194*. https://www.semanticscholar.org/paper/06fa3137c7bf9d0c9b2347bdbcc5fba4c793c654 (accessed on 27 May 2025).

12. Charoenvicha, C., Sirimaharaj, W., Khwanngern, K., Chattipakorn, N., & Chattipakorn, S. C. (2022). Alterations in DNA methylation in orofacial clefts. *International Journal of Molecular Sciences, 23*, 12727. https://doi.org/10.3390/ijms232112727.

13. Chen, X., Ma, J., & Zhang, T. (2024). Genetics and epigenetics in the genesis and development of microtia. *The Journal of Craniofacial Surgery, 35*, e261–e266. https://www.semanticscholar.org/paper/bfcfb2d1408acd97ed74c459fde46c5813c1276a (accessed on 27 May 2025).

14. Chocholata, P., Kulda, V., & Babuška, V. (2019). Fabrication of scaffolds for bone-tissue regeneration. *Materials, 12*(4), 568. https://doi.org/10.3390/ma12040568.

15. Corsi, A. K. (2015). A transparent window into biology: A primer on *Caenorhabditis elegans*. *WormBook*. https://doi.org/10.1895/wormbook.1.177.1.

16. DeLaurier, A., Dowd, J., Eames, B. F., Huycke, T. R., et al. (2013). FishFace: Interactive atlas of zebrafish craniofacial development at cellular resolution. https://core.ac.uk/download/28945948.pdf (accessed on 27 May 2025).

17. Eppig, J. T. (2017). Mouse Genome Informatics (MGI) resource: Genetic, genomic, and biological knowledgebase for the laboratory mouse. *ILAR Journal, 58*(1), 17–41. https://doi.org/10.1093/ilar/ilx013.

18. Erbel, R., Aboyans, V., Boileau, C., Bossone, E., Di Bartolomeo, R., Eggebrecht, H., et al. (2014). 2014 ESC Guidelines on the diagnosis and treatment of aortic diseases. *European Heart Journal, 35*, 2873–2926. https://doi.org/10.1093/eurheartj/ehu281.

19. Farran, W. H., Tarabzouni, K. W., Almuqati, T., Khawaji, N., Alasmari, M. M. F., AlMoqbel, R. M., Alahmed, R. M., et al. (2024). The growing role of genetics in orthodontic diagnosis and treatment planning. *Journal of Healthcare Sciences*. https://www.semanticscholar.org/paper/80b6ee5bcbeb51b8a9beb30e9a1e23a841f16657 (accessed on 27 May 2025).

20. Gallagher, E. R., Chow, P., Mills, M. R., Perry, H., Tam, A. C., Rosenbluth, G., Matthews, M., et al. (2024). Genetic testing in craniofacial care: Development of algorithms for testing patients with orofacial clefting, branchial arch anomalies, and craniosynostosis. *The Cleft Palate–Craniofacial Journal*. https://www.semanticscholar.org/paper/80e2a68752a3a3adb554a81cfae43acf87482dbf (accessed on 27 May 2025).

21. Jabeen, K., Rehman, K., & Akash, M. (2021). Genetic mutations of APOEε4 carriers in cardiovascular patients lead to the development of insulin resistance and risk of Alzheimer's disease. *Journal of Biochemical and Molecular Toxicology, 36*(1). https://www.semanticscholar.org/paper/18b6d2caa8f527fdcdd51cdac987e29a768998ca (accessed on 27 May 2025).

22. Jaruga, A., Ksiazkiewicz, J., Kuźniarz, K., & Tylżanowski, P. (2022). Orofacial cleft and mandibular prognathism—Human genetics and animal models. *International Journal of Molecular Sciences, 23*, 953. https://doi.org/10.3390/ijms23020953.

23. Jiang, H., Vimalesvaran, S., Wang, J. K., Lim, K. B., Mogali, S. R., & Tudor Car, L. (2021). Virtual reality in medical students' education: Scoping review. *JMIR Medical Education, 8*, e34860. https://doi.org/10.2196/34860.

24. Juhi, D. (2023). Exploring the evolution, development, and trends in craniofacial biology. *International Journal of Orofacial Biology*. https://www.semanticscholar.org/paper/281381a446b3c7e712f0e934734a21ef8e62b521 (accessed on 27 May 2025).

25. Khouri-Farah, N., Winchester, E. W., Schilder, B. M., Robinson, K., Curtis, S. W., Skene, N. G., Leslie-Clarkson, E. J., et al. (2025). Gene expression patterns of the developing human face at single cell resolution reveal cell type contributions to normal facial variation and disease risk. *bioRxiv*. https://www.semanticscholar.org/paper/235a69cbcea75965a89566c5e6e76ce2e7bf30c6 (accessed on 27 May 2025).

26. Köhler, S., Gargano, M., Matentzoglu, N., Carmody, L., Lewis-Smith, D., Vasilevsky, N., Daniš, D., et al. (2020). The Human Phenotype Ontology in 2021. *Nucleic Acids Research, 49*(D1), D1207–D1217. https://doi.org/10.1093/nar/gkaa1043.

27. Lajis, A. F. B. (2018). Systematic review on the effect of chemical compounds on craniofacial development of a zebrafish embryo. *Journal of Bioinformatics and Systems Biology, 1*. https://doi.org/10.26502/jbsb.5107001.

28. Liu, S., Xu, L., Kashima, M., Narumi, R., Takahata, Y., Nakamura, E., Shibuya, H., et al. (2024). Expression analysis of genes including Zfhx4 in mice and zebrafish reveals a temporospatial conserved molecular basis underlying craniofacial development. *Developmental Dynamics, 254*, 257–271. https://www.semanticscholar.org/paper/42466d615bffc1b4b6a724feffc74c082c388c57 (accessed on 27 May 2025).

29. Liu, Z., & Teng, L. (2023). Focuses, trends, and developments in craniofacial microsomia from 1992 to 2022: A bibliometric analysis. *The Journal of Craniofacial Surgery, 34*, 2291–2296. https://www.semanticscholar.org/paper/7677b77e3ff125427020f214808be7a3a2f7f198 (accessed on 27 May 2025).

30. Luo, S., Liu, Z., Bian, Q., & Wang, X. (2023). Ectomesenchyme Six1 controls mandibular skeleton formation. *Frontiers in Genetics, 14*. https://www.semanticscholar.org/paper/f64f2b49072273b8ea0caa6d1f01c19faa7c53a4 (accessed on 27 May 2025).

31. Lyons, M. M., Bhatt, N., Pack, A. I., & Magalang, U. J. (2020). Global burden of sleep-disordered breathing and its implications. *Respirology, 25*(7), 690–702. https://doi.org/10.1111/resp.13838.

32. Ma, L., Zhou, X., Yao, S., Zhang, X., Mao, J., Vona, B., Fan, L., et al. (2024). METTL3-dependent m6A modification of PSEN1 mRNA regulates craniofacial development through the Wnt/β-catenin signaling pathway. *Cell Death & Disease, 15*(1). https://www.semanticscholar.org/paper/b7c09a32da8ac14ea952046542d355f22dae6bde (accessed on 27 May 2025).

33. Mathijssen, I. M. J. (2015). Guideline for care of patients with the diagnoses of craniosynostosis. *Journal of Craniofacial Surgery, 26*, 1735–1807. https://doi.org/10.1097/scs.0000000000002016.

34. Mathijssen, I. M. J. (2020). Updated guideline on treatment and management of craniosynostosis. *Journal of Craniofacial Surgery, 32*(3), 371–450. https://doi.org/10.1097/scs.0000000000007035.

35. Mincer, S., Niethamer, T., Teng, T., Bush, J., & Percival, C. (2021). Effects of EPHB receptors on facial morphology: Non-additive interactions during mouse facial development. *The FASEB Journal, 35*(2). https://www.semanticscholar.org/paper/59cfaefdd5fa0b9fe232f929872fd105122b1c8e (accessed on 27 May 2025).

36. Morikawa, M., Derynck, R., & Miyazono, K. (2016). TGF-β and the TGF-β family: Context-dependent roles in cell and tissue physiology. *Cold Spring Harbor Perspectives in Biology, 8*(5), a021873. https://doi.org/10.1101/cshperspect.a021873.

37. Morriss-Kay, G. (2024). A journey in the world of craniofacial development: From 1968 to the future. *Journal of Anatomy, 245*, 816–828. https://www.semanticscholar.org/paper/1d04adddddc91e1d9866005b26524946859a0773 (accessed on 27 May 2025).

38. Pierpont, M. E., Brueckner, M., Chung, W. K., Garg, V., Lacro, R. V., McGuire, A. L., Mital, S., et al. (2018). Genetic basis for congenital heart disease: Revisited: A scientific statement from the American Heart Association. *Circulation, 138*(21), e653–e711. https://doi.org/10.1161/cir.0000000000000606.

39. Pini, J., Kueper, J., Hu, Y., Kawasaki, K., Yeung, P., Tsimbal, C., Yoon, B., et al. (2020). *ALX1*-related frontonasal dysplasia results from defective neural crest cell development and migration. *EMBO Molecular Medicine, 12*(12). https://doi.org/10.15252/emmm.202012013.

40. Riggs, K., Chen, H. S., Rotunno, M., Li, B., Simonds, N. I., Mechanic, L. E., & Peng, B. (2020). On the application, reporting, and sharing of *in silico* simulations for genetic studies. *Genetic Epidemiology, 45*(2), 131–141. https://www.semanticscholar.org/paper/4c36ff81ea96de58d3fc13189714a3d2476e0d59 (accessed on 27 May 2025).

41. Silva, R. S., Kraft, K., Arno, G., Cipriani, V., Heinrich, V., Pontikos, N., Puech, B., et al. (2019). Abstracts of papers presented at the 29th Genetic Society's Mammalian Genetics and Development Workshop held at the UCL Great Ormond Street Institute of Child Health, University College London on Thursday 29th November 2018. *Genetics Research, 101*, e15. https://www.semanticscholar.org/paper/51e0bd7c20c112904b2e6aba9aba2cedaca3be59 (accessed on 27 May 2025).

42. Smarius, B., Loozen, C. S., Manten, W., Bekker, M. N., Pistorius, L. R., & Breugem, C. C. (2017). Accurate diagnosis of prenatal cleft lip/palate by understanding the embryology. *World Journal of Methodology, 7*, 93–100. https://doi.org/10.5662/wjm.v7.i3.93.

43. Smith, T. D., Wagner, F., & DeLeon, V. (2025). Introduction and review of cartilage and craniofacial growth. *Anatomical Record*. https://www.semanticscholar.org/paper/c7a7e38bf7c4a7af634990a6f3d5c6b0ada32560 (accessed on 27 May 2025).

44. Sun, Q., Huang, J., Tian, J., Lv, C., Li, Y., Yu, S., Liu, J., et al. (2024). Key roles of Gli1 and Ihh signaling in craniofacial development. *Stem Cells and Development*. https://www.semanticscholar.org/paper/353f1723369b7b51a9b536fdcebba42377bdaf04 (accessed on 27 May 2025).

45. Tajan, M., Paccoud, R., Branka, S., Édouard, T., & Yart, A. (2018). The RASopathy family: Consequences of germline activation of the RAS/MAPK pathway. *Endocrine Reviews, 39*(6), 676–700. https://doi.org/10.1210/er.2017-00232.

46. Trainor, P. A., Cox, T. C., Clouthier, D., Fantauzzo, K. A., Harris, M. P., Jeong, J., Stottmann, R. W., et al. (2025). The Society for Craniofacial Genetics and Developmental Biology 47th Annual Meeting. *American Journal of Medical Genetics Part A*. https://www.semanticscholar.org/paper/8808ea0bf2f4f9d3ed8db9b5f99d59333f77fdbb (accessed on 27 May 2025).

47. Varma, P. K. V. V., Bai, P., Panda, S., Patil, S., Goutham, G. N., & Kumar, N. (2025). Comparative evaluation of craniofacial morphology between monozygotic and dizygotic individuals and zygosity determination by microsatellites–A dermatoglyphic study. *Journal of Neonatal Surgery*. https://www.semanticscholar.org/paper/b08684337a1ea330f030f10b111f8d68839f3545 (accessed on 27 May 2025).

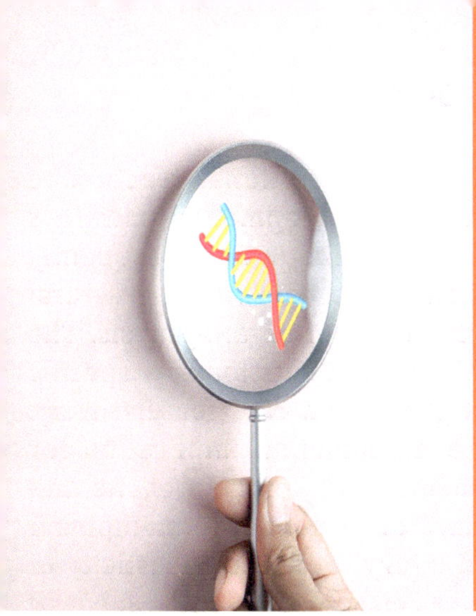

Chapter 8

GENETIC REGULATION OF ORGANOGENESIS

Contents

Introduction

The intricate process of organogenesis, the formation of organs during embryonic development, is an important aspect of life that shows the significance of gene control. Coordination of a set of genes and their interaction not only governs differentiation of stem cells into specific organ shapes but also integration of spatial and temporal growth. Genetic control is a complex network of signal cascades and transcription factors that communicate with one another to give cells the proper response to internal genetic signals and external environmental stimuli. Identification of these mechanisms of control is significant because disruptions of organ formation are a causative agent in congenital disabilities, which underscores the need for a comprehensive investigation of the molecular scaffolds that regulate organogenesis. Of prime importance in organogenesis are definitive transcription factors and signaling pathways that control cellular decisions during development. Regulatory proteins, including members of the nuclear factor-kappa B (NF-κB) family, are pivotal in functions such as inflammation, survival, and differentiation. NF-κB, for instance, is pivotal to the transcriptional reaction to stress signals, and the regulation of which has a generalized effect on developmental pathways critical to organogenesis and maturation of function. Because NF-κB signaling may subsequently influence the expression of those genes that are accountable for cellular response and structural organization, it is exceedingly important to examine its role in the context of organogenesis. The dynamic relationship between genetic elements and signaling pathways accounts for how specific organ structures emerge and function, and thus the interactions are a field ripe for discovery. Moreover, understanding of organogenesis gene regulation has a monumental implication for regenerative medicine and therapeutic intervention. With an understanding of the genetic and molecular pathways underlying organ development, researchers have the potential to manipulate such pathways to promote repair and regeneration in response to injury or disease. Plasticity of the stem cell, particularly when obtained through the modulation of genes, has potential for new therapies. Besides, the determination of ways through which cellular microenvironments and macrophage contacts facilitate or prevent organ maturation heightens insight of critical relevance to tissue engineering treatment innovations. As reflected in current studies, the intricate roles played by macrophages in tissue remodeling underlie the importance of insight into the cell-cell contacts during organogenesis (Mantovani et al., 2012). Also, continued scrutiny of NF-κB emphasizes its central position within many different biological processes, underlining its significance in pathologic disease and the generation of therapeutic agents (Ghosh et al., 2012) (Figure 8.1).

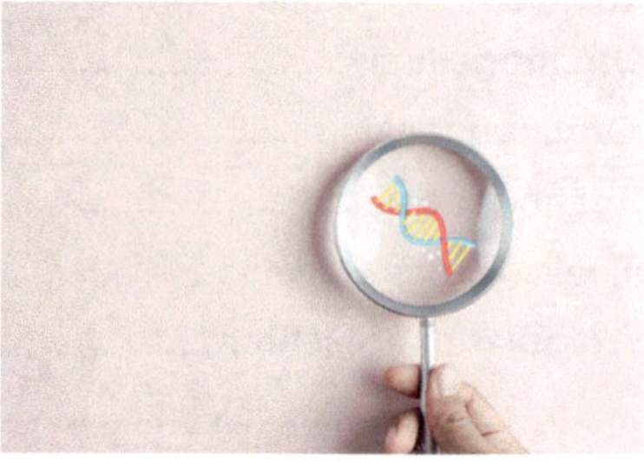

Figure 8.1. The role of genetic regulation in organogenesis.

Source: https://d1g9yur4m4naub.cloudfront.net/images/Article_Images/ImageForArticle_1352_17236430633296744.jpg.

Definition of Organogenesis

The process of organogenesis is the establishment of the particular organs and structures that occur in animal embryonic development. It's a tightly regulated process that is a part of morphogenesis, wherein cells assemble and reach particular spatial arrangements to develop functional tissues. Organogenesis starts after gastrulation, when there is distinct germ layer formation—the endoderm, mesoderm, and ectoderm. Each cell layer forms organ systems, and the timing and position of gene expression are controlled by complex pathways of signals important in organ formation. Organogenesis is relevant to study because it gives a model through which it is possible to understand congenital malformations due to disruption in development, an indication of the extensive interaction of the environmental and genetic factors that influence organ systems. At the molecular level, organogenesis is regulated by an extremely ordered cascade of transcription factors and signal molecules that decide cell fate decisions. Such molecules induce certain cells to acquire appropriate identity in order to become specific tissues or organs, thereby regulating organ size, shape, and function. Genomic technological advances have significantly transformed our understanding of such regulatory networks so that researchers today can investigate the gene expression dynamics at different stages of organogenesis. Chromatin accessibility analyses of embryonic tissues, for instance, identify important regulating factors accountable for the regulation of gene expression in developing tissues and offer insights into the complexity of organ development (and tissue specificity) (Cao et al., 2020). As scientists unravel these genetic underpinnings, the potential to apply this information in regenerative medicine and developmental biology becomes increasingly clear. Organoid technology has also made it possible to open up the study of organogenesis, with a significant focus on human development modeling. Organoids, in turn, are three-dimensional stem cell structures that emulate the organization and physiology of native organs and therefore are great resources for studying developmental phenomena and mechanisms of disease (Qian et al., 2019). Through culturing brain organoids, for instance, researchers can study cerebral development complexity such as neurogenesis and cortical layering, which are integral to the investigation of diseases such as autism and schizophrenia. Though they have excellent attributes, current organoid systems lack, in that they are merely capable of mimicking aspects of the process of organ development. Upcoming advances by organoid methods will not only be capable of defining the genetic regulation of organogenesis but offer novel therapies for an extensive array of developmental abnormalities, ultimately bridging the gap between research and clinical application (Figure 8.2).

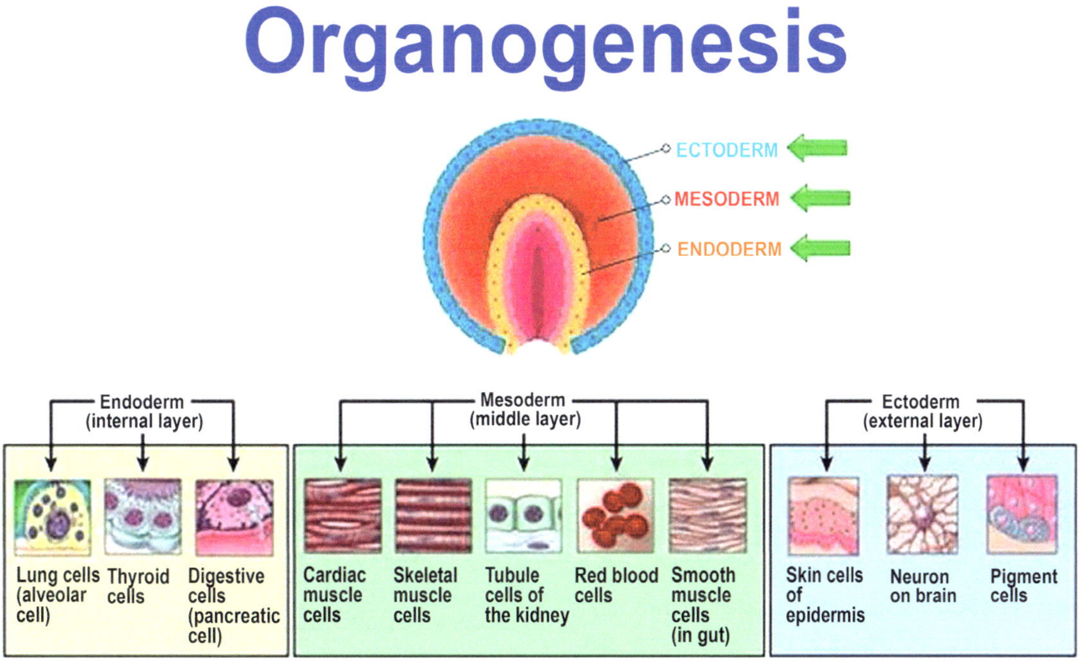

Figure 8.2. The process of organogenesis.

Source: https://i.ytimg.com/vi/t-86dB3JkBw/hq720.jpg?sqp=-oaymwEhCK4FEIIDSFryq4qpAxMIARUAAAAAGAElAADIQj0AgKJD&rs=AOn4CLAR20Qz-oMd_QX-HQPwqoS1kQN90A.

Importance of Genetic Regulation in Development

The function of genetic regulation during development, and organogenesis specifically, is not as emphasized as it should be. As organismal development proceeds, temporal regulation of gene expression ensures that cells contribute to specific tissues and organs at specific times. Such refined coordination of gene action is the hallmark of such events as stem cell differentiation and organ system formation. Gene dysregulation may lead to developmental deformities, which illustrate the requirement of closely regulated genetic mechanisms. For instance, dynamic cross-talk among different molecules of signaling and transcription factors is a central feature in specification of cell fate and patterning and creates a network of gene regulation that is not only necessary for normal development but also has resistance to environmental stress. Therefore, the understanding of genetic mechanisms can open the door to the future in agriculture and medicine by demonstrating the potential target for intervention. Further, studies on individual genetic factors involved in organogenesis reveal the complexity of the regulatory pathways. For example, in plant biology, adventitious root formation provides a model system to explore these regulatory pathways. Genetic regulation of AR development varies from that of lateral roots, suggesting an evolutionary adaptation of the plant in response to environmental stimulation that demands differential rooting response. Geelen et al. (2014) explains how AR development is regulated by a variety of factors involving auxin concentration and other hormonal cues. The differential gene expression following these stimuli indicates that the regulation of AR development by genes is tightly regulated, corresponding to the need to respond to environmental cues. Such information not only contributes to the advancement of botanical science but also facilitates the development of stress-tolerant plant lines that can withstand climatic stress. Apart from that, the role of regulatory factors during organogenesis extends beyond the single organogenesis of the roots to include vital processes of economic importance, i.e., grain development of rice. OsCEO1 has been a primary regulatory factor for endosperm organogenesis according to studies, suggesting the degree to which gene expression controls vital biological processes like starch biosynthesis and protein deposition in rice plants. Itoh et al. (2009) highlights the link of OsCEO1 activity with the abiotic stress response of the crops, showing the function of genetic regulation in preserving yield in adverse environment conditions. Identification of genes like OsCEO1 establishes a platform to improve the hardness and productivity of crops and thus makes contribution to the food security scenario in the backdrop of global climate change. Lastly, interaction among developmental mechanisms and genetic control inevitably determines the viability of organisms together with their ability to respond to the surrounding environment.

8.1. The Role of Genes in Organogenesis

The intricate process of organogenesis is innately controlled by the expression and regulation of specific genes, which orchestrate the development of various organs from embryonic tissue. Spatial and temporal transcription factor expression at this core stage are crucial to cell fate and differentiation. For instance, in the model organism *Caenorhabditis elegans*, the genetic network for regulation of vulval development is a case study on how certain transcription factors collaborate to modulate the identity of vulval cell types. Surprisingly, the like of egl-38 has been found to stabilize the vulf fate and thereby enable correct gene expression patterns to be maintained during organ development. This highlights the necessity of gene regulation to produce functional organ systems, showing the precision of genetic control is imperative in an effort to ensure successful organogenesis in multicellular organisms (Bach et al., 2008). Efficient interaction of diverse transcription factors with differential gene expression allows for the intricate balance of developmental pathways required to develop organs. The case of nhr-113, proven to be a novel member of the vulval GRN, also highlights the complexity of such gene interactions. nhr-113, as well as other transcription factors lin-11 and cog-1, are implicated in defining distinct cell types by regulating target gene expression. This shows how more than one genetic input synergistically converges to produce the diverse cellular identities needed for function of mature organs.

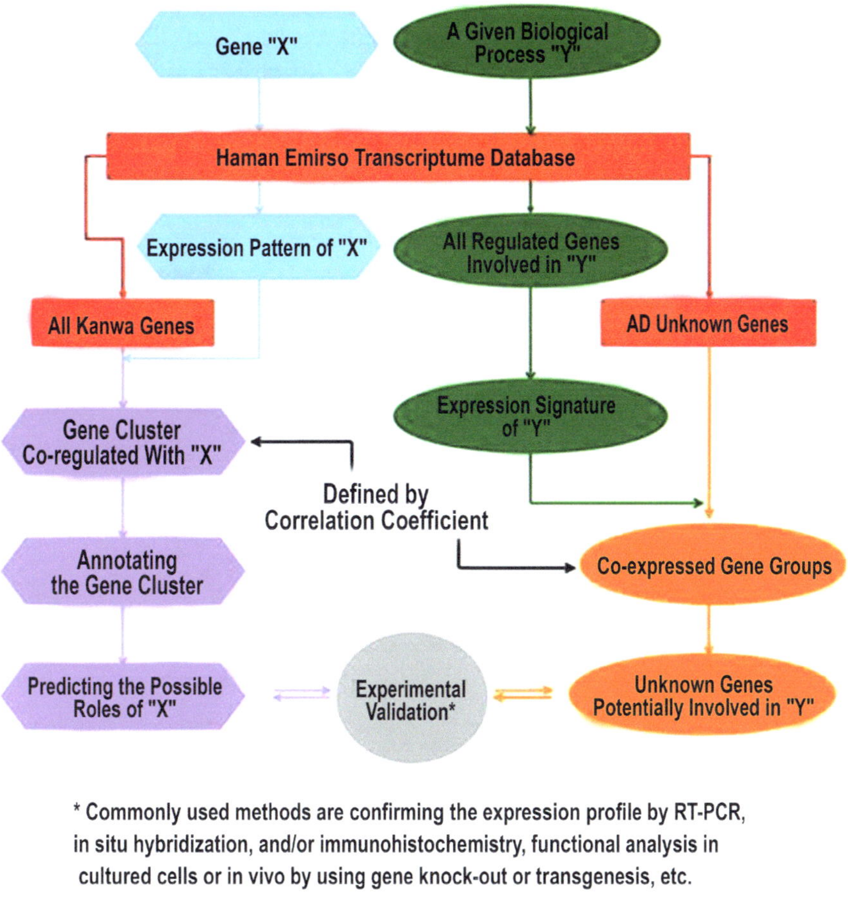

Figure 8.3. The role of genes in organogenesis.

Source: https://www.ijbs.com/ms/getimage.php?name=ijbsv07p1068g02.jpg.

Elucidation of these gene interactions not only sheds light on organogenesis mechanisms in *C. elegans* but also provides insights applicable to more complex organisms, in which identical regulatory paradigms are purportedly at work (Bach et al., 2008). Gene regulation significance even transcends model organism research into biotechnology applied to agriculture, plant organogenesis manipulation in particular. Plant genetics developments emphasize the role of single gene functions towards processes such as genetic transformation and tissue regeneration. For example, research has been interested in the potential role of KNOTTED1-like homeobox (KNOX) transcription factors, known to regulate hormonal homeostasis—a crucial element in plant morphogenesis. By disclosing molecular mechanisms regulating development from juvenile to adult plant phases, genetic regulation can be employed to improve crop yield and genetic diversity. Thus, as fundamental ideas of gene regulation in organogenesis continue to be studied intensely within model organisms, uses in agronomic genetics reveal broader meanings for food production and sustainability (Figure 8.3).

8.1.1. Key Genes Involved in Organ Development

Organogenesis is finally regulated by a complicated network of significant genes that guide various patterns of development. Among these, the Notch signaling pathway has emerged as a major player. This mechanism of intercellular communication regulates cell fate decisions and thereby affects cell differentiation and organization in organogenesis. Notch signaling is involved in epithelial-mesenchymal transition (EMT), a process by which the epithelial cells acquire mesenchymal properties, allowing them to move and reorganize into diverse organ structures. By regulating target genes that are involved in cell adhesion and cytoskeletal remodeling,

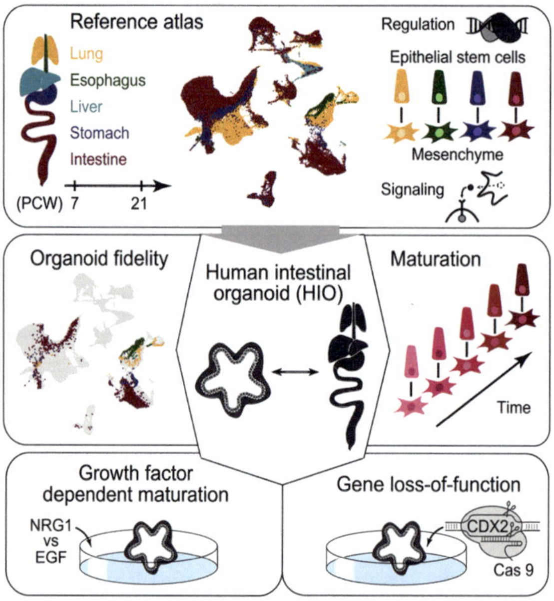

Figure 8.4. Genes involved in organ development.

Source: https://www.cell.com/cms/10.1016/j.cell.2021.04.028/asset/ca1ba8b6-5f86-44ca-9cee-c490729c6c54/main.assets/fx1_lrg.jpg.

Notch influences the structure and function of the organ and also the manner in which the organs are properly formed. These intricate regulation of genes underscore the significance of pathway interactions in determining the fate of progenitor cells, as Notch dysregulation can lead to developmental abnormalities or be involved in disease like cancer, that could hijack such pathways for metastatic activity (Yu et al., 2020). No less vital during organ development are the transcription factors that control the expression of downstream target genes. For instance, the SRY (Sex-determining Region Y)-related

HMG-box (Sox) protein family of proteins plays a central role in organogenesis at various stages, primarily in neural and kidney development. Sox transcription factors facilitate the transition from pluripotent stem cells to differentiated cell types through the induction of specialized gene expression programs. They also play roles in key events such as nephron patterning and mesenchymal condensation during kidney development. These correct developmental pathways can be interrupted by Sox factor misexpression, leading to functional impairment or organ malformations. Hence, the Sox family explains how control of transcription is central to effective execution of the developmental plan for structure and function of organs (Moustakas et al., 2017). In addition to the Notch and Sox pathways, the interaction between growth factors also significantly influences organogenesis. TGF-β signaling, for example, is crucial for EMT and subsequent differentiation of mesenchymal cells during organ development. TGF-β regulates expression patterns leading to structural integrity as well as biochemical properties of developing organs, which influence organ functionality. The role of TGF-β signaling is particularly important in fibrosis and organ regeneration, where its aberrant regulation will result in an abnormal process at the expense of normal organ function. These signaling pathways are informative about genetic control manifested in organ development and show the complexity and interconnectivity of genes involved. Through mapping these avenues, scientists are able to improve their understanding of the basic mechanisms of normal development and of the diseases' pathogenesis (Yu et al., 2020) (Figure 8.4).

8.1.2. Mechanisms of Gene Expression Regulation

Regulation of gene expression is one of the critical determinants of the complicated processes of organogenesis, controlling the utilization of genetic information within the developing tissues and structures. Gene expression regulation takes place at various levels, including epigenetic regulation, transcriptional regulation, and post-transcriptional regulation. Epigenetic modification, such as DNA methylation and histone modification, serves to activate or repress gene expression and is an active response to environmental cues. In plants, some transcription factors can bind to promoter regions, activating or inhibiting the transcription of target genes that are required for organ development. This complex interaction ensures that genes appropriate to specific tissues or developmental stages are expressed at the right time and place, and thus enables proper maturation of organ form and function required for plant survival and reproduction. Spatial and temporal regulation of gene expression is extremely critical in organogenesis, as highlighted in the latest research studies, which have utilized spatial transcriptome technologies.

The technologies allow quantitative estimation of the spatial pattern of gene expression, showing the cell dynamics in the development of floral organs in plants such as Phalaenopsis Big Chili. By mapping active gene expression patterns in developing tissues, it is clear that specific cell types, i.e., meristematic cells, possess continuous roles during various developmental stages. This understanding of such spatial regulation enables a greater appreciation of flower development, considering that flower identity and structure genes are expressed in a highly coordinated manner in different cellular contexts, one that is predominantly mediated by MADS-box genes and other downstream regulators, as captured in advanced genetic mapping techniques (Liu et al., 2022). Furthermore, the function of chloroplasts in genetic regulation extends the classical paradigms of gene expression, emphasizing their application in biotechnology and applied genetics. Recent advances in chloroplast genome engineering have demonstrated mechanisms for high-level expression of transgenes, which can be exploited not only for improved crop traits but also for pharmaceutical and bioproduct synthesis. The promise of chloroplasts as expression systems is underscored by the fact that they can sustain life while allowing the alteration of metabolic pathways through the introduction of transgenes. By using systems such as Gateway/modular vectors, researchers can circumvent the challenges of transgene expression in these organelles and attain greater specificity in gene expression in response to specific environmental or developmental cues (Jin et al., 2015). This accounts for the intricacy of the regulation of genes and its pivotal role in the coordination of organogenesis in plants (Figure 8.5).

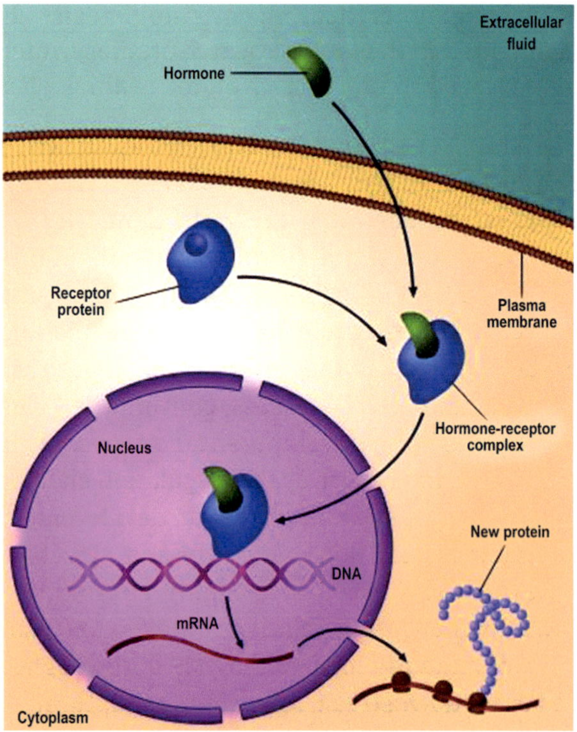

Figure 8.5. Regulation of gene expression.

Source: https://upload.wikimedia.org/wikipedia/commons/e/e6/Regulation_of_gene_expression_by_steroid_hormone_receptor.svg.

8.1.3. Interaction Between Different Genes During Organogenesis

The intricate coordination of several genes during organogenesis is essential for normal organ and organ structure development. Gene regulatory networks (GRNs) orchestrate this complex concert by regulating the expression and activity of genes involved in the development of different tissues and cell types. For instance, in the model organism *Caenorhabditis elegans*, studies have demonstrated how transcription factors such as lin-11, lin-29, cog-1, egl-38, and nhr-67 act in concert to pattern the different vulval cell types through precise spatial and temporal gene expression. These interactions not only show the need for many genes to act in concert but also the multidimensionality of gene regulation that occurs during organ development. The study of *C. vulval* GRN of elegans is a good illustration of the manner in which several factors act together to define the unique characteristics of each cell, pointing towards the complexity of genetic control during organogenesis (Bach et al., 2008). Organogenesis is also not a straightforward linear sequential expression of individual genes but is rather based on an elaborate feedback system that controls gene interactions based on internal and external signals. The OsCEO1 gene, which occurs in rice endosperm organogenesis, is a case in point for regulatory complexity. OsCEO1, being an orchestra leader of endosperm development, also communicates with proteins, demonstrating a network of regulatory components that must coordinate to buffer stresses like high temperatures. The exploration of these interactions reveals that the regulation of gene expression is not only involved in the structural formation of the organ but also establishes a framework of resistance to environmental adversity. This delicate balance of interaction and regulation underscores the intricacy of genetic networks in governing organogenesis (Itoh et al., 2009). The significance of being aware of gene interactions in organogenesis is not merely academic but also of practical relevance for agriculture, biotechnology, and developmental biology. By helping to understand how genes communicate and regulate one another across various organisms, researchers are able to devise strategies that render crops more resilient against environmental stress or regenerative medicine treatments more efficient. Furthermore, insights gained from investigating networks, such as those in *C. elegans* and rice be extrapolated into broader biological contexts, revealing universal principles of gene interaction. As scientists unravel the complexity of genetic regulation, the evolutionary advantages provided by these interactions can form the basis for future advancements in some of the most significant ecological and health issues (Bach et al., 2008; Itoh et al., 2009) (Figure 8.6).

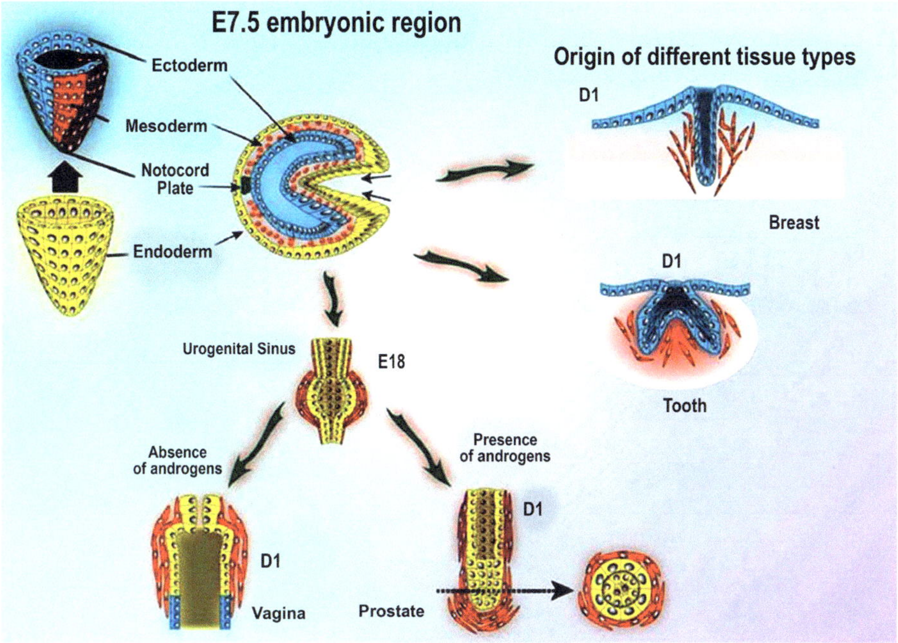

Figure 8.6. Interaction between different genes during organogenesis.

Source: https://www.researchgate.net/profile/Douglas-Strand/publication/41806323/figure/fig1/AS:394243907571712@1471006480180/Fig-1-Cell-Origins-in-Organogenesis-The-interacting-tissues-that-induce-pattern.png.

8.2. Signaling Pathways in Organogenesis

Signaling pathways provide the foundations for organogenesis, dictating cellular communication that coordinates complex organ and tissue construction. Among various molecular mechanisms, purine and pyrimidine metabolism has been center stage due to the crucial roles played during embryonic and fetal development. These metabolic pathways are interconnected with the signaling molecules that dictate cellular interactions during organ formation. For instance, fluctuations in the expression of purine-metabolizing enzymes regulate the stepwise release of signaling molecules that activate particular membrane receptors important for cell growth and differentiation. More notably, the purinergic receptors, adenosine and various P2 receptor subtypes, exhibit differential expression depending upon the developmental stage of the cells. Any disruption of such tightly regulated purinergic transmissions can result in severe developmental disorders, and this underscores the vital role of metabolic regulation in the coordination of cell activities during organogenesis (Fumagalli et al., 2017). Besides purine metabolism, planar cell polarity (PCP) signaling is also another major pathway that has a crucial role to play in organogenesis. First identified in *Drosophila*, the core Wnt-Frizzled PCP pathway has been studied extensively in several vertebrate models such as the mouse and zebrafish. The pathway directs the orientation and patterning of tissue cells and hence organ morphogenesis. The complexity of pathways is further heightened by the involvement of new factors and genes such as *Van Gogh* and *Vangl* that are involved in PCP regulation. PCP signaling disruption can lead to anatomical deformities and functional impairments, illustrating how cell orientation and behavior are specifically regulated in order to ensure normal organ formation. The interaction of the above factors exhibits a multilayer network of interactions that define the maturation of organogenesis (Yang et al., 2015).

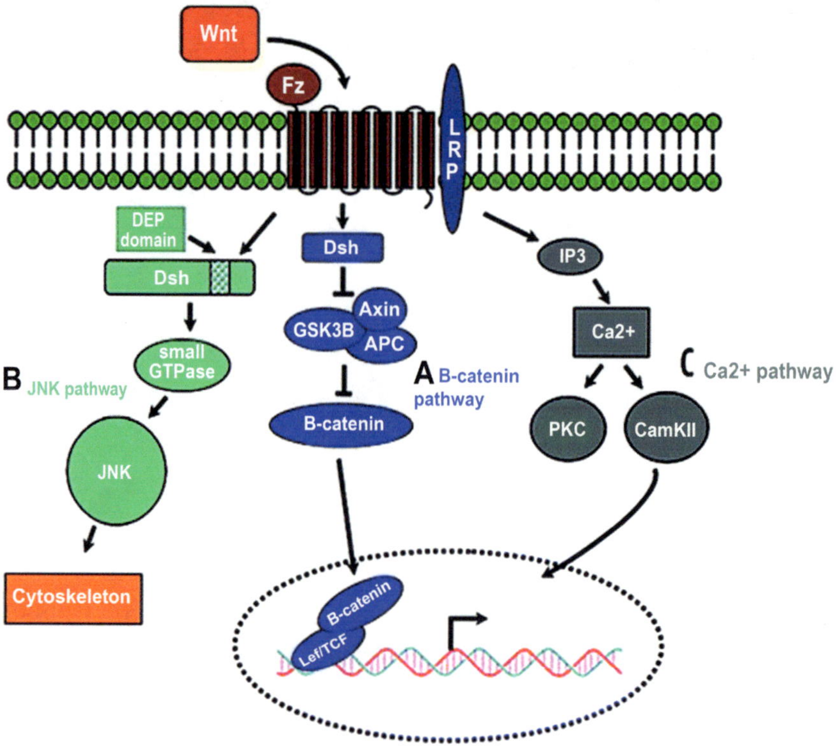

Figure 8.7. Wnt signaling in limb organogenesis.

Source: https://www.tandfonline.com/cms/asset/64a3123a-a519-4510-8d07-a14bd9fe0d23/kogg_a_10905857_f0001.gif.

The interaction between purinergic signaling and PCP pathway illustrates the multilayered regulatory mechanism governing organ development. These signaling pathways interact in a dynamic manner to produce organized regulation of various cellular processes such as differentiation, migration, and tissue patterning. The subtleties of these interactions need to be understood for the appreciation of how genetic regulation controls organogenesis. As our knowledge progresses, it becomes more and more clear that alterations within any element of these pathways can lead to considerable developmental defects, highlighting the requirement for accurate genetic regulation. Thus, this data gives new directions for particular therapeutic intervention that can reverse or mitigate the effect of such perturbations, offering promise of treatment of congenital disease due to faulty organogenesis. Further investigation of these pathways holds out the potential to unveil the intricate complexity of developmental biology (Fumagalli et al., 2017; Yang et al., 2015) (Figure 8.7).

8.2.1. Overview of Major Signaling Pathways (e.g., Wnt, Hedgehog)

The intricate process of organogenesis is under the stringent regulation of a multitude of signaling pathways, of which the Wnt and Hedgehog (Hh) pathways are of supreme significance. Wnt signaling is a key regulator of the processes of cell fate determination, proliferation, and differentiation throughout embryonic development. The pathway functions via a cascade of interactions that eventually influence the transcription of target genes required for the formation of various organ structures. Experiments have shown that strict control of canonical Wnt signaling is particularly important during the development of the pancreas, and perturbations lead to defects such as pancreatic hypoplasia. Experiments also show that ectopic activation of Wnt signaling leads to inappropriate expression of gut markers in the pancreatic epithelium, highlighting the importance of coordinated signaling in the control of correct organ morphogenesis (Cano et al., 2016). Similarly, the Hedgehog signaling pathway plays a role in organogenesis through the control of cell differentiation and tissue patterning.

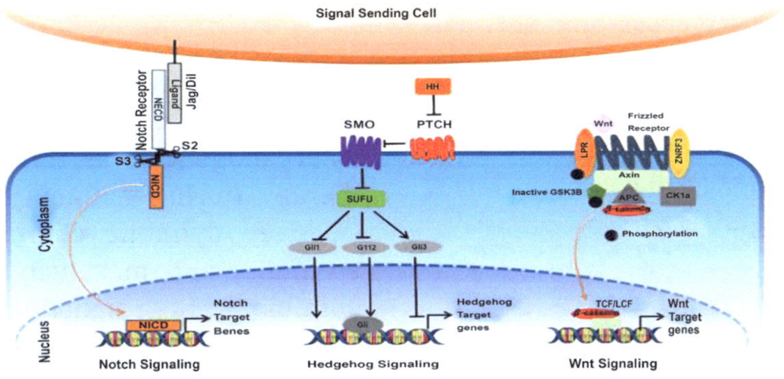

Figure 8.8. The role of notch, hedgehog, and wnt signaling pathways.

Source: https://www.frontiersin.org/files/Articles/650772/fcell-09-650772-HTML/image_m/fcell-09-650772-g001.jpg.

The Hh pathway also interacts with other major signaling pathways, including Wnt and Notch, demonstrating the complexity of embryonic development. Such integration is necessary, as defective signaling is responsible for a spectrum of developmental defects. For instance, canonical Hh signaling not only influences growth and patterning of the embryonic central nervous system (CNS) but also intersects with Wnt signaling to attain a balance that is necessary for organogenesis. When these pathways indulge in uncontrolled crosstalk, it may result in significant developmental defects or toward the pathogenesis of tumors later on in life, indicating the critical need for tightly controlled signaling mechanisms throughout the various stages of organ development (Bellavia et al., 2019). The functional interaction of Wnt and Hedgehog signaling pathways illustrates a fundamental principle of developmental biology: the balance and coordination of more than one signaling mechanism are required for successful organogenesis. Misregulation of either pathway can annihilate this delicate balance, with catastrophic consequences in the form of organ malformations or predispositions to cancer. For example, β-catenin's involvement in the Wnt pathway was shown to interfere with pancreatic development by interacting with Hedgehog signaling, indicating how these pathways control each other's activity during critical stages of embryogenesis. Thus, it is essential to comprehend the intersecting functions and regulatory cross-talk between these pathways to grasp the genetic control of organogenesis, which can also provide an avenue for therapeutic interventions to treat developmental disorders (Bellavia et al., 2019; Cano et al., 2016) (Figure 8.8).

8.2.2. Role of Signaling Pathways in Cell Differentiation

The intricate cell differentiation process of organogenesis is kept firmly in control through numerous distinct signaling pathways. These pathways serve as key regulators in guiding the development of specialized cell types from pluripotent stem cells. As a model, interaction between growth factors, morphogens, and extracellular matrix constituents directs progenitor cell fate towards adopting particular lineages required for organ development. Wnt, Notch, and Hedgehog signaling are pivotal wherein they facilitate intercellular communication between neighboring cells and act as a proliferation counterbalance to differentiation. A study of the interactions between these pathways and how they control gene expression not only unravels simple biological processes but also offers an option on developmental pathology and organogenetic disorder brought about by impaired signaling. Sophistication of cell signaling is observed in some organ systems, where it governs large differentiation processes. In the vertebrate kidney, for example, nephrogenesis pathways are reiterated with regeneration, suggesting differentiated cells still possess the capacity to revert to a progenitor-like cell state under certain conditions. This process illustrates cellular identity plasticity and the regenerative capacity, and both are governed by the identical molecular mechanisms as embryonic development. These regeneration mechanisms show the potential of applying embryonic signaling pathways to enhance tissue regeneration in adult organs. The reactivation of developmental genes in kidney regeneration, as described in (Cirio et al., 2013), is proof demonstrating how signaling pathways can cross construction and reconstruction and enhance their function in organogenesis as well as potential use in therapy. During mammary gland development, two-way dynamic communication between epithelial and mesenchyme tissues is made possible through signaling pathways, reflecting the importance of two-way communication during differentiation. Specifically, hormone-independent fetal development relies on such pathways, which orchestrate cell processes such as specification, proliferation, and migration. Advances through observations in mouse and human genetics are revealing some of the signals that control these intricate processes, which have more to say about how tissue interactions are responsible for creating organs. Surprisingly, according to (Yang et al., 2004), the degree of application of such signaling processes is not only restricted to organogenesis but also enlightens routes that are involved in tumorigenesis. The characterization of these interactions is not only of potential significance to developmental biology but also to cancer therapeutic therapy for tumors resulting from aberrant differentiation signaling (Figure 8.9).

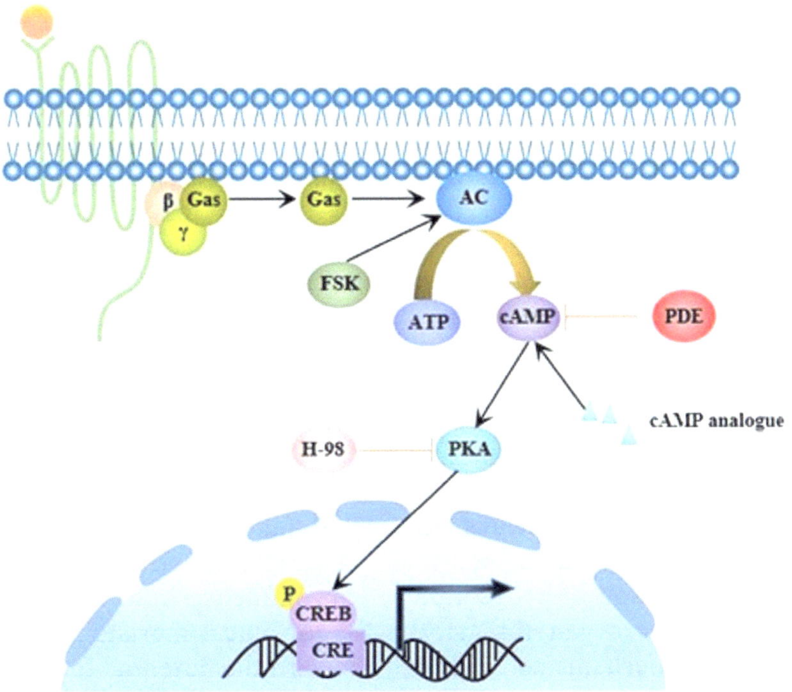

Figure 8.9. Role of signaling pathways in cell differentiation.

Source: https://www.cusabio.com/manage/upload/201905/PKA-Cell-differentiation.jpg.

8.2.3. Impact of Signaling Pathway Disruptions on Organ Development

Abnormalities in critical signal pathways have significant implications for organogenesis, illustrating the intricate interaction between genetic regulation and morphological outcome. Among the numerous signal pathways, the Wnt, Hedgehog, and Notch signal pathways are all essential to regulating cell differentiation and tissue pattern formation in organogenesis. For instance, aberrant Wnt signaling has been implicated in improper endodermal specification leading to developmental abnormalities of organs such as the pancreas and liver. The highly tuned regulation of Wnt pathway activity is essential for the maintenance of proliferation-differentiation balance; thus, disruptions can lead to congenital malformations or even cancer. Understanding these processes of signaling is very significant for organogenesis's underlying mechanisms and potential therapeutic targets for disorders related to organs (Spencer et al., 2016). Furthermore, perturbation of Hedgehog pathway signaling has been identified to induce spectacular developmental anomalies, particularly in limb and CNS formation. Hedgehog pathway signaling plays a vital role in the specification of boundaries during embryogenesis, regulation of organ system growth and differentiation. Aberrations in components of the Hedgehog pathway, for instance, can lead to holoprosencephaly, a situation where the forebrain fails to properly split into hemispheres. Hedgehog signaling is not just involved in patterning but also in cellular proliferation and survival, emphasizing its multi-faceted role in organogenesis. With further development in the field, the necessity for distinguishing these signaling pathways remains on the rise, emphasizing their potential as therapeutic targets in avoiding or reversing developmental defects (Ghosh et al., 2012). Notch signaling pathway, together with Wnt and Hedgehog, is crucial in cell fate specification during organ development. Notch signaling usually mediates cell-cell interactions between adjacent cells to provide the coordination for communication that enables the balance between differentiation and proliferation. The disrupted Notch signaling can lead to a wide range of developmental disorders, including cardiovascular malformations and neurogenic defects. Involvement of the pathways in maintaining stem cell niches ensures quality maintenance and differentiation of progenitor cells that is paramount for organ integrity. By further exploring the mechanisms behind Notch signaling, researchers can obtain better understanding of tissue homeostasis and regenerative medicine potential. The compounded understanding obtained by studying such defective signaling pathways not only brings us closer to understanding healthy organ development but also offers avenues towards novel therapy in developmental and regenerative biology (Spencer et al., 2016).

8.3. Genetic Mutations and Organogenesis

Organogenesis is a very complex process that requires rigorous genetic control to proceed normally. The process is so highly regulated that genetic mutations can make a great difference, leading to structural defects and functional abnormalities of various organs. For instance, mutations of key transcription factors, such as p63, are associated with a wide range of clinical disorders affecting epithelial organs like the skin, limbs, and craniofacial tissues. Studies have determined that p63 is a central regulator of gene expression in the differentiation of keratinocytes, influencing the proliferation and maturation of epidermal cells, which are essential to the skin barrier integrity. Disruption of the activity of p63 through genetic mutations can lead to ectrodactyly and ectodermal dysplasia, and this indicates how critical genetic integrity is to organogenesis and how transcription factors have a general function in developmental processes (Evelyn et al., 2015). Genetic mutations can also work together with other mechanisms of control to affect organogenesis from various fronts. For instance, the intersection between hormonal signaling and genetic control is exemplified in plant root nodulation. The tricot (tco) mutation in Lotus japonicus illustrates how genetic alterations can influence both nodule organogenesis and shoot apical meristem maintenance, pointing toward the potential for shared genetic control of developmental processes that are distinct. This kind of interaction between genetic disruption and developmental processes emphasizes the sensitive balance required for successful organ development to be completed. By explaining the interconnection between the various genetic factors and how they contribute to organogenesis, such studies improve our knowledge of how breakdowns in these processes lead to developmental abnormalities and associated disorders (Suzaki et al., 2012). Furthermore, research into genetic mutations and how they impact organogenesis improves our knowledge of evolutionary biology and genetics. It has been discovered that some genes, e.g., TCO of Lotus japonicus, not only regulate particular developmental processes, i.e., nodule formation, but also maintain other developmental processes, illustrating the multifunctionality of genetic elements. This dual role suggests that genetic mutations influencing one developmental process can have a cascade effect on others, rendering developmental biology all the more complicated to decipher. In human beings, the identification of these intricate roles for genes involved in organogenesis can be transformed into improvements in medical science, such as in genetic counseling and therapeutic intervention of congenital disorders caused by gene mutations. Complete information about such genetic networks holds the secret to understanding the molecular basis of development along with potential pathways for remedial measures (Evelyn et al., 2015) (Figure 8.10).

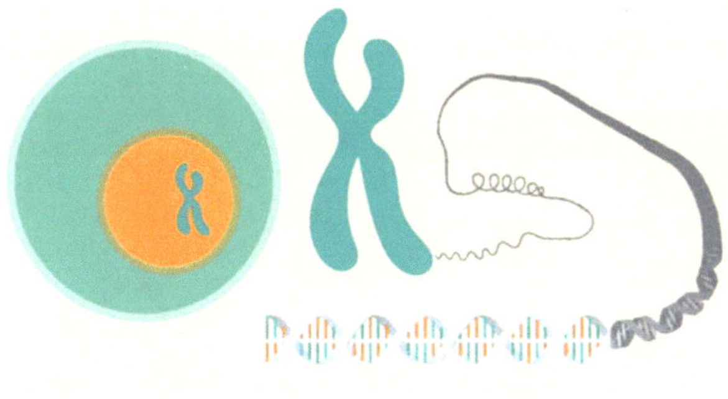

Figure 8.10. Genetic Mutations and Organogenesis.

Source: https://knyamed.com/cdn/shop/files/genetics-and-embryology-708x364.jpg?v=1716623619&width=600.

8.3.1. Types of Genetic Mutations Affecting Organogenesis

Genetic mutations play an important role in organogenesis, with most contributing to the formation and development of organs during embryonic growth. Mutations can be classified into different types, each affecting the process of organogenesis in a different way. Point mutations, involving a mutation of one nucleotide, can have an effect highly on proteins encoded in genes for organ formation. For instance, mutations in genes that code for signaling pathways disrupt proper cell fate determination, and this leads to congenital defects such as defects in the heart. Nucleotide insertions and deletions also lead to disruptions of reading frames in genes, leading to dysfunctional proteins that disrupt organogenesis. The impacts of such mutations lead to a range of developmental disorders, and severity varies with the time at which the mutation takes place during embryonic development. Moreover, structural mutations, such as duplications or rearrangements of the chromosomes, can also significantly contribute to the process of influencing organogenesis. These mutations could lead to an altered dosage of gene expression that can result in unbalances of the genetic pathways that guide organ development. For example, duplication can result in hyperplasia of organs due to overexpression of certain development genes that can lead to malformation. Conversely, deletion can rid a cell of vital regulatory components, leading to underdevelopment or absence of an organ. Studies on the above mutations have been supported by advances in genomic technologies that provide for more in-depth exploration of the correlation between genetic variation and organ health. Recent studies illustrate how mutations that act on cell division and differentiation genes have their impact compounded into broader effects on whole organism development as discovered within several model organisms. In addition to structure and point mutations, epigenetic modification is a major amount of genetic control that regulates organogenesis. Epigenetic modifications can modify gene expression without altering the DNA sequence and thus design the pattern of gene activation or repression during development. Environmental cues are known to induce epigenetic changes that might interact with genetic predispositions to generate intricate phenotypes as seen in organ development. An example of the interaction between epigenetic changes and genetic mutations would be as seen in pathways associated with reproductive health as cited in recent research. These investigations identified genetic risk factors for reproductive lifespan that share an association with those in organogenesis, again emphasizing the complexity of gene regulation during the process of development. Overall, understanding the interaction of various types of genetic mutation is important in unlocking mechanisms of organogenesis and potential therapeutic intervention in congenital conditions (Isabelle et al., 2021; Zhernakova et al., 2024) (Figure 8.11).

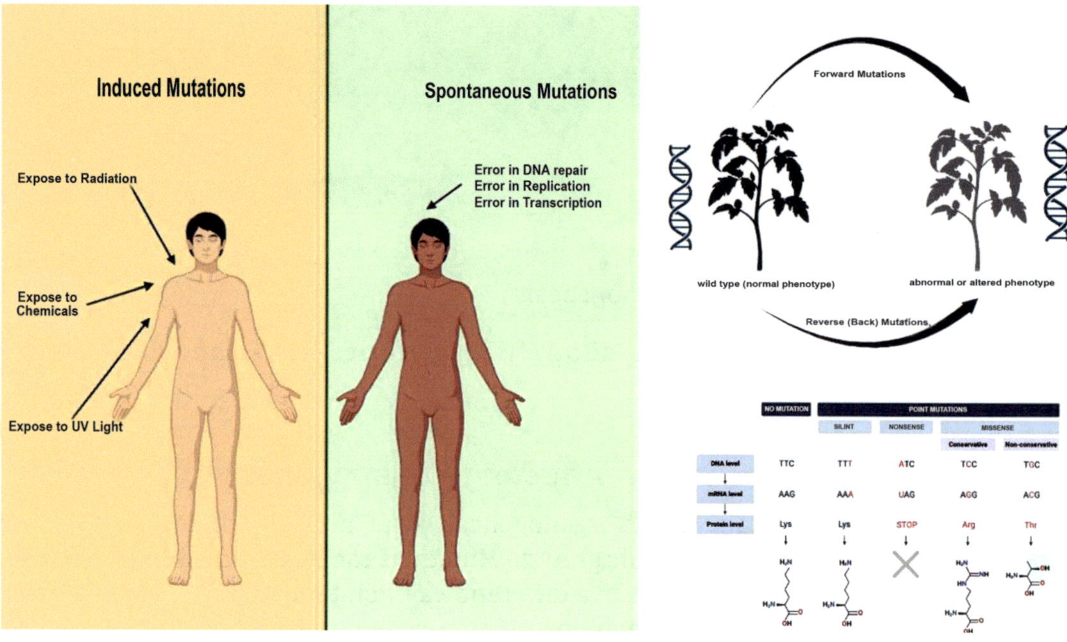

Figure 8.11. Types of genetic mutations affecting organogenesis.

Source: https://biologynotesonline.com/wp-content/uploads/2024/09/Types-of-Mutations.jpg.

8.3.2. Case Studies of Specific Mutations and Their Effects

Relative to previous knowledge, the recognition of the influence of isolated genetic mutations has an important effect on organ development genetic control, as seen by several case studies. The myelofibrosis case shows the role of mutations in essential genes such as JAK2, CALR, MPL in initiating defects during the development of blood cells. The mutations have wide-ranging implications both in the activation of the signaling pathways and the treatment response of patients under consideration. Myelofibrosis in approximately 80% of the cases has other associated additional mutations impacting the regulatory pathways of gene expression, which further decide the progression and presentation of the disease. Identification of these types of mutations has been a critical factor in the development of prognostic scoring systems that inform clinical decision, a significant step towards individualized medicine in haematologic disease. By studying mutations in such contexts, researchers can gain further insights into cellular processes involved in organogenesis in health and disease (Verma et al., 2024). Another example is cortical development malformations (MCD), where some somatic mTOR pathway mutations have been linked with childhood epilepsy. These induce dysregulation of neuronal function, producing hyperexcitability and the development of seizure disorders. In a comparison of 35 children, mutations were linked with alteration of cation–chloride cotransporters (CCCs), which play the key role of regulating intracellular chloride concentrations, having a direct impact on GABAergic transmission. The research illustrated that the KCC2/NKCC1 ratio was greatly decreased in MCD patients, portraying the disrupted inhibitory signaling in the brain. Additionally, treatment was also promising as blocking the pathological signaling cascade with mTOR inhibitors resulted in the restoration of CCC function. This not only shows the central role of certain genetic mutations in organogenesis but also their general role in cellular excitability and the treatment of epilepsy (Bakouh et al., 2024). Finally, the study of genetic mutations gives us basic information that is needed to unravel organogenesis complexities. Case studies of the mutations teach us about the regulatory circuits controlling organ development and on the developmental effects of their disruption. For instance, dysregulating JAK-STAT and mTOR pathways illustrate how derangement may find its expression in dramatic phenotypic manifestations, from cancers to neurologic disorders. By characterization of such kinds of mutations and their effects, researchers are able to formulate more precise interventions that modulate the involved genetic processes. The strategy promotes better recognition of human development and disease, and the consequent need for individualized treatment regimens based on the specific genetic makeup of the patients. With more being understood regarding such mutations, expectations of developing novel therapeutic approaches to eliminate or reduce the effects of genetic aberrations continue to increase, eventually to enhance organogenesis-based areas (Bakouh et al., 2024; Verma et al., 2024).

8.3.3. Implications of Genetic Mutations for Developmental Biology

Genetic mutation research gives profound insights into developmental biology, particularly organogenesis. Genetic mutations can result in extreme alterations in developmental processes, patterning the form and function of numerous organs. For instance, mutations in regulatory genes can disrupt the ordered processes during tissue differentiation and organogenesis. Understanding how these mutations influence development not only reveals the mechanisms of congenital anomalies but also highlights the evolutionary implications of changes at the genetic level. Thus, understanding how genetic mutations work allows scientists to connect genotype, phenotype, and the environment developmental processes interact with. This intricate interaction serves to underscore the necessity of evolutionary theory in the realm of developmental biology, such that the search for an expanded framework—apart from the traditional Modern Synthesis—that can grapple with such complexities becomes increasingly pertinent (Kevin et al., 2015). Furthermore, the implications of genetic mutations are experienced in the concept of developmental plasticity, in that certain mutations can enable or inhibit an organism's capacity to adapt to environmental change. The interaction between genetic mutation and developmental environment can yield an extremely broad range of phenotypic outcomes, a reflection of the dynamic equilibrium of evolutionary and biological development. This is a deviation from the strict definitions of adaptation to look toward a more dynamic evolutionary synthesis that addresses the dynamism of developmental processes. Scientists can reveal why some mutations foster resistance or susceptibility to environmental stressors and, in so doing, enrich the debate of organogenesis and adaptive evolution.

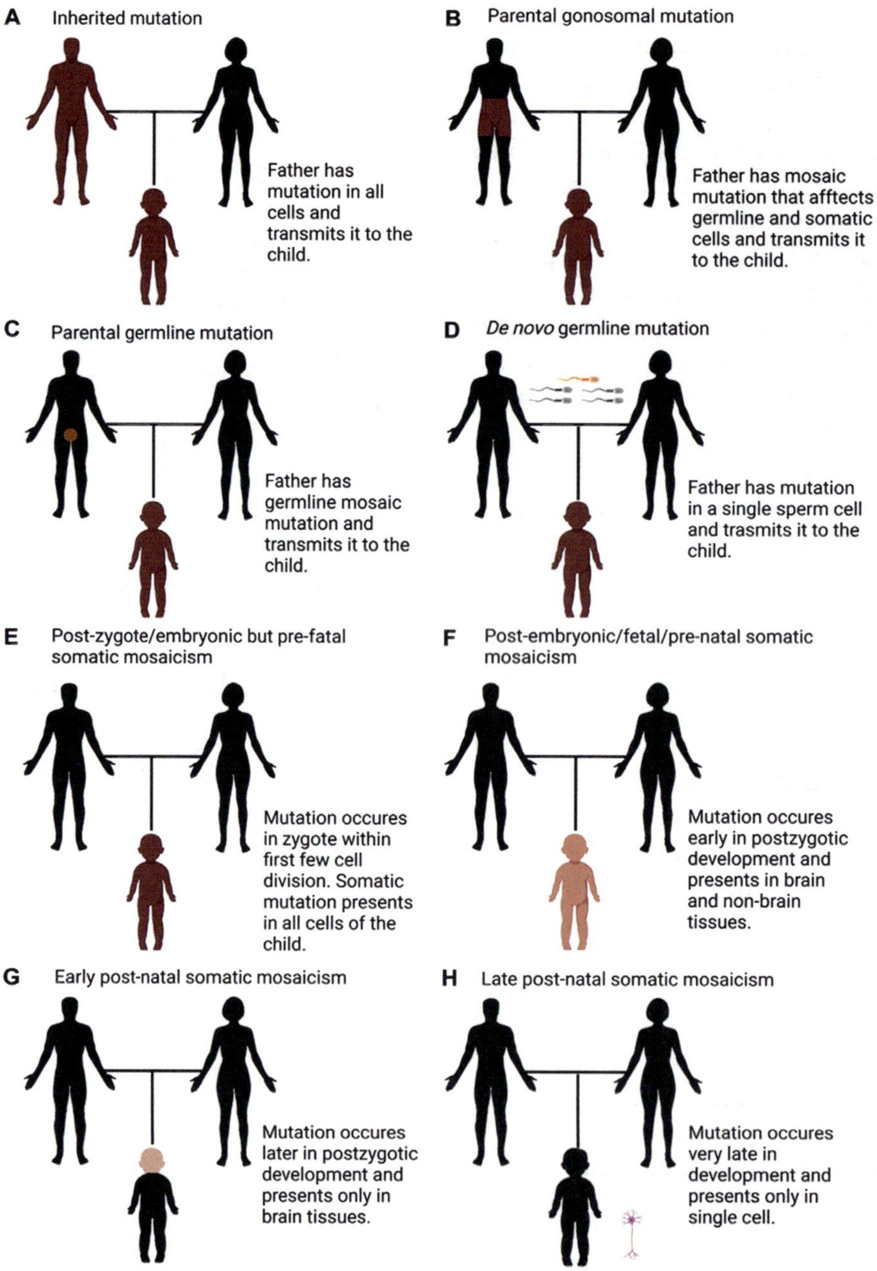

Figure 8.12. Implications of genetic mutations for developmental biology.

Source: https://images-provider.frontiersin.org/api/ipx/w=1200&f=png/https://www.frontiersin.org/files/Articles/983668/fgene-13-983668-HTML-r1/image_m/fgene-13-983668-g001.jpg.

Global exploration of genetic mutations offers a context from which developmental biologists and evolutionary theorists both can appreciate the multifaceted implications of genetic change in creating organismal diversity and functional capacity (Kevin et al., 2015). In developmental biology, genetic mutation is of significant medical relevance. In the case of cancer pathogenesis, for instance, mutations disrupting normal developmental signaling pathways can contribute to abnormal growth and tumor formation in cells. This association of organogenesis with disease state reflects the relevance of understanding how genetic regulation works not just in terms of normal development but also towards an understanding of potential therapeutic strategies in the treatment of cancer. Recent advances in cancer biology have enabled comparisons to be drawn between mechanisms of organogenesis and processes that regulate tumor development and progression. Establishing the effect of different mutations on developmental pathways allows scientists to identify more about what causes various cancers, as was evidenced through results from investigating cancer models and the nature of cancer stem cells. The effects of gene mutations thus extend over a broad range, giving us critical information on both the underlying mechanism of developmental biology and human health issues (Figure 8.12).

8.4. Epigenetic Factors in Organogenesis

The role of epigenetic elements throughout organogenesis is increasingly being considered as a vital part of explaining the complex genetic control of development phenomena. Epigenetic regulation, such as DNA methylation and histone modification, governs gene expression without altering the underlying DNA sequence. Control is required to confer cell identity and proper functioning of organ systems during development. Experiments have indicated that changes in DNA methylation patterns can play a significant role in the transcriptional destiny of individual genes involved in organogenesis. For instance, in shoot organogenesis in hybrid poplar, genome-wide levels of DNA methylation are considerably reduced and correlate with gene activity needed for organ development. These epigenetic mechanisms are more capable of describing the manner in which cells interpret developmental signals and respond to intrinsic as well as extrinsic stimuli during organogenesis and hence reinforce current understanding in developmental biology (Guo et al., 2024). The dynamics between environmental influence and epigenetic control also mark the adaptability of organogenesis gene expression. Hormones such as thyroid hormones play crucial roles in mediating epigenetic changes that are entirely necessary for the formation of certain organs. In the case of cerebellar development, thyroid hormones bind to specific receptors found within the nucleus and initiate a series of transcriptional events that culminate in cell division, cell migration, and cell differentiation. Their removal may result in gross developmental malformations, showing the importance of epigenetic mechanisms for the definition of organ development. This tightly controlled system underlines the importance of intrinsic genetic programs and extrinsic environmental influences in defining developmental processes. Therefore, the epigenetic landscape is not a passive background but an active scaffold through and in which genetic information is used in response to various developmental cues (Ishii et al., 2021). Generally, epigenetic effects on organogenesis highlight the intricacy of genetic control in development. Epigenetic marks are significant mediators that integrate both genetic and environmental information, which drive gene expression and developmental pathways. The cross-talk between plant DNA methylation reactions and hormonal regulation in mammals demonstrates the broad array of mechanisms through which epigenetic factors function between organisms. Through continuing studies in this direction, it is increasingly apparent that knowledge of the role of these epigenetic factors is at the forefront of demystifying organogenesis complexity and attaining conceivable insight into developmental disease and regenerative medicine. By combining both epigenetic and genetic studies, scientists are now able to construct a more complete understanding of the mechanisms that control organ growth (Guo et al., 2024; Ishii et al., 2021) (Figure 8.13).

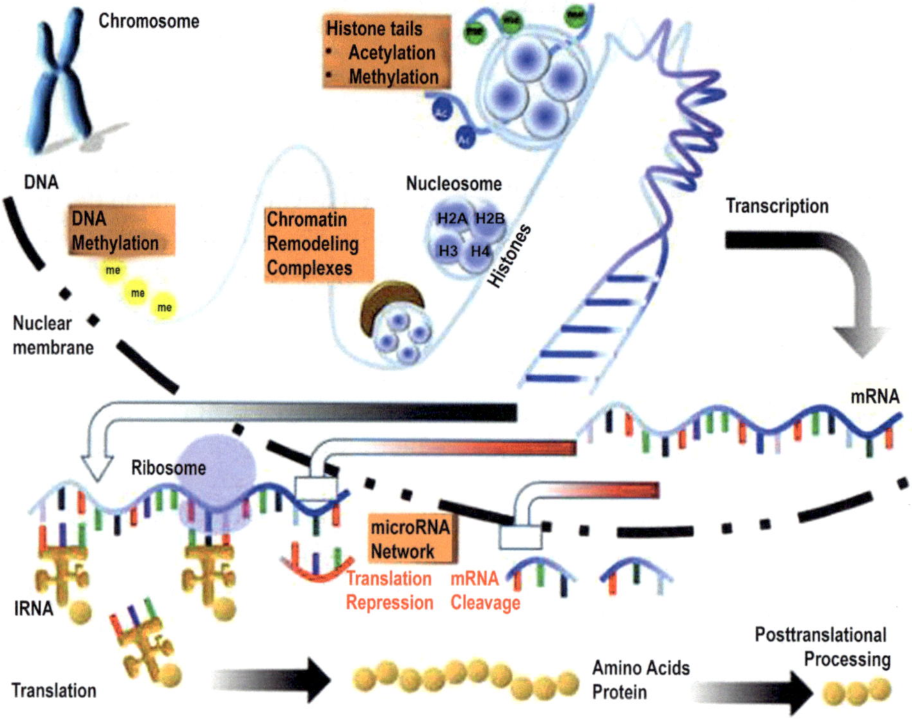

Figure 8.13. Epigenetic factors in organogenesis.

Source: https://www.mdpi.com/jdb/jdb-10-00026/article_deploy/html/images/jdb-10-00026-g001-550.jpg.

8.4.1. Definition and Significance of Epigenetics

Epigenetics refers to the investigation of heritable gene-expression changes that are not a result of alterations in the underlying DNA sequence. Epigenetics is crucial for understanding how external exposures and lifestyle influence lead to gene-behavior change with implications for development and function. During organogenesis, these epigenetic mechanisms like DNA methylation and histone modification play a key role in regulating stem cell differentiation into organ-forming cells. By such regulation of gene expression, some genes are triggered or repressed at specific times to coordinate complex developmental events resulting in normal development and function of organ systems. The significance of epigenetics also encompasses its role in health and disease, particularly during the process of organogenesis. It is demonstrated that certain of these epigenetic alterations predispose a person to noncommunicable disease through the process of programming, whereby early life conditions are linked to long-term health outcomes. For instance, exposure to toxic environmental stress during critical stages of development has been shown to cause epigenetic changes which manifest as metabolic syndromes or other diseases in adulthood. This emphasizes the importance of understanding how epigenetic control during organogenesis may influence not just the disease course of an individual but also factor into inheritance patterns of traits across generations, as emphasized in lifestyle effects on disease susceptibility research findings (Al-Za'abi et al., 2019). Furthermore, the dynamic character of the epigenetic modifications implies reversibility in response to environmental inputs, and reversible changes as well as challenges and opportunities for therapeutic interventions become open. As studies progress, it is becoming clear that the targeting of epigenetic pathways could possess the ability to reverse harmful changes brought about by disease, thus regaining optimal gene function. This is specifically pertinent within the realm of regenerative medicine, where the leverage of epigenetics' potential could potentially improve the efficacy of stem cell treatments and organ repair methods. For instance, understanding how epigenetic mechanisms interact with developmental signals can lead to new methods for regulating stem cell behavior towards regenerative organ targets, thereby facilitating advances in organ failure and birth defect therapies. An understanding of epigenetics is thus critical to unravel the complexities associated with organogenesis and develop successful medical therapies (Mikhailov et al., 2012).

8.4.2. Mechanisms of Epigenetic Regulation During Organ Development

Epigenetic regulation plays a key role in the coordination of organ development with profound effects on gene expression, but not through altering the DNA sequence, rather through different modifications involving DNA methylation and histone modification. Such modifications have the potential to activate or repress gene function, regulating cellular differentiation and organogenesis. In particular, coordination of environmental signals with epigenetic modifications supports adaptation during development. The relationship between epigenetic modifications and reactive oxygen species (ROS) has been under active research, revealing the capability of ROS to modulate gene expression at the epigenetic level. By orchestrating such molecular events, organisms can hone their developmental processes in order to respond to internal and external stimuli, resulting in successful organogenesis amidst a dynamic environment (Huang et al., 2019). MicroRNAs (miRNAs) also emerge as principal actors in the epigenetic stage of organogenesis. These small noncoding RNAs possess the ability to post transcriptionally regulate gene expression by destabilizing messenger RNAs (mRNAs) or suppressing their translation. They are not only regulators but also involved in complex networks that determine cell fate, differentiation, and organ identity. Also, miRNA expression is epigenetically controlled, meaning they must have a complex feedback loop between them. By controlling such networks, miRNAs are involved in coordinating spatial and temporal gene expression that is crucial for organogenesis. With further research continually elucidating the complex function of miRNAs in development, their therapeutic use increases more evident, particularly in understanding disorders due to deranged organ development (Saliminejad et al., 2018). Clarification of the epigenetic regulation of organ development not only increases our knowledge of the process but is also relevant to regenerative medicine and developmental disease. As scientists identify the particular epigenetic regulation and how they interact during vulnerable phases of organogenesis, the ability to modulate these pathways may be near. Implementing this knowledge would create new channels of therapeutic processes for repairing or regenerating damaged tissues and organs. Clarity of the impact of environmental stimuli on epigenetic modifications would also make a way for the prevention of congenital malformations. Lastly, the inclusion of epigenetic data in the organogenesis paradigm emphasizes the requirement for an integrative process that considers the complex interplay of genetics, environment, and epigenetics in defining organismal development and health (Figure 8.14).

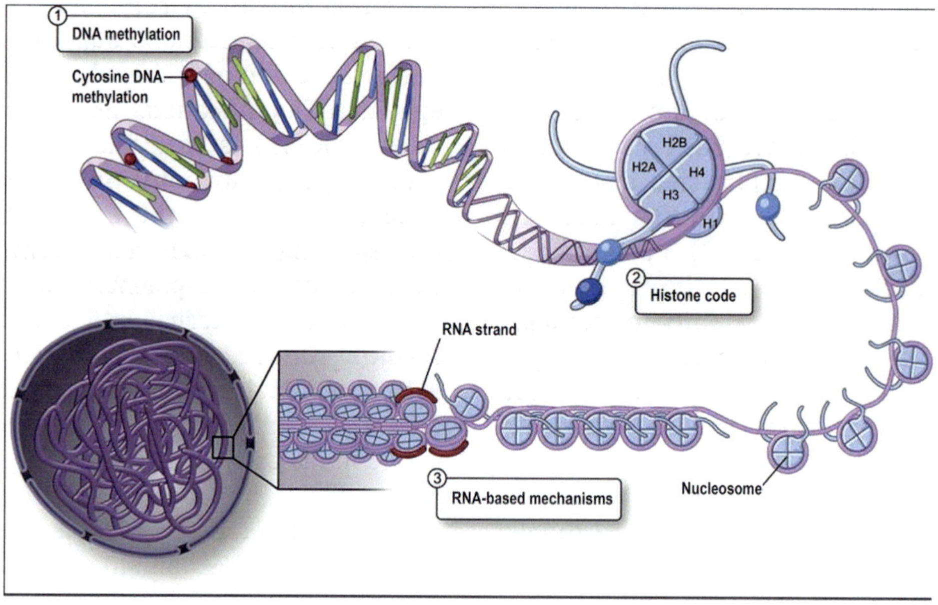

Figure 8.14. Mechanisms of epigenetic regulation during organ development.

Source: https://www.researchgate.net/profile/Charles-Matouk/publication/43299038/figure/fig1/AS:601788541579264@1520488977260/Three-fundamental-mechanisms-of-epigenetic-gene-regulation-Epigenetic-mechanisms-of-gene.png.

8.4.3. Examples of Epigenetic Modifications Influencing Organogenesis

Epigenetic marks significantly influence organogenesis since they regulate gene expression without the modification of the underlying DNA sequence. Such modifications, e.g., DNA methylation and histone marks, are significant during various development stages and enable differentiation of pluripotent stem cells into specialized cell types necessary for organ formation. For instance, during the early phase of mammalian development, ESCs undergo extensive epigenetic reprogramming, which is essential in establishing the appropriate gene expression patterns necessary for organ-specific lineage commitment. Single-cell technologies have enhanced our understanding of such dynamic processes, allowing separation of the precise epigenetic landscapes from which cell fate determination is governed during organogenesis. As the subject matter here, integration of *in vivo* perturbation methods and sophisticated *in vitro* systems provides avenues for comprehending the complicated roles of epigenetic regulators in embryonic development (Bolondi et al., 2022). Hormonal regulation, in this case estrogen, introduces an additional level of complication to epigenetic regulation of organogenesis. The hormone has a central position in arranging embryonic development since it regulates various pathways involved in cell growth and differentiation. Estrogen acts through specific receptors which speak to the genomic environment, eliciting changes in the transcription profile of developing tissues. These changes may trigger epigenetic alterations that can modulate gene expression leading to genes necessary for organ development. For example, abnormally high or low levels of estrogen during pregnancy will disrupt the delicate balance between gene expression, which finally influences organogenesis and yields long-term health effects. Studying the estrogen regulatory networks and their potential epigenetic impacts throws valuable insight into the way external forces can intersect with genetic control to form organs (Arifzai et al., 2024). Furthermore, epigenetic modifications also extend to the response of cells to external stimuli, again determining organogenesis. Nutrient availability and toxins represent environmental forces that can induce epigenetic changes impacting gene expression and developmental outcomes. For example, under stress or malnutrition, epigenetic reprogramming is induced, leading to altered organ development during embryonic stages. This highlights the malleability of the epigenome and its capacity to respond to external stimuli, thus rechanneling the trajectory of organogenesis. Contemporary studies focus on such interaction, revealing the significance of context-dependent epigenetic regulation in ensuring proper organ development. Through the identification of how environmental pressures and epigenetic control interact, researchers are better positioned to comprehend processes that underpin organogenesis as well as their implications for long-term health and disease (Bolondi et al., 2022).

8.5. Comparative Organogenesis Across Species

The comprehension of the comparative organogenesis across different species heightens our understanding of genetic regulation in the development of organs. Different organisms have unique pathways and mechanisms that propel the differentiation and formation of organs, creating fertile soil for investigation. For instance, studies involving model organisms, such as zebrafish and mouse embryos, establish that, although these organisms share basic genetic elements, they vary in the spatiotemporal regulation of organogenesis. That variation is not just governed by gene sequences but also by epigenetic means of controlling the expression of genes within varied environmental situations. These developments are crucial to the study of evolutionary processes that control organ development in order to provide a more complete picture of the genetic determinants of organogenesis across a range of species. Organoid technology has enhanced the comparative organogenesis science considerably, making it possible for scientists to rebuild tissue architecture resembling native organs closely. Brain organoids, for example, are derived from pluripotent stem cells and exhibit characteristics akin to early human brain development (Qian et al., 2019). Despite their revolutionary method, however, such organoids might not fully reproduce the intricate processes in phenomena like cortical layering and the development of neuronal circuitry. Such limitations reflect the complications involved in recapitulating organ development and highlight the necessity of continuous refinement of organoid methods. By observing these organoids along with embryonic development, scientists can better characterize the key genetic factors and signaling pathways required for organogenesis and thereby reduce the gap between *in vitro* and *in vivo* studies. In addition, research on wound healing has revealed a number of important insights into cellular dynamics and interactions that are involved in organ regeneration and repair in various species (Mélanie Rodrigues et al., 2018). The finding of stem cell subsets in various tissues illustrates cellular plasticity during organogenesis, particularly as a reaction to injury. In addition, the understanding of these phenomena is comparative and considers how various species structurally and functionally react to wounds. By borrowing from knowledge based on varied organisms, researchers can identify conserved genetic mechanisms that facilitate tissue regeneration and improve therapy. This comparative study not only enhances our understanding of the genetic regulation of organogenesis but also uncovers the potential of translational use to regenerative medicine (Figure 8.15).

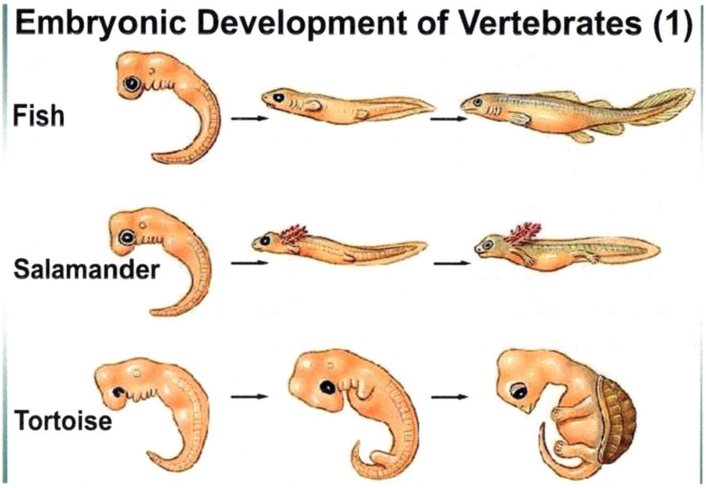

Figure 8.15. Comparative organogenesis across species.

Source: https://external-content.duckduckgo.com/iu/?u=https%3A%2F%2Fslidetodoc.com%2Fpresentation_image_h%2F30853fc53e932a1794acb2ed7dfcf521%2Fimage-29.jpg&f=1&nofb=1&ipt=a8fbc08528ef30da118d9fe7e5680a2611b5be155330a90afd2f0cde3162722e.

8.5.1. Similarities in Genetic Regulation Among Different Organisms

The intricate process of organogenesis is regulated by a multitude of genetic mechanisms showing unparalleled similarities in different organisms, attesting to evolutionary conservation of developmental processes. Signaling molecules regulating odontogenesis in vertebrates, such as those described in a comparative study of leech and mouse teeth, highlight the similarity of genetic control despite anatomical variation. 4113 genes were found to be expressed similarly in embryonic tooth germs in both species, suggesting conserved genetic blueprints on which tooth development may occur. The results only add to the significance of conserved signaling pathways in organogenesis, when analogous morphological patterns arise from a shared genetic inheritance. Appreciation of these similarities not only advances our understanding of evolutionary biology but also sheds light on the underlying genetic networks that coordinate organogenesis across different taxa (Aryal et al., 2024). Furthermore, epigenetic regulation adds more layers of complexity to the genetic similarities seen in organogenesis. Plants have been under investigation where narrow-endemic plants have shown less epigenetic variation, spatially structurally, than their widely distributed counterparts, showing the same degree of epigenetic reaction to environmental factors by all organisms with the same ecological requirements. This shows the prospect of preservation of epigenetic mechanism with a possible influence on organ development depending on differences in environments. Specifically, the lack of congruence between genetic and epigenetic information in closed environments might be a sign of directed adaptations that permit survival and effective reproduction. Not only do the patterns of epigenetic regulation observed supplement those of genetic regulation, but they form a broader evolutionary system through which different organisms cope with developmental processes within the uncertainty of the environment (Valverde et al., 2023). The shared genetic control among organisms underscores the potential for interdisciplinary application in developmental and regeneration biology.

The conservation of genetic elements in organogenesis provides researchers with the opportunity to discover potential therapeutic targets in regenerative medicine. The shared pathways of signaling, such as the ones present in leech dental development and mice, provide insights into the organ formation molecular mechanisms. Besides, epigenetic regulation knowledge can also offer clues on how to speed up tissue regeneration by modulating these pathways. Therefore, the intersection of genetic regulation across various taxonomic classes not only enlightens us on organogenesis evolution mechanisms but also raises the horizon for innovative approaches to treating developmental disorders and optimizing regenerative therapies in different species (Aryal et al., 2024; Valverde et al., 2023) (Figure 8.16).

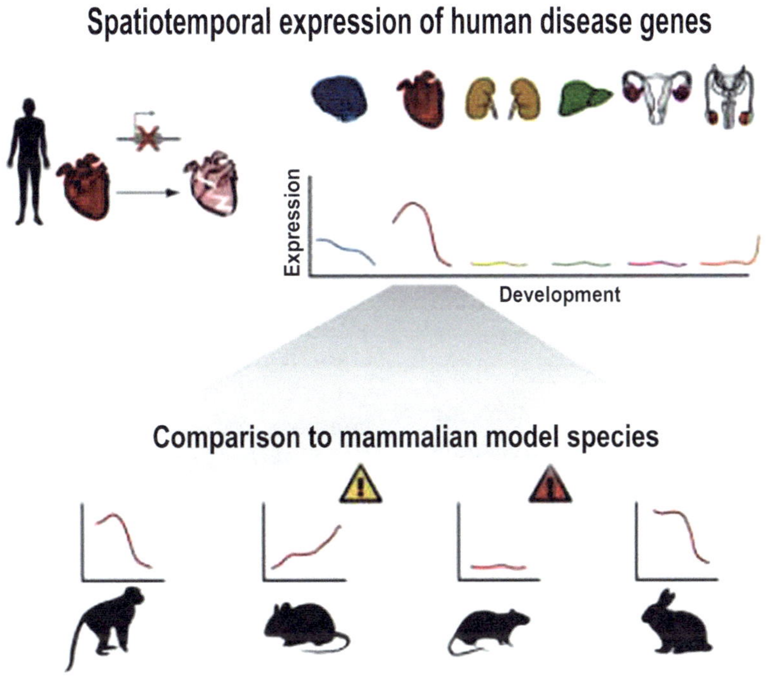

Figure 8.16. Similarities in genetic regulation among different organisms across species.

Source: https://ars.els-cdn.com/content/image/1-s2.0-S2211124720312973-fx1.jpg.

8.5.2. Differences in Organogenesis Processes Across Species

The organogenesis difference between species lies fundamentally in the regulation and differentiation of those genes involved in organ development. Floral organ development in flower plants, for instance, is well regulated by a well-characterized set of gene families like MADS-box and AP2/ERF clusters. These genes act by a complex interplay of interactions that not only determine floral organ identity but also their positioning and morphology. The specificity and functionality of the genes lead to extreme diversity of floral characters, which may differ immensely even in close relatives. This developmental genetic model and its influence on organogenesis reinforce the dependence of development on evolutionary adaptations and demonstrate how genetic regulation establishes the phenotypic range of plant species across generations.

In contrast, the processes of organogenesis in more complex multicellular organisms like animals are usually regulated by a different set of evolutionary pressures and developmental pathways. The genetic control of animal organogenesis—i.e., limb, organ, and body plan formation—is one way that individual variability is created through patterns of gene expression. As one example, studies have shown that genes that are most variable for their expression levels between individuals are more likely to be associated with organ function and environmental responsiveness. This heterogeneity can occur due to evolutionary pressures such as stochastic variation, epigenetic modification, and the environment, thus rendering the organ traits' patterns difficult to inherit. The dynamics of these gene expression dynamics provide a window into the evolution and adaptation of animal lineages' organ systems as an index of idiosyncratic evolutionary histories. In addition, variation in the process of organogenesis among species is not only determined by genetics but also by evolutionary forces that condition heterogeneity in gene expression in relation to organ function. For instance, research has demonstrated that organ-specific genes tend to have patterns of expression that are differentially regulated based on their broad function in certain tissues. This disparity signals a selective pressure for stability in certain organ systems and enhanced flexibility in others. These findings document the nuances of genetic control, demonstrating that organogenesis is not simply an issue of gene expression and suppression, but also of an organism's evolutionary heritage. Lastly. These URLs bring to the fore the intricate interplay between organogenesis and gene regulation, thereby elucidating how life organisms have evolved to adapt to their environments using intricate developmental strategies, as hypothesized by gene expression levels in various taxa (Bucao et al., 2024; Zhou et al., 2025).

8.5.3. Insights Gained from Comparative Studies in Developmental Biology

Comparative developmental biology has significantly contributed to understanding genetic control of organogenesis across various species. With the model organisms such as *Drosophila*, zebrafish, and mice, researchers have identified conserved genetic pathways that determine organ development. Such studies reveal that despite evolutionary divergence among species, a few genes and networks of regulation preserve similar activities, highlighting the idea of evolutionary conservation. For instance, studies of embryonic lethal mutant mice facilitated through the DMDD programme underscore the utility of gene knockout studies in delineating gene function with organogenesis. Because embryonic development in these systems is incomplete, they are valuable tools for developmental biologists interested in linking certain genetic mutations with abnormalities of organ form, important to the understanding of the genetic causes of congenital human maladies (Adams et al., 2013). Comparative approaches have also illuminated basic regulatory processes guiding morphogenetic processes in different organisms. Plant gene regulation, for example, has employed *in vitro* techniques to analyze the role of KNOTTED1-like homeobox (KNOX) transcription factors. The factors are significant in the maintenance of stem cell populations and contribute significantly to organogenesis by influencing hormonal signaling pathways as well as cell differentiation. By analogy between animal and plant systems, scientists have developed a better understanding of how the same genetic pathways might have different morphological outcomes. The identification of such regulatory factors not only enriches our conceptual model but provides practical use in agricultural biotechnology in the form of enhancing crop yields by optimizing organ formation and tissue regeneration (Caretto et al., 2019). Finally, the integration of new tools such as transcriptomics and imaging has revolutionized the field of developmental biology to permit extensive study of gene expression patterns in organogenesis. The cooperative work of the International Mouse Phenotyping Consortium, as in collaboration with the DMDD programme, shows how comparative studies thrive on shared data and resources, yielding deeper insight into embryonic development. By contrasting embryonic lethal mutant line gene expression profiles, scientists are able to identify genes that govern critical developmental processes. The resulting emerging database not only represents a useful tool for the understanding of gene-function relationships during organogenesis but also facilitates interdisciplinary interaction among developmental biologists, clinicians, and geneticists. Ultimately, such integrated approaches will advance our knowledge of the genetic basis of organogenesis and its potential for human disease (Adams et al., 2013).

8.6. Applications of Genetic Regulation Research

The research in genetic regulation has significant implications in the progress of agriculture, particularly in enhancing yields and tolerance in crops. Some of the most significant areas include the use of *in vitro* plant cell and tissue culture. These technologies exploit certain genetic traits that can lead to enhanced metabolite production and genetic diversity. If researchers are aware of what genes, particularly those regulated by *Agrobacterium rhizogenes* rol genes, do to plant growth and development, they can engineer genetically modified organisms (GMOs) that can grow well in unfavorable environments. These innovations not only contribute to food security but also provide the potential for coming up with sustainable agriculture practices that can mitigate the effects of climate change. This plan of action highlights the place of genetic regulation research as the foundation of modern agricultural biotechnology, with findings pivotal to future innovations (Caretto et al., 2019). Tissue culture techniques, particularly the use of thin cell layers (TCLs), have maximized the investigation of plant genetics through the enabling of the observation of cellular differentiation directly. By isolating tiny numbers of cells from various organs of plants, researchers can localize marker molecules within specific responding cells effectively. This enables more accurate studies of gene control and the process involved in organogenesis. The versatility of TCL systems has led them to become a crucial tool for applied research as well as for theoretical research. For instance, such systems facilitate investigations into hormone signaling pathways exclusive to the KNOX transcription factors, which are known to control crucial aspects of plant morphogenesis. In totality, these advancements confirm the pivotal role of TCL systems in the development of our understanding of plant biology and gene regulation and with ramifications for crop enhancement and breeding processes (Giraldo et al., 2015). The scientific development that comes from studies of genetic control also makes possible the study of evolutionary processes in plants. By knowing how various genetic factors control the phase shift from juvenile growth to adult growth in such plants as *Prunus*, researchers can discover more about evolutionary adjustments that have occurred over time. This research does not only improve information on plant growth but also helps in conservation attempts at endangered species. Moreover, knowledge attained from genetic regulation may be applied to enhance genetic transformation processes, especially in traditionally recalcitrant legume crops. Understanding the complexity of genetic regulatory networks positions researchers to conceive more effective breeding programs, ultimately resulting in creating improved crop varieties. Thus, the application of genetic regulation research is a critical component of theory building as well as practical applications in agriculture and conservation, reinforcing its central role in ongoing research into organogenesis (Caretto et al., 2019) (Figure 8.17).

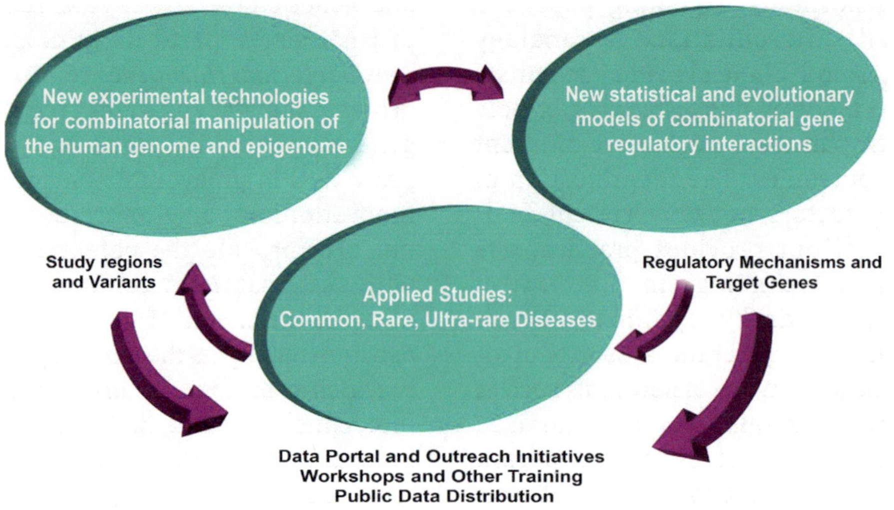

Figure 8.17. Genetic regulation research.

Source: https://biostat.duke.edu/sites/default/files/2022-05/figure_4_aims_relationships_2020_updated_for_website_green-1-1920x1066.png.

8.6.1. Implications for Regenerative Medicine

The advances in the genetic regulation of organogenesis have far-reaching effects on regenerative medicine, particularly in the development of therapeutic strategies in organ repair and regeneration. By the elucidation of the pathways and gene networks that regulate the differentiation and proliferation of stem cells, scientists can make use of these mechanisms to improve tissue regeneration. For instance, studies on epithelial stem cell niches provide insight into the ways that extracellular signaling molecules can be designed to sustain stem cell populations effectively. The recognition of Activin, BMP, and FGF operating in a complex regulatory network to control stem cell dynamics suggests targets for therapies to enhance regenerative capacities in other tissues. Given that regenerative medicine is increasingly focusing on repairing or replacing impaired organs, knowledge of such signaling pathways can lead to developments in stem cell therapies with the potential to revolutionize treatment of numerous degenerative diseases (Alonso et al., 2007). In addition, the implications of sexual dimorphism, as highlighted in current organogenesis studies, extend the range of potential applications for regenerative medicine. Understanding hormonal influences, in this case, the influence of estrogen on embryonic development and organogenesis, emphasizes the importance of gender consideration in therapy. In addition, the intricate relationship between hormones and genes affects not just organ development but also long-term health in individuals. Through the integration of findings from studies that have focused on hormonal control, such as those investigating estrogens' roles in embryonic development, regenerative medicine is able to develop more complex treatment models that are tailored to the needs of different patient populations. This in-depth understanding of organogenesis can pave the way for personalized medicine, with the effectiveness of stem cell therapies enhanced based on an individual's hormonal and genetic profile (Arifzai et al., 2024). Moreover, the latest results on the asymmetrical growth patterns observed during organogenesis provide fascinating insights into the regenerative potential of various organs. Clarification of the key regulatory factors, i.e., Follistatin, implicated in the internal asymmetry of structures such as the mouse incisors can drive the innovation of new regenerative strategies. Insight into the ways that differential signaling pathways give rise to a range of regenerative capacities in tissues may inform the development of targeted therapies that draw upon nature's own strategies. For instance, studies showing that selective stem cell proliferation can be achieved through specific manipulation of signaling molecules invite exploration of how similar principles can be applied to human tissue regeneration. This not only enhances our scientific understanding but also positions regenerative medicine to replicate these complex biological processes in clinical settings, ultimately improving treatment outcomes for patients requiring organ repair or replacement (Alonso et al., 2007).

8.6.2. Potential for Genetic Engineering in Organ Development

The potential for genetic engineering in organogenesis is a new frontier in the field of regenerative medicine and organogenesis. With the application of advanced gene editing tools such as CRISPR-Cas9 and TALENs, researchers can iteratively manipulate gene expression to design organs with precise spatial and temporal characteristics. This kind of manipulation involves unraveling the intricate networks of transcriptional regulation of organ development with implications for therapeutic applications as well as fundamental insight into developmental biology. Genetic manipulations enable control over the cellular signaling pathways and transcription factors necessary for the specification of stem cells to desired organ lineages. These advances are key to resolving tissue engineering obstacles and organ transplant rejection, and thus offer a way to create functional organs that are patient-specific, which will ultimately improve patient outcomes and reduce the need for donor organs. As genetic engineering techniques are developed, new opportunities for the treatment of organ disease and condition are unveiled. The incorporation of spatiotemporal molecular medicine into organ development allows for a deeper understanding of disease progression through the investigation of the interaction between genetic and cellular microenvironmental factors. Investigations of the phenotypic variation in genetically modified organ structures can inform the roles that specific genes and signaling pathways play during organogenesis. The coupling of genetic engineering with sophisticated imaging modalities allows researchers to visualize the precise alterations that are occurring at the molecular level, which can lead to the identification of novel therapeutic targets. Moreover, the generation of genetically manipulated organogenesis models provides unparalleled windows into pathology with a huge influence on the field of personalized medicine and paving the way for the evolution of new modalities of treatment according to individual genetic configuration, as substantiated by advances in wound healing research and tissue regeneration. The future of organ fabrication through genetic engineering is also reliant upon the advancement of biomaterial and scaffolding technologies that merge engineered tissues and cells. Emerging strategies focus on the design of biocompatible scaffolds that not only support cell attachment and growth but are also biofunctionalized with genetic molecules capable of triggering organ-specific differentiation and vascularization. These scaffolds can also be designed to release growth factors and other bioactive molecules to enhance the regenerative process and expedite tissue repair. As pointed out in recent research, the use of genetically modified cells in combination with such advanced scaffolds can significantly improve skin regeneration and chronic wound healing, which is just one use in the broader scheme of organ development (Tottoli et al., 2020; Wang et al., 2021). Looking ahead, the therapeutic potential of these genetic engineering innovations is enormous, emphasizing the need for continued partnership among geneticists, biomedical engineers, and clinicians to move the potential of genetic engineering into clinically useful therapeutic approaches to organ development and repair (Figure 8.18).

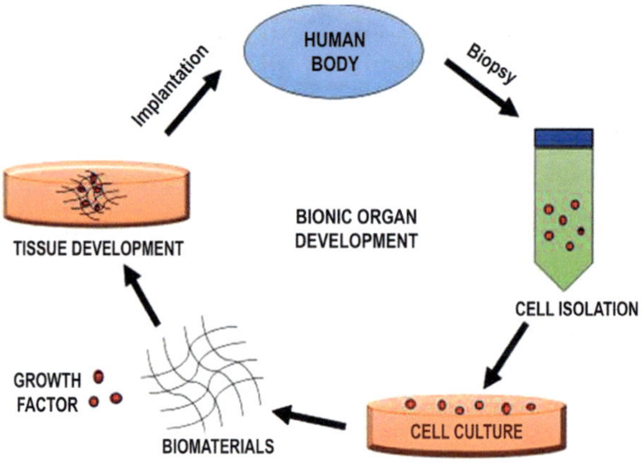

Figure 8.18. Genetic engineering in organ development.

Source: https://www.tandfonline.com/cms/asset/825f786b-9f77-452b-b339-59d9f0bef3c7/ymte_a_2242732_f0002_oc.jpg.

8.6.3. Ethical Considerations in Manipulating Genetic Regulation

Genetic control has strong ethical consequences, particularly with the processes of organogenesis. As scientists move to utilize gene editing and stem cell therapy in controlling developmental patterns, there are possibilities of unintended consequences. The manipulation towards editing genes precisely has the consequence that there might be conditions where undesirable characteristics are removed, and there would be ethical concerns in the direction of eugenics and the commodification of human life. This commodification is viewed as scientists develop advanced therapy medicinal products (ATMPs), which have the capability of addressing congenital and genetic illness. Such potential, however, brings along with it the responsibility to ensure that such innovations do not exacerbate social inequalities. The pressure is to meet a balance between scientific progress and the ethical imperative to maintain respect for human dignity as well as ensure equitable access to such revolutionizing technologies (Tottoli et al., 2020). Moreover, economic ramifications of changing genetic control further complicate the ethical dilemma. Manufacture and subsequent sale of ATMPs are typically accompanied by very high costs, making them inaccessible to the majority of patients who would significantly benefit from them. The differential access not only perpetuates existing health inequalities but also calls into question the equity in utilizing public funds in creating therapies that benefit largely affluent parts of society. As noted, the prices of gene therapy have been approximated to be, on average, $1 million or higher, setting policymakers into a sudden imperative to determine how these drugs will be funded and distributed (Seoane et al., 2019). Ethical argumentation needs to address the fiscal cost to health care systems and the possible effect on patients' right to receive fair treatment, highlighting the fundamental nature of health care as a human right, not a marketable commodity. Lastly, there is a serious philosophical concern about the implications of altering organisms through genetics, especially with regards to what is meant by human life. The power to manipulate genetic material poses profound questions about the nature of individuality and the coherence of human identity. As researchers advance to be able to programme genes to produce specific phenotypic outcomes during organogenesis, society must reconcile what these capabilities mean. Such manipulation could eventually give rise to individuals who are inherently different from the norm and shatter previous ideas of what it is to be human. These ethical issues call for consideration of the scientists' and policymakers' role in ensuring that advances in genetic control are based on a vision for respect for human values and the natural order of living (Tottoli et al., 2020). Such issues need to be part of the broader story of genetic technologies and their application in medicine and beyond.

SUMMARY

The controversy surrounding genetic organogenesis control, it is important to understand the intricate patterns of gene interactions that orchestrate developmental processes. The experiment on the *Caenorhabditis elegans* vulva illustrates how a single transcription factor coordinates cellular fates within a limited spatial plan, thus highlighting the precision of genetic control over organ development. Such recognition of vulval GRN elements not only illuminates the nuances of how individual cell types are formed but also emphasizes the complexity of transcription factor interactions. These findings suggest that, beyond the abilities of isolated genes, total genetic interaction dynamics are crucial in specifying organ form and function, justifying further research into the regulatory representations inherent in other development models (Bach et al., 2008). Moreover, comparative genetic process analysis across species reveals convergences and divergences that guide organogenesis. Analysis of E-cadherin expression in zebrafish teeth, for example, illustrates the complexity of cell adhesion molecule patterning needed in morphogenesis. This comparison is also important because it creates avenues for debate on how different evolutionary histories may influence the genetic models guiding development. The ongoing expression of E-cadherin in tooth development implies that different species may have adapted their regulatory mechanisms to fulfill similar developmental purposes. These observations do not only add to a broader view of dental morphogenesis but also call for a broader view of the evolutionary perspectives in organ development, highlighting the robustness of genetic regulation and its contingency in all organisms (Huysseune et al., 2010). Lastly, the integration of findings between *C. elegans* vulval GRN and zebrafish tooth development points to an important juncture of convergence for developmental biology and genetics. The regulatory patterns laid down provide a foundation for subsequent work to establish more intricate features of organogenesis in other organisms. The uses even extend beyond the simple biological perspective since understanding genetic regulation is applied to the design of regenerative medicine and therapeutic treatments for organ regeneration. As scientists proceed to unravel the complexity of these genetic networks, it is essential to maintain an integrated view that considers findings from numerous biological models. The continued study of genetic control not only reveals developmental key principles but can also have the power to revolutionize strategies relative to health and disease related to organ function and regeneration (Bach et al., 2008; Huysseune et al., 2010).

Organogenesis is regulated by a complex interplay of hormonal and genetic elements that order the specific temporal and spatial organization of cellular differentiation. It incorporates many transcription factors and hormones, which regulate gene expression and ultimately result in the development of organs and tissues in embryonic development. Among those transcription factors, p63 is one of the most significant, proven to be essential for the formation of epithelial tissues in a wide range of species. The role of p63 is explicitly demonstrated in the epidermis, where it regulates keratinocyte proliferation and differentiation, indicating the significance of spatial and temporal regulation of genes during organogenesis. Genetic as well as hormonal signals must harmoniously integrate to achieve appropriate organ development, indicating the intricate interministering scheme behind developmental biology (Wang et al., 2018). In addition, the study of shoot architecture gives valuable insights into genetic regulation of organogenesis, but in plants. Plant architectural organization relies on meristem activity and the genetic control of hormones like auxins and strigolactones. New advances into the understanding of the roles played by some genes like Ideal Plant Architecture1 and Teosinte Branched1 demonstrate how developmental consequence may be defined by genetic pathways. These findings show that gene control is not specific to the animal system but is general in the plant kingdom, revealing a more widespread theme of biology in which gene expression regulates the morphological characteristics of significance for survival and reproduction. Understanding these regulatory mechanisms enables us to fine-tune plant architecture for crop production and sustainability (Wang et al., 2018). Furthermore, organogenesis is controlled by genes, and thus the role of enhancer regions in controlling gene transcription during development comes to light. Enhancers that are bound by transcription factors like p63 tend to be responsible for determining the activity of nearby genes in differentiation processes. According to research, it has been shown that the control of enhancer activity dynamics, which is characterized especially by the pattern of histone marks like H3K27ac, is strongly correlated with gene expression levels. This finding reveals that although transcription factors are needed, their regulation is heavily supported by the epigenetic environment of genes. The observation that enhancer dynamics directly correlates with transcription highlights the importance of further research on epigenetic regulators as central components of the genetic network responsible for organogenesis (Evelyn et al., 2015).

CLOSER LOOK

CAENORHABDITIS ELEGANS

Caenorhabditis elegans (*C. elegans*) is a small, transparent nematode (roundworm) that has become one of the most extensively studied model organisms in biological research. Measuring approximately 1 millimeter in length, *C. elegans* has a simple anatomy and a short life cycle of about three days from egg to adult, making it ideal for genetic and developmental studies. First introduced as a model system by Sydney Brenner in the 1960s, *C. elegans* has provided invaluable insights into fundamental biological processes such as cell division, differentiation, development, aging, and neurobiology. One of the organism's most notable features is its invariant cell lineage—each of its approximately 959 somatic cells in the adult hermaphrodite follows a highly predictable pattern of development, allowing researchers to trace cell fates with remarkable precision. In addition, the entire genome of *C. elegans*, which contains around 20,000 genes, has been fully sequenced, and the complete neural connectome (map of its 302 neurons and their synaptic connections) has been mapped, making it the first multicellular organism to be so thoroughly characterized at both genetic and anatomical levels.

C. elegans exists primarily as a self-fertilizing hermaphrodite, although males occur naturally at a low frequency and can be used for genetic crosses. This reproductive simplicity allows for controlled genetic experiments, and powerful tools such as RNA interference (RNAi) and CRISPR-Cas9 gene editing have been effectively employed in this organism. Because of its transparency, researchers can observe cellular and developmental processes in living worms under a microscope in real time. The simplicity of *C. elegans*, however, does not limit its usefulness. Many of its genes and molecular pathways are highly conserved with those in humans, including those involved in apoptosis, insulin signaling, and stress responses, making it a valuable model for studying human diseases, including neurodegenerative disorders, cancer, and metabolic syndromes.

In the field of neurobiology, *C. elegans* has been instrumental in uncovering mechanisms of neural development, behavior, and sensory processing. Although it has a simple nervous system, the worm exhibits complex behaviors such as chemotaxis, thermotaxis, learning, and memory. The Nobel Prize in Physiology or Medicine was awarded in 2002 to researchers who used *C. elegans* to identify key genes involved in programmed cell death, and again in 2006 for discoveries related to RNAi. In 2008, research involving *C. elegans* contributed to the Nobel Prize awarded for discoveries in green fluorescent protein (GFP), which revolutionized live imaging of gene expression.

Furthermore, *C. elegans* has become a popular model in aging research due to its short lifespan of about 2–3 weeks and its well-characterized aging pathways, such as insulin/IGF-1 signaling. Its use in high-throughput genetic and drug screens continues to expand, offering promise for discovering treatments for age-related and genetic diseases. In summary, *C. elegans* is a powerful and versatile model organism that has significantly advanced our understanding of molecular and developmental biology, and it remains at the forefront of biomedical research.

REFERENCES

1. Adams, D. J., Aijö, T., Airik, R., Anders, S., Brown, S. D. M., Dorr, A., Geyer, S., et al. (2013). Deciphering the Mechanisms of Developmental Disorders (DMDD): A new programmed for phenotyping embryonic lethal mice. https://core.ac.uk/download/16257083.pdf (accessed on 27 May 2025).
2. Alonso, M. T., Chuong, C. M., Felszeghy, S., Maas, R., et al. (2007). An integrated gene regulatory network controls stem cell proliferation in teeth. https://pmc.ncbi.nlm.nih.gov/articles/PMC1885832/.
3. Al-Za'abi, A., Kilani, A., Kilani, H., Kilani, R., et al. (2019). Fetal-neonatal lifestyle basis of the adult metabolic syndrome patients. https://core.ac.uk/download/322444282.pdf (accessed on 27 May 2025).
4. Arifzai, R., & Hewadmal, T. K. (2024). The impact of estrogen on embryonic development: A review paper. https://core.ac.uk/download/603903664.pdf (accessed on 27 May 2025).
5. Aryal, Y. P., Neupane, S., Kwak, H. J., An, C. H., Sohn, W. J., Yamamoto, H., Kwon, T. Y., et al. (2024). Unraveling the structure, chemical composition, and conserved signaling in leech teeth. *Animal Cells and Systems, 28*, 272–282. https://www.semanticscholar.org/paper/0a9ccd20cfd8e39bc7ade4dd8c797d4f109a27c3 (accessed on 27 May 2025).
6. Bach, M., Bettinger, J. C., Burdine, R. D., Cai, D., Chamberlin, H. M., Chang, C., Clark, S. G., et al. (2008). The *Caenorhabditis elegans* vulva: A post-embryonic gene regulatory network controlling organogenesis. https://www.pnas.org/doi/10.1073/pnas.0806377105.
7. Bakouh, N., Castaño-Martín, R., Métais, A., Dan, E. L., Balducci, E., Chhuon, C., Lepicka, J., et al. (2024). Chloride deregulation and GABA depolarization in MTOR-related malformations of cortical development. *Brain, 148*(2), 549–563. https://www.semanticscholar.org/paper/4ee5b075f8e516a870e65b8f20f58fdbe8b98078 (accessed on 27 May 2025).
8. Bellavia, D., Checquolo, S., Nardozza, F., Pelullo, M., et al. (2019). Wnt, Notch, and TGF-β pathways impinge on Hedgehog signaling complexity: An open window on cancer. https://core.ac.uk/download/231747363.pdf (accessed on 27 May 2025).
9. Bolondi, A., Kretzmer, H., & Meissner, A. (2022). Single-cell technologies: A new lens into epigenetic regulation in development. https://core.ac.uk/download/533535970.pdf (accessed on 27 May 2025).
10. Botero Giraldo, C., Della Rovere, F., Dhir, S., Dobránszki, J., Falasca, G., Gomes, G. M., et al. (2015). The untapped potential of plant thin cell layers. https://core.ac.uk/download/188822800.pdf (accessed on 27 May 2025).
11. Bucao, C. F., Aletti, C., Moretti, S., Thompson, A. W., Racicot, B. L., Wilson, C., Bobe, J., et al. (2024). Inter-individual gene expression variability implies stable regulation of brain-biased genes across organs. *bioRxiv*. https://www.semanticscholar.org/paper/bae3441fc7f69de97d18458cb71329f2fa4d201d (accessed on 27 May 2025).
12. Cano, D. A., Flores Martínez, Á., Hebrok, M., Herrero Martín, J. E., et al. (2016). Loss of pancreas upon activated Wnt signaling is concomitant with emergence of gastrointestinal identity. https://core.ac.uk/download/186618050.pdf (accessed on 27 May 2025).
13. Cao, J., O'Day, D. R., Pliner, H. A., Kingsley, P. D., Deng, M., Daza, R. M., Zager, M., et al. (2020).

A human cell atlas of fetal gene expression. *Science, 370*(6518), eaba7721. https://doi.org/10.1126/science.aba7721.

14. Caretto, S., Frugis, G., Giannino, D., Iannelli, M. A., et al. (2019). Plant cellular and molecular biotechnology: Following Mariotti's steps. https://core.ac.uk/download/188831409.pdf (accessed on 27 May 2025).

15. Cirio, M. C., Davidson, A. J., de Caestecker, M. P., de Groh, E. D., et al. (2013). Kidney regeneration: Common themes from the embryo to the adult. https://core.ac.uk/download/159296304.pdf (accessed on 27 May 2025).

16. Fumagalli, M., Lecca, D., Abbracchio, M. P., & Ceruti, S. (2017). Pathophysiological role of purines and pyrimidines in neurodevelopment: Unveiling new pharmacological approaches to congenital brain diseases. *Frontiers in Pharmacology, 8*, 941. https://doi.org/10.3389/fphar.2017.00941.

17. Geelen, D., Schotte, S., & Verstraeten, I. (2014). Hypocotyl adventitious root organogenesis differs from lateral root development. https://core.ac.uk/download/55765422.pdf (accessed on 27 May 2025).

18. Ghosh, S., & Hayden, M. S. (2012). Celebrating 25 years of NF-κB research. *Immunological Reviews, 246*(1), 5–13. https://doi.org/10.1111/j.1600-065x.2012.01111.x.

19. Guo, Y., Feng, Y. F., Yang, G., Jia, Y., He, J., Wu, Z. Y., Liao, H. R., et al. (2024). Allele-specific DNA methylation and gene expression during shoot organogenesis in tissue culture of hybrid poplar. *Horticulture Research, 11*. https://www.semanticscholar.org/paper/cb490e7aa7ee61c29029cff0d83d362aa84d0ef4 (accessed on 27 May 2025).

20. Huang, H., Ullah, F., Zhou, D. X., Yi, M., & Zhao, Y. (2019). Mechanisms of ROS regulation of plant development and stress responses. *Frontiers in Plant Science, 10*, 800. https://doi.org/10.3389/fpls.2019.00800.

21. Huysseune, A., Sanders, E., van Hengel, J., Verstraeten, et al. (2010). Zebrafish teeth as a model for repetitive epithelial morphogenesis: Dynamics of E-cadherin expression. https://core.ac.uk/download/55797288.pdf (accessed on 27 May 2025).

22. Ishii, S., Amano, I., & Koibuchi, N. (2021). The role of thyroid hormone in the regulation of cerebellar development. *Endocrinology and Metabolism, 36*(4), 703–716. https://www.semanticscholar.org/paper/8f569e2c9949824071d4095ab9e05e3348a92d71 (accessed on 27 May 2025).

23. Itoh, E., Satoh, H., Kusano, H., Shimada, H., Yamakawa, H., Yazaki, J., She, K. C., et al. (2009). A novel superior factor widely controlling the rice grain quality. https://core.ac.uk/download/pdf/288519.pdf (accessed on 27 May 2025).

24. Jin, S., & Daniell, H. (2015). The engineered chloroplast genome just got smarter. *Trends in Plant Science, 20*, 622–640. https://doi.org/10.1016/j.tplants.2015.07.004.

25. Kouwenhoven, E. N., Oti, M., Niehues, H., van Heeringen, S. J., Schalkwijk, J., Stunnenberg, H. G., van Bokhoven, H., et al. (2015). Transcription factor p63 bookmarks and regulates dynamic enhancers during epidermal differentiation. *EMBO Reports, 16*(7), 863–878. https://doi.org/10.15252/embr.201439941.

26. Laland, K. N., Uller, T., Feldman, M. W., Sterelny, K., Müller, G. B., Moczek, A. P., Jablonka, E., et al. (2015). The extended evolutionary synthesis: Its structure, assumptions and predictions.

Proceedings of the Royal Society B: Biological Sciences, 282(1813), 20151019. https://doi.org/10.1098/rspb.2015.1019.

27. Liu, C., Leng, J., Li, Y., Ge, T., Li, J., Chen, Y., Guo, C., et al. (2022). A spatiotemporal atlas of organogenesis in the development of orchid flowers. *Nucleic Acids Research, 50*, 9724–9737. https://doi.org/10.1093/nar/gkac773.
28. Mantovani, A., Biswas, S. K., Galdiero, M. R., Sica, A., & Locati, M. (2012). Macrophage plasticity and polarization in tissue repair and remodeling. *The Journal of Pathology, 229*, 176–185. https://doi.org/10.1002/path.4133.
29. McGrath, I. M., Mortlock, S., & Montgomery, G. (2021). Genetic regulation of physiological reproductive lifespan and female fertility. *International Journal of Molecular Sciences, 22*(4), 1–20. https://www.semanticscholar.org/paper/34eaaa896d1d3dd96b345ddcdd88b121bf6a574c (accessed on 27 May 2025).
30. Mikhailov, A. T. (2012). Russian comparative embryology takes form: A conceptual metamorphosis toward "evo-devo." https://core.ac.uk/download/61920109.pdf (accessed on 27 May 2025).
31. Moustakas, A., & García de Herreros, A. (2017). Epithelial–mesenchymal transition in cancer. *Molecular Oncology, 11*, 715–717. https://doi.org/10.1002/1878-0261.12094.
32. Qian, X., Song, H., & Ming, G.-l. (2019). Brain organoids: Advances, applications and challenges. *Development, 146*. https://doi.org/10.1242/dev.166074.
33. Rodrigues, M., Kosaric, N., Bonham, C. A., & Gurtner, G. C. (2018). Wound healing: A cellular perspective. *Physiological Reviews, 99*(1), 665–706. https://doi.org/10.1152/physrev.00067.2017.
34. Saliminejad, K., Khorram Khorshid, H. R., Soleymani Fard, S., & Ghaffari, S. H. (2018). An overview of microRNAs: Biology, functions, therapeutics, and analysis methods. *Journal of Cellular Physiology, 234*(6), 5451–5465. https://doi.org/10.1002/jcp.27486.
35. Seoane-Vazquez, E., Shukla, V., & Rodríguez-Monguió, R. (2019). Innovation and competition in advanced therapy medicinal products. *EMBO Molecular Medicine, 11*, e9992. https://doi.org/10.15252/emmm.201809992.
36. Shen, M. M., & Abate-Shen, C. (2010). Molecular genetics of prostate cancer: New prospects for old challenges. *Genes & Development, 24*(18), 1967–2000. https://doi.org/10.1101/gad.1965810.
37. Suzaki, T., Kim, C. S., Takeda, N., Szczygłowski, K., & Kawaguchi, M. (2012). *TRICOT* encodes an AMP1-related carboxypeptidase that regulates root nodule development and shoot apical meristem maintenance in *Lotus japonicus*. *Development, 140*, 353–361. https://doi.org/10.1242/dev.089631.
38. Tottoli, E. M., Dorati, R., Genta, I., Chiesa, E., Pisani, S., & Conti, B. (2020). Skin wound healing process and new emerging technologies for skin wound care and regeneration. *Pharmaceutics, 12*(8), 735. https://doi.org/10.3390/pharmaceutics12080735.
39. Valverde, J., Medrano, M., Herrera, C. M., & Alonso, C. (2023). Comparative epigenetic and genetic spatial structure in Mediterranean mountain plants: A multispecific comparison. *bioRxiv*. https://www.semanticscholar.org/paper/7f630aadf6774a0dec2f91c98c8a1e58824e24e1 (accessed on 27 May 2025).

40. Verma, T., Papadantonakis, N., Barclift, D. P., & Zhang, L. (2024). Molecular genetic profile of myelofibrosis: Implications in the diagnosis, prognosis, and treatment advancements. *Cancers, 16.* https://www.semanticscholar.org/paper/dd75e317999a7cce24210e788488000e549a6a17 (accessed on 27 May 2025).

41. Wang, B., Smith, S. M., & Li, J. (2018). Genetic regulation of shoot architecture. *Annual Review of Plant Biology, 69*, 437–468. https://doi.org/10.1146/annurev-arplant-042817-040422.

42. Wang, X., & Fan, J. (2021). Spatiotemporal molecular medicine: A new era of clinical and translational medicine. *Clinical and Translational Medicine, 11.* https://doi.org/10.1002/ctm2.294.

43. Willet, S. G., & Mills, J. C. (2016). Stomach organ and cell lineage differentiation: From embryogenesis to adult homeostasis. *Cellular and Molecular Gastroenterology and Hepatology, 2*, 546–559. https://doi.org/10.1016/j.jcmgh.2016.05.006.

44. Yang, A., Mailleux, A. A., Mill, A. A., van Genderen, C., Chapman, D. L., Robinson, G. W., van Bokhoven, H., et al. (2004). Identification of signaling pathways in early mammary gland development by mouse genetics. https://pmc.ncbi.nlm.nih.gov/articles/PMC400673/.

45. Yang, Y., & Mlodzik, M. (2015). Wnt-Frizzled/Planar Cell Polarity signaling: Cellular orientation by facing the wind (Wnt). *Annual Review of Cell and Developmental Biology, 31*, 623–646. https://doi.org/10.1146/annurev-cellbio-100814-125315.

46. Yu, H., Lin, L., Zhang, Z., Zhang, H., & Hu, H. (2020). Targeting NF-κB pathway for the therapy of diseases: Mechanism and clinical study. *Signal Transduction and Targeted Therapy, 5*, 209. https://doi.org/10.1038/s41392-020-00312-6.

47. Zhernakova, D., Wang, D., Liu, L., Andreu-Sánchez, S., Zhang, Y., Ruiz-Moreno, A., Peng, H., et al. (2024). Host genetic regulation of human gut microbial structural variation. *Nature, 625*, 813–821. https://www.semanticscholar.org/paper/22c469e9731b919b4a69fafc1709032a6814bd1c (accessed on 27 May 2025).

48. Zhou, L., Iqbal, A., Yang, M., & Yang, Y. (2025). Research progress on gene regulation of plant floral organogenesis. *Genes, 16*(1), 1–16. https://www.semanticscholar.org/paper/9bfae1c52983dcab12c230b6200610c01eb44ca2 (accessed on 27 May 2025).

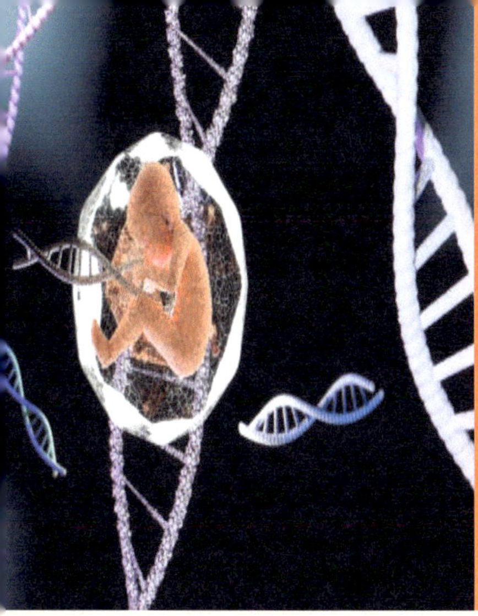

Chapter 9
EPIGENETICS IN EMBRYONIC DEVELOPMENT

Contents

Introduction

The study of epigenetics in embryonic development is a paradigm change in the understanding of the intricate processes that govern organismal construction. Epigenetics has been defined as heritable gene expression changes caused by phenomena other than modifications to the DNA sequence. This process is important in embryonic development, where it regulates cellular differentiation and tissue establishment. The interaction of environmental and genetic factors in the modulation of epigenetic alterations is a sign of the intricacy of developmental biology. Various studies have validated the means by which such alterations can present in phenotypic consequences, hence initiating the hypothesis that epigenetic mechanisms can account for developmental defects and diseases. As researchers probe these mechanisms, it is more evident that epigenetic regulation is at the heart of embryonic health and development, facilitating the interface between genetic susceptibility and environment. At the heart of comprehending epigenetic regulation in embryonic growth is maternal nutrition, which exerts a profound impact on the forming embryo. Maternal components such as nutritional components are paramount to establishing epigenetic landscapes during periods of opportunity in growth. For instance, methionine, an essential sulfur amino acid, is involved in many metabolic pathways critical to methylation reactions that affect gene expression. Methionine deficiency or excess anomalies would hinder such pathways and produce unwanted effects during pregnancy as well as impact embryonic development (Yan et al., 2025). Besides, maternal nutrition can modulate the availability of key metabolites that potentiate effective epigenetic modifications. These results underscore the importance of optimizing maternal nutrition for embryonic development and preventing potential developmental malformations. In addition to maternal nutrition, epigenetic intervention timing and nature during embryogenesis can lead to significant differences in development and health. Studies on in ovo nutrition of key nutrients, such as vitamin C, illustrate the possibility for nutritional enhancement during incubation in order to optimize the growth results and metabolic signatures of embryos in development. For example, vitamin C supplementation has been shown to improve hatching success and metabolic health in avian embryos, suggesting that specific nutrients have the capability to modulate epigenetic programs enhancing successful development (Du et al., 2025). This is evidence that strategic nutritional intervention at embryonic stages has beneficial impacts but can have long-term consequences for the offspring's health. Thus, understanding the epigenetic effects of maternal nutrition and the timing of them is an appealing area for the treatment of developmental problems and improving the viability of offspring (Figure 9.1).

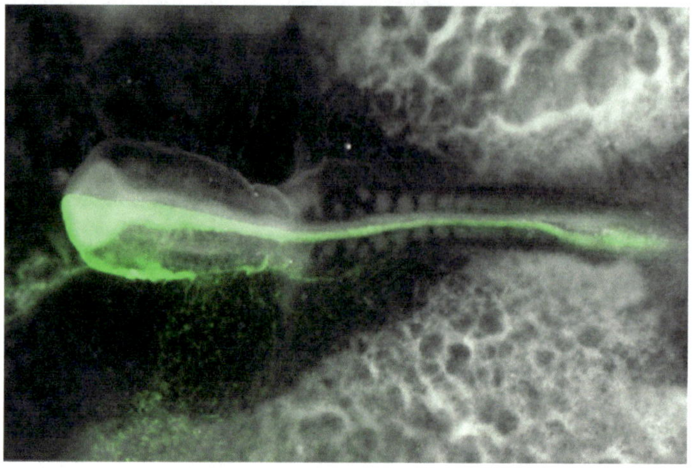

Figure 9.1. Epigenetics and embryonic development.

Source: https://www.conicet.gov.ar/wp-content/uploads/divulgacion/2014/04/Embrion.jpg.

Definition of Epigenetics

Epigenetics is about the ways genes are controlled without changing the DNA sequence. It studies how environmental conditions, signals from cells and developmental signals can change the epigenome which involves chemical changes to DNA and histone proteins. Such modifications, for example DNA methylation and histone acetylation, can either turn on or turn off genes which affects how cells behave and what they become during development. Epigenetic regulation is vital during embryonic development because it decides how stem cells become different types of tissue. The way cells navigate the epigenetic landscape is important for their identity, so understanding epigenetics is essential for understanding developmental biology. The regulation of embryonic development is mainly done by epigenetic mechanisms. In the beginning of development, different signaling pathways and outside factors can cause epigenetic changes that direct the expression of genes related to specific lineages. This process is particularly evident in studies involving somatic cell nuclear transfer (SCNT), where researchers observed significant deviations in DNA methylation profiles. These anomalies were linked to disorders such as XY disorder of sex development (DSD), indicating that improper epigenetic regulation can alter developmental outcomes (Jeong et al., 2016). They point out that epigenomics is important for normal growth and development and can explain some congenital anomalies that happen because of epigenetic problems. Additionally, the integration of gene regulatory networks (GRNs) within the context of epigenetics provides a quantifiable approach to understanding stem cell differentiation. New models have shown that gene regulation is random and that transcription factors play a key role in its dynamics. For example, the role of the master regulator Nanog in preserving pluripotency illustrates the impact of epigenetic modifications on gene expression stability (Zhang et al., 2014). Since epigenetic factors can affect stem cells, the study of stem cells is made more complex by the fact that their state can change with changes in the epigenetic environment. Consequently, a rigorous exploration of epigenetics in embryonic development not only illuminates the mechanisms governing differentiation but also offers insights into potential therapeutic interventions for developmental disorders (Figure 9.2).

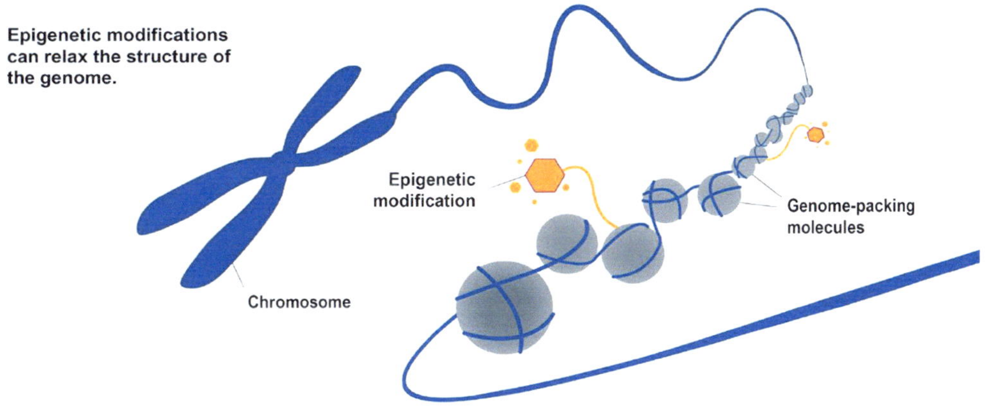

Figure 9.2. Epigenetics.

Source: https://www.genomicseducation.hee.nhs.uk/wp-content/uploads/2021/07/Carousel_1-01.png.

Importance of Embryonic Development

Embryonic development is important because it helps create the structure of complex organisms. At this important time, strict genetic and epigenetic rules control the process of cell differentiation, organ formation and growth. This phase is very important because any problems during embryonic development can result in many congenital anomalies and developmental disorders. New studies have pointed out that epigenetic changes such as those in DNA methylation and histones, are important for influencing gene expression. To find out what causes developmental issues, it is important to understand these modifications which helps with both prevention and treatment of congenital disorders. By studying these layers of regulation, developmental biologists are making it more likely that methods to address these complications will be developed. During embryonic development, epigenetic mechanisms help mediate how the environment affects gene expression and development. For example, the nutrition of the mother, the environment around the embryo and exposure to toxins can cause epigenetic changes in the embryo that last. As a result, public health is greatly influenced, since it highlights the importance of maternal health for the development and future health of children. Changes in epigenetic reprogramming caused by stress in the environment can upset the balance needed for healthy development which may result in problems that appear later in life. So, studying these interactions points out the strong connection between environmental factors and embryonic epigenetics, making it a key area for more research that could lead to better intervention strategies for reproductive and developmental health. The way epigenetic regulation works during embryonic development is essential for guiding cells to their proper roles and for the success of development. It has been found that DNA demethylation in early development is important for making the genome less methylated which is necessary for the blastocyst stage. Disruptions in this process, as observed with *in vitro* fertilization (IVF), can lead to aberrant developmental outcomes, emphasizing the importance of epigenetic integrity during early embryogenesis. Specifically, the activity of ten-eleven translocation (TET) enzymes is fundamental to active DNA demethylation, with emerging evidence suggesting that small molecules, such as vitamin C, can ameliorate deficiencies in this pathway. By highlighting the significance of proper epigenetic reprogramming, current research outlines a viable strategy for enhancing IVF success rates while reinforcing the critical importance of healthy embryonic development to prevent long-term epigenetic errors (Chu et al., 2021; Wang et al., 2024).

Overview of the Relationship Between Epigenetics and Development

How organisms change from a single-cell zygote to a multicellular body depends on the interaction between epigenetics and development. During embryonic development, DNA methylation and histone modifications are important for controlling gene expression. They do not change the DNA sequence but help create a flexible environment that affects cell identity and function. For example, turning on or off certain genes with epigenetic marks is what creates the different cell types needed for building tissues and organs. As such, the study of epigenetics provides insights into how developmental processes are finely tuned, ensuring that the right genes are expressed at the correct time, a phenomenon that has been observed across numerous model organisms, including yeast and zebrafish, which continue to reveal the complexity of these processes (Baruah et al., 2020). While the embryo is developing, different environmental influences can change the epigenetic pattern which may affect both cell differentiation and health in the future. Studies have shown that what we eat and the toxins we are exposed to can change DNA methylation which then influences how our genes function. Such changes might be a result of epigenetic plasticity which allows individuals to adapt to different environments but could also make them more likely to develop complex diseases in the future. Moreover, studies suggest that the compound ten-eleven translocation 1 (TET1) plays a significant role in mediating such epigenetic modifications, suggesting a specific pathway through which environmental exposures can exert their effects (Brown et al., 2020). It is important to understand these relationships, as they explain how epigenetics links the environment and the development of an organism. In addition, the effects of epigenetic marks can be passed down through generations, affecting the development of future generations. It raises interesting questions about how genes are affected by both heredity and the environment which can last for generations. As scientists study these mechanisms further, it is clear that epigenetic changes can react to the environment and also be passed on to future generations, affecting their development. Epigenetics is complex which suggests it may play a part in how organisms adapt to their environment. This area of research continues to unveil new dimensions of developmental biology and has significant implications for understanding evolution, disease susceptibility, and the potential for therapeutic interventions (Baruah et al., 2020) (Figure 9.3).

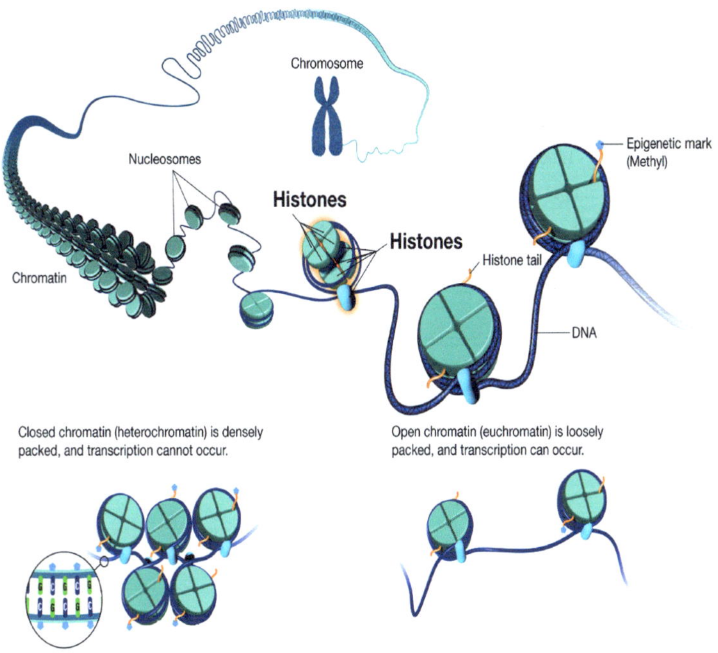

Figure 9.3. Relationship between epigenetics and development.

Source: https://external-content.duckduckgo.com/iu/?u=https%3A%2F%2Fwww.genomicseducation.hee.nhs.uk%2Fgenotes%2Fwp-content%2Fuploads%2F2023%2F04%2FEpigenetics_Figure-1.jpg&f=1&nofb=1&ipt=eef8d8f734e989f5ab34a47bd4a50372d9af0dbe95d4bf2f41c9fb17d339dfcb.

9.1. Mechanisms of Epigenetic Regulation

Epigenetic regulation includes several ways that affect gene expression without changing the DNA sequence. DNA methylation is one of the mechanisms that has been studied the most. The process adds methyl groups to cytosine in DNA, usually at CpG dinucleotides. DNA methylation is crucial during embryonic development for setting up cell identity and regulating when genes are turned on or off. When methylation patterns are not normal, it can cause developmental disorders, so understanding how DNA methylation works is necessary to learn about successful embryonic development. Because DNA methylation and histone modifications interact, it is more difficult to understand these regulatory networks which is why we need to study them in detail during important stages of development. Another important aspect of epigenetics, histone modifications, greatly affect how chromatin is structured and functions which in turn affects which genes are accessible and active. Acetylation, methylation, phosphorylation and ubiquitination of histones cause different changes in gene transcription. Histone acetylation during embryonic development usually leads to gene activation, but histone methylation can either activate or repress transcription depending on the situation. The levels of histone marks are controlled and can respond to the signals the embryo experiences during development. Being responsive is necessary for creating the right epigenetic environment needed for proper cell differentiation and growth. New studies have pointed out that histone modifications are important for cells to respond to stresses from the environment, making it harder to understand how epigenetic regulation supports strong development. More and more, scientists are seeing that nutritional and environmental factors play a key role in epigenetic regulation during embryogenesis. For instance, methionine, an essential amino acid, is integral to methyl metabolism and has been linked to various epigenetic modifications through its role in providing methyl groups for DNA and histone methylation processes (Yan et al., 2025). In addition, the environment inside the embryo, especially the mother's nutrition, is very important for controlling gene expression through epigenetic processes. It points out that embryonic development depends on both genetic information and the influence of external and internal factors. As such, interventions targeting nutritional and pharmaceutical strategies may hold promise for mitigating developmental defects, suggesting that understanding epigenetic regulation opens new avenues for enhancing embryonic health and outcomes in various species, including humans (Kisliouk et al., 2024) (Figure 9.4).

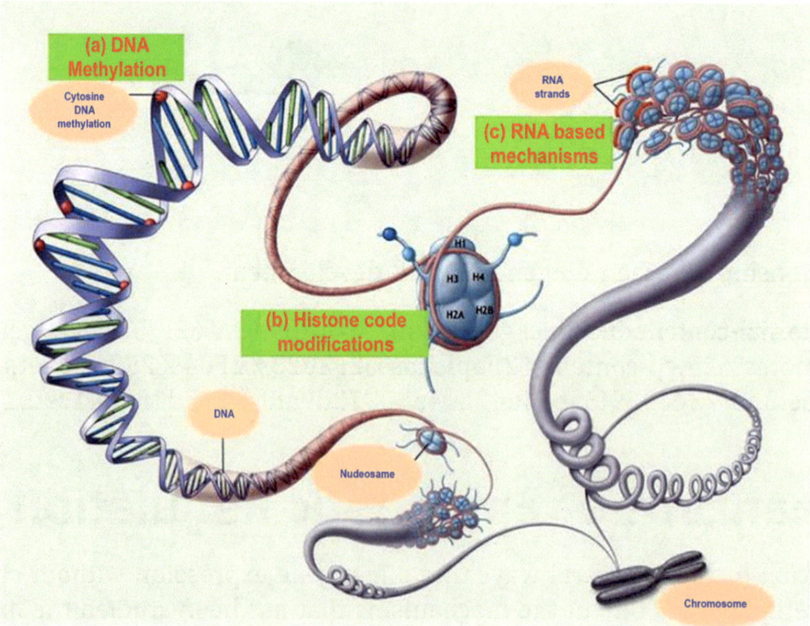

Figure 9.4. Mechanisms of epigenetic regulation.

Source: https://ars.els-cdn.com/content/image/1-s2.0-S1052305721000938-gr1.jpg.

9.1.1. DNA Methylation

DNA methylation is a key way epigenetic changes help guide the development of the embryo. The process adds methyl groups to the cytosine in DNA, mainly at CpG dinucleotides. It is primarily mediated by a family of enzymes known as DNA methyltransferases (DNMTs), which catalyze the covalent modification. It is necessary for controlling gene activity, turning off transposable elements and keeping the structure of chromatin during development. If DNA methylation is not at the right level, it may disrupt these processes and cause developmental problems or diseases in the future. The early phases of embryogenesis are particularly sensitive to methylation patterns, underscoring the necessity of tightly regulated methylation processes during critical stages of development, where proper gene expression is essential for outcomes such as cell differentiation and tissue patterning (Yan et al., 2025). More research on DNA methylation and diet shows that metabolic factors play a major role in shaping the epigenetics of embryos. Methionine which is an essential amino acid, is needed to donate methyl groups in many metabolic processes, including DNA methylation. What a woman eats during the periconceptional period can affect the supply of substances needed for methylation. It has been found that not having enough or too much methionine can lead to problems with methylation, regulating genes and the health of the embryo. It is important to understand how methionine metabolism works with folate metabolism and other pathways to get a better picture of epigenetics during embryonic development.

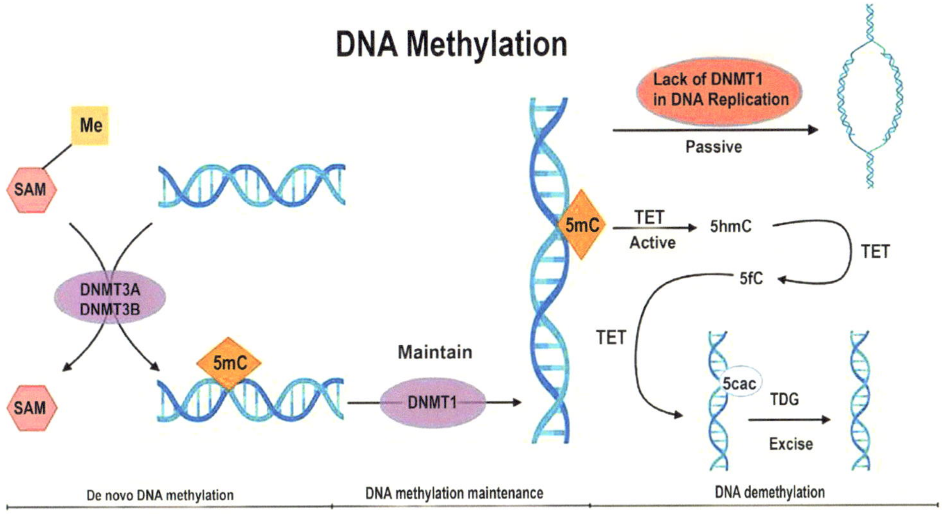

Figure 9.5. Mechanism of DNA methylation.

Source: https://www.researchgate.net/publication/381488030/figure/fig2/AS:11431281252394868@1718688052049/Mechanism-of-DNA-methylation-DNA-methylation-under-the-catalytic-action-of-DNA.tif.

Methylation modifications influenced by nutritional status may play direct roles in maintaining genomic stability and regulating gene expression throughout the developmental trajectory, highlighting an intricate connection between diet and epigenetic regulation (Yan et al., 2025). Problems with DNA methylation during embryonic development can also influence health later in life. When methylation is not normal, it can cause oncogenes to be turned on and tumor suppressor genes to be turned off which raises the risk of diseases such as cancer. It is clear from the link between early methylation and cancer that epigenetic changes in early life can have lasting effects. Furthermore, the involvement of non-coding RNAs, such as microRNAs (miRNA), in modulating DNA methylation and gene expression introduces an additional layer of complexity to these regulatory processes. As research in epigenetics continues to unravel the tightly woven relationships between environmental factors, dietary influences, and genetic regulation, it becomes evident that understanding DNA methylation is central to addressing both immediate embryonic development and long-term health outcomes (Shukla et al., 2023) (Figure 9.5).

9.1.2. Histone Modification

Histone modification is a key way epigenetics controls gene expression during the development of an embryo. Chemical groups are added or removed from histone proteins which together make up the framework of chromatin.

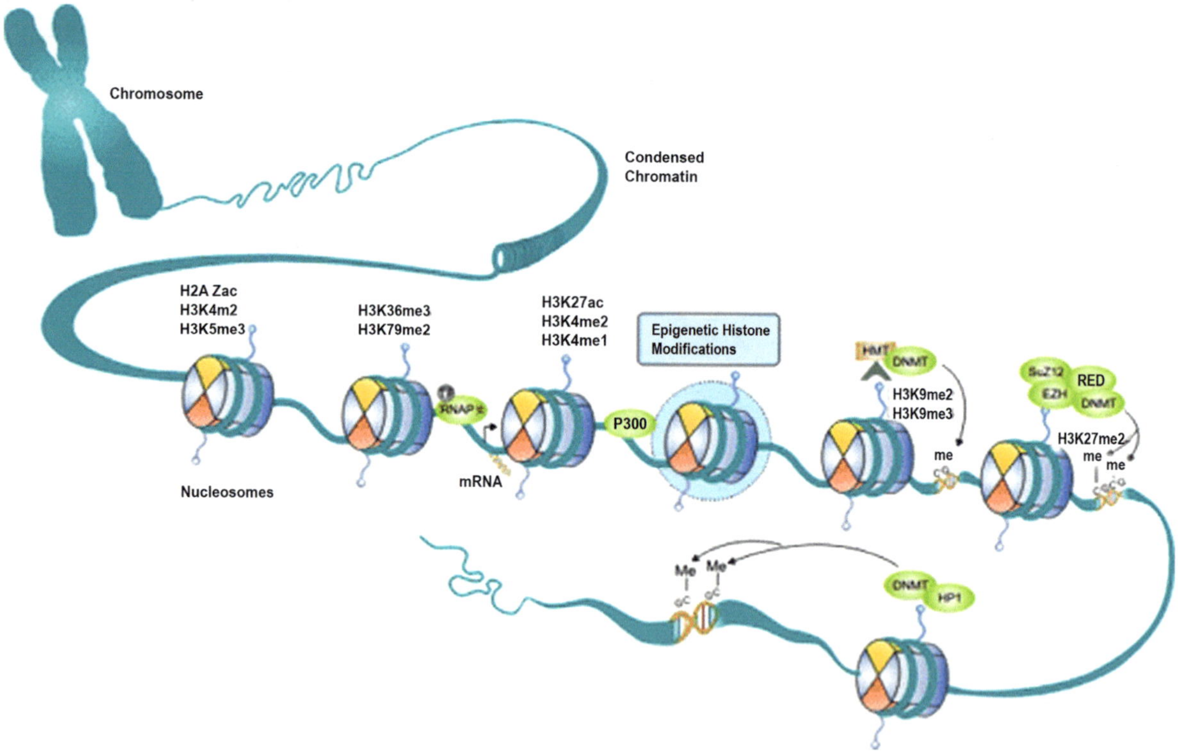

Figure 9.6. Epigenetic histone modifications.

Source: https://www.cusabio.com/manage/upload/201901/histone_pathway_img1.png.

Methylation, acetylation, phosphorylation and ubiquitination can change the structure of chromatin which allows or prevents transcriptional machinery from reaching DNA. For embryonic development to work properly, it is important to control these modifications to direct the expression of genes that determine how cells differentiate and what lineage they belong to. Experiments have shown that making such changes is necessary, since disturbances can result in abnormal development and a lower chance of the embryo surviving, proving the importance of epigenetic regulation through histone modification in normal development. Besides affecting chromatin structure, histone modification also plays a role in interacting with important signaling pathways involved in embryogenesis. For example, some changes have been found to influence the genes responsible for how cells react to their environment and to nutrients. Methionine, a necessary amino acid, has become a key factor in epigenetics. Methionine's role in methyl metabolism influences histone methylation patterns, which, when disrupted, can result in detrimental effects on embryonic development as indicated in recent studies (Yan et al., 2025). Moreover, the way histone modifications affect important metabolic pathways highlights a complex network that links nutrition with gene expression, proving that epigenetic changes depend on both genes and the environment. Furthermore, the way histone methyltransferases and demethylases change histone modifications is essential for the correct regulation of gene expression in embryos. They help maintain the right balance of histone methylation, controlling how accessible chromatin is and how much transcription happens. Research has shown that aberrations in these enzymatic processes can lead to significant implications in various diseases, including cancer, where epigenetic reprogramming plays a pivotal role (Dong et al., 2023). Thus, it is important to study the ways these demethylases function and what roles they play in embryonic development and disease. The complexity of histone modifications reflects a rich tapestry of regulation that highlights their importance in controlling developmental outcomes and ensuring proper organismal growth and function (Figure 9.6).

9.1.3. Non-Coding RNA Involvement

The role of non-coding RNAs (ncRNAs) in embryonic development represents a significant area of investigation within the broader field of epigenetics. Unlike the usual coding RNAs, ncRNAs do not make proteins but are important for controlling gene activity. Specifically, miRNAs have emerged as crucial regulators by targeting messenger RNAs (mRNAs) for degradation or translational repression, thereby influencing gene expression without altering the underlying DNA sequence. During embryogenesis, it is especially important for genes to be expressed at the right time and place and this is made possible by regulatory capacity. Furthermore, the intricate interplay between miRNAs and other epigenetic modifications illustrates a complex regulatory network that underscores the importance of non-coding RNAs in maintaining developmental fidelity (Shukla et al., 2023). Studies have pointed out that DNA methylation and ncRNAs can affect each other's regulatory processes. When DNA methylation is not normal, it can change the activity of ncRNAs which may then affect the methylation of other genes. This interaction is very important during different stages of embryonic development, influencing cell fate and the formation of organs. Some recent studies indicate that ncRNAs might help set up genome-wide epigenetic patterns as embryos change from being pluripotent to differentiated. This dynamic interaction between ncRNAs and DNA methylation highlights the necessity of understanding these multifaceted relationships to grasp the complexities of embryonic development fully (Gan et al., 2022). Moreover, the diversity of ncRNAs extends beyond miRNAs to include long non-coding RNAs (lncRNAs) and circular RNAs, which have shown promising roles in embryonic regulation. For example, lncRNAs may help organize transcriptional complexes or act as decoys for transcription factors which affects how genes are expressed. The fact that they help organize chromatin highlights their role in setting up and sustaining GRNs during development. As researchers continue to unravel the diverse functions of ncRNAs, it becomes increasingly clear that these molecules are integral to the epigenetic landscape that orchestrates embryonic development, necessitating a more nuanced understanding of their contributions to both normal and aberrant developmental processes (Shukla et al., 2023) (Figure 9.7).

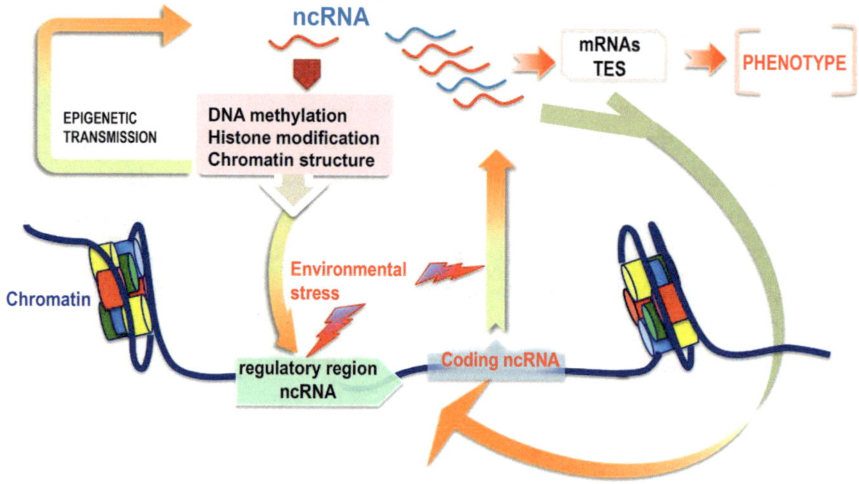

Figure 9.7. Epigenetic non-coding RNA involvement.

Source: https://www.mdpi.com/ijms/ijms-17-00452/article_deploy/html/images/ijms-17-00452-g001.png.

9.2. Role of Epigenetics in Cell Differentiation

Epigenetics helps control how genes are expressed which is key to the process of cell differentiation in the embryo. Specific epigenetic modifications, such as DNA methylation and histone acetylation, influence which genes are activated or silenced, thereby dictating the fate of embryonic stem cells (ESCs). As soon as these undifferentiated cells react to different signals, epigenetic changes direct them to specific lineages, so that each cell type gets the right functions in tissues and organs. Because of these modifications, the regulatory system is flexible and supports the growth of the embryo. It is important to understand these epigenetic mechanisms, since any problems with their regulation can result in developmental disorders or birth defects, highlighting the need for accurate epigenetic processes at this time. It has been found by recent studies that epigenetic factors are important for the regeneration of some cell types after embryonic development. For example, research on auditory hair cells indicates that epigenetic changes help these cells develop and regenerate which is important for hearing. In humans, the inability to regenerate auditory hair cells after damage presents a significant challenge, prompting investigations into the potential for targeting epigenetic modifications to stimulate regeneration (Khalaily et al., 2024). It demonstrates that studying how epigenetics works in differentiated cells can lead to new ways to repair damaged tissues, showing that epigenetics plays an important role in regenerative medicine. Moreover, the role of signaling pathways, particularly those involving the aryl hydrocarbon receptor (AHR), showcases the intricate relationship between epigenetics and cell differentiation. AHR's interaction with certain regulatory sequences changes both how genes are expressed and the structure of chromatin which affects different body functions and growth. Research indicates that these epigenetic modifications orchestrated by AHR can profoundly impact cellular responses to environmental stimuli, including differentiation and regeneration (Claudia et al., 2022). While scientists study these interactions, new ways to treat diseases are discovered, mainly by boosting the ability of tissues to heal. Ultimately, unraveling the epigenetic landscape in cell differentiation not only deepens our understanding of development but also paves the way for innovative treatments for degenerative diseases and injuries (Figure 9.8).

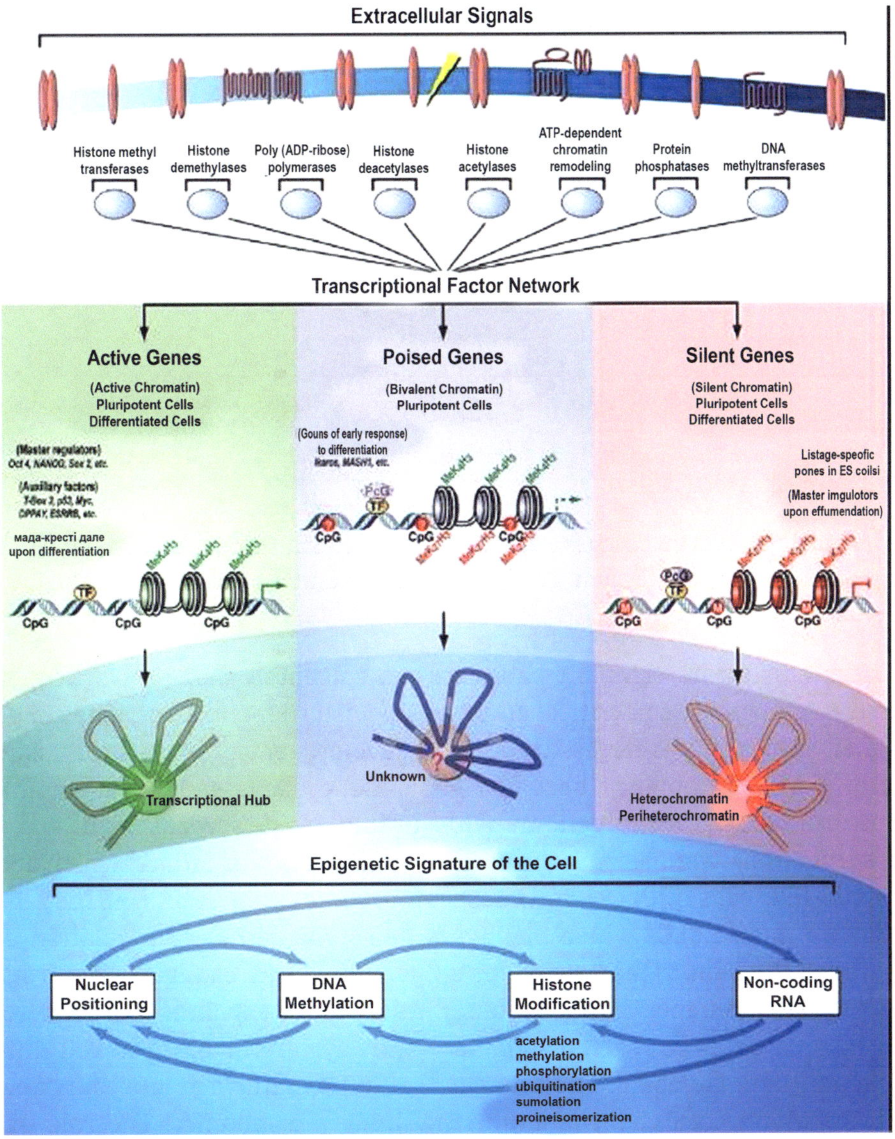

Figure 9.8. Stem cell epigenetics.

Source: https://www.creative-diagnostics.com/upload/image/Stem-Cell-Epigenetics-1.jpg.

9.2.1. Stem Cell Pluripotency

The ability of stem cells to be pluripotent is important for understanding embryonic development, since it allows them to become any type of cell in the organism. Initially, the cells in the embryo are totipotent which means they can become any type of cell, including those needed for extra-embryonic tissues. With development, there is a change in regulation, resulting in pluripotency which allows cells to differentiate but not to become every cell type.

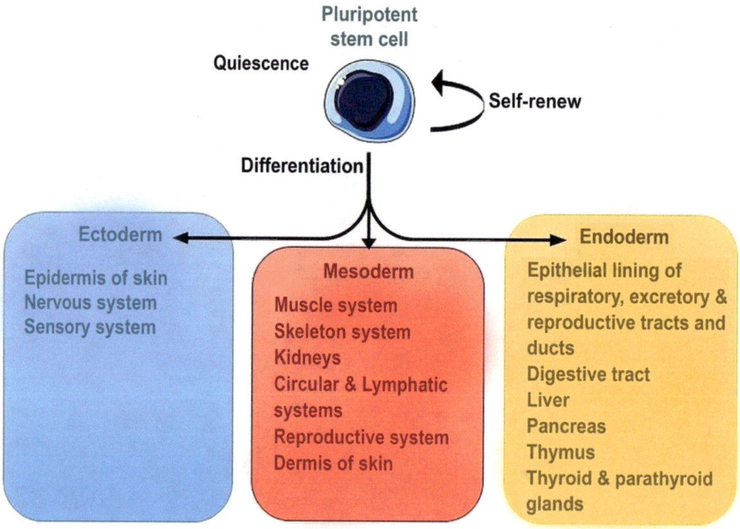

Figure 9.9. Pluripotent stem cells.

Source: https://static.wixstatic.com/media/dfb214_e5e53579ff514fe4b2aeec4933bc4933~mv2.jpg/v1/fill/w_980,h_586,al_c,q_85,usm_0.66_1.00_0.01,enc_avif,quality_auto/dfb214_e5e53579ff514fe4b2aeec4933bc4933~mv2.jpg.

Many transcription factors, signaling pathways and epigenetic changes work together to manage this transition. It is shown through critical analyses that cells depend on changes in gene expression to determine their fate which is necessary for the development of important tissues in the body. Investigations into how totipotency becomes pluripotency have shown important details about epigenetic control. Research using genome-wide CRISPR/Cas9 screens identifies key regulators influencing this transition, emphasizing the role of proteins such as Mdm2, which acts as a negative regulator of 2-cell-like cells (2CLCs) in mouse embryonic stem cells (mESCs). When Mdm2 is disturbed, there are more 2CLCs which highlights its role in cell cycle regulation and H3K27me3 changes. They reveal that the right balance of epigenetic marks changes the chromatin structure which supports the maintenance of pluripotency. As a result, explaining these mechanisms helps us understand how carefully controlled signaling pathways are involved in cell differentiation for development. In addition, the epigenetic changes that happen during embryonic development play a major role in regulating cell changes and maintaining pluripotency. The role of the transgene activation suppressor (TASOR) within the human silencing hub (HUSH) complex exemplifies this idea. When TASOR is reduced during the change from naive to primed pluripotency, it is obvious that it is needed to maintain cell health at this point. When TASOR is missing, replication stress increases and H3K9me3 heterochromatin is not formed which disturbs the process of silencing transposable elements. Such disruption may lead to an immune response which causes naive cells to die as they become primed. Such insights underline the importance of maintaining a tightly regulated epigenetic landscape to support pluripotency, emphasizing how epigenetics dictate the trajectory of cell fate decisions throughout development (Figure 9.9).

9.2.2. Epigenetic Changes During Differentiation

During the development of an embryo, esoteric epigenetic changes are important for turning stem cells into specialized types of cells. These changes are mainly about changing DNA methylation and histone modifications which control gene expression without changing the genetic code. As the embryo develops, the epigenome is actively changed which helps certain genes become active or inactive depending on the embryo's growth.

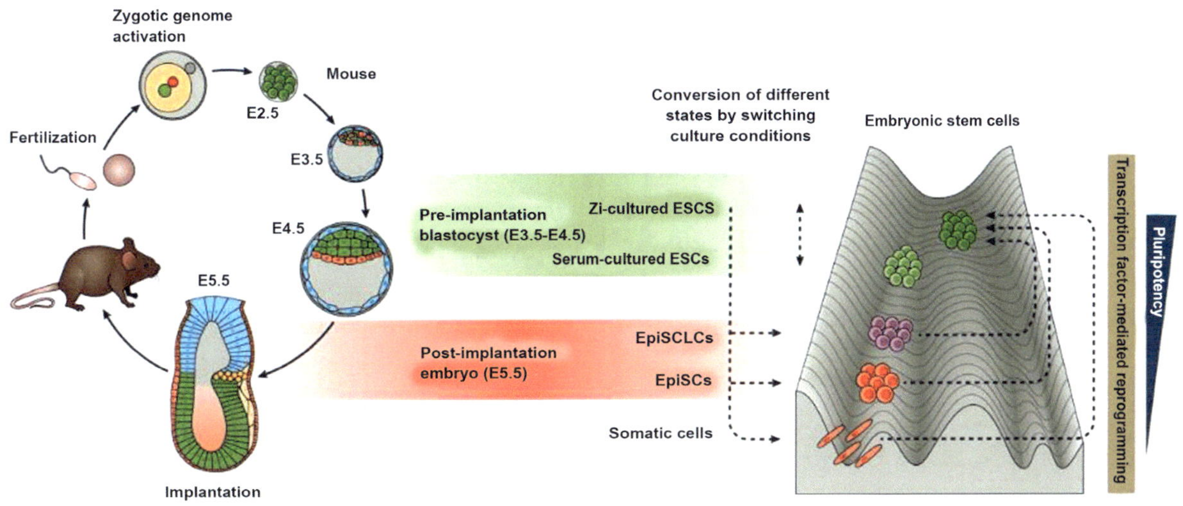

Figure 9.10. Epigenetic changes during differentiation.

Source: https://media.springernature.com/lw1200/springer-static/image/art%3A10.1038%2Fnrg.2017.57/MediaObjects/41576_2017_Article_BFnrg201757_Figa_HTML.jpg.

Thanks to epigenetic regulation, cells can take on the identity needed to do their specialized tasks well. Notably, studies have revealed that genes involved in critical processes such as cellular proliferation and differentiation are influenced by these regulatory pathways during the early stages of embryonic development, underscoring the complexity of epigenetic control mechanisms that facilitate differentiation (Zhang et al., 2023). Examining epigenetic changes during differentiation, it has been found that several environmental factors play a major role in influencing them. For example, being exposed to opioids or similar substances can cause major changes in the methylation of ESCs. Research indicates that morphine exposure results in hypomethylation of the genomic landscape, ultimately delaying differentiation and preserving pluripotency in mESCs (Araolaza et al., 2023). This points out that the developing embryo's epigenome can be easily affected by the environment which raises worries about the possible long-term effects of environmental exposures on development. It is important to understand how environmental factors affect epigenetics to spot risks from prenatal exposure and to support the best health of the fetus. Changes in epigenetics during differentiation can influence the whole development of an organism and its health. If these epigenetic processes are not properly regulated, it can cause cells to differentiate incorrectly which may result in developmental problems or higher risk of diseases in the future. For example, the identification of key hub genes linked to early embryonic arrest sheds light on crucial epigenetic regulatory networks that may govern embryogenesis (Zhang et al., 2023). As scientists learn more about how genes and epigenetic changes work together during differentiation, this knowledge will help develop treatments for preventing or treating developmental problems. Consequently, further investigation into the interplay between epigenetics and cellular differentiation is integral to advancing the field of developmental biology and enhancing our grasp of human health (Figure 9.10).

9.2.3. Impact on Tissue-Specific Gene Expression

During embryonic development, the expression of genes in different tissues is carefully controlled by epigenetic changes that guide the differentiation needed for forming different types of cells. At important times in embryogenesis such as when cells move from being pluripotent to having specific tissue roles, the pattern of gene expression changes a lot. For example, the way transcription factors are activated is often controlled by changes in histones and DNA methylation at promoter regions which can either allow or prevent the expression of important genes for tissue function and structure. This is especially clear in studies focusing on the Nrf2 pathway, where turning on Nrf2 in zebrafish embryos led to changes in gene expression that are important for different tissues. The regulation of Nrf2 demonstrates the importance of considering not only the activation of gene networks but also how those networks function uniquely across various tissues during development (Marques et al., 2024). The difficulty of tissue-specific gene expression is further shown by looking at how germline genes are turned off in somatic cells at the beginning of embryonic development.

The presence of a soma-germline boundary which separates genes needed for germ cells from those needed for somatic cells, highlights the need for accuracy in keeping cells different from each other. In particular, KDM5C which is a histone demethylase, explains how epigenetic factors can influence gene expression in both males and females at different stages of development. In Kdm5c knockout mice, many tissues in the body turned on germline genes that are usually kept silent, showing that the mechanisms that keep cells healthy are not working properly. The findings suggest that a combination of transcriptional repression and epigenetic regulation, including DNA methylation, dictates the landscape of tissue-specific gene expression throughout embryogenesis (Katherine et al., 2024). Studying gene expression in different tissues reveals the role of epigenetics and may point to the causes of developmental disorders and cancer. When developmental pathways are turned on in the wrong cells, genes involved in choosing a cell's identity may be expressed incorrectly. Such pathways, when dysregulated, may result in tumorigenesis or various neurodevelopmental disorders (NDD) by fostering an environment conducive to inappropriate cellular plasticity and differentiation. So, it is important to understand how epigenetic regulation affects tissue-specific gene expression to better understand the many issues found in developmental biology and diseases caused by epigenetic errors. Core to this understanding is the need to explore the precise timing and context of gene regulation, as these factors lay the foundational groundwork for both normal embryonic development and its associated anomalies (Katherine et al., 2024).

9.3. Environmental Influences on Epigenetic Changes

During embryonic development, the way environmental factors and epigenetic changes interact is very important, as it can determine results that last for many generations. Nutrition, stress and toxins can lead to epigenetic changes which can alter how genes are expressed without changing the DNA itself. This happens through several methods such as DNA methylation and histone modification and these are affected by the environment.

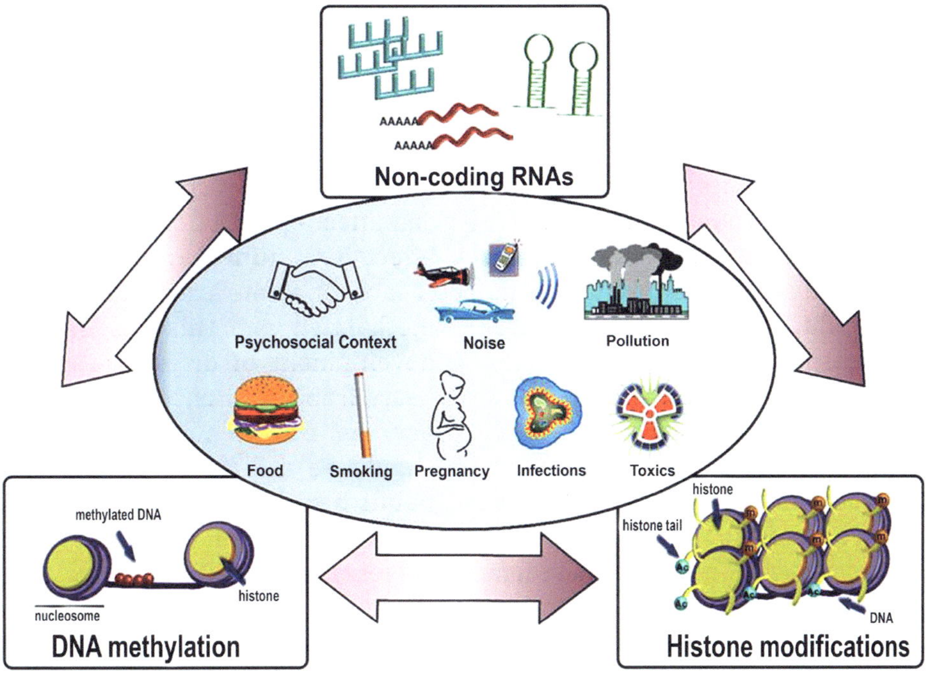

Figure 9.11. Environmental factors and epigenetic modifications.

Source: https://www.researchgate.net/publication/336854335/figure/fig1/AS:819031984582658@1572283850692/Environmental-factors-and-epigenetic-modifications-Several-environmental-stimuli-are.jpg.

For instance, what a mother eats during pregnancy can change the epigenetic pattern of the embryo which can affect the embryo's metabolism. As the embryo grows, these epigenetic marks may shape both present traits and future health in later generations, showing that environmental factors can have a lasting effect on how epigenetic inheritance works in embryos. It is especially interesting that epigenetic information can be passed down through generations which makes us question how heredity works. New studies suggest that changes in small non-protein-coding regulatory RNAs can be affected by the environment the father experiences. Such changes may then affect how the embryo develops and the health of the offspring when the sperm with these marks fertilizes an egg. Epididymosomes also play a part in changing the sperm sRNA profile during storage which highlights how complex epigenetic inheritance can be. Epididymosomes which contain RNAs and proteins, may help transfer changes caused by the environment during spermatogenesis. Consequently, understanding these mechanisms provides insight into how external factors may shape not only individual development but also the health of lineage over time, contributing to intergenerational epigenetic landscapes that can affect future generations (Natalie et al., 2019). In short, studying how our environment affects epigenetic changes reveals the close link between our environment and how we develop. They demonstrate how outside factors can strongly affect the expression of genes that are important for development. Epigenetic changes have been found to cause immediate changes in traits and also to influence the health of future generations. The results suggest that lifestyle, changes in society and climate are all important for public health. This knowledge about how the environment can cause epigenetic changes suggests new research and policy paths to support healthier outcomes by acting early in development. Factors, such as maternal nutrition and paternal stress, therefore remain integral to the comprehension of epigenetics in embryonic development and beyond (Jennifer et al., 2019) (Figure 9.11).

9.3.1. Nutritional Factors

The food and nutrients available to the embryo are very important for both the short-term health of the fetus and the long-term health of the child. The presence of important vitamins, minerals and macronutrients in the diet can affect epigenetic changes, mainly by altering DNA methylation and histones. Such changes are necessary for controlling gene expression at important times in development. For example, not getting enough important nutrients can cause problems with genomic imprinting and cell differentiation which may result in various developmental problems and chronic diseases in the future. Studies suggest that maternal nutrition significantly impacts fetal programming, reinforcing the notion that a well-balanced diet is not merely a source of energy, but a determinant of genetic and epigenetic stability across generations (Lubanzi, 2024). Also, the relationship between nutrients and epigenetic regulation highlights the need for a complete approach to maternal health during pregnancy. Essential vitamins and trace elements are needed as cofactors in biochemical reactions and also help control the activity of DNMTs and TETs which are important enzymes in epigenetics. The fact that micronutrients regulate these enzymes means that nutrition can affect epigenetics and epigenetics can also affect how nutrients are absorbed and used. A lack of folate can change the way DNA is methylated and this has been linked to the development of diseases such as cancer and heart problems. Hence, the intricate relationship between nutrition and epigenetic mechanisms should be a focal point in prenatal care and public health strategies (Leesang et al., 2024). In the end, knowing how nutrition affects epigenetics during embryonic development can guide interventions that help both the mother and the fetus. By integrating knowledge from the Developmental Origins of Health and Disease (DOHaD) theory, healthcare providers can assess environmental and nutritional exposures to provide personalized dietary recommendations. For example, giving pregnant women advice on eating a wide range of nutritious foods can help reduce harmful changes in their epigenetics. In addition, pushing for public policies that ensure nutritious food and a safe environment for pregnant women will help them have healthier children. Given the potential long-lasting effects of nutritional factors on gene expression and cellular function, a proactive approach to maternal nutrition emerges as crucial for enhancing both present and future health trajectories of populations (Lubanzi, 2024) (Figure 9.12).

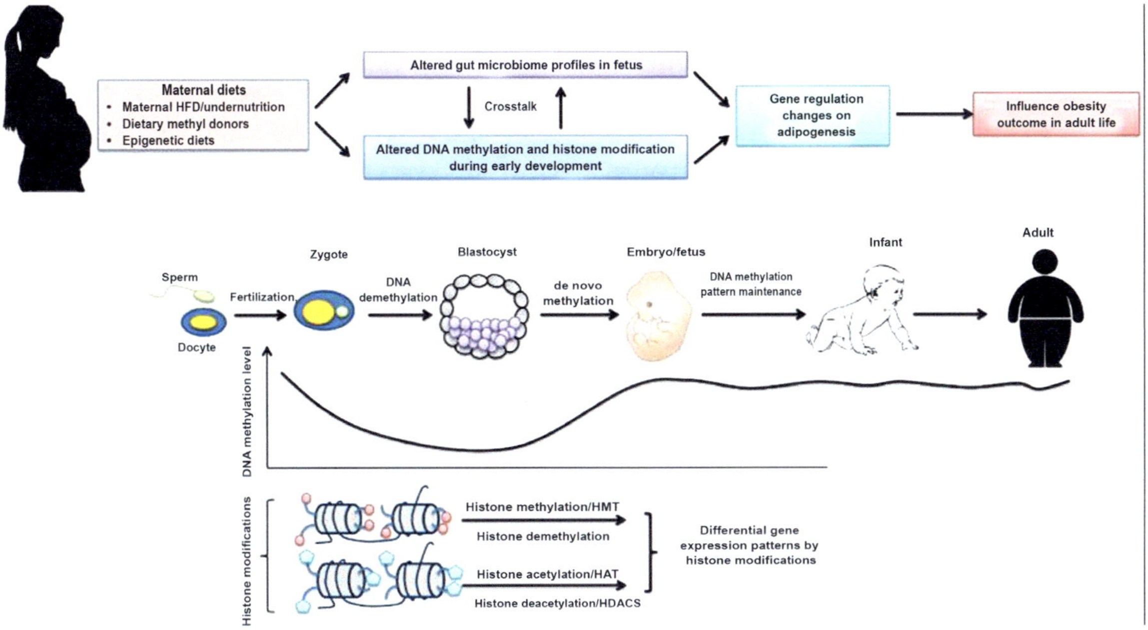

Figure 9.12. The interaction of maternal dietary factors with early-life epigenetic mechanism and the gut microbiome in regulation of obesity in adult life.

Source: https://www.frontiersin.org/files/Articles/390209/fgene-09-00342-HTML/image_m/fgene-09-00342-g001.jpg.

9.3.2. Chemical Exposures

Recently, there has been a lot of focus on chemical exposures during embryonic development because they can seriously affect health in the future. Environmental pollutants, heavy metals and endocrine disruptors are able to affect epigenetic processes like DNA methylation, changes in histones and the expression of non-coding RNAs. The exact ways these exposures work are often not clear, but they can disrupt important developmental processes in the organism. As Brown et al. (2020) highlights, understanding the modulation of epigenetic markers due to chemical exposures is paramount, especially considering the potential for these alterations to result in chronic diseases later in life. This points out that thorough research is needed to describe these relationships and guide future efforts to prevent them. It is now clear that even small amounts of chemicals can lead to major epigenetic changes in the embryo at important stages. Mild environmental influences, as mentioned in recent studies, can change epigenetic markers which may increase a person's risk of neurodegenerative disorders and cancers. Such exposures are very important for understanding the causes of these conditions, especially because they have a big impact on society. Certain substances such as pollutants and nutritional deficiencies, have been found to change how genes function in the embryo through epigenetics. Such insights affirm the importance of revisiting current regulations surrounding permissible exposure levels to protect both vulnerable populations and future generations, as evidenced by findings within (Fuso et al., 2015). Also, the relationship between chemicals and nutrition in influencing the epigenome during embryonic development is a promising area to study. Essential nutrients, especially B vitamins, are important for metabolic processes that control DNA methylation and epigenetic health. If environmental pollutants are present, the chance of harmful epigenetic changes rises. In particular, when nutritional deficiencies are combined with low-level exposure to harmful chemicals, it seems that several factors may contribute to the development of complex diseases later in life. As Fuso et al. (2015) indicates, even subtle imbalances in nutrient intake can have significant and enduring effects on the epigenetic landscape, necessitating a comprehensive approach to both dietary recommendations and environmental health policies. The way chemicals and nutrition affect epigenetics highlights how complicated epigenetics can be and why we should reconsider the safety limits for various environmental factors.

9.3.3. Maternal Stress and Its Effects

The effects of stress on a mother during pregnancy are a major focus of epigenetics research. Higher stress levels in pregnant women can cause important changes in their bodies which might harm the growth and development of the fetus. Stresses in the environment such as money problems or loneliness, can cause changes in gene expression through epigenetics.

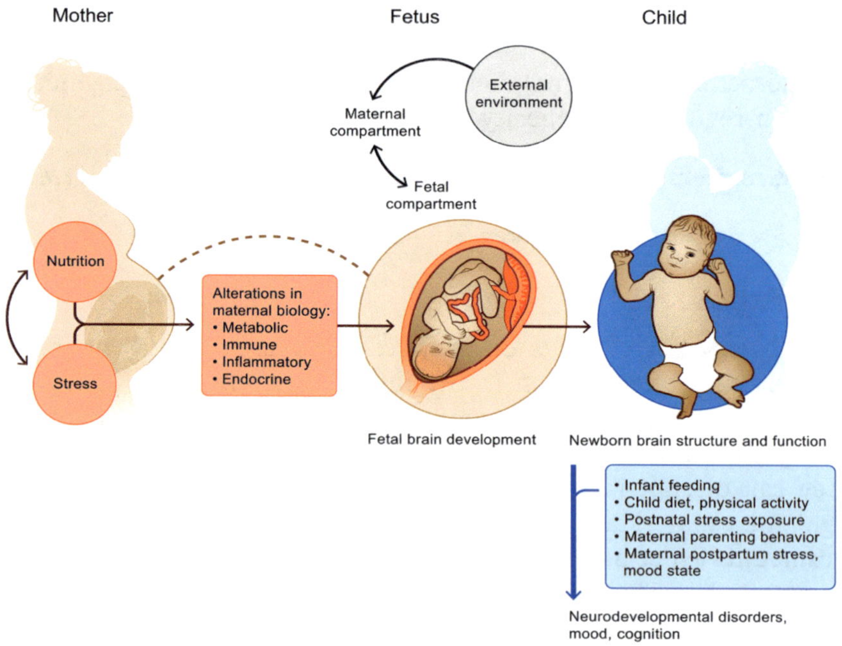

Figure 9.13. The impact of maternal stress on embryonic development.

Source: https://external-content.duckduckgo.com/iu/?u=https%3A%2F%2Fels-jbs-prod-cdn.jbs.elsevierhealth.com%2Fcms%2Fattachment%2F400ea37b-9fc5-4262-9ed8-420c7983337b%2Fgr1_lrg.jpg&f=1&nofb=1&ipt=5c03b1617e9a1912ba9b9d497371a2222c8dc14e2732a8fb9836626d8c582de7.

In particular, stress can lead to changes in DNA methylation which may then influence how the offspring develop, stay healthy and behave. It highlights the role of maternal experiences in guiding embryonic development through epigenetic processes which shows the link between a mother's health and the health of her baby. In addition, the link between a mother's lactation and epigenetic changes is important for learning about embryonic development. It has been found that when mothers are lactating, the nutrients and energy provided to the fetus are affected which adds another level of complexity to their relationship. Calves born to nonlactating heifers had different methylation patterns than those born to lactating cows, suggesting that the mother's physiological state can change fetal epigenetic marks. Such findings emphasize that maternal lactation not only influences nutrient delivery but also has profound ramifications on the epigenetic landscape of the embryo, revealing an important axis of maternal-fetal communication that warrants further investigation (López-Catalina et al., 2024). Maternal stress also has lasting effects on the health of the offspring, not just on the fetus. It has been found that environmental stresses such as poor nutrition and exposure to pollutants, are linked to adverse development in children and these changes in the fetus may increase the risk of health issues throughout life. They may change important biological activities such as how cells function and which genes are expressed and are affected by various environmental factors, including the stress experienced by the mother. The DOHaD theory posits that the prenatal environment, enriched by the biological underpinnings of maternal experiences, shapes an individual's health trajectory across the lifespan (Lubanzi, 2024). Thus, recognizing the multifaceted effects of maternal stress is crucial for promoting healthier pregnancy outcomes and informing public health strategies (Figure 9.13).

9.4. Epigenetic Reprogramming in Early Development

Epigenetic reprogramming in early embryonic development starts as soon as fertilization occurs. After sperm and egg fuse, the genomes from both parents are extensively changed which affects their epigenetic landscape. They are necessary to reset the epigenetic markers that control gene activity, making sure the embryonic genome works properly. Maternal oocyte-specific reprogramming factors are important because they help remove the inherited epigenetic marks. It supports the change from gamete to zygote and also prepares for the next steps in development such as embryonic genome activation. The way chromatin changes during development supports cell differentiation which affects the embryo's growth and the ability of its cells to become different types of cells. Epigenetic reprogramming becomes even more complex because the genomes of the father and mother are handled differently during early embryonic growth. DNA methylation and histone modifications which are epigenetic marks, can change quickly due to factors from the oocyte that interact with the parental genomes. TET3 which is part of the TET family, is responsible for demethylating the paternal genome by converting 5-methylcytosine to 5-hydroxymethylcytosine. The enzyme action decreases DNA methylation and prepares the paternal genome for more changes. Alternatively, the maternal genome is guarded from these oxidative changes mainly because of maternal factors like STELLA which prevent harmful epigenetic changes. It is important to understand these mechanisms, since unequal epigenetic reprogramming in parents' genomes can result in developmental problems or disorders. Besides its role in development, epigenetic reprogramming is also very important for clinical applications. If epigenetic reprogramming is not correct during early development, it can cause serious problems that appear as epigenetic disorders in the offspring. New research has pointed out that changes in epigenetic modulators can lead to clinical conditions, so it is important to study how these changes happen. Many embryos produced in vitro have epigenetic issues which makes people worry about their ability to survive and stay healthy. By understanding the mechanistic actions of epigenetic modulators and their influence on embryonic development, researchers can foster improvements in assisted reproductive technologies, potentially leading to strategies that rectify epigenetic errors, thereby enhancing individual well-being and reproductive outcomes in future generations (Figure 9.14).

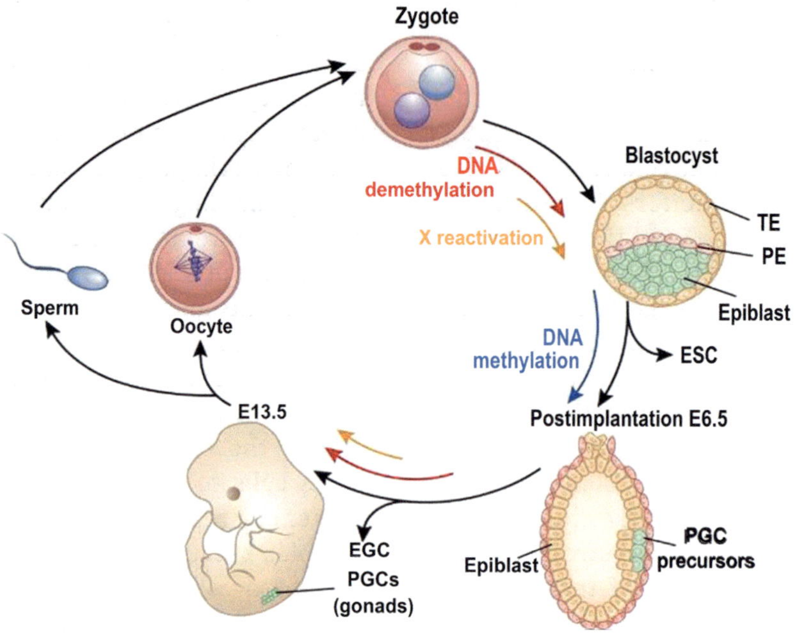

Figure 9.14. Epigenetic reprogramming in early development.

Source: https://media.springernature.com/full/springer-static/image/art%3A10.1038%2Fnsmb.2489/MediaObjects/41594_2013_Article_BFnsmb2489_Fig1_HTML.jpg.

9.4.1. Reprogramming During Fertilization

During fertilization, the zygote undergoes reprogramming which involves many epigenetic changes that alter the way genes are expressed. After the sperm and oocyte fuse, the environment changes and the epigenetic marks from both gametes start to change a lot. It is important for the zygotic genome to be activated and for the embryo to develop correctly. The maternal-to-zygotic transition (MZT) encapsulates this transformative phase, during which maternal factors are degraded and zygotic genome activation (ZGA) occurs, enabling the embryo to transition from dependence on maternal RNA and proteins to its intrinsic genetic programming. As a result, fertilization and the growth of the embryo depend on the precise control of these reprogrammed epigenetic events which are important for creating a viable pathway for development. It is clear from studies that certain histone modifications are important for reprogramming, as they are either kept or removed during the early stages of embryonic development. According to studies, in nonmammalian vertebrates,

H3K27ac and H3K9me3 are partially retained even though H3K4 methylation is almost completely removed after fertilization. These changes are not only left over from the parental epigenome; they are important for the early development of the embryo. For instance, H3K27ac is found to mark promoters important for gene expression during cleavage, suggesting it helps prepare the chromatin for later activations. Such findings highlight the many ways epigenetic reprogramming works and the different mechanisms that help guide development in the early stages of life, pointing out the connection between inherited epigenetic marks and new ones. In addition, when reprogramming is disrupted during fertilization, it can seriously affect embryonic development and may result in failures. If the processes of MZT are not accurate such as when epigenetic changes go wrong, it can lead to early death of the embryo or reduced chances of survival. Advances in low-input epigenome profiling have revealed that different epigenetic changes are important during MZT and have shown new details about how normal and abnormal development occurs. If histone modifications are not properly controlled, they may cause abnormal development and sometimes lead to miscarriage. These findings not only enhance our understanding of epigenetic reprogramming in the context of natural fertilization but also bear significant implications for the effectiveness of assisted reproductive technologies, where a keen awareness of epigenetic integrity is essential for optimizing outcomes and ensuring healthy embryonic development (Figure 9.15).

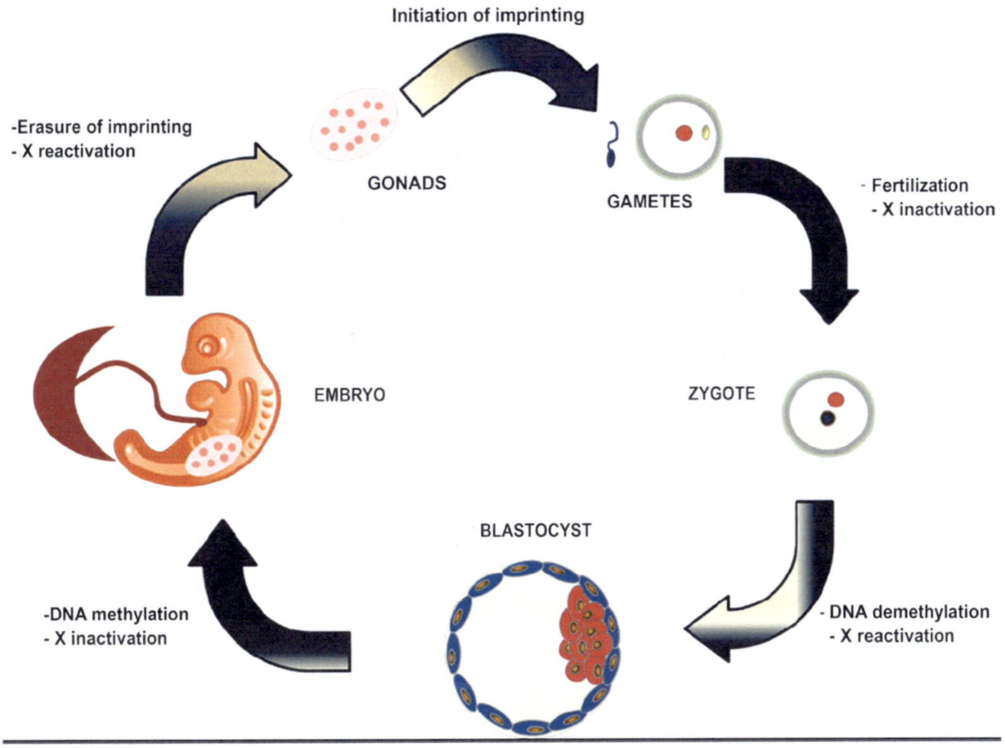

Figure 9.15. Epigenetic reprogramming during fertilization.

Source: https://www.researchgate.net/profile/Md-Mostofa-Kamal/publication/235901490/figure/fig5/AS:299657478590471@1448455318841/The-epigenetic-reprogramming-cycle-showing-the-two-major-waves-of-epigenetic.png.

9.4.2. Epigenetic Resetting in the Zygote

The resetting of epigenetic marks in the zygote is important for the cell to regain totipotency which means it can become any cell type in the organism. After fertilization, the germ cells which are sperm and oocytes, go through a major process of epigenetic reprogramming. Reprogramming happens when epigenetic marks are changed which allows cells to move from a differentiated state to one that can become an embryo. As these changes happen, they help create an epigenetic environment that supports the correct development and specialization of embryonic cells, proving the importance of epigenetics in early embryogenesis.

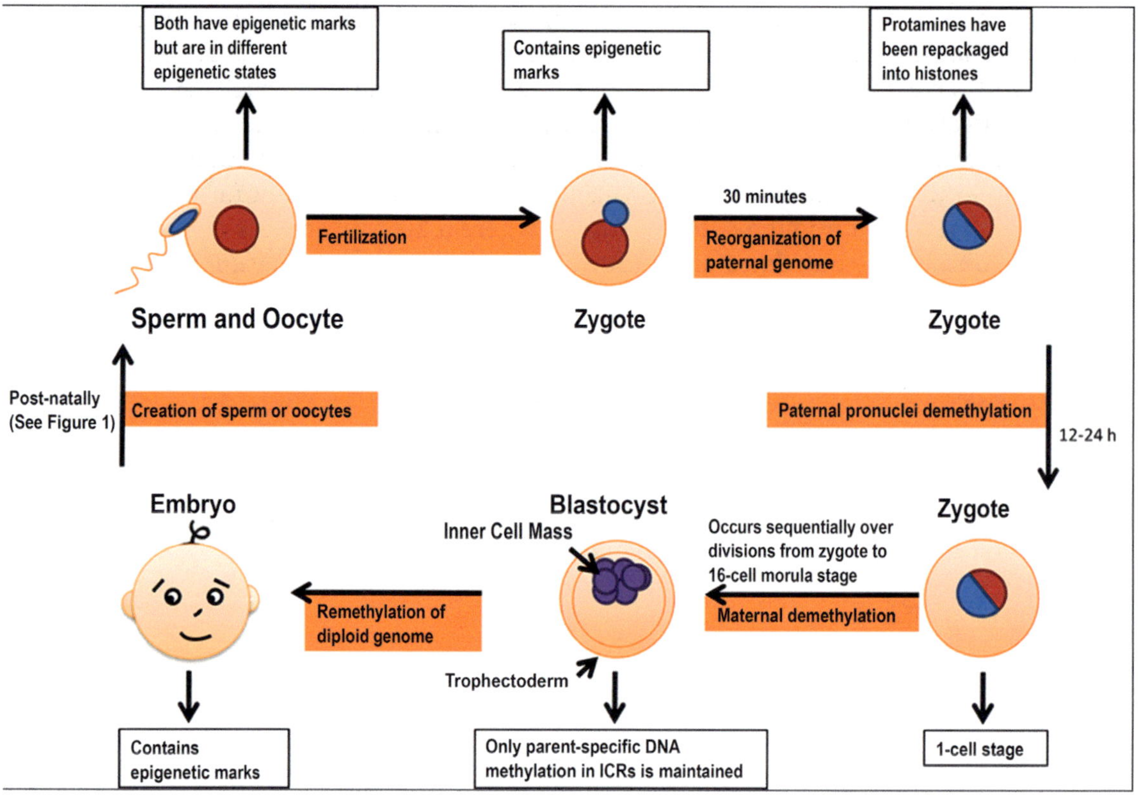

Figure 9.16. Epigenetic resetting in the zygote.

Source: https://www.researchgate.net/publication/221804020/figure/fig2/AS:11431281241153635@1714976344639/Second-round-of-epigenetic-reprogramming-occurs-following-fertilization-sequentially-from.tif.

The study of epigenetic resetting has improved a lot due to new genomic technologies. Next-generation sequencing (NGS), for instance, has allowed scientists to obtain comprehensive epigenomic profiles of germ cells and zygotes, fostering a deeper understanding of the molecular processes at play during the early stages of development. It is shown by these studies that the zygotic epigenome is marked by significant demethylation and changes in histones which together reset the embryonic developmental program. This resetting not only erases parental imprints but also prepares the zygote for subsequent cellular divisions and differentiation processes (Brown et al., 2018). The results show that epigenetic states play a major role in shaping how an organism develops. In addition, epigenetic resetting is important in evolution, helping us understand why species can adapt and survive. Because epigenetic marks can be reset at conception, organisms may be able to quickly react to changes in their environment and developmental signals over many generations. As highlighted in studies contrasting epigenetic and cumulative DNA damage models of aging, the transient nature of epigenetic modifications presents a viable pathway for rejuvenation and developmental integrity (Brown et al., 2018). Understanding these principles is essential for addressing not only basic biological inquiries but also for potential applications in regenerative medicine and therapeutic interventions targeting developmental anomalies associated with disrupted epigenetic regulation (Figure 9.16).

9.4.3. Implications for Genetic Inheritance

When we look at epigenetics in embryonic development, genetic inheritance goes beyond the usual ideas about DNA sequences. Epigenetic changes, for example DNA methylation and histone modifications, can affect the expression of genes without changing the DNA sequence. It means that environmental and developmental factors can cause epigenetic changes that can be passed on to future generations. For example, research has found that stress or poor nutrition in parents can change the epigenetic patterns of their children which may result in health problems. The implications of these findings challenge the classic Mendelian view of inheritance by highlighting the dynamic interplay between genes and the environment in shaping phenotypes (Nishiyama et al., 2021). In addition, environmental epigenetics highlights that we should pay attention to the environment and society when studying how genes are passed down. It has been found by recent studies that what a mother eats, the toxins she is exposed to and her stress levels during pregnancy can change the epigenome of the embryo which may result in health problems later in life. It is now clear that epigenetic changes can happen because of outside factors which means we need to consider both biological and environmental influences when studying inheritance. This interplay also aligns with broader discussions in public health and social policy, wherein addressing environmental disadvantages may mitigate hereditary health outcomes linked to epigenetic changes, thereby advocating for prevention strategies rooted in social equity considerations (Ruth Müller et al., 2017). In general, these findings about epigenetics and genetic inheritance have major effects on both personal health and the makeup of populations. Seeing that inheritance includes both fixed genes and flexible epigenetic changes encourages a broader view of development. It suggests that actions taken to improve the environment for mothers and young children can change how genes are expressed, leading to better health for their children and grandchildren. As this field continues to evolve, it is crucial to integrate epigenetic perspectives into medical and educational frameworks, thereby promoting awareness of how lifestyle and environmental choices can lead to profound implications in genetic inheritance and public health initiatives (Nishiyama et al., 2021).

9.5. Epigenetics and Developmental Disorders

Epigenetics is very important in controlling gene expression during embryonic development, since accurate control of these processes is necessary for cells to differentiate and organs to form. Problems in epigenetic processes such as DNA methylation and histone modification, may result in developmental disorders. For example, changes in methylation have been linked to syndromes such as Beckwith-Wiedemann syndrome and Prader-Willi syndrome, demonstrating that epigenetic imbalances can cause different physical features. The Encyclopedia of DNA Elements (ENCODE) project has elucidated the regulatory landscapes of the genome, revealing how epigenetic modifications coordinate developmental pathways crucial for morphogenesis and cellular identity (Abascal et al., 2020). It shows that epigenetic regulation is not just a minor process, but is essential for the development of the embryo and for preventing related disorders. Also, the effects of environmental factors on epigenetic regulation during important stages of development should be carefully studied to understand developmental disorders. Teratogens, nutritional shortages or stress experienced by the mother can cause epigenetic changes that may affect the health of her children for a long time. The gut-brain axis which is a key way the brain and gut microbiota communicate, adds another level of complexity. Studies suggest that early-life microbiota influence key neurodevelopmental processes, with microbial metabolites potentially impacting the epigenetic regulation of brain development (John et al., 2019). As a result, the link between environmental factors and epigenetics points out that good maternal health and nutrition during pregnancy can help prevent developmental disorders. Epigenetic therapies are gaining attention as a possible solution for developmental disorders. New discoveries about epigenomes flexibility make it possible to consider interventions that could correct harmful epigenetic changes. For instance, approaches that focus on certain histone deacetylases or small molecules that change DNA methylation could be used to treat diseases caused by epigenetic problems. Because of these approaches, more research is needed to see if epigenetic modulation can be used to treat common developmental disorders. As ongoing studies continue to elucidate the complexities of epigenetic regulation in embryonic development, they promise to enhance our capacity to devise early interventions that could mitigate or prevent the manifestation of these debilitating conditions (Figure 9.17).

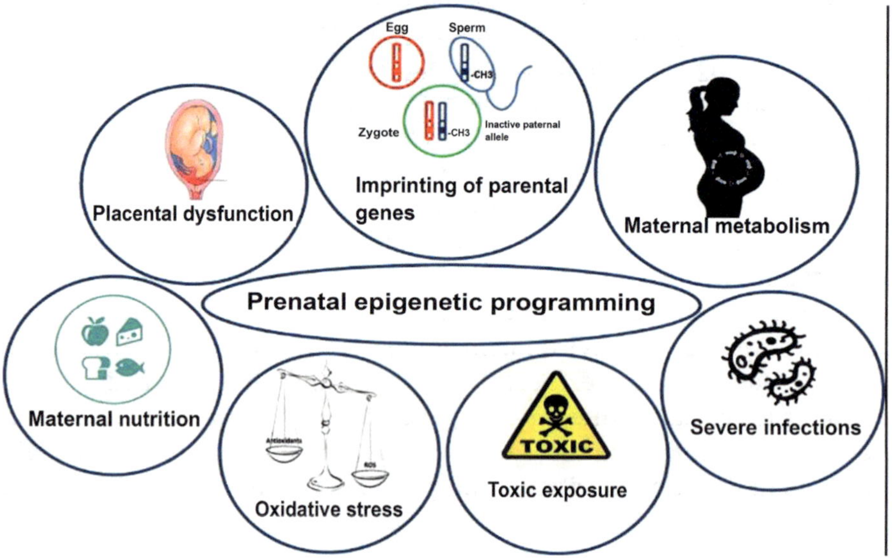

Figure 9.17. Epigenetics and developmental disorders.

Source: https://media.springernature.com/lw1200/springer-static/image/art%3A10.1038%2Fs41398-017-0062-x/MediaObjects/41398_2017_62_Fig1_HTML.jpg.

9.5.1. Role in Congenital Anomalies

The complex interplay between epigenetics and embryonic development is a significant determinant of the manifestation of congenital anomalies. Epigenetic changes, including DNA methylation and histone modification, profoundly influence gene expression by way of not being involved in any alteration of the DNA sequence itself. To be more precise, alterations in the methylation status of genomic areas have been implicated in developmental processes and susceptibility to congenital defect. For example, abnormal patterns of methylation within regions involved in embryonic development can interfere with the expression of morphogenesis genes for normal development.

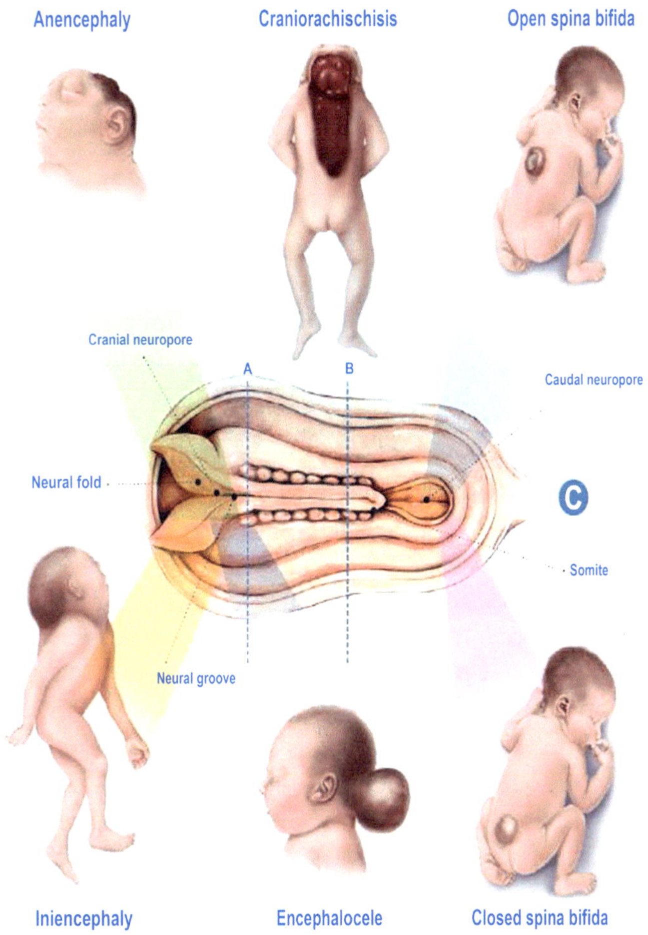

Figure 9.18. Role in congenital anomalies.

Source: https://archive.cdc.gov/www_cdc_gov/ncbddd/birthdefects/surveillancemanual/chapters/chapter-4/chapter4-2_html_files/01-002.png.

The ribosomal DNA (rDNA) locus, though more notably involved in encoding rRNA, is under strong epigenetic control during development. Studies have established that methylation of rDNA affects diverse biological processes, with consequences for ESC pluripotency and lineage specification, and thereby highlighting the central role of epigenetics in specifying developmental fates and, possibly, the etiology of congenital defects (Yang et al., 2024). Congenital defects are usually the result of a complex interaction between genetic predispositions and environmental exposures during vulnerable windows of embryonic development. More recent studies on chromosomal microdeletion syndromes, such as 22q11.2 deletion syndrome, have uncovered mechanisms for specific congenital heart defects (CHDs). The Slc25a1 gene deletion in the region 22q11.2 demonstrates how epigenetic regulation—more specifically, histone modifications—can prespecify developmental trajectories.

This gene was shown to control trophoblast and placental morphogenesis by affecting histone H3K27 acetylation of key regulatory regions. These alterations in such epigenetic marks can therefore result in structural defects in the heart, showing how epigenetic dysregulation can result in serious congenital disorders (Fan et al., 2024). Clarifying the role of epigenetics in congenital defects not only gives knowledge about their etiology but also identifies opportunities for therapy. As an example, understanding how epigenetic modifiers exert their action on development could unlock new therapies directed toward the causes of such disorders. In 22q11.2 deletion syndrome, for example, treatments that reverse trophoblast function, such as the administration of recombinant human pregnancy-specific glycoprotein 1, have shown promising results in amelioration of cardiac defects. Such findings suggest the more general use of epigenetic modulation in the clinic, with the hope that by modulating epigenetic landscapes with greater specificity, it will be possible to prevent or ameliorate certain congenital anomalies. As the science unfolds, the incorporation of epigenetic data into prenatal care can radically alter the practice of congenital anomaly prevention and treatment (Figure 9.18).

9.5.2. Epigenetic Factors in Neurodevelopmental Disorders (NDDs)

The complex interplay of neurodevelopmental disorders with epigenetic mechanisms highlights the significance of epigenetics in embryonic development. Epigenetic modifications are key regulators of gene expression, orchestrating the differentiation processes required for normal neural development. Notably, the timing and magnitude of such epigenetic impacts can affect the susceptibility of the developing nervous system to a broad spectrum of environmental stimuli. For example, dysregulation of the typical patterns of gene activation and inactivation can result in aberrant neuronal differentiation and synaptic formation, which have been linked to conditions like autism spectrum disorder (ASD) and schizophrenia. Thus, the analysis of the particular epigenetic signatures that are linked to particular NDDs identifies common pathways that can be targeted for preventative or therapeutic intervention to reduce risks associated with environmental exposures during this vulnerable period of development (Juga et al., 2022). An accumulating body of evidence points to the adverse effect of environmental toxins on epigenetic regulation, especially during the susceptible window of embryonic development. A case in point is provided by polybrominated diphenyl ethers (PBDEs), which are ubiquitous flame retardants employed in a number of consumer items. Evidence exists that human PBDE exposure correlates with behavioral disturbances characteristic of neurodevelopmental disorders (NDDs), thus prompting concern regarding the mechanisms by which these toxins impinge on biological endpoints. Vulnerability of developing nervous systems to environmental stimulus is habitually attributed to their dependence on specific epigenetic alterations regulating developmental processes. The interference with these processes, specifically by chemicals such as PBDEs, has been associated with alterations in the DNA methylation patterns and chromatin dynamics, further complicating the already complex interplay between epigenetics and neurodevelopmental well-being (Poston et al., 2019). Ultimately, clarifying the interplay between epigenetic factors and neurodevelopmental disorders (NDDs) is of noteworthy importance to future research and therapeutic applications. An enhanced knowledge of the ways in which epigenetic disruptions affect neural development can guide the creation of directed interventions that restore normal epigenetic function and counteract the detrimental actions of environmental agents. By creating associations between biochemical pathways included in neurodevelopment and those included in psychiatric illness, scientists are able to create the possibilities for new genetic counseling approaches and epigenetic treatments. This holistic strategy not only deepens our understanding of the etiological underpinnings of neurodevelopmental disorders (NDDs) but also promotes a preventive strategy to protect vulnerable populations from harmful environmental insults at embryonic stages of development (Juga et al., 2022) (Figure 9.19).

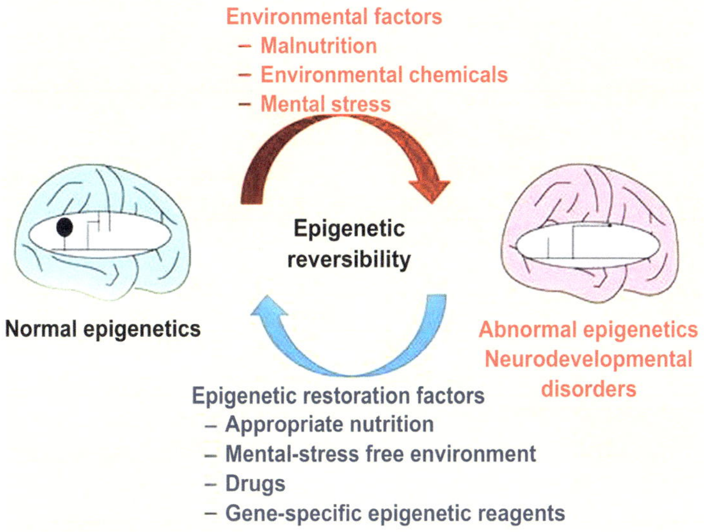

Figure 9.19. Epigenetic factors in neurodevelopmental disorders.

Source: https://www.tandfonline.com/cms/asset/a0b4b768-2e96-4694-a4a2-114aa6603fd8/iero_a_925805_f0005_b.jpg.

9.5.3. Potential for Therapeutic Interventions

The complex interaction of epigenetic factors during embryonic development has great therapeutic potential for treating a range of diseases. Epigenetic processes like DNA methylation and histone modifications regulate gene expression patterns that play fundamental roles in cell differentiation and developmental processes. Dysregulation of these processes routinely results in congenital abnormalities and developmental disease, making the need for targeted therapeutic approaches urgent. For example, the ECM's regulatory role in modulating cellular behavior has been associated with anoikis, a critical type of programmed cell death that may affect embryonic tissue integrity. Elucidating these mechanisms paves the way to potential interventions that can correct or mitigate the consequences of aberrant epigenetic regulation during development, underlining the necessity for appropriate modulation of epigenetic marks in enhancing desirable outcomes in affected populations (Mei et al., 2024). Aside from these, therapeutic applications derived from epigenetic research may also encompass regenerative medicine and stem cell therapy. The alteration of epigenetic factors has the potential to increase the effectiveness of stem cells dramatically by regulating their differentiation into specialized cell types necessary for tissue repair and regeneration. For example, recent research has revealed that the modulation of mitochondrial processes by the mitochondrial carrier homolog 2 (MTCH2) has the potential to influence metabolic processes and cell fate, which are central during embryonic development and in pathological states such as cancer and neurodegenerative diseases. Through the use of epigenetic editing technologies, scientists hope to create stem cell therapies that perfectly match developmental processes and, as such, generate improved treatments for various disorders caused by epigenetic dysregulation (Peng et al., 2024). Further, the incorporation of epigenetics into treatment methods is indicative of the requirement for an interdisciplinary method to treat developmental disorders, as well as other disorders. The cross-talk between anoikis and ECM signaling facilitates a more comprehensive understanding of cell death mechanisms that are important not only for development but also for homeostasis in adult tissues. Therapeutic interventions that interfere with such pathways will ultimately lead to novel therapies that inhibit or reverse the deleterious effects of epigenetic changes. Such strategies can usher in breakthroughs in personalized medicine, in which medications are tailored to the specific epigenetic profile of the patient. As the advances keep unfolding, the therapeutic promise of epigenetics remains a key focus, driving innovation in basic and translational biomedical research (Mei et al., 2024).

9.6. Current Research and Future Directions

Contemporary studies of epigenetics in embryonic development are progressively emphasizing the complex interaction between the environment and gene expression. Emerging evidence has accentuated how conditions such as nutritional state, psychological stress, and chemical exposure are able to alter the epigenetic landscape during sensitive periods in development, with long-lasting effects on health and susceptibility to disease. Gene expression during embryonic development is not only regulated by the genetic code but is also affected by epigenomic changes, such as DNA methylation and histone modifications. These changes enable scientists to comprehend mechanisms whereby embryos acclimatize to their surroundings, a postulation backed by facts linking bioprocesses and quantum effects, explained in the context of obligatory recapitulation that can be applied across all eukaryotes, emphasizing the significance of this developmental phase (Miller et al., 2016). As investigations of epigenetic mechanisms unfold, the directions of future studies are bound to reveal more about how the same genomic information can lead to the development of diverse cell types. By examining chromatin-modifying enzymes and noncoding RNAs, scientists aim to explain how such factors lead to specific functional consequences during embryogenesis. One of the most promising is the combination of high-throughput sequencing with epigenomic analysis to map these modifications across a range of cellular types and developmental stages. This has the potential not only to advance our knowledge of embryonic development but also to guide therapeutic intervention for congenital anomalies. The continued evolution of epigenomic methods means that their incorporation into classical research practice has the ability to address intricate inquiries into cellular differentiation and heterogeneity across individuals in developmental outputs (TA et al., 2018). The possible translational potential of this work is also immense, specifically in devising new therapeutic methods for dampening developmental disorders resulting from epigenetic changes. Based on the knowledge derived from recent studies, researchers can create interventions founded on precise epigenetic markers for those diseases that arise at initial development stages. The curiosity regarding environmental influences and their contribution to epigenetic alteration paves the way for the discussion of collaborative efforts between the fields of genetics, environmental science, and clinical medicine. Additional studies will be aimed at the long-term consequences of prenatal epigenetic changes, enhancing our knowledge of how maternal lifestyle during pregnancy can exert profound effects on offspring health. Integrative approach to knowledge suggests that surmounting these hurdles will move the field forward and enhance outcomes based on action in a timely manner during embryonic development, thus enhancing the usefulness of epigenetics in research and clinical practice (Miller et al., 2016; TA et al., 2018).

9.6.1. Advances in Epigenetic Technologies

Epigenetic technologies have rapidly advanced our knowledge of embryonic development and uncovered intricate mechanisms of regulation controlling cellular differentiation. Recent advances in technologies like CRISPR-Cas9 gene editing, single-cell RNA sequencing, and high-throughput methylation assays have empowered researchers with the tools to decipher the dynamic processes through which epigenetic alterations influence developmental outcomes. They provide unparalleled visibility into how the environment interacts with the epigenome during embryogenesis, stressing the importance of precise epigenetic regulation in the formation of functional tissues. The capacity to manipulate epigenetic marks and examine their effect on gene expression not only improves our understanding of developmental biology but also for possible therapeutic uses in future reproductive medicine. In this instance, some epigenetic changes have the capacity to improve embryo viability or rectify developmental abnormalities that are associated with epigenetic changes (Zhang et al., 2025). The inclusion of sophisticated epigenomic profiling methods has encouraged research into how metabolic substrates affect embryonic development, in this case, their role in energy metabolism and epigenetic control. Researchers have initiated work to investigate the specific effects of metabolites such as glucose on the epigenetic alterations that take place during oocyte maturation and early embryonic development. Through the application of metabolomics together with genomic strategies, researchers have deciphered how substrates influence the plasticity of the epigenome directly, which is an important consideration for cellular fate decisions. This novel insight has the potential to transform strategies in assisted reproductive technologies, with the possibility of creating noninvasive methods that optimize embryo selection according to metabolic profiles, with an associated enhancement in viable pregnancies (Zhang et al., 2025). Aside from metabolic processes, the investigation into environmental influences such as microgravity represents an especially interesting avenue of epigenetic research. The effects of space travel defy conventional hypotheses regarding embryonic development, showcasing the effects of changed gravitational forces on cell differentiation and tissue organization. Research suggests that microgravity can interfere with critical signaling pathways such as the WNT and Notch pathways, thereby influencing both gastrulation and cardiovascular development in embryos. By applying a suite of high-resolution imaging techniques coupled to cutting-edge omics instrumentation, scientists are starting to decipher the molecular and epigenetic landscapes supporting such disruptions. Such knowledge has profound implications for the discipline of space biology, as well as delivering valuable insights applicable to regenerative medicine and tissue engineering, thereby informing the discipline about adaptation of physiological state to enhance growth in diverse environments (Figure 9.20).

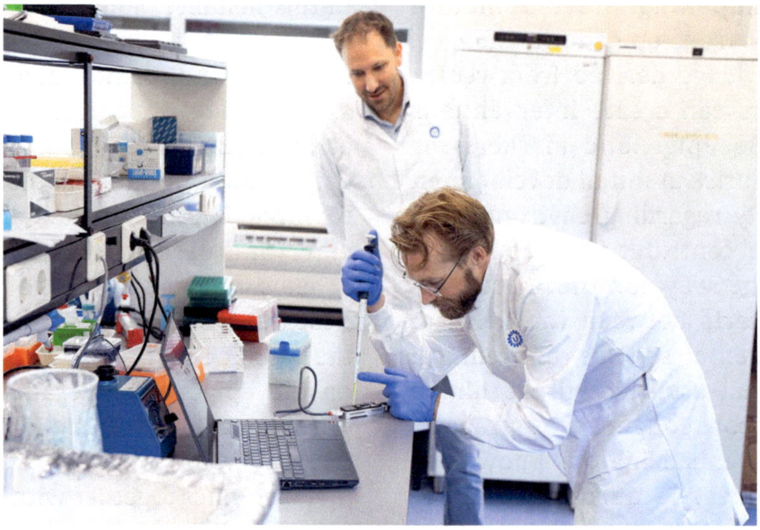

Figure 9.20. Epigenetic technologies of embryonic development.

Source: https://www.genengnews.com/wp-content/uploads/2024/04/Epigenetics_UMCUtrecht_Pic1.jpg.

9.6.2. Potential Applications in Regenerative Medicine

The convergence of epigenetics and regenerative medicine offers a significant promise for the advancement of therapeutic interventions toward tissue function and integrity recreation. Epigenetic control of gene expression that doesn't alter the intrinsic DNA sequence has been very significant in the fields of development and differentiation. Evidence has established that epigenetic instability can result in pathological conditions, including cancer or degenerative disease, thus necessitating the development of strategies capable of rectifying such aberrancies. Therapeutic strategies taking advantage of this reversibility have the potential to bring about novel treatments for disorders once thought to be irreversible. Through the use of compounds such as histone deacetylase inhibitors, scientists are able to alter epigenetic states in order to restore normal cell behavior, an especially important consideration for regenerative purposes where normal cell function is essential (Pandian et al., 2012). One of the more important considerations in regenerative medicine is being able to leverage cellular pathways for rejuvenation and repair. Extracellular vesicles (EVs) have been identified as new carriers for delivering epigenetic modifiers that can induce regenerative processes in cells. Through the transfer of bioactive molecules, EVs are able to alter the epigenetic landscape of target cells, thus inducing tissue regeneration. Clinical use of EVs highlights the significance of the relationship between epigenetics and cellular regeneration. The regulation of epigenetic factors by extracellular vesicles (EVs) not only pertains to the process of biological aging but also to preventing age-associated diseases, thereby enhancing health span. Elucidation of EV biology thus seems to be an important sector for the formulation of efficient cell-free therapeutic strategies in regenerative models (Neytchev et al., 2018). As the realm of regenerative medicine advances, increasing acknowledgment of the contribution of epigenetics as a significant area of research is being realized. The potential future uses of epigenetic modulation involve personalized medicine, in which therapy can be individualized according to the specific epigenomic signature of a patient. Such personalized therapy has the potential to enhance therapeutic efficacy by targeting specific epigenetic alterations linked to different diseases. Additionally, interactions among molecular biologists and regenerative medicine scientists can enable novel applications of gene editing tools in conjunction with epigenetic modulators. Such interdisciplinary research has the potential to create novel therapies that not only heal injured tissues but also effectively restore their functional properties at the molecular level, rendering regenerative medicine more effective overall. Ongoing research on epigenetic mechanisms will undoubtedly play a fundamental role in the future of regenerative medicine, providing new possibilities in the treatment of challenging health disorders (Pandian et al., 2012) (Figure 9.21).

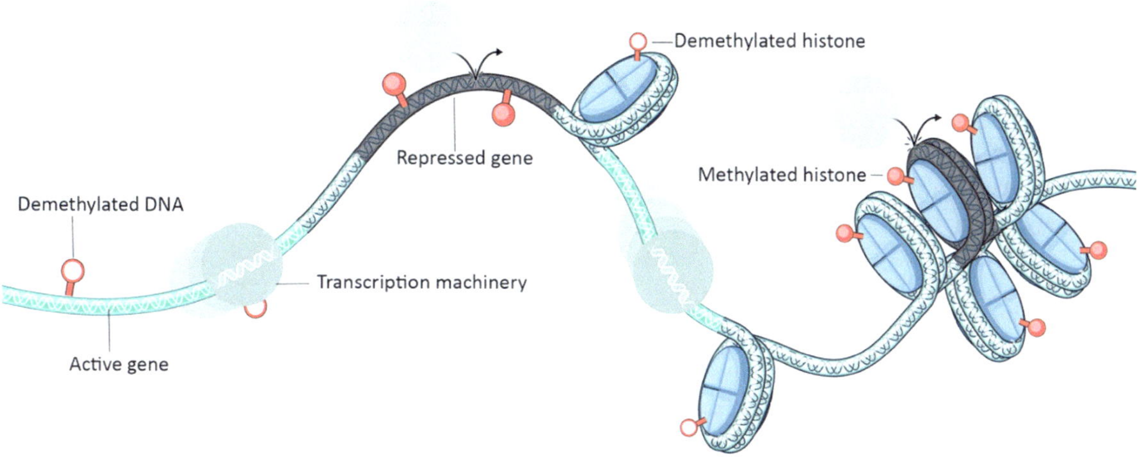

Figure 9.21. Developing epigenetic drugs for genetic and regenerative medicine.

Source: https://www.genengnews.com/wp-content/uploads/2023/08/Radar_TuneTherapeutics_Epigenetics.jpg.

9.6.3. Ethical Considerations in Epigenetic Research

Ethical implications are foremost in epigenetic studies, particularly in embryonic development. As scientists explore the heritable changes in gene expression that happen without alteration to the DNA sequence, the implications of manipulating the epigenetic mechanisms become more complex. For instance, research on long noncoding RNAs (lncRNAs), such as GATA6-AS1, highlights the need for ethical consideration in studying their role in essential processes like cardiogenesis. Though such molecules are promising to provide insights into congenital heart diseases and potential therapeutic intervention, they also call into question the ethical concerns implicated in their manipulation in embryonic tissues. Scientists are obligated to reconcile the twin role of advancing medical knowledge with preventing unwanted effects and ethical violation that may emanate from trespassing the natural limits of human development (Kim et al., 2025). In the field of epigenetics, the possibility in gene editing poses great ethical concerns in regard to how far human intervention should go. With the breakthrough in technology making it possible to introduce precise changes to the epigenome, the possibility of designing embryos with genetically designed characteristics emerges, thereby bringing up ethical concerns over the same. For instance, in the scenario of Klinefelter syndrome (KS), treatments may enable individuals to become biological parents via assisted reproductive technologies by means of alterations in their epigenetic profiles. Such activities require complete deliberations of the ethical obligations of practitioners and researchers, especially with regards to issues of consent, equity, and long-term consequences for society. The nexus between epigenetic interventions and personal autonomy underscores the need for developing comprehensive ethical frameworks for addressing the complex challenges entrenched in embryonic research (Chen et al., 2024). In addition, ethical ramifications encompass not just thorough case studies and personal health outcomes but also initiate significant societal concerns about fairness and accessibility of emerging technologies. The potential future gains of epigenetic research in embryonic development must be carefully balanced against the risk of increasing existing health inequities. If access to the epigenetic advances is limited to certain socioeconomic groups, there is a risk of an increasing differential in health outcomes influenced by privilege. Mechanisms for facilitating equitable access to such advances must thus be evolved. It is imperative that researchers, policymakers, and ethicists work together to make sure that epigenetics research benefits every sector of society and does not add to existing inequalities. The complexity of ethics that is involved in this science must be scrutinized continuously as it evolves, making sure that everyone's voice is heard and that ethical guidelines are steering the future of epigenetic research in embryonic development (Chen et al., 2024).

SUMMARY

The epigenetic mechanism research in embryonic development offers a breakthrough insight into genetic regulation over and above the paradigms of classical inheritance. The understanding developed through the study of phenomena such as X chromosome inactivation (XCI) reveals the highly complex interaction between developmental outcomes and epigenetic changes. Experiments also pointed to the elaborate process of keeping epigenetic states, such as in the instance of female mammalian cells, wherein factors such as ATF7IP act with both long non-coding RNAs and DNA methylation, such as the Xist, in order to enable appropriate silencing of the inactive X chromosome. This exchange underscores the important function of epigenetics in the course of cellular differentiation, illustrating that alterations in these pathways can have important developmental repercussions (Bonora et al., 2014). Further, the development of transgenic technologies has equipped the research community with sophisticated tools to investigate epigenetic regulation at the embryonic development levels. By utilizing techniques that allow for specific manipulation of epigenetic marks, scientists are able to examine the consequences of such alterations on gene expression and subsequently on developmental processes. Meetings like the 11th Transgenic Technology meeting most accurately reflect the current collaboration and exchange of information between scientists committed to the implementation of these techniques for human disease modeling and the refinement of biotechnological methods. As scholars advance their comprehension of epigenetic influences, they are able to replicate intricate interactions and identify key transitions that are essential for successful embryonic development (Strathdee et al., 2013). Ultimately, the ramifications of epigenetics within the realm of embryonic development transcend mere biological knowledge; they possess considerable implications for medical practice and therapeutic strategies. As studies reveal the intricate epigenetic mechanism underlying numerous developmental disorders, new approaches to intervention can be formulated with epigenetic modifiers targeting aberrant patterns. Future therapeutic interventions based on this understanding may try to correct or ameliorate epigenetic regulation defects that cause conditions. This potential highlights the urgent need for further investigation of the epigenetic mechanisms at work during the initial phases of development, thereby underlining their significance not just for developmental biology, but also for practical application in regenerative medicine and fertility therapy.

The complex interplay between epigenetics and embryonic development has been a major area of interest in the recent past, citing the involvement of a broad array of metabolic pathways influencing developmental processes and genetic control. One of the key facets of this interaction is the significance of glucose metabolism, which has been found to be essential for effective oocyte maturation to blastocyst formation. This metabolism provides the metabolic substrates and energy that control cell proliferation and differentiation and govern major epigenetic marks. It is important to understand how these processes of metabolism coordinate during early embryogenesis to advance fertility therapy and reproductive medicine. These observations point to the promise of noninvasive metabolic testing for the enhancement of embryo selection procedures and improved success rates in assisted reproductive technologies, thereby placing metabolic pathways as important drivers in embryonic growth processes and reproductive success (Zhang et al., 2025). A central aspect of epigenetic processes in embryonic development regards the influence of micronutrients, in particular Vitamin B12, which are components of critical metabolic pathways, such as One-Carbon Metabolism. The dysregulation of vitamin B12 has been involved in a range of developmental defects, from congenital abnormalities and neural tube defects, underpinning its importance in maintaining correct embryonic development. Studies have shown that changes in B12 transport, specifically the knockout of transcobalamin 2 (tcn2) in animal models, can result in profound phenotypic variation as well as a rise in embryonic death rates. Interestingly, vitamin B12 treatment has shown promise in reversing such developmental perturbations, highlighting a potential modulatory role of B12 in epigenetic transcriptional events. Screening for DEGs and their enrichment in significant biological pathways under B12 deficiency highlights the complex interplay between nutritional status, gene expression, and epigenetic modifications during early development (Ajay et al., 2023). Finally, the general message of epigenetics in relation to embryonic development underscores the critical importance of both energetic and nutritional determinants in shaping developmental trajectories. The insight gained from studies of glucose metabolism and control by vitamins offers insight that environmental and metabolic status can modify expression of genes and cellular response to a profound extent. Such insight requires further exploration of the mechanisms by which epigenetic changes are set, read, and possibly reset according to metabolic status. By the incorporation of metabolic pathway-related knowledge with epigenetic mechanisms, scientists can develop better-integrated approaches aimed at optimizing embryo health and viability. Progress toward understanding these relations is on the verge of transforming reproductive practices and providing promise for increased facilitation in fertility treatments with an expanded range for optimal embryonic development (Ajay et al., 2023; Zhang et al., 2025).

CLOSER LOOK

TEN-ELEVEN TRANSLOCATION (TET)

TET refers to a family of enzymes—TET1, TET2, and TET3—that play a crucial role in the epigenetic regulation of gene expression through the process of DNA demethylation. These enzymes are named for their discovery in a chromosomal translocation involving the TET1 gene in acute myeloid leukemia (AML). TET proteins function by catalyzing the oxidation of 5-methylcytosine (5mC), a common DNA modification involved in gene silencing, to 5-hydroxymethylcytosine (5hmC) and further oxidized derivatives. This process initiates active DNA demethylation, allowing for dynamic regulation of gene expression without altering the underlying DNA sequence. By influencing methylation patterns, TET enzymes are critical for numerous biological processes, including embryonic development, stem cell pluripotency, hematopoiesis, neural differentiation, and immune function.

Among the TET family, TET2 is the most studied, especially in the context of hematological malignancies. Loss-of-function mutations in the TET2 gene have been identified in a variety of blood cancers, including myelodysplastic syndromes (MDS), AML, and chronic myelomonocytic leukemia (CMML). These mutations are associated with impaired DNA demethylation, leading to abnormal gene expression and dysregulation of hematopoietic stem cell differentiation and proliferation. TET2 mutations are also found in clonal hematopoiesis of indeterminate potential (CHIP), a condition where blood-forming cells acquire mutations associated with leukemia but without overt disease. This suggests that TET2 dysfunction may represent an early event in cancer development, highlighting its role as a tumor suppressor. In addition to cancer, alterations in TET activity have been linked to NDDs, cardiovascular diseases, and immune dysfunction, underscoring the broad physiological significance of these enzymes.

Regulation of TET enzyme activity is tightly controlled and influenced by various factors, including the availability of cofactors such as α-ketoglutarate (aKG) and iron, which are essential for TET catalytic function. Environmental factors, metabolic changes, and inflammation can affect these cofactors and, in turn, modulate TET activity. Interestingly, vitamin C has been shown to enhance TET activity, promoting DNA demethylation and offering potential therapeutic applications, particularly in cancer therapy. Research into pharmacological modulation of TET enzymes is ongoing, aiming to correct aberrant DNA methylation patterns in diseases where TET function is compromised. TET proteins also interact with other epigenetic regulators and transcription factors, forming complex networks that fine-tune gene expression in a cell-type-specific and context-dependent manner. For example, TET1 and TET3 are more involved in early development and neural differentiation, whereas TET2 plays a predominant role in hematopoietic cells. Disruption of this balance through mutation or altered expression can lead to widespread epigenetic dysregulation, contributing to disease pathogenesis.

The TET enzymes are vital players in the epigenetic landscape, mediating active DNA demethylation and regulating gene expression across diverse biological contexts. Their dysfunction is implicated in various diseases, particularly hematological cancers, and represents a promising target for therapeutic intervention. As research advances, a deeper understanding of TET enzymes will likely lead to novel strategies for diagnosing and treating epigenetically driven disorders.

REFERENCES

1. Abascal, F., Acosta, R., Addleman, N. J., Adrian, J., Afzal, V., Ai, R., Aken, B., et al. (2020). Expanded encyclopedias of DNA elements in the human and mouse genomes. *Nature, 583*, 699–710. https://doi.org/10.1038/s41586-020-2493-4.
2. Araolaza, M., Muñoa-Hoyos, I., Odriozola, A., & Subirán, N. (2023). P-799: Morphine causes global hypomethylation through active and passive demethylation mechanisms in mESCs hindering optimal embryonic development. *Human Reproduction*. https://www.semanticscholar.org/paper/e6277cbe3920d8d8eb7a53c6bb163e302c5d5a43 (accessed on 27 May 2025).
3. Baruah, S. K., Bossier, P., Norouzitallab, P., & Vanrompay, D. (2020). Non-mammalian model organisms in epigenetic research: An overview. https://core.ac.uk/download/322829180.pdf (accessed on 27 May 2025).
4. Bonefas, K. M., Venkatachalam, I., & Iwase, S. (2024). KDM5C is a sex-biased brake against germline gene expression programs in somatic lineages. *bioRxiv*. https://www.semanticscholar.org/paper/4b6ca82d739eda98255fede09a6bf7335b693d55 (accessed on 27 May 2025).
5. Bonora, G., Minkovsky, A., Patel, S., & Plath, K. (2014). The Mbd1-Atf7ip-Setdb1 pathway contributes to the maintenance of X chromosome inactivation. https://pmc.ncbi.nlm.nih.gov/articles/PMC4099106/.
6. Brown, A. P., Ji, H., & Zhu, T. (2020). The emerging role of Ten-Eleven Translocation 1 in epigenetic responses to environmental exposures. https://core.ac.uk/download/323070431.pdf (accessed on 27 May 2025).
7. Brown, O. A., Canatelli Mallat, M., Chiavellini, P., & Goya, R. G. (2018). Rejuvenation by cell reprogramming: A new horizon in gerontology. https://core.ac.uk/download/287880771.pdf (accessed on 27 May 2025).
8. Chen, X., Zhang, X., Jiang, T., & Xu, W. (2024). Klinefelter syndrome: Etiology and clinical considerations in male infertility. *Biology of Reproduction*. https://www.semanticscholar.org/paper/bb3717b752dc967493e4fb5cb4266b215266e11a (accessed on 27 May 2025).
9. Chen, Y., Wang, L., Guo, F., Dai, X., & Zhang, X. (2023). Epigenetic reprogramming during the maternal-to-zygotic transition. *MedComm, 4*. https://www.semanticscholar.org/paper/c77019f999c54b3e7662256030a8c356886e0cf5 (accessed on 27 May 2025).
10. Chu, M., Yao, F., Xi, G., Yang, J., Zhang, Z., Yang, Q., Tian, J., et al. (2021). Vitamin C rescues *in vitro* embryonic development by correcting impaired active DNA demethylation. *Frontiers in Cell and Developmental Biology, 9*. https://www.semanticscholar.org/paper/360a9ad4f63060a3437a32e61bdf668bbbceba45 (accessed on 27 May 2025).
11. Cryan, J. F., O'Riordan, K. J., Cowan, C. S. M., Sandhu, K. V., Bastiaanssen, T. F. S., Boehme, M., Codagnone, M. G., et al. (2019). The microbiota-gut-brain axis. *Physiological Reviews, 99*, 1877–2013. https://doi.org/10.1152/physrev.00018.2018.
12. Dong, L., Zhu, J., Deng, A., Wei, J., Li, J., Mao, X., & Jia, Z. (2023). Relationship between histone demethylase LSD family and development and prognosis of gastric cancer. *Frontiers in Immunology, 14*. https://www.semanticscholar.org/paper/02b084508cfa32b81c638f9e1dcb0c6b8ec4529b (accessed on 27 May 2025).
13. Du, S., Zhou, J., Ao, X., & Zhu, Y. (2025). Effects of in ovo feeding of vitamin C on embryonic development, hatching process, and chick rectal temperature of broiler embryos. *Frontiers*

in Veterinary Science, 11. https://www.semanticscholar.org/paper/994baf6bd43ee87584ce05b6e1693b99157d162a (accessed on 27 May 2025).

14. Fan, W., Li, Z., He, X., Wang, X., Sun, M., & Yang, Z. (2024). SLC25A1 regulates placental development to ensure embryonic heart morphogenesis. *Development, 151*(22). https://www.semanticscholar.org/paper/3ba754d72ce07af69855ef53e870f89c7ff29049 (accessed on 27 May 2025).
15. Fukushima, H. S., Takeda, H., & Nakamura, R. (2023). Incomplete erasure of histone marks during epigenetic reprogramming in medaka early development. *Genome Research, 33*, 572–586. https://www.semanticscholar.org/paper/2d68c7d56bc01f37bca9cb239992d32f96970332 (accessed on 27 May 2025).
16. Fuso, A., Lucarelli, M., & Nicolia, V. (2015). Environment, epigenetics and neurodegeneration: Focus on nutrition in Alzheimer's disease. https://core.ac.uk/download/54507601.pdf (accessed on 27 May 2025).
17. Gan, J., Zhang, X., Lu, Y., Wu, Z., Cai, G., & Hong, L. (2022). A unique glimpse into the crosstalk between different epigenetic mechanisms in porcine embryonic development. *Biology of Reproduction, 107*, 1411–1424. https://www.semanticscholar.org/paper/41e6b8a07982201ea67c277f33c31cf1cc88da92 (accessed on 27 May 2025).
18. Gao, C., Gao, X., Gao, F., Du, X., & Wu, S. (2024). A CRISPR/Cas9 screen in embryonic stem cells reveals that Mdm2 regulates totipotency exit. *Communications Biology, 7*. https://www.semanticscholar.org/paper/ac57fc3852f4e168d66236506c1da4f107212ec1 (accessed on 27 May 2025).
19. Jeong, Y., Lu, H., Park, C. H., Li, M., Luo, H., Kim, J. J., Liu, S., et al. (2016). Stochastic anomaly of methylome but persistent SRY hypermethylation in disorder of sex development in canine somatic cell nuclear transfer. *Scientific Reports, 6*. https://www.semanticscholar.org/paper/30bb86b2b7ebc23d322668157cf730b4c9681e7f (accessed on 27 May 2025).
20. Juga, L. (2022). Epigenetic pathogenesis of neurological disorders *in utero* and considerations for genetic counseling. https://core.ac.uk/download/516439925.pdf (accessed on 27 May 2025).
21. Khalaily, L., & Avraham, K. (2024). Insights into the regulation of hearing regeneration. *Frontiers in Audiology and Otology*. https://www.semanticscholar.org/paper/49107708edf8ccbc0a529e0b102a09664ca2ca98 (accessed on 27 May 2025).
22. Kim, N. J., Moon, E. H., Oh, J. H., Kim, H. M., Sung, S. H., Kim, H. S., Kim, C. Y., et al. (2025). Tissue-specific lncRNA GATA6-AS1 and its ortholog Moshe as essential regulators of aortic valve development. *BMB Reports, 58*, 175–182. https://www.semanticscholar.org/paper/eb26a2ababa912f6dec94af42e86366cb820adb9 (accessed on 27 May 2025).
23. Kisliouk, T., Ravi, P., Rosenberg, T., & Meiri, N. (2024). Embryonic manipulations shape life-long, heritable stress responses through complex epigenetic mechanisms: A review. *Frontiers in Neuroscience, 18*. https://www.semanticscholar.org/paper/4c31313edbbaa5bd094bb4f4eb502722041e8b68 (accessed on 27 May 2025).
24. Leesang, T., Lyon, P. D., Pinzone, J., & Cimmino, L. (2024). Micronutrient regulation of the DNA methylome. *Frontiers in Epigenetics and Epigenomics*. https://www.semanticscholar.org/paper/7eba748d43f459aa7cb21ee04dd45ad6f5662482 (accessed on 27 May 2025).

25. López-Catalina, A., Reverter, A., Alexandre, P. A., Nguyen, L. T., & González-Recio, O. (2024). Stress-induced epigenetic effects driven by maternal lactation in dairy cattle: A comethylation network approach. *Epigenetics, 19*. https://www.semanticscholar.org/paper/672ee0fafe157da1563e1cb637ac74b144b2fa3c (accessed on 27 May 2025).

26. Lubanzi, M. (2024). Influence of environmental factors on embryonic development and fetal programming in South Africa. *International Journal of Biology*. https://www.semanticscholar.org/paper/14725cfc8d3167b0f73410acd255dd4ca582da4a (accessed on 27 May 2025).

27. Marques, E., Severance, E. G., Arsenault, P., Zahn, S. M., & Timme-Laragy, A. (2024). Activation of Nrf2 at critical windows of development alters tissue-specific protein S-glutathionylation in the zebrafish (*Danio rerio*) embryo. *Antioxidants, 13*. https://www.semanticscholar.org/paper/cbb28eb99a5abf7dca70787300dc800399df09ec (accessed on 27 May 2025).

28. McKinsey, T. A., Morimoto, T., Poller, W., Turner, B. M., & Wang, Y. (2018). Epigenomes in cardiovascular disease. https://pmc.ncbi.nlm.nih.gov/articles/PMC5976233/.

29. Mei, J., Jiang, X. Y., Tian, H. X., Rong, D. C., Song, J. N., Wang, L., Chen, Y. S., et al. (2024). Anoikis in cell fate, physiopathology, and therapeutic interventions. *MedComm, 5*. https://www.semanticscholar.org/paper/409b00eeeb94e3b223bc9378e744a359d3d17f26 (accessed on 27 May 2025).

30. Miller, W. B., & Torday, J. S. (2016). The unicellular state as a point source in a quantum biological system. https://www.mdpi.com/2079-7737/5/2/25.

31. Montgomery, T., Uh, K., & Lee, K. (2024). TET enzyme driven epigenetic reprogramming in early embryos and its implication on long-term health. *Frontiers in Cell and Developmental Biology, 12*. https://www.semanticscholar.org/paper/5beb821a20b8cb5a1300665bdd87966da21e680a (accessed on 27 May 2025).

32. Müller, R., Hanson, C., Hanson, M. A., Penkler, M., Samaras, G., Chiapperino, L., Dupré, J., et al. (2017). The biosocial genome? *EMBO Reports, 18*, 1677–1682. https://doi.org/10.15252/embr.201744953.

33. Neytchev, O., Panagiotou, N., Selman, C., & Shiels, P. G. (2018). Extracellular vesicles, ageing, and therapeutic interventions. https://pmc.ncbi.nlm.nih.gov/articles/PMC6115766/.

34. Nishiyama, A., & Nakanishi, M. (2021). Navigating the DNA methylation landscape of cancer. *Trends in Genetics, 37*, 1012–1027. https://doi.org/10.1016/j.tig.2021.05.002.

35. Pandian, G., & Sugiyama, H. (2012). Strategies to modulate heritable epigenetic defects in cellular machinery: Lessons from nature. https://core.ac.uk/download/39296150.pdf (accessed on 27 May 2025).

36. Pankammoon, P., Qing, Y., Zhao, H., Jiao, D., Li, H., Wang, F., Wiriyahdamrong, T., et al. (2025). Transcriptomic insights into developmental arrest in fluorescent labeling transgenic Asian elephant (Elephas maximus) embryos via inter-order cloning. *Frontiers in Cell and Developmental Biology, 13*. https://www.semanticscholar.org/paper/9e61520f3578fa22a60fb3305c3597c67abde2e8 (accessed on 27 May 2025).

37. Peng, X., Yang, Y., Hou, R., Zhang, L., Shen, C., Yang, X., Luo, Z., et al. (2024). MTCH2 in metabolic diseases, neurodegenerative diseases, cancers, embryonic development and reproduction. *Drug Design, Development and Therapy, 18*, 2203–2213. https://www.semanticscholar.org/paper/e0b036088d4a32daaf9818076bceae2ac9987f83 (accessed on 27 May 2025).

38. Pinzon-Arteaga, C. A., O'Hara, R., Mazzagati, A., Ballard, E. D., Hu, Y., Pan, A., Schmitz, D. A., et al. (2024). TASOR expression in naive embryonic stem cells safeguards their developmental potential. *Cell Reports, 43*, 114887. https://www.semanticscholar.org/paper/9f9102fc37b377ff513b242c522519e042c15ba3 (accessed on 27 May 2025).

39. Poston, R. G., & Saha, R. N. (2019). Epigenetic effects of polybrominated diphenyl ethers on human health. https://pmc.ncbi.nlm.nih.gov/articles/PMC6695782/.

40. Rejano-Gordillo, C. M., Marín-Díaz, B., Ordiales-Talavero, A., Merino, J., González-Rico, F. J., & Fernández-Salguero, P. (2022). From nucleus to organs: Insights of Aryl Hydrocarbon Receptor molecular mechanisms. *International Journal of Molecular Sciences, 23*. https://www.semanticscholar.org/paper/256e12fc85088c1a160586b6487ce1c6ca25439e (accessed on 27 May 2025).

41. Shukla, V., & Tyagi, A. (2023). Editorial: DNA & RNA methylation: Impact on cancer progression. *Frontiers in Genetics, 14*. https://www.semanticscholar.org/paper/baffd59f93c7d949841ae328124ccc62d703abb3 (accessed on 27 May 2025).

42. Strathdee, D., & Whitelaw, C. B. A. (2013). TT2013 meeting report: The transgenic technology meeting visits Asia for the first time. https://core.ac.uk/download/16459953.pdf (accessed on 27 May 2025).

43. Trigg, N. A., Eamens, A. L., & Nixon, B. (2019). The contribution of epididymosomes to the sperm small RNA profile. *Reproduction, 157*, R209–R223. https://doi.org/10.1530/rep-18-0480.

44. Tuscher, J. J., & Day, J. J. (2019). Multigenerational epigenetic inheritance: One step forward, two generations back. *Neurobiology of Disease, 132*, 104591. https://doi.org/10.1016/j.nbd.2019.104591.

45. Varnika, S., Arunasri, P. M., Jelina, K. J., & Parakunni, P. S. (2025). Microgravity-induced alterations in embryonic development and stem cell differentiation. *International Research Journal on Advanced Engineering Hub (IRJAEH)*. https://www.semanticscholar.org/paper/1783a5fe5e8ee251aac4f2eb02a7983842895faa (accessed on 27 May 2025).

46. Verma, A. D., Nongmaithem, S. S., Mounika, C., Ramachandran, S., Umesh, A., & Chandak, G. (2023). Zebrafish model of *tcn2* deletion reveals new molecular insights into the role of vitamin B12 in embryonic development. *bioRxiv*. https://www.semanticscholar.org/paper/a214b6e634d1e9500de41975a7360c34e5074b1d (accessed on 27 May 2025).

47. Wang, X., Jin, X.-Y., & Cheng, L. (2024). Recent advance in the study on 5-formylcytosine (f5C) RNA modification. *Israel Journal of Chemistry*. https://www.semanticscholar.org/paper/7899e2d0afdef61c0163a0084f2a8d8df35c05c5 (accessed on 27 May 2025).

48. Yan, C., He, B., Wang, C., Li, W., Tao, S., Chen, J., Wang, Y., et al. (2025). Methionine in embryonic development: Metabolism, redox homeostasis, epigenetic modification and signaling pathway. *Critical Reviews in Food Science and Nutrition*. https://www.semanticscholar.org/paper/3cca7781304fbc3258f652000aba2db6b1e8b9c0 (accessed on 27 May 2025).

49. Yang, F., Guo, X., Bao, Y., & Li, R. (2024). The role of ribosomal DNA methylation in embryonic development, aging and diseases. *Epigenetics & Chromatin, 17*. https://www.semanticscholar.org/paper/addc7db29e74077945c05141098a7dc6f40ec3ae (accessed on 27 May 2025).

50. Zhang, B., & Wolynes, P. (2014). Stem cell differentiation as a many-body problem. *Proceedings*

of the National Academy of Sciences, 111, 10185–10190. https://www.semanticscholar.org/paper/594249f9a58f7733604bb3e012ffc5ad7d1e9a77 (accessed on 27 May 2025).

51. Zhang, W., Li, K., Li, S., Lv, R., Ma, J., Yin, P., Li, L., et al. (2023). High-throughput sequencing reveals hub genes for human early embryonic development arrest *in vitro* fertilization: A pilot study. *Frontiers in Physiology, 14*. https://www.semanticscholar.org/paper/60bbb3bf0e217a1c0bc9406cbef0d596bfebaa31 (accessed on 27 May 2025).

52. Zhang, Y., Li, T., Wang, Y., & Yu, Y. (2025). Key glucometabolic during oocyte maturation and early embryonic development. *Reproduction, 169*. https://www.semanticscholar.org/paper/9106e2734328c48f404dc0d16d94a067867cbe01 (accessed on 27 May 2025).

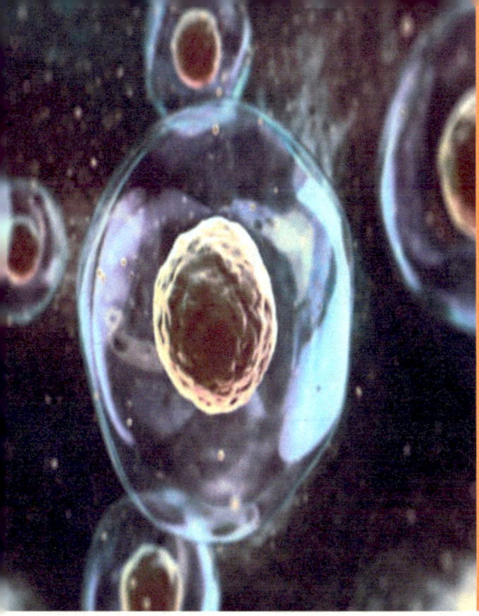

Chapter 10

PRENATAL GENETIC DIAGNOSIS AND SCREENING

Contents

Introduction

The development of prenatal genetic screening and diagnosis has become a critical field in contemporary reproductive medicine, greatly influencing the way potential parents comprehend the genetic risks. In the past, genetic diseases like beta-thalassemia and cystic fibrosis went undiagnosed in carriers until their children presented with advanced health problems. Recent reports indicate that a large number of couples learn about their carrier status after they have given birth, highlighting the urgency with which extensive screening programs are needed. The continuous evolution of genetic testing technologies is directed towards providing future parents with significant information to allow them to make reproductive decisions and consequently decrease the incidence of genetic disorders in newborns. Furthermore, the use of proactive strategies in prenatal screening can facilitate earlier interventions and more informed counseling, which is also in line with the moral obligation to offer informed decisions on family planning (Castaldo et al., 2013). The utility of prenatal genetic screening is also enhanced by targeted awareness and education campaigns that seek to enhance uptake across all demographic groups. For example, while some couples at high risk readily take up genetic screening, the majority of the population does not know their carrier status until a health emergency strikes. The need for targeted informational campaigns becomes evident, as these programs can inform prospective parents about the existence and applicability of prenatal testing. In addition, the findings of the Delphi technique with respect to HTA stress the importance of feedback from a broad spectrum of experts in deciding what questions and issues need to be given priority in the area of prenatal genetic testing (Freeman et al., 2005). The method guarantees that the aggregated information reflects the complexity involved in genetic disorders and adequately responds to societal and individual needs. As developments continue in the debate surrounding prenatal genetic diagnosis, it is imperative to consider the ethical implications and psychological effects on families who are confronted with possible genetic disorders. Diagnosis of an individual as a carrier for a genetic disorder can bring about varied feelings, such as worry and fear for a child's future health. Hence, it is imperative to incorporate extensive genetic counseling within the screening, giving families adequate guidance and care so that they may accept their choices with confidence. In addition, the emphasis on developing standard screening protocols will not only simplify procedures but also increase the accessibility of these crucial tests within varied demographic backgrounds. In conclusion, as our knowledge of genetics increases, it is our obligation to keep assessing and refining our practices of prenatal screening and diagnosis (Castaldo et al., 2013), so that they remain responsive, inclusive, and sensitive to all future parents' needs (Figure 10.1).

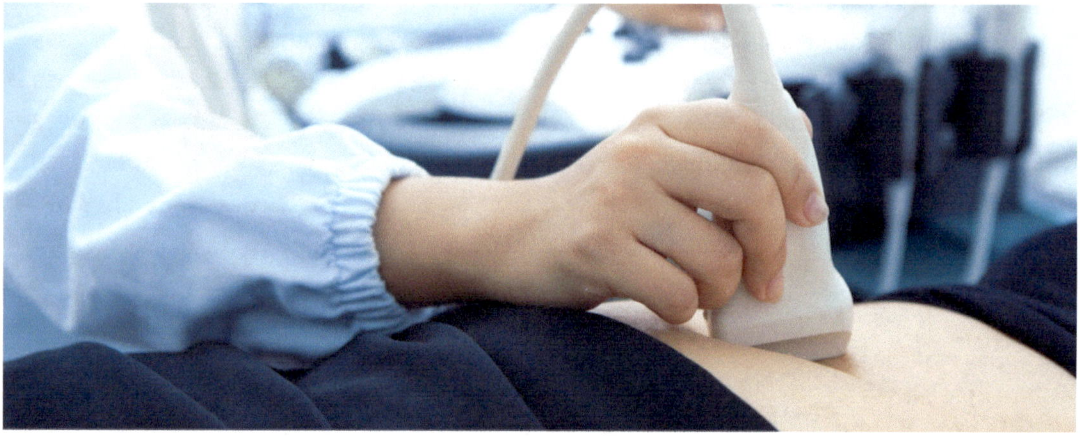

Figure 10.1. Prenatal genetic screening.

Source: https://external-content.duckduckgo.com/iu/?u=https%3A%2F%2Fwww.ucsfhealth.org%2F-%2Fmedia%2Fproject%2Fucsf%2Fucsf-health%2Feducation%2Fhero%2Fprenatal-screening-tests-2x.jpg%3Fh%3D1112%26w%3D2880%26hash%3D762FA98D1875328EDFCD59F6589669D1&f=1&nofb=1&ipt=4973bc3af2dac3c7b8b7aba3ac2e0c39f031d21795049ed8df8777e46198229a.

Definition of Prenatal Genetic Diagnosis and Screening

Prenatal diagnosis and genetic screening are significant developments in the fields of genetics and obstetrics, where fetal well-being can be assessed before birth. These technologies encompass a range of procedures aimed at detecting genetic or chromosomal defects within the developing fetus. Prenatal screening generally employs non-invasive procedures, such as blood work and ultrasound scan, which try to ascertain the risk for a specific disorder, i.e., Down syndrome and neural tube defects. Whereas, prenatal diagnostic tests usually employ more invasive procedures, like amniocentesis or CVS, that yield definitive information pertaining to the fetal genotype. This difference between screening and diagnostic testing accentuates the need to comprehend the underlying technology and its clinical ramifications for pregnant couples as they navigate potential health issues concerning their child. One of the most significant applications of prenatal genetic diagnosis includes the identification of certain genetic disorders such as uniparental disomy (UPD)-related imprinting disorders. These inherited diseases may be caused by the abnormal establishment of genomic imprinting, which may cause inappropriate parental gene expression and thus catastrophic congenital abnormalities.

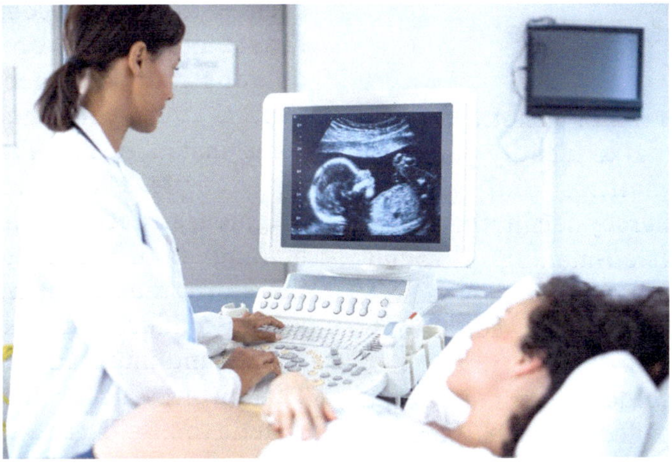

Figure 10.2. Prenatal genetic testing.

Source: https://external-content.duckduckgo.com/iu/?u=http%3A%2F%2Fcdn.shopify.com%2Fs%2Ffiles%2F1%2F1407%2F3324%2Farticles%2Fprenatal-genetic-testing_1300x%402x.jpg%3Fv%3D1663020056&f=1&nofb=1&ipt=1e7e49f7cb9edc2579037b107716c2446f438b89321af1a25da348494d8f511c.

As techniques in genetic testing improve, prenatal diagnosis of UPD-related disorders has become more of a routine clinical practice. Yet, the complex mechanisms of such conditions deserve an accurate comprehension, definite diagnosis, and firmly established management. Modern guidelines emphasize the importance of standardized procedures in prenatal counseling and genetic testing and therefore strengthen the support system for parents facing the likelihood of genetic defects in their fetuses (Reproductive Health Branch of China Maternal and Child et al., 2024). These innovations underscore the increasing applicability of precision medicine to the concerns of prenatal health. Technological development, as exemplified by non-invasive prenatal testing (NIPT), has dramatically changed the dynamics of prenatal genetic screening and diagnosis. The advent of NIPT 2.0 has remarkably enhanced the detection of fetal chromosomal aneuploidies and dominantly inherited monogenic disorders through high-throughput sequencing techniques. The latest edition of testing technologies avoids the pitfalls of earlier approaches, allowing for improved accuracy and broader detection of fetal diseases (Reproductive Health Branch of China Maternal and Child et al., 2024). However, the use of such advanced testing technologies in clinical practice provokes valid questions about optimal practices, including proper scope, targeted conditions, and protocols for genetic counseling. As stakeholders come together to craft consensus guidance for NIPT 2.0, it is extremely important that pregnant individuals are provided with credible information and support, which will eventually facilitate informed decision-making during prenatal care (Figure 10.2).

Importance of Prenatal Genetic Testing

The significance of prenatal genetic testing lies largely in its potential to identify potential chromosomal abnormalities and genetic disorders prenatally, thereby facilitating early intervention and decision-making. Through procedures such as NIPT and CVS, the medical practitioner is able to diagnose conditions like Down syndrome, Turner syndrome, and other such genetic disorders that may affect fetal growth. Such knowledge allows parents to prepare themselves for the upcoming challenges that can range from specialized medical treatment to lifestyle adjustments, even difficult choices regarding the continuation of pregnancy. Due to this, prenatal genetic testing has come to be known as a crucial tool in modern obstetrics, providing valuable information on fetal health and allowing prospective measures to take care of identified conditions. In addition, prenatal genetic screening also has significant implications for families with a history of genetic disease or habitual miscarriage. These families might harbor chromosomal abnormalities that put them at risk of transmitting harmful traits to their children. According to the investigation of recurrent pregnancy loss, detection of these types of chromosomal structural abnormalities by pre-implantation genetic testing can significantly affect future pregnancy outcomes. The capacity to identify such risks at an earlier stage not only allows for more informed reproductive decisions but also improves the prospects for achieving successful and healthy pregnancies. By utilizing technologies such as pre-implantation genetic testing for structural rearrangements (PGT-SR), couples are better placed to manage the challenges linked to genetic predispositions, thus making a compelling argument for extensive genetic assessment for personalized pregnancy care (Mahalingam et al., 2024). While prenatal genetic testing provides a list of benefits, it also has some challenges, particularly in how test results are interpreted. Uncertain results, such as those from complicated chromosomal rearrangements or mosaic embryos, demonstrate the necessity for thorough genetic counseling and additional testing. In some instances of unbalanced translocations, for example, erroneous interpretations may heighten anxiety and inappropriate decision-making among potential parents. As it is, therefore, the job of health providers is not just to conduct tests, but to also communicate results and implications to families effectively. This involves a coordinated plan incorporating genetic counseling as a component of diagnostic testing with the ultimate objective of improving patient comprehension and care in the prenatal process (Daghsni et al., 2024).

10.1. Historical Background

The history of prenatal genetic diagnosis and screening traces its roots to enormous medical advancements in the late 20th century. With the improved understanding of genetics, reproductive medicine began to apply molecular biology. The advent of techniques such as amniocentesis and CVS during this period allowed the analysis of fetal DNA during pregnancy. Initially, these methods were used mainly to detect chromosomal abnormalities and certain genetic diseases. The incorporation of these techniques into clinical use was motivated by the increased awareness of the public about genetic disorders, which made prenatal diagnosis more broadly accepted. Consequently, this set the stage for more complex screenings, aimed at informing prospective parents about potential genetic illnesses that can affect the health of their newborns. As research continued, targets for prenatal genetic testing expanded, reflecting a growing demand for more extensive screening. Importantly, the development of NIPT through the utilization of cell-free fetal DNA has revolutionized the field, offering significant enhancement in precision and safety compared to alternative approaches. The non-invasive method avoids risks associated with invasive methods while yielding precise information regarding chromosomal disorders such as Down syndrome and additional aneuploidies. Furthermore, NIPT has facilitated the exploration of more complex genetic disorders, thereby shaping the discussion on reproductive choice and parental responsibility. The implications of such developments are far-reaching in that they challenge conventional ethical issues of selective abortion and informed consent in the prenatal context. Recent studies have also highlighted the potential benefits and challenges linked to prenatal genetic screening, widening the discourse on its implementation within modern healthcare. For instance, advances in understanding diseases like gestational diabetes have necessitated a critical review and optimization of screening practices, as these conditions are increasingly recognized for their long-term health implications for the mother and the child. In addition, the discovery of circulating biomarkers, such as cell-free EBV DNA, illustrates the potential for prenatal screening to expand to cover various cancers and other major health conditions, which can further influence intervention strategies. As prenatal genetic diagnosis improves, ethical considerations come into play about access to the testing, social pressures in decision-making, and the necessity of proper communication among healthcare professionals and patients. Such complexities point to the continuing necessity of weighing medical progress against the ethical burden entailed in reproductive decision-making (Figure 10.3).

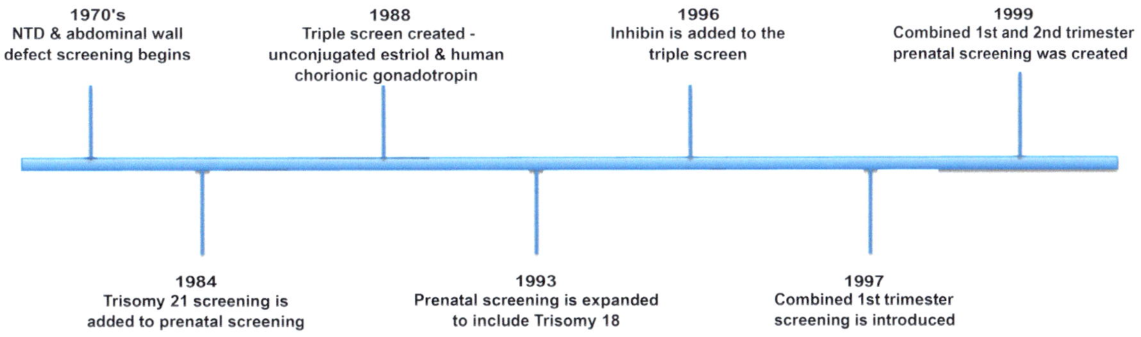

Figure 10.3. History of prenatal screening tests.

Source: https://www.researchgate.net/publication/281846413/figure/fig1/AS:614012681203724@1523403439200/History-of-prenatal-screening-tests-7-10.png.

10.1.1. Development of Prenatal Genetic Testing Techniques

The evolution of techniques in prenatal genetic testing has revolutionized the field of reproductive medicine through the early and accurate diagnosis of genetic disease. Amniocentesis and CVS have been the older techniques of sampling fetal genetic material for analysis. However, these are invasive procedures with risks such as miscarriage and potential harm to the mother and fetus. Recent developments in Non-Invasive Prenatal Testing (NIPT) through maternal blood sampling have dramatically lessened risks involved while simultaneously improving detection rates of chromosomal abnormalities. With the growing availability of these newer methods, the field of prenatal genetic diagnosis is evolving at a rapid pace, enabling clinicians to provide timely and informed decisions for pregnant couples. This, in turn, enhances perinatal care and postnatal clinical management (Purwin et al., 2024).

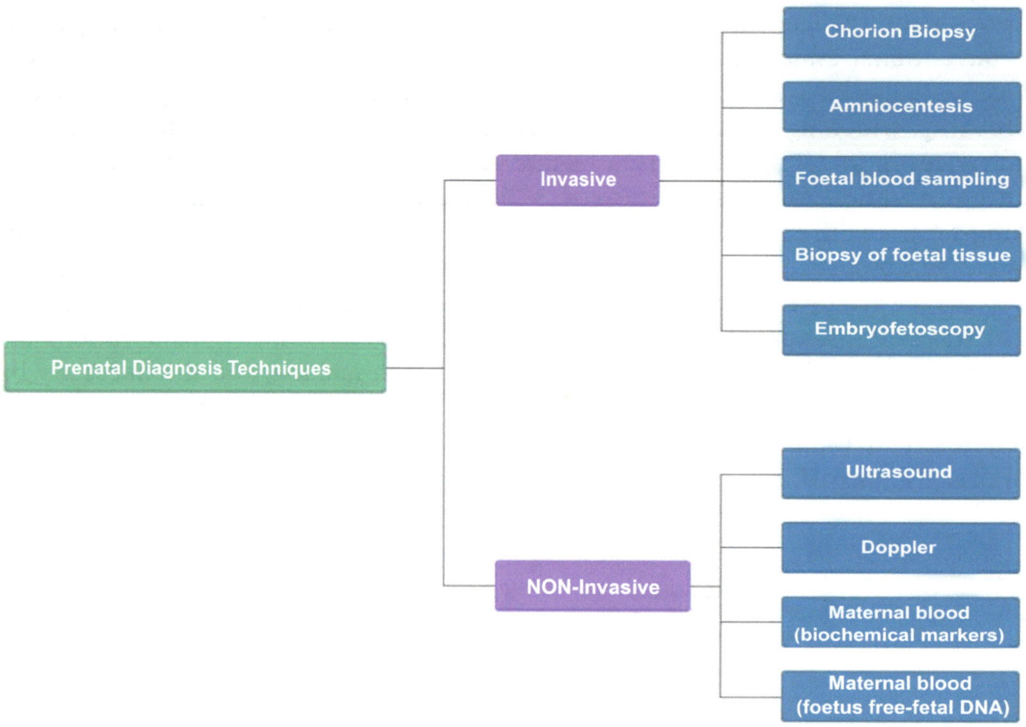

Figure 10.4. Prenatal diagnosis techniques.

Source: https://lagenetica.info/wp-content/uploads/2014/10/esquema-tecnicas-diagnostico.en_1.jpg.

Also, the advent of next-generation sequencing (NGS) has provided a very broad arena for prenatal genetic testing beyond screening for common chromosomal disorders, and it has enabled detection of a far greater number of genetic diseases. With NGS, it is possible to get large genomic data, thus facilitating the screening of multiple conditions concurrently. This has enhanced the accuracy of diagnosis and also facilitated genetic counseling for the parents, so that they receive proper information regarding any probable genetic disorder that their child is likely to inherit.

Furthermore, the application of these sophisticated techniques into clinical use has promoted the creation of specific guidelines and protocols that address the requirements of different populations. With the advancing field, the emergence of genetic testing technologies can be expected to advance preventive medicine and address a variety of medical necessities (Gao et al., 2023). In addition to this, prenatal genetic testing is an important measure in reducing the burden of genetic disease on affected families. Disorders like Prader-Willi syndrome (PWS) illustrate the tremendous significance of early diagnosis through advanced screening protocols. PWS can be significantly affected by early diagnosis, allowing for early intervention to optimize quality of life and long-term outcomes. Given the complexities of genetic disorders, research into ideal diagnostic workflows and the efficacy of novel techniques is continuous. The combination of classical methodologies with new technologies has the potential to form more comprehensive and efficient prenatal screening workflows. Consequently, the continued advancement of prenatal genetic testing procedures is an important way forward towards effective and knowledgeable prenatal care (Gao et al., 2023) (Figure 10.4).

10.1.2. Milestones in Genetic Research and Technology

Significant advances in genetic studies and technological advances have contributed immensely to the science of prenatal genetic diagnosis and screening. Of particular note was the successful completion of the Human Genome Project in 2003, which fully mapped the entire human genome. This remarkable feat has made it possible for a variety of genetic testing methods to be employed, enabling medical practitioners to identify genetic diseases before birth with unprecedented accuracy. Since the advent of NGS technologies, fetal DNA processing has become faster and less expensive, revolutionizing screening protocols. Such advances allow future parents to make fully informed choices regarding their pregnancies, and consequently save lives, highlighting the value of genetic information in perinatal medicine. The ramifications of these developments are extensive, opening the door to progress in maternal-fetal medicine while also bringing up ethical concerns about the possibility of selective termination based on genetic information. Furthermore, the introduction of genetic technology has led to an expansion of prenatal diagnostic testing offered to pregnant women. NIPT was among the most significant recent developments, making it possible to screen for conditions such as Down syndrome through the analysis of cell-free fetal DNA in the blood of a mother. The new technology is less risky to both mother and fetus than the traditionally used invasive methods with potential complications. The groundbreaking nature of NIPT is depicted by its rapid adoption in various healthcare systems and has significantly influenced maternal-fetal medicine. This extensive use mirrors a paradigm shift to safer, more precise prenatal screenings. As medical centers persist in exploring multifarious genetic methodologies, the prenatal screening discipline is transforming with sophisticated advancement, providing patients with more comprehensive information about their unborn children's health. While the trajectory of genetic research and its ensuing technologies has been encouraging, it is crucial to consider the various social and ethical implications that accompany such advancements. As a consequence of increased access to genetic information, privacy concerns, discrimination, and informed consent in the context of prenatal genetic testing have attracted increased scrutiny. For example, the possibility of stigmatization of fetuses identified with genetic disorders raises ethical questions about the application of technology that could facilitate selective abortion. Moreover, there remain inherent difficulties of conveying genetic information to parents, particularly in relation to clear and compassionate presentation of complicated results. To properly deal with these challenges, a requirement exists to embrace multidisciplinary interventions with scientific progress in mind as well as psychosocial considerations. As such, prenatal genetic testing and screening must go hand in hand with ethics discussions to prepare parents to make choices that reflect their beliefs and values (Blank et al., 2019; Cools et al., 2018) (Figure 10.5).

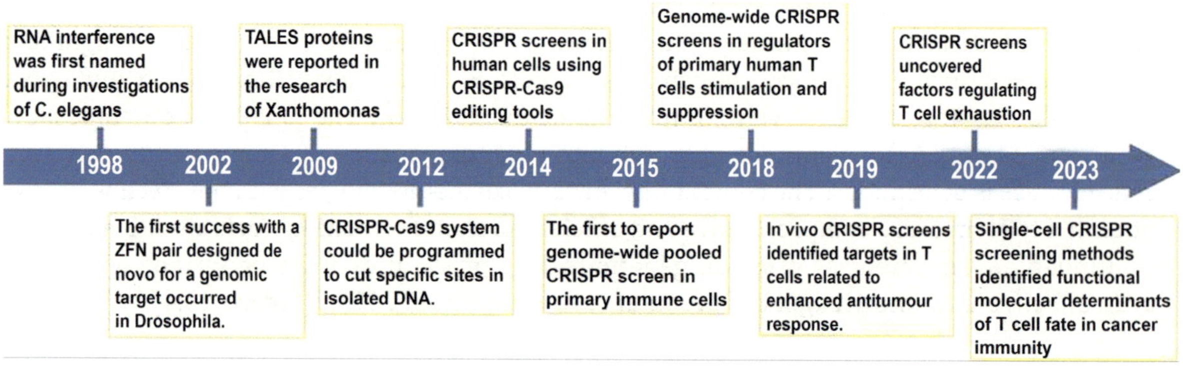

Figure 10.5. Milestones in genetic research and technology.

Source: https://www.researchgate.net/publication/379602073/figure/fig2/AS:11431281234685593@1712370734525/Timeline-of-major-milestones-in-researches-of-genetic-engineering-and-T-cell-associated.png.

10.1.3. Evolution of Public Perception Regarding Genetic Testing

The development of public attitude towards genetic testing has undergone remarkable changes during the past couple of decades because of scientific advances and increased awareness. Initially, genetic testing was viewed with suspicion and ethical apprehensions regarding its implications for confidentiality and discrimination. People were concerned that genetic information would fall into the wrong hands of employers or insurance organizations, and result in social stigma or exclusion. As awareness increased, facilitated especially by campaigns of advocacy and education, the discourse started moving towards embracing the possible advantages, for example, early detection of disease and informed reproductive decision-making. The growing practice of genetic testing in medicine has, in turn, promoted a greater appreciation of its application in prenatal diagnosis, where it is regarded as an important tool for prospective parents who want to know the genetic status of their embryos and fetuses. Cultural and geographical differences have also significantly influenced public perceptions of genetic testing, underlining the complex relationship between societal values, ethical concerns, and health practices. In countries such as Serbia, parliamentary measures such as the 2015 "Zoja's Law" have been crucial to public sensitization while addressing ethical concerns, thereby promoting acceptance not only within the medical community but even among prospective patients. Not only did the law define rights and obligations concerning genetic services, but it also guaranteed access to essential genetic tests, with the government's contribution towards shaping public opinion being particularly noteworthy. Such legislative action can have the power to both mirror and influence public opinion, as it gives legitimacy to genetic testing practices, thus stimulating debate regarding the social and ethical ramifications of reproductive health advances. In addition, recent public opinion polls indicate increasing public openness to prenatal genetic testing. Research carried out in different areas, particularly in the Jazan region of Saudi Arabia, demonstrates favorable attitudes toward premarital and prenatal genetic screening. This shows that uptake is high with individuals realizing the benefits of such procedures in the prevention of genetic disorders. About 79.1% of the respondents were in favor of mandatory government genetic screening prior to marriage, with a high percentage showing readiness to accept testing during pregnancy, portraying a pragmatic attitude towards genetic risk. These changes in opinion reflect growing acceptance of genetic testing as part of responsible reproductive decision-making, demonstrating that public opinion is not fixed but fluid, being sensitive to developments within the practice of medicine and the trajectory of social norms. Generally, the greater acceptability of genetic testing within the general population is a reflection of the debate that continues to surround its place in contemporary healthcare, especially as it pertains to prenatal screening and diagnosis.

10.2. Types of Prenatal Genetic Testing

The terrain of prenatal genetic screening involves constructing a range of methodologies aimed at examining genetic factors for health conditions prior to birth. Of these, NIPT has become a favored option through its use of a mere blood test from the mother to screen fetal DNA present in her blood. This method has high rates of accuracy for detecting chromosome conditions like Down syndrome and is praised for having a reduced risk factor compared to invasive procedures like amniocentesis or CVS. Amniocentesis, involving the extraction of amniotic fluid, and CVS, which collects placental tissue, are both considered diagnostic tests. They provide definitive results on chromosomal abnormalities but pose threats like miscarriage and are therefore less desirable to many expecting parents. By being thoroughly aware of the numerous available options, couples can make informed choices regarding their prenatal care and genetic testing plans. Elaborating on the range of prenatal testing options, carrier screening is significant in determining the risks associated with inherited genetic diseases. This form of testing is especially valuable for parents with a known family history of genetic illness or those belonging to particular ethnic groups that make them prone to particular illnesses. Carrier screening is employed to identify if one or both parents are carriers of mutations for various conditions, including cystic fibrosis, Tay-Sachs disease, and sickle cell disease. The results of this screening are helpful in allowing the couple to discover their risk of having a child with the condition, thereby assisting them in exploring the reproduction options available to them, such as IVF in conjunction with PGT. But it is crucial to ponder over the social and ethical implications of the knowledge acquired through carrier screening since they can significantly affect familial relationships and decision-making processes (Boardman et al., 2013). Ultimately, decision-making concerning prenatal genetic testing is usually guided by experiential knowledge of the conditions under inquiry among the family members. Understanding derived from relatives who are carriers of genetic disorders also significantly influences future parents' knowledge and attitudes towards testing. Qualitative interviewing has shown that some individuals derive a sense of empowerment from this knowledge within the family, which allows them to deal with the intricacies of reproductive choice. For others, there is a tension because their awareness of the consequences of a condition clashes with their aspiration to safeguard the welfare of their family. The ensuing emotional and ethical landscape foretells that knowledge of a genetic disorder should not be considered only positive; it may also generate intricacies that get in the way of decision-making during prenatal testing (Freeman et al., 2005). If we reflect on these personal stories, the more evident it becomes that the decision about prenatal genetic testing encompasses not only medical aspects but also intensely personal ones (Figure 10.6).

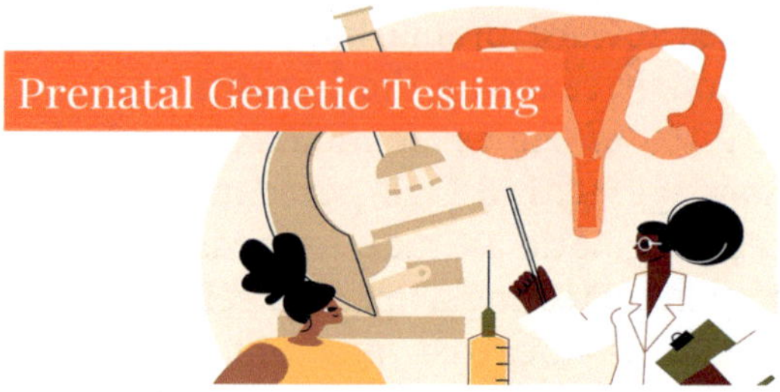

Figure 10.6. Prenatal Genetic Testing.

Source: https://external-content.duckduckgo.com/iu/?u=https%3A%2F%2Fi.ytimg.com%2Fvi%2F__oEeGl1Uik%2Fmaxresdefault.jpg&f=1&nofb=1&ipt=f449d79924de95da684a56432677a927f8576a7c7a696b0ea63a92f4188e3342.

10.2.1. Non-Invasive Prenatal Testing (NIPT)

The introduction of NIPT has revolutionized the area of prenatal genetic screening and diagnosis. A non-invasive test, NIPT involves the screening for common fetal aneuploidies, mainly trisomy 21, trisomy 18, and trisomy 13 using cell-free fetal DNA derived from maternal plasma. A safer test than more invasive testing methods such as amniocentesis, which carries a risk of miscarriage, NIPT combines accuracy with safety in prenatal testing. The introduction of NIPT has been shown to have an extremely good rate of specificity and sensitivity in the diagnosis of the conditions, lessening some of the anxiety of prospective parents and enabling effective early intervention where necessary, as shown in the large evaluation of 1081 clinical samples reported in the study (Smet et al., 2016). As much as NIPT holds a lot of promise, it is also worth considering its limitations within the area of prenatal screening.

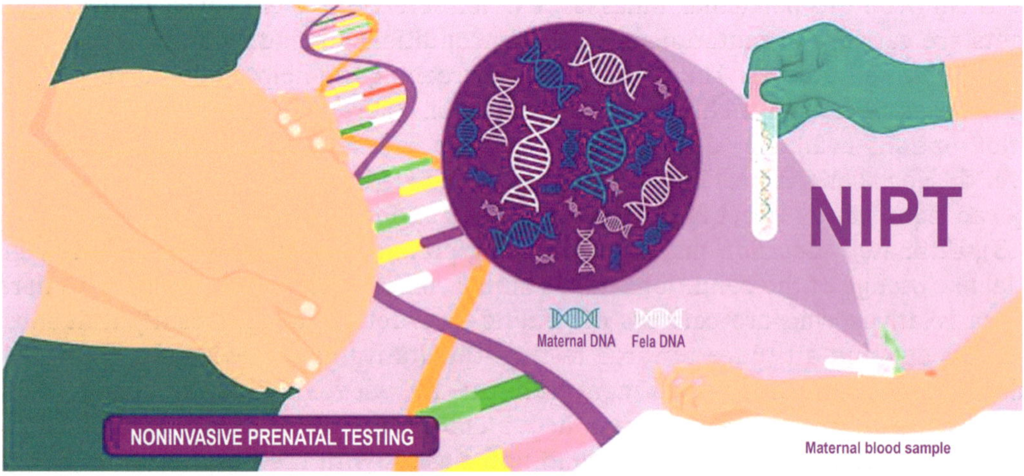

Figure 10.7. Non-invasive prenatal testing (NIPT).

Source: https://d2jx2rerrg6sh3.cloudfront.net/images/Article_Images/ImageForArticle_22565_16530523002333360.jpg.

Although the technique dramatically improves detection over conventional screening techniques, it is also significant to note that Non-Invasive Prenatal Testing (NIPT) is not a diagnostic test. The possibility of false positives and false negatives explains the necessity of follow-up invasive testing for abnormal results. A recent publication indicated that a large percentage of patients might overestimate the residual risk of aneuploidy after a negative NIPT result (Wittman et al., 2016). This misunderstanding can be attributed to the lack of thorough education on the implications of the screenings, emphasizing the need for broad genetic counseling in order to allow future parents to efficiently utilize the complicated outcomes of NIPT. Moreover, the view of NIPT's limitation appears to be linked with the level of patients' education. Female participants who had at least four years of college were shown to have a better grasp of the subtlety present in NIPT, specifically in the residual risks that stem from negative results for disorders like trisomy 13 or sex chromosome abnormalities (Wittman et al., 2016). This disparity highlights the need for effective communication in genetic counseling. Health care providers need to modify their approach to communicate the implications of NIPT results to all patients, especially those with less education. By promoting a greater appreciation of the consequences surrounding NIPT, health care providers can aid expectant parents in making knowledgeable choices regarding their prenatal care and genetic testing (Figure 10.7).

10.2.2. Chorionic Villus Sampling (CVS)

CVS is a foundation procedure in prenatal genetic screening and diagnosis. The invasive test, which is typically performed between the 10th and 13th weeks of pregnancy, allows for the testing of chorionic villi, tiny projections of the placenta that have genetic material. By sampling the villi, physicians can identify chromosomal abnormalities such as Down syndrome, cystic fibrosis, and other genetic diseases. The ability to conduct these tests early during pregnancy offers parents critical information that can be used in making decisions regarding the pregnancy's future. In this way, CVS is a significant option for individuals carrying greater risks for genetic diseases, successfully integrating sophisticated genetic technology into prenatal care. With CVS's benefits, it is essential to balance its risks, such as miscarriage risk. Though the procedure is overall considered safe when performed by experienced practitioners, evidence supports that the rate of complications can be a problem. One comparative study of outcomes among various prenatal diagnostic procedures found no overall association between chorionic villus sampling (CVS) and the onset of hypertensive disorders of pregnancy, leading researchers to suspect that the procedure itself would not lead to poor maternal outcomes (Ghazal et al., 2009).

This is comforting news that helps to dispel some of the concerns regarding the safety of CVS. Therefore, thorough counseling prior to the procedure is essential so that the expectant parents can make a decision based on a balanced understanding of the risks and benefits involved. The application of CVS is not only for common genetic disorders, but it has also revolutionized the diagnosis of rare genetic diseases. A retrospective study from a tertiary care center highlights that significant numbers of patients who had CVS were exposed to screening for disorders like muscular dystrophies and cystic fibrosis (Dileep et al., 2020). Advances in laboratory techniques and DNA banking have made it possible to enhance the detection of these less common but clinically significant disorders. In addition, the integration of specialist care teams—fetal medicine specialists, pediatric geneticists, and laboratory personnel—makes genetic counseling and diagnosis more effective. This multi-disciplinary approach ensures that families receive individualized care, thus increasing the need for invasive testing options like CVS while enhancing patient satisfaction in prenatal genetic diagnosis (Figure 10.8).

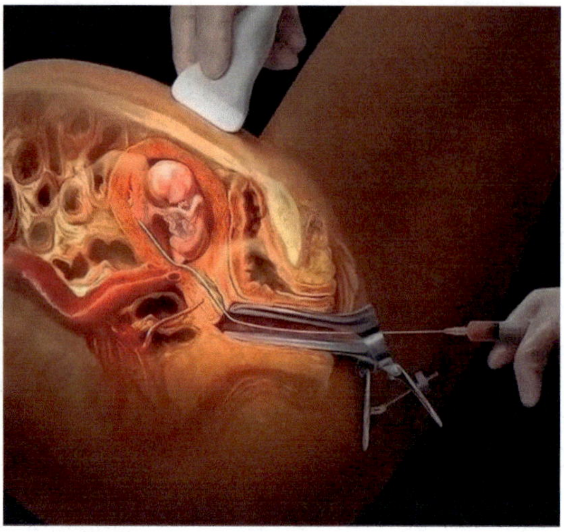

Figure 10.8. Chorionic villus sampling (CVS).

Source: https://www.parvathihospital.com/wp-content/uploads/elementor/thumbs/Chorionic-Villous-Sampling-qscvob47p9h9cwyjwvglj5t3ixew87khblwvpsdwno.jpg.

10.2.3. Amniocentesis

Amniocentesis is an essential procedure within the field of prenatal genetic diagnosis and screening that is performed primarily to evaluate genetic abnormalities in the developing fetus. The invasive diagnostic procedure entails the extraction of amniotic fluid from the amniotic sac that encloses the fetus, typically carried out between the 15th and 20th week of pregnancy. The amniotic fluid also has fetal cells along with a range of biochemical markers, which can be tested for chromosomal disorders, i.e., Down syndrome, cystic fibrosis, and other genetic disorders. As a valuable option for prospective parents who are under hereditary risk, amniocentesis has its pros and cons. Though it yields a definite diagnosis that may dictate medical as well as personal choice, the test is associated with a minor risk of miscarriage, which is estimated to be about 1%. This risk requires careful consideration and direction for parents before proceeding with the test. The role of amniocentesis in prenatal genetic screening is particularly vital for pregnancies that pose a high risk of genetic disorder. For instance, maternal age and family medical history are key considerations in determining whether amniocentesis is a viable option. This practice is fundamentally unlike non-invasive prenatal screening, which often cannot achieve comparable diagnostic precision. The capacity to detect specific mutations associated with conditions like Marfan syndrome demonstrates the value of amniocentesis for facilitating informed parental choice in terms of management and care following birth, as evidenced by recent developments in genetic testing (Aragon-Martin et al., 2016).

By implication, amniocentesis not only enables timely diagnosis but also provides a platform for improved healthcare planning designed to respond to the specific needs of the child found. Beyond this, ethical implications surrounding amniocentesis warrant careful scrutiny. The choice to obtain such a procedure involves weighing the possible benefits against the ethical implications of genetic knowledge and the consequent decisions prompted by such knowledge. Whereas parents might recognize the value of having the ability to prepare for the arrival of a child with special needs, they also might be confronted with the high emotional toll of such decisions, including the possibility of pregnancy termination due to test outcomes. With advancement in prenatal genetic screening, a separation of prenatal and genetic screening is essential because labeling these two tests as the same may result in confusion regarding their interpretation and scope. Proper communication and counseling by health practitioners, therefore, remain essential for parents while they make the involved decision regarding amniocentesis and prenatal genetic diagnosis (Figure 10.9).

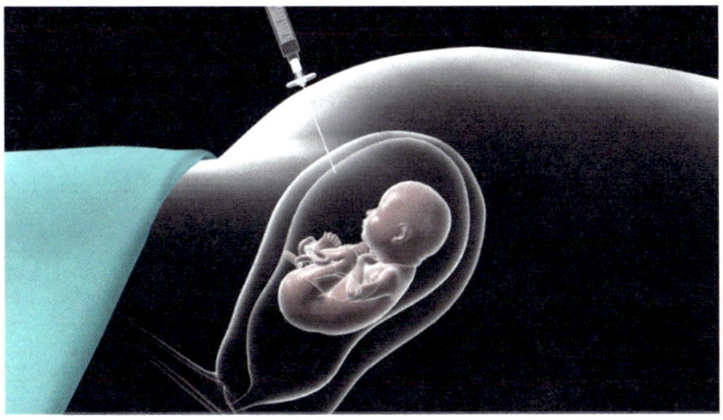

Figure 10.9. Amniocentesis.

Source: https://d2yjegym0lbr1w.cloudfront.net/thumbs/amniocentesis_1280.jpg?v=201406114.

10.3. Ethical Considerations

The ethical issues involved in prenatal genetic screening and diagnosis are complex, involving autonomy, informed consent, and the possibility of discrimination. Informed consent demands that patients be made completely aware of the implications of genetic testing as well as the potential results of such testing. This is especially complicated when factoring in NIPT, as it offers both a possibility of less risk to the fetus and a complicated set of ethical issues. As highlighted by Mahesh et al. (2024), there is a necessity to make the accuracy of test outcomes, factors affecting these outcomes, and internal limitations involved in the testing process explicit to prospective parents. Not only does this uphold the value of autonomy but also enhances trust between healthcare providers and families who are grappling with such life-changing decisions. Further, there are ethical implications of the possible misuse of genetic information for discriminatory reasons. The development of advanced screening technologies such as NIPT has been accompanied by concerns about the possibility of identifying genetic defects that can lead to stigmatization in society or an eugenics-driven philosophy. The need to make certain that genetic information is being utilized ethically and equitably cannot be overemphasized. As outlined in Lugo (2023), healthcare providers should carry out prenatal genetic diagnosis under the principles of beneficence—doing good for patients—and non-maleficence—doing no harm. Preventive steps would have to be instituted to prevent misuse of genetic information so that decisions of future parents are in line with fully informed choices rather than cultural pressure or genetic determinism. The moral framework within which prenatal genetic diagnosis is utilized also relies upon multicultural, social, and legal views. Societies classify the interpretation of genetic information on the basis of various ethical considerations that can hinder the provision of universal healthcare guidance. Genetic counseling professionals have to work through such complexities with respect for given cultural norms as well as maintaining ethical principles in practice. The guidelines articulated by Lugo (2023) indicate that such adherence is to be brought about through conformity to basic bioethical principles, with a focus on respect for autonomy and informed consent, and a lack of discrimination. It is this balance that will be required to preserve ethical standards and promote equal access to prenatal genetic care, thereby enabling a broader model of reproductive health.

10.3.1. Informed Consent and Patient Autonomy

The principle of informed consent is extremely significant in the area of prenatal genetic screening and diagnosis since it is closely related to the autonomy of the patient. The principle requires that patients be aware of the full implications of being subjected to different genetic tests, such as possible risks and results. The process, however, is usually incomplete since most patients are likely to be overwhelmed with too much information. In spite of recommendations for thorough discussion before screening, empirical evidence supports the fact that the majority of patients do not like to engage in profound moral reflection on their decisions. This observation identifies a significant gap in making sure the informed consent process is fulfilling the function of confirming medical decisions with patients' values and goals of care (Megan et al., 2025). It is therefore important that practitioners achieve a balance between providing necessary information and enabling patients to make choices that are consistent with their own beliefs and situation. The ethical aspect of informed consent is especially important in the practice of prenatal screening, where implications include both fetal outcome and maternal health. Individuals confronting the prospect of a positive screening result frequently demonstrate considerable anxiety, exacerbated by a perceived deficiency in support following the screening process. Present strategies highlight a consent process that is heavily laden with information; however, this model may prove unfeasible, especially in contexts where resources are constrained. A different framework, known as just-in-time consent, suggests that essential dialogues should take place precisely when they are most necessary—namely, when families obtain their screening results. This transition seeks to maximize support provided to patients while concurrently maintaining ethical principles, thereby allowing patients to engage in values-based decision-making in accordance with individual circumstances (Megan et al., 2025). It recognizes the emotional intricacies involved in prenatal care and seeks to offer rapid guidance in dealing with them. Incorporation of artificial intelligence (AI) technologies within prenatal genetic testing also forces further complexity on the issues of informed consent and patient autonomy. Though artificial intelligence has potential advantages like personalized diagnostic information, it also comes with important ethical issues in the form of algorithmic bias, data privacy, and decision-making transparency. The use of uninterpretable black box AI systems has the potential to subvert the fundamental principle of informed consent by obscuring the decision-making process and the reasons why particular decisions are arrived at. Furthermore, biased algorithms may reinforce health disparities, thereby nullifying the principle of equal care. Therefore, medical education must evolve to prepare the next generation of healthcare professionals to engage with these technologies responsibly so that informed consent procedures are not only a question of technical understanding but an exercise also devoted to patient-centered values and ethical regard (Figure 10.10).

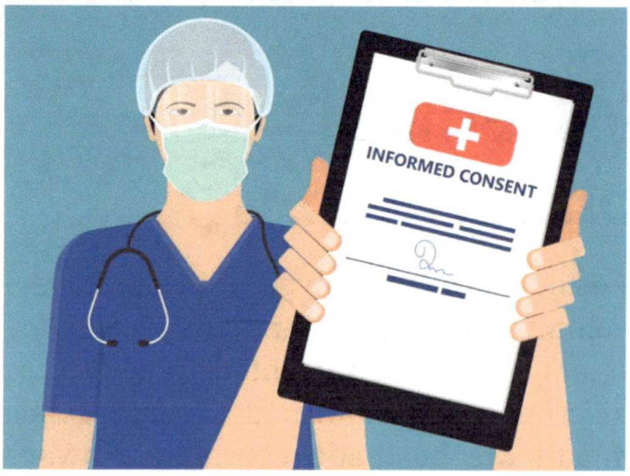

Figure 10.10. Informed consent and patient autonomy.

Source: https://d2jx2rerrg6sh3.cloudfront.net/images/Article_Images/ImageForArticle_22535_16528938764304702.jpg.

10.3.2. Potential for Discrimination Based on Genetic Information

The possibility of discrimination on the basis of genetic information is a significant issue in the context of prenatal genetic screening and diagnosis. As genetic testing technologies improve, making identification of a range of conditions possible, so too does the possibility of stigmatization associated with such findings increase. The discrimination can take many forms, ranging from individual prejudices within the healthcare sector to societal implications such as employment and insurance discrimination. These consequences threaten to entrench existing inequalities, especially for marginalized communities who are already more likely to receive unequal care in healthcare facilities. The ethical implications of the use of genetic information, as well as the availability of such data, require careful examination to limit the possibilities of discriminatory practices against individuals grouped by special genetic indicators. It is also important to develop environments that prioritize patient secrecy and ensure that genetic data is used solely for therapeutic purposes without punitive repercussions. The opinions held by some communities towards prenatal screening might even complicate the genetic discrimination dynamics further. For instance, a study conducted with Black and South Asian parents establishes commonality in the acceptance of prenatal screenings among them, driven by the desire to gain essential health information about their unborn children. However, there is widespread anxiety regarding invasive testing due to the very risks involved, as well as fear of the use of genetic information on the part of healthcare providers and societal institutions. The need for culturally sensitive care is paramount; healthcare systems have to establish trust with these populations in order to encourage open discussions regarding genetic risk free of fear of discrimination or negative repercussions. As suggested by Peter et al. (2025), learning the distinctive viewpoints of these populations is critical to forging fair healthcare policy that respects personal choice and protects against genetic discrimination threat. Also, alongside ethical issues associated with genetic information utilization, the construction of guideline structures is necessary to avert discrimination in actual practice. A healthcare workforce that is well-educated can offer better guidance on prenatal screening alternatives, simultaneously emphasizing the importance of ethical concerns about genetic information. As noted by Pande et al. (2025), the development of standard protocols for prenatal screening will be capable of contributing significantly to primary healthcare providers making informed choices in the area of genetic testing, thereby reducing concerns related to discrimination. By raising the importance of genetic counseling in addition to extensive education for both patients and healthcare professionals, it is possible to reduce the negative impacts that come with the abuse of genetic information. Finally, well-thought-out policies that protect individuals from discrimination based on genetic susceptibility are key to developing a more equitable healthcare environment where each individual feels a sense of safety and guidance in prenatal care decisions.

10.3.3. The Moral Implications of Selective Termination

The procedure of selective termination following prenatal genetic diagnosis brings up grave ethical considerations, inviting an examination of social norms regarding disability and the role of parenthood. While genetic screening advances allow parents to make informed choices regarding the health of their possible offspring, pregnancy termination due to genetic abnormalities offers a contentious moral terrain. Empirical studies, such as the study that established the critical role of perceived morality in shaping attitudes toward genetic testing, demonstrate that individuals examine the consequences of their decisions in relation to their moral values and societal norms (Maftei et al., 2022). The intricacy of the dilemma is compounded when one takes into account the diverse elements that enter the picture in such decisions, such as demographic factors and individual beliefs, thereby underscoring the complex nature of defining a "desirable" life and to whom the right of choice belongs. The ethical case for selective abortion is commonly argued on utilitarian grounds, weighing the perceived advantages to the family and society against the intrinsic worth of every human life. Women who participated in research investigating their decisions about future disabilities indicated that disabilities such as Down syndrome triggered long discussions about termination, with societal biases about quality of life prevailing (Maftei et al., 2022). Moreover, parents who experienced the emotional toll of having to make such decisions highlight an even bigger ethical dilemma: does the availability of selective termination perpetuate ableist ideology, that the lives which are found to be less than ideal are not worth living? The inevitable tensions in such arguments point to the imperative of cautious consideration of the repercussions of such choices, not only on the individual but also on society as a whole, thus challenging whether it is right to pre-judge the value of a future life. The legal and ethical foundations of prenatal testing and selective abortion continue to evolve, and this further compounds the challenges of decision-making for prospective parents.

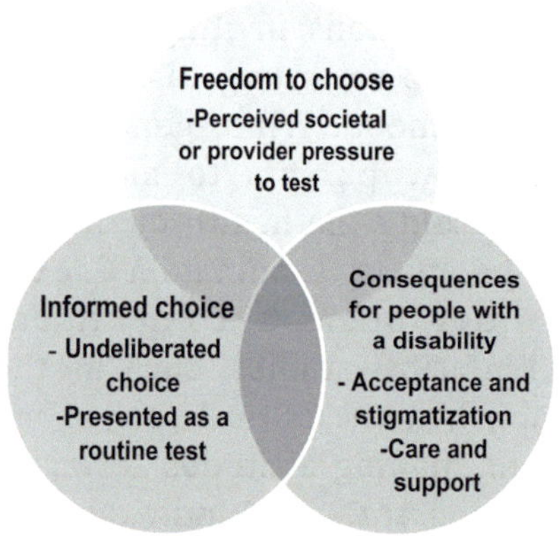

Figure 10.11. The moral implications of selective termination in prenatal genetic diagnosis.

Source: https://media.springernature.com/m685/springer-static/image/art%3A10.1038%2Fs41431-021-00940-8/MediaObjects/41431_2021_940_Fig1_HTML.png.

As technology progresses, so do the policies and procedures associated with it, usually remaining behind the advancements in society and bringing about confusion within the ethical standards. Such disparity gives rise to serious concerns about the ethical accountability of healthcare professionals to provide non-directive counseling while navigating through the complexities of personal values and social norms. The moral principle of non-directiveness, which is at the heart of genetic counseling practice, is subject to question as counselors grapple with their own biases as well as with the requirement to preserve parental autonomy. The new reproductive terrain demands continued argument over the ethical issues of selective termination, compelling society to face difficult truths about disability, value, and the human condition (Figure 10.11).

10.4. Benefits of Prenatal Genetic Diagnosis

The use of prenatal genetic diagnosis presents various benefits that significantly increase the potential for good outcomes in pregnancies. By identifying genetic disorders, like cystic fibrosis, early, potential parents can make informed choices regarding how to proceed with their pregnancies. Genetic screening can potentially determine illnesses that are asymptomatic until later in life, hence giving parents as well as medical practitioners a chance to prepare for possibly extensive medical interventions. Greater focus on early detection of problems via genetic screening can also result in immense savings in medical expenses, since early treatment tends to avert the development of illnesses requiring long-term medical care in the future. This preventive strategy underlines the practical advantages contained in prenatal genetic diagnosis, and it is one of the most important aspects of modern maternal-fetal medicine. Aside from this, prenatal genetic diagnosis is also an important instrument for facilitating parents' empowerment by increasing autonomy in reproductive decision-making. On being informed of potential genetic disorders, parents can benefit from seeking consultations with medical practitioners in order to understand the extensive range of options available to them. These options can include anticipatory preparation for likely medical interventions or, in some cases, the possibility of considering terminating the pregnancy if serious conditions are discovered. The openness provided by this clarity aids in making informed choices, so that families are not caught off guard by the problems that may develop after the birth of a child with genetic disorders. Better communication between parents and healthcare providers can result in better psychological outcomes, as parents can feel more in charge of their reproductive choices through informed consent and planned parental decision (Freeman et al., 2005). Additionally, prenatal genetic diagnosis can serve as a stimulus for broad social and ethical debate regarding genetic testing and its consequences. While developing these test technologies, it is necessary to debate the ethical issues that will most likely be generated, specifically with regard to how fetuses identified with genetic diseases will be managed. Detailed examination of the pros and cons of such tests can inform health policy, thereby ensuring it addresses the ethical dimensions. Greater public awareness of such issues can also stimulate debate that, in turn, can contribute towards finer definitions of healthy reproductive options. As society grapples with the implications of genetic diagnosis, discussions about the responsibilities of medical practitioners, the rights of parents, and the implications for people with disabilities come to the fore, highlighting the need for large-scale ethical frameworks as prenatal genetic diagnosis becomes a routine practice (Figure 10.12).

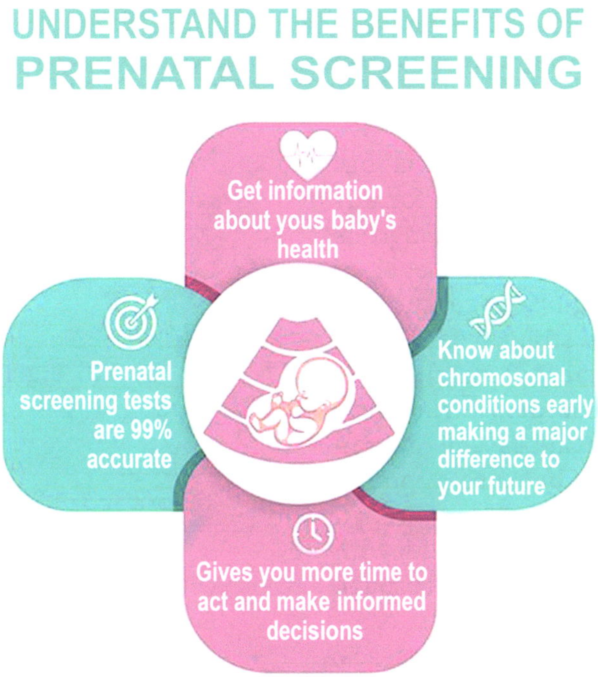

Figure 10.12. Benefits of prenatal genetic diagnosis.

Source: https://www.gargfetalmedicinecentre.com/wp-content/uploads/2020/10/Ist-trimester-screening.png.

10.4.1. Early Detection of Genetic Disorders

Early detection of genetic diseases has been an essential part of prenatal genetic screening and diagnosis. With advancements in technology, techniques like noninvasive prenatal testing (NIPT) and cell-free DNA (cfDNA) screening have revolutionized the field of prenatal care. These new techniques enable the identification of chromosomal disorders and specific genetic disorders with greater precision than conventional screening tests. Notably, cfDNA testing can also identify not only aneuploidies but also sub-chromosomal copy number variations. While these advances are in place, application of cfDNA for dominant single-gene disorders is still not optimized within the general obstetric population, which marks a need for more extensive dissemination and integration of such technologies into the routine prenatal care (Liao et al., 2025). The inclusion of noninvasive genetic screening as a part of standard prenatal testing has significant implications for prospective parents, as it gives them important information before they give birth. This enables decision-making about potential interventions or preparation for any illness that may arise. Previously, numerous families have experienced a high level of uncertainty about undiagnosed conditions, which has caused emotional strain in addition to expense. The capacity of current prenatal genetic screening to detect some disorders during early pregnancy not only maximizes the overall management of pregnancy but also supports improved mental well-being of parents through the minimization of anxiety associated with undiagnosed congenital abnormalities. Through NIPT and cfDNA screening, medical professionals can initiate early intervention on health issues, thereby providing a favorable family atmosphere (Shiekedien et al., 2024). Yet, notwithstanding the encouraging potential presented by these prenatal diagnostic tests, numerous challenges remain that preclude the general use of early detection of genetic disorders. Some of the key challenges are disparities in access to testing, access to unbiased genetic counseling services, and ethical issues in prenatal genetic diagnosis. As health systems rush to implement these new testing techniques, there is a necessity to establish strong mechanisms guaranteeing informed consent, adequate counseling, and fairness in access for disparate groups. Moreover, the introduction of these tests also demands ongoing training for healthcare professionals to ensure the quality and precision of genetic screening tests. Overcoming these challenges will not only improve the efficacy of early diagnosis of genetic disorders but also support the overall objective of healthy pregnancies and favorable results for families (Liao et al., 2025) (Figure 10.13).

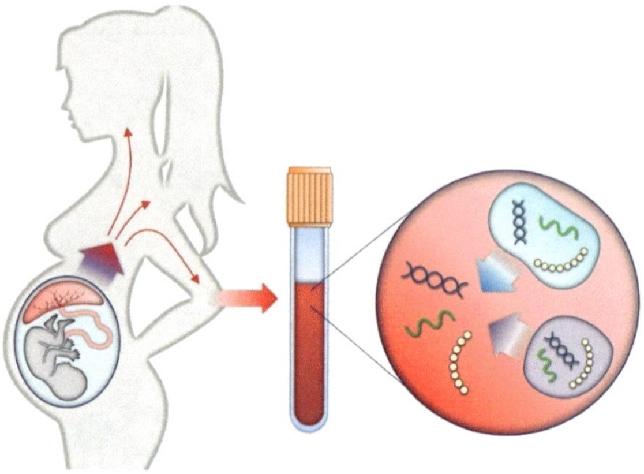

Figure 10.13. Early detection of genetic disorders.

Source: https://d7xvj3qn4ee4u.cloudfront.net/img/blog/230811_NIPT.webp.

10.4.2. Informed Decision-Making for Prospective Parents

The decision-making process for potential parents in the event of prenatal genetic screening and diagnosis is beholden to an appropriate comprehension of medical, psychologic, and social determinants. After receiving a prenatal diagnosis (PND), parents are frequently confronted with a range of possibilities, the choice being conditional on the interaction of anomalies identified by ultrasound, karyotype results, and the success of prenatal counseling. Research confirms that successful genetic counseling has the potential to enable parents to carefully weigh their alternatives, and hence achieve a more informed decision-making process with respect to potential interventions. The need exists to deal with the numerous complex determinants of parental choice; hence, the application of patient-centered and non-directive approaches to counseling can considerably strengthen parents' capacities for making value-consistent and situation-specific choices, ultimately resulting in improved outcomes for both parents and children (Dorf et al., 2025). The importance of tailoring information and resources to specific families cannot be overstated. Demographic factors, such as age, reproductive history, and socio-cultural status, are shown to have a powerful impact on parents' attitudes towards prenatal screening and testing. Even more so in Black and South Asian groups, participants expressed a strong desire for information, showing how personal, cultural, and religious values mediate their perceptions of genetic testing (Peter et al., 2025). Knowledge of the specific factors influencing various populations can aid healthcare providers in the development of those factors required to obtain trust and deliver equal care. Through the provision of a collaborative atmosphere in which parents feel free to express their opinions and concerns, healthcare providers can help ensure that the information given facilitates informed choices considerate of the cultural circumstances and personal needs of families. Decision-making while being informed is not only about obtaining medical information but is also largely reliant on emotional and social support networks available for the prospective parents. The impact of family dynamics, in addition to the dynamic of their respective groups of friends, is a critical factor in decision-making processes that entail prenatal testing. The vast majority of parents turn to close family members and friends for comfort and advice prior to reaching important medical decisions. This highlights the necessity for healthcare providers to manage the family as a unit, understanding that decisions by prospective parents frequently involve advice and feelings of multiple stakeholders. Through the adoption of a holistic model acknowledging the familial and social dimensions of decision-making, healthcare systems can enhance the support provided to pregnant parents in order to develop an environment where informed choices are made confidently (Peter et al., 2025) (Figure 10.14).

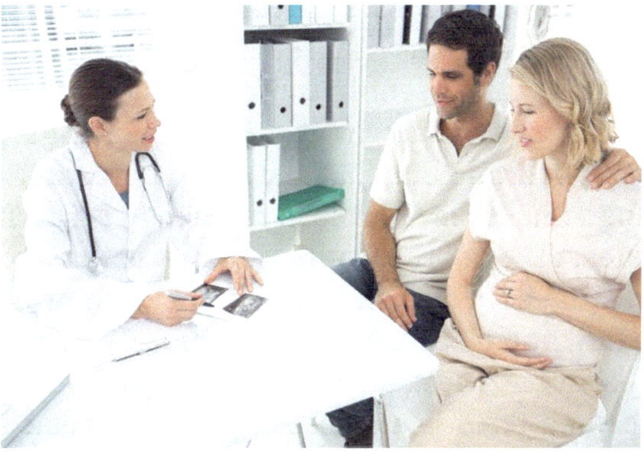

Figure 10.14. Informed decision-making for prospective parents.

Source: https://ambadyscan.com/wp-content/uploads/2024/09/gynaecologist-explaining-reports-expectant-couple_13339-97179.jpg.

10.4.3. Potential for Improved Health Outcomes for the Child

The promise of better health status in children using prenatal genetic diagnosis and screening functions at various levels, more so when it comes to the prevention of genetic disorders that have a hereditary nature. Using techniques like Preimplantation Genetic Testing for Monogenic disorders (PGT-M), parents are able to avoid transferring established genetic diseases to their offspring, effectively lowering the occurrence of genetic disorders within families. This targeted approach not only protects the child's near-term health but also lessens the long-term medical burden on families and healthcare systems. For example, as noted in research specific to assisted reproductive technologies, the integration of preimplantation genetic testing (PGT) is more clearly recognized as a normative practice, emphasizing the idea that parents' informed choices can result in improved health for the next generation and support overall public health goals (Turrini et al., 2025). Also, economic considerations that come into play with genetic testing provide a significant contribution to its advantages, making a strong case for incorporating it into standard prenatal care procedures. Research on thalassemia control in Thailand demonstrates how normal screening combined with genetic testing can result in significant savings in costs, pointing out that the early detection of genetic risks plays a role in reducing healthcare expenses over the course of the child's life. Investment in diagnostic technologies improves health outcomes by enabling more informed reproductive decisions and, meanwhile, reduce the long-term health costs of unmanaged or poorly managed genetic illnesses. Such a preventive approach proves genetic testing is more than a clinical instrument but also a fundamental public health program aimed at optimizing health gains for both individuals and the entire society (Malasai et al., 2025). Moreover, the discussion about prenatal genetic diagnosis underlines the role and power of future parents to make well-informed decisions in a way that can enhance their children's health. In the wake of developments in genetic screening technology, the shifting storyline within assisted reproduction offers new possibilities for parents to rectify risks of genetic disorders. The increased dependency on genetic data fosters a moral and ethical environment in which the onus for a healthy child increasingly shifts to the parents. This tendency may give rise to an anticipatory strategy, in which parents are motivated to take prophylactic interventions founded on genetic data, developing the overall health of the future generation. The provision of information and choice to parents strongly enhances the prospects of achieving better health outcomes for children, thereby underlining the central role of prenatal genetic screening and diagnosis within current reproductive healthcare practice (Turrini et al., 2025).

10.5. Risks and Limitations

Application of prenatal genetic screening and diagnosis involves various risks and limitations that can significantly influence patient outcomes and decisions. Among the problems is the risk of experiencing false-positive or false-negative results from tests, which may initiate unnecessary distress or, on the contrary, provide a false assurance of the health of the fetus. This inconsistency is certain to result in emotional stress and affect decision making in prospective parents. Additionally, the invasiveness of certain diagnostic procedures, such as amniocentesis or CVS, is attended by risks of complications, i.e., miscarriage and infection. Fear of such complications generally leads to low uptake of these potentially life-saving tests, particularly in disadvantaged populations. Culturally grounded discussions that acknowledge these concerns are instrumental to the establishment of trust between healthcare providers and patients, as seen in research with Black and South Asian populations citing invasive procedure concerns (Peter et al., 2025). A further significant limitation of prenatal genetic testing is that research investigations do not have adequate diversity in populations, which affects the applicability of results across various cultural and ethnic populations. For instance, the majority of prenatal screening protocols have been established using data from predominantly White populations, which can lead to the exclusion of genetic variations that are more likely to occur in Black, South Asian, or other underrepresented populations. This underrepresentation has the potential to generate disparities in both access to, and the effectiveness of, prenatal care. In addition, caregivers might not have the requisite education to appropriately interpret results for these varied populations, making inappropriate clinical choices. Greater awareness and comprehension of the intricacies in varied populations is central to improving both the availability and quality of prenatal care, as noted in recent research exploring parental attitudes toward prenatal screening (Pande et al., 2025). Furthermore, the moral implications of prenatal genetic screening and diagnosis increase their complexity of use. The problem of selective abortion following genetic testing raises especially grave ethical concerns for pregnant women and healthcare providers. Compulsion to undertake testing and follow-up interventions according to perceived desirable genetic characteristics is also bound to generate societal pressures surrounding what is deemed a desirable birth outcome. Furthermore, privacy issues and the possibility of misuse of genetic information intensify these ethical issues. Informed consent and transparency become paramount as parents have to traverse complicated emotional paths in deciding about prenatal screening. As the profession develops, it is essential that medical professionals uphold ethical principles and foster an atmosphere where future parents are supported in their decisions, while simultaneously acknowledging the constraints that are implicit in the present prenatal screening system (Pande et al., 2025; Peter et al., 2025).

10.5.1. False Positives and False Negatives

The occurrence of false positives and false negatives for prenatal genetic diagnosis and screening is a major concern for both medical practitioners and expectant parents. False positives are the results obtained when a diagnostic test indicates the existence of a genetic disorder when in fact there is none, potentially causing needless emotional upset as well as unneeded medical procedures. On the other hand, false negatives show that a diagnostic test is unable to identify an existing condition, and this can lead to the loss of early treatment and proper intervention. Such inaccuracy is of great concern, particularly in screening for such diseases as cystic fibrosis, where the implications of false diagnosis can seriously impact family dynamics as well as decision-making. As there is a development in the technology of genetic tests, their accuracy and reliability must be evaluated to help guarantee that parents are provided with meaningful results that are not complicated by unwarranted distress or false reassurance. New genetic tests based on methods such as restriction fragment length polymorphisms (RFLPs) have enhanced the prospects for prenatal diagnosis of genetic disease such as cystic fibrosis. Risks of false positives and false negatives need to be carefully considered. The use of tests with lower specificity for universal prenatal screening leads to a significant rise in the likelihood of false positives, which can cause unnecessary worry and even lead to the elective termination of normal fetuses. It is, therefore, important that prenatal testing programs prioritize the development of highly specific tests in order to reduce the chances of false positives while at the same time minimizing the rate of false negatives. Current debate on prenatal testing highlights the importance of examining ethical issues of such technologies to avoid coercive utilization and parental choice-making informed about reproductive issues. The significance of examining issues concerning false positives and false negatives is applicable to developing new prenatal genetic testing technologies' technology assessment process. Delphi technique used by the health technology assessment professionals stresses the need for incorporating major questions into the evaluation of such tests, more precisely with the emphasis on their accuracy and practical implications. This enables the development of consensus among an interdisciplinary group of professionals to define what elements of false positive and false negative rates are most vital to incorporate in HTA reports. By a methodical approach to such concerns, stakeholders can minimize the adverse outcomes related to incorrect test results, increase the utility of genetic screening, and facilitate fully informed decision-making for families. As prenatal genetic diagnosis technologies advance, it will be essential to deal with the technical and ethical aspects of false positives and negatives, which will be central to the ethical application of these breakthrough technologies (Freeman et al., 2005) (Figure 10.15).

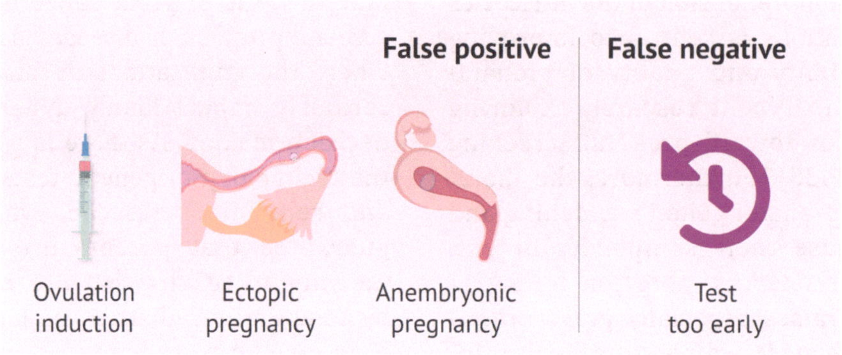

Figure 10.15. False positives and false negatives.

Source: https://www.invitra.com/en/wp-content/uploads/2017/10/false-negative-false-positive.png.

10.5.2. Psychological Impact on Parents

The process of prenatal genetic screening and diagnosis usually generates a lot of emotional stress in parents. The event, especially when it comes with unforeseen results like congenital heart disease (CHD), might seem like a life-altering occurrence that would alter the dynamics and future of the family. Parents primarily grapple with anxiety, fear, and uncertainty as they face the possibility of their child having difficulties after birth. The emotional implications are also exacerbated by the demands of making instantaneous decisions concerning caregiving and parenting styles. This stress response is not just a temporary reaction but, rather, one that has the potential of developing into long-term emotional difficulties, underscoring the necessity for robust psychological support systems. This type of support is necessary to help parents manage their emotional responses as they deal with the situation they face, highlighting the fact that the psychological effect of prenatal diagnosis goes well beyond short-term responses (Mutti et al., 2024). Moreover, how genetic counselors deliver prenatal results significantly influences parents' experiences. A study targeting the resources utilized by the National Society of Genetic Counselors (NSGC) pointed out the correlation between guideline adherence in communication and the psychological state of parents who were diagnosed with Down syndrome (DS). Parents expressed varied feelings depending on the level of guideline adherence by genetic counselors, where greater perceived adherence was associated with better emotional reactions. The results imply that the manner in which sensitive information is delivered has a profound impact on the psychological adjustment of parents, highlighting the importance of having qualified professionals talk to families in a compassionate way. This further highlights the central role of health care providers, not only as providers of information, but also as central agents in guiding parents through their emotional process (Maryam et al., 2024). Finally, the compounding psychological effect of these diagnoses is witnessed in parents' long-term emotional well-being and in the health of their interpersonal relationships. The stress of navigating a prenatal diagnosis can come with stressors that intrude on marital interaction and family unity, commonly resulting in parental feelings of isolation. Couples will differ in their coping styles in that one will be more inclined to pursue information and the other will withdraw emotionally. Such disconnection can heighten feelings of loneliness and isolation, thus the need to facilitate open communication and coping mechanisms. In addition, integrating psychological support services into prenatal care models can help create more positive discussions and coping mechanisms, ultimately reducing the possibility of suffering emotional distress associated with the loss. Such efforts are essential in fostering resilience among parents confronted with the issues of prenatal genetic diagnosis (Maryam et al., 2024; Mutti et al., 2024) (Figure 10.16).

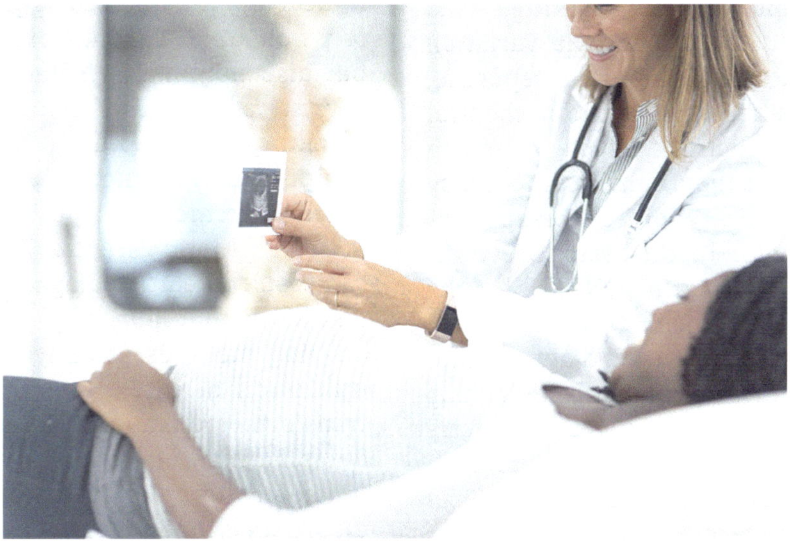

Figure 10.16. Process of prenatal genetic screening.

Source: https://www.pretrm.com/wp-content/uploads/2023/03/early-pregnanyc-blood-test-pretrm-test.jpg.

10.5.3. Limitations in the Scope of Detectable Conditions

The practice of prenatal genetic screening and diagnosis is characterized by intrinsic limitations, particularly with regard to the quantity of conditions that can be diagnosed. Despite tremendous technological innovation that has radically improved the capacity to detect specific genetic aberrations, a multitude of conditions cannot be detected by existing screening procedures. An example is that cfDNA screening shows higher efficacy in screening for major aneuploidies, including trisomies 21, 18, and 13, but it cannot detect structural abnormalities or chromosomal disorders that are rare. This thus provides a false reassurance to the parents, who tend to think that a low-risk label is synonymous with having a normal fetus. In addition, the constraints of ultrasound imaging, specifically in identifying conditions that become evident during the late stages of pregnancy, highlight the deficiencies in our diagnostic capacity. These constraints make prenatal screening an inadequate answer and therefore require continuous study and enhancement to resolve the existing disparities in identifiable conditions (Caterina et al., 2023). In addition, a fundamental limitation is the variability that is experienced in the interpretation and implementation of screening guidelines in various clinical environments. No standard screening procedures observable has been widely accepted, causing variable reporting of what information is made available to prospective parents. For example, though clinical practice guidelines guide healthcare providers, local guidelines and available resources can significantly shape decision-making. This variability can lead to considerable variation in the assessment, diagnosis, and reporting of conditions to patients. In addition, medical providers can also confront issues related to equipment quality, sonographer competency levels, and accessibility of follow-up care for abnormal results. To this extent, even if the condition is potentially detectable, the healthcare delivery and clinical competency nuances can undermine accurate diagnosis and early intervention, thereby further complicating the practice of prenatal genetic screening (Melamed et al., 2021). Finally, there is a significant limitation with regards to ethical considerations concerning prenatal genetic screening and diagnosis. The possibility of conditions not being detected raises ethical concerns about parental choice, but also wider societal consequences of selective abortion. Parents who have negative screening may subsequently have to deal with the distress of finding out unexpectedly after birth, resulting in emotional feelings of upset and regret. Also, pressure to go ahead with invasive tests when abnormalities are suspected can endanger fetal well-being and complicate maternal well-being. These ethical considerations point to the necessity of adequate counseling in the course of screening so that parents receive a realistic picture of the risks and limitations of screening. With advancements made in prenatal genetic diagnosis, there is a need to integrate ethical paradigms with clinical practice to enable well-informed decision-making for families awaiting the birth of a child (Caterina et al., 2023).

10.6. Future Directions in Genetic Screening

The future prospects of genetic screening, particularly as they apply to prenatal diagnosis, rest on methodological and technological progress. As prenatal cfDNA screening begins to develop, it is increasingly feasible to screen for not only chromosomal abnormalities, but also dominant single-gene diseases. The current cfDNA tests are designed to detect primarily aneuploidies; however, as more comprehensive genomic panels are included, there is tremendous potential to screen for de novo genetic variants. These developments can result in earlier diagnosis of most genetic disorders that normally evade conventional imaging methods at early gestation. Effective utilization of extended cfDNA screening can transform prenatal care by allowing informed decision-making among pregnant women, ultimately improving fetuses at risk for genetic disorders. Nonetheless, the shift towards an increasingly integrated screening paradigm requires additional investigation to confirm its clinical relevance and the complexities involved with these emerging technologies (Liao et al., 2025). Moreover, the ethical dimensions of prenatal genetic screening must be tackled as the landscape continues to change. Although emerging technologies yield useful information, they also present challenges in terms of informed consent, access, and genetic counseling. This complexity is also added to by the possibility of identifying variants of uncertain significance, which will make family counseling harder. As cell-free DNA pregnancy screening is extended to include screening for more conditions, the development of standard protocols for genetic counseling is essential. These protocols must include pre-test and post-test counseling so that parents are adequately prepared to comprehend their options and interpret the test results accurately. Genetic counselors' roles are expected to change alongside these developments, requiring ongoing education and training in order to be able to deal with the complexities involved in widening genetic screening (Liao et al., 2025). Meanwhile, besides ethical considerations, the application of artificial intelligence in the process of genetic screening is promising to improve accuracy in prenatal diagnosis. Artificial intelligence technologies can improve the accuracy of genomic data interpretation, enabling the recognition of patterns associated with specific genetic risks more effectively than traditional techniques. Additionally, the utilization of machine learning algorithms can optimize screening protocols by streamlining data analysis and minimizing the chances of human error. As researchers explore the use of artificial intelligence in combination with liquid biopsy and multiomics approaches, the possibility of developing comprehensive, patient-centered screening strategies becomes more realistic. These techniques should enhance the detection of genetic defects while simultaneously customizing interventions according to the unique profiles of each patient, thus enhancing the quality of prenatal care across the globe (Figure 10.17).

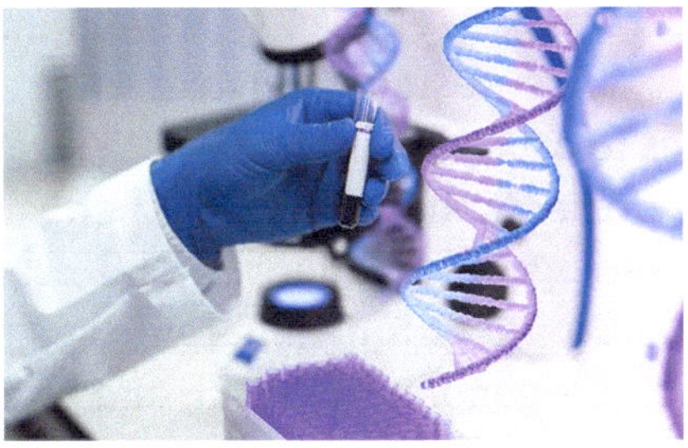

Figure 10.17. Advancements in genetic testing.

Source: https://erayafertility.com/wp-content/uploads/elementor/thumbs/Advancements-in-Genetic-Testing-qpz3mdq0h0k4tilum43hfh50jgcirnd117yxjs9i14.webp.

10.6.1. Advances in Technology and Methodology

Advances in prenatal genetic screening and diagnosis using technology have significantly improved accuracy and dependability in identifying fetal abnormalities and irreversibly changed clinical practices. Specifically, the creation of NIPT with cfDNA has completely changed screening technologies. This novel approach enables the examination of fetal genetic material present in a mother's blood, thereby making it possible to detect trisomies like Down syndrome at an early period with much better detection rates than other conventional screening techniques. The cfDNA test is more sensitive than serum marker screening, which translates to fewer false positives and less need for invasive testing. Consequently, the couples are now able to make better-informed decisions regarding their pregnancies, representing a significant enhancement in the level of prenatal care. Moreover, cfDNA testing is progressing to include more conditions pertinent to multifetal pregnancies, thereby tackling some of the clinical dilemmas of complicated gestational cases (Melamed et al., 2021). Besides NIPT, innovations in imaging modalities, especially in ultrasound methodologies, have significantly influenced prenatal screening and diagnostic procedures. Advanced ultrasonographic technologies, such as three-dimensional (3D) and four-dimensional (4D) imaging systems, enable health professionals to obtain improved visualization and evaluation of fetal anatomy and placental growth. These technologies permit the early identification of possible growth restriction and structural defects that may signify fetal distress or genetic abnormalities. In addition, the use of Doppler ultrasound allows for the real-time evaluation of blood flow patterns in fetal vessels, which plays a critical role in the suspected FGR diagnosis. Not only does this multi-dimensional method improve diagnostic sensitivity but also directs management decisions aimed at optimizing perinatal outcomes, illustrating the active intersection of technology and maternal-fetal medicine in augmenting prenatal diagnostic capability (Melamed et al., 2021). The continuous development of technologies for prenatal genetic screening and diagnosis highlights the urgent need for constant research and coordination among health professionals. FIGO and other bodies have stressed the need for adherence to evidence-based guidelines in the introduction of such high-technology, recognizing the variation in resource levels between regions as well. Efforts to translate achievements in high-resource environments into low-resource environments are needed to bridge disparities in access to care. Synthesis of emerging data and standardization of evidence-based practices offer maximal management of at-risk pregnancies for FGR, for example. Sustainability of healthcare innovations in the long term depends on increased education and training of practitioners, in addition to the creation of standard operating procedures for the integration of emerging technologies. These efforts are essential in fostering an innovative ecosystem that supports maternal and fetal health outcomes (Glenn et al., 2020).

10.6.2. Integration of Artificial Intelligence in Genetic Analysis

The application of artificial intelligence in genetic testing holds great promise for the future development of prenatal genetic screening and diagnosis practices. As reproductive medicine continues to develop, AI algorithms—particularly those utilizing deep learning methods—have been shown to be exceptionally proficient in deciphering multifaceted genomic information. Through the utilization of convolutional neural networks and various machine learning models, AI is capable of detecting and categorizing genetic disorders with great precision. This capability is especially important in the area of prenatal diagnoses, where early and accurate detection of abnormalities like neural tube defects is essential to enhance outcomes for both infants and mothers. The literature indicates that artificial intelligence-augmented ultrasound technologies have greatly enhanced diagnostic precision, outperforming conventional techniques in sensitivity and specificity rates, with direct implications for enhanced patient care and health outcomes for mothers (Yeganegi et al., 2025). Furthermore, artificial intelligence not only improves the precision of genetic testing but also optimizes the general workflow in clinical environments. Having the capability to review high volumes of fetal ultrasound images alongside genetic data at high speed enables healthcare providers to prioritize timely interventions while maintaining quality. For example, studies indicate that there is a decreased median scan time owing to the incorporation of AI, thereby enhancing the efficiency of prenatal screening workflows. The saving of time on each evaluation, in turn, enhances healthcare organizations' operational efficiency, whereas it lowers waiting times for patients, thus decreasing anxiety and enhancing the overall patient experience.

Additionally, health messages generated by artificial intelligence can enhance public knowledge of genetic disease, thus promoting informed decision-making among prospective parents (Yeganegi et al., 2025). The future direction of artificial intelligence in terms of genetic analysis for prenatal screening demonstrates an emerging development in its ability. As the technological environment continues to evolve, multimodal data fusion in AI systems presents the possibility of unparalleled understanding of genetic risk and associated outcomes. By integrating different categories of information—genomic, clinical, and image—AI is able to provide a unifying evaluation that guides personalized healthcare approaches. The exploration of large medical language models and generative AI can even further enhance diagnostic precision, elucidating the molecular characteristics of developmental disorders.

Ethical factors must be incorporated, nonetheless, so that the implementation of AI in prenatal diagnosis is supported by foundations of transparency and fairness, and eventually gives rise to trust by patients and clinicians as well (Figure 10.18).

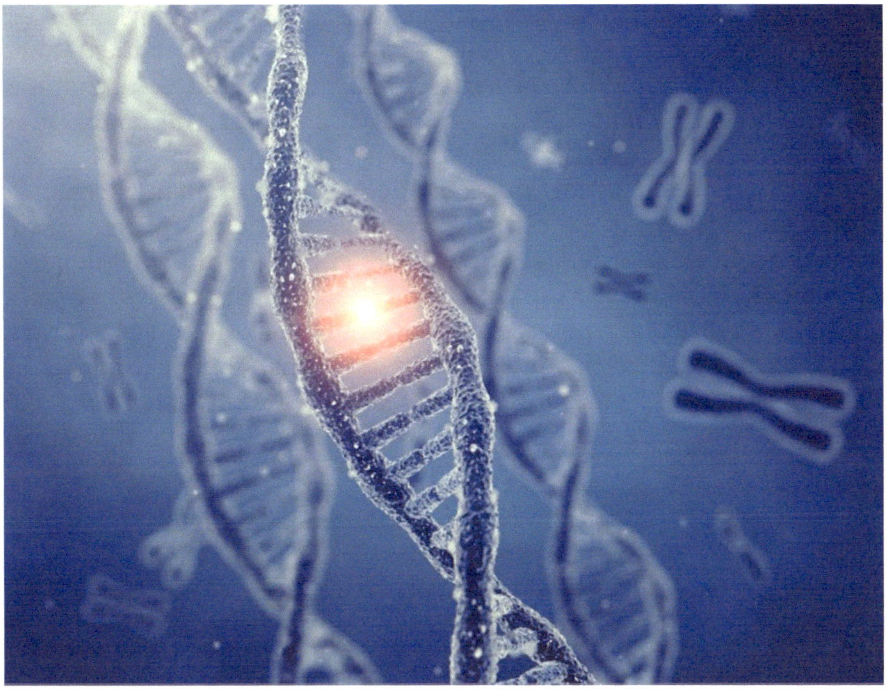

Figure 10.18. Artificial Intelligence in Genetic Analysis.

Source: https://d2jx2rerrg6sh3.cloudfront.net/images/Article_Images/ImageForArticle_23907_16994605155791811.jpg.

10.6.3. Potential for Expanded Screening Panels

The prospect of better screening panels within the framework of prenatal genetic diagnosis is a significant development in the field of reproductive health care. Utilization of a series of genetic tests can grant extensive knowledge regarding the genetic composition of a fetus, resulting in the identification of numerous genetic disorders. The conventional screening techniques are being supplemented more and more by Next Generation Sequencing (NGS) technologies, which facilitate the simultaneous identification of various genetic abnormalities. Not only does this method improve the accuracy of diagnosis, but it also helps to inform prospective parents of possible health dangers involved in their pregnancies. The possibility of delivering instant and dependable genetic data could empower early intervention and the creation of more effective health care plans for those affected individuals and families. The incorporation of expanded screening panels into clinical care reflects the changing potential of genetic testing and the need for genetic counseling along the way (Cunniff et al., 2019). As expanded screening panels continue to develop, they also introduce special challenges and ethical dilemmas into the landscape of prenatal genetic diagnosis. One of the significant worries is concerning the consequences of the finding of variants of unknown significance (VUS), which complicate clinical decision-making and patient counseling.

The presence of these VUS can generate ambiguous information concerning their possible effect on fetal development, resulting in stress and uncertainty among parents. The broader extent of testing also gives rise to ethical issues in terms of informed consent and test result reporting. As healthcare professionals strive to balance the merits of cutting-edge screening modalities against the sophistication of genetic data, sustained communication among clinicians is essential. In this case, genetic counseling serves an imperative function by facilitating patients' understanding of their test results while promoting informed decision-making (Chacon-Camacho et al., 2017). Also, the application of enhanced screening panels can dramatically affect public policy, especially in the control of genetic disorders. Through the promotion of an anticipatory strategy for prenatal care, the panels assist future parents in making informed decisions about their pregnancy. The potential to detect inherited disorders prenatally can allow for the creation of personalized interventions, including customized monitoring or surgery, ultimately enhancing the well-being of both parents and children. Additionally, the utilization of extended screening panels may have an important part in reducing the incidence of certain genetic disorders in the population since informed reproductive decisions are also expected to affect family planning decisions. This dual impact summarizes the twofold potential of expanded screening panels: enhancing the treatment of individual patients while, at the same time, advancing the objectives of public health (Cunniff et al., 2019).

SUMMARY

A critical examination of prenatal genetic diagnosis and screening highlights the extensive consequences this discipline has on reproductive choice and the ethical concerns it raises. Prenatal genetic testing has revolutionized the art of maternal-fetal medicine through the introduction of new technologies. Being able to make a diagnosis of genetic disease as well as chromosomal abnormalities prenatally offers parents important information that can be used to make pregnancy choices. Yet, their accuracy is of the utmost importance because serious differences may occur, and this could result in poorly informed choices. This is echoed in the research regarding sex chromosome aneuploidies, where difficulties in the false-positive rates require intensive genetic counseling so that parents are aware of both the limitations and the implications of the findings, as noted by (Howell et al., 2024). The discrepancy observed between test results and real phenotypic expressions necessitates further advances in techniques involving genetic counseling. The variability of disorders like the 22q11.2 microduplication syndrome also brings into focus the intricate nature of prenatal genetic testing and its results. The phenotypic variability linked with this microduplication presents difficulties that may hinder diagnostic precision. In most instances, the lack of specific ultrasound features requires a prudent and informed strategy for prenatal decision-making. A study of fetuses with 22q11.2 microduplications showed that more than half lacked intrauterine presentation, thereby making the counseling process greatly challenging. Under such circumstances, highlighting the importance of offering sophisticated genetic counseling is essential as it allows parents to make a decision with increased awareness of possible long-term outcomes. The takeaway from such research is the need for robust support mechanisms in the offering of prenatal genetic testing, as established in the results of (Jiang et al., 2024). In summary, the incorporation of prenatal genetic screening and diagnosis into obstetric care needs to be done carefully and with ethical consideration. As the discipline evolves, ensuring that professionals are more aware of the limitations and possible results of genetic testing is of utmost significance. Parents need to be adequately informed about the consequences of prenatal test results in order to properly guide them in their decision-making. Beyond its clinical nature, the emotional toll experienced by parents who must make such choices highlights the importance of holistic counseling and ongoing support from medical professionals. By fostering a setting conducive to informed choice, the medical profession can more effectively assist families in dealing with the complexities of pregnancy amidst genetic abnormalities, leading to a more compassionate model of reproductive health.

Prenatal genetic screening and diagnostic recent advances have significantly transformed the practice of reproductive medicine, offering prospective parents' valuable information about fetal well-being. Carrier screening, especially, has become a primary technique of interest, with recommendations from organizations like ACOG and ACMG backing its implementation, preferably before conception. The scope of carrier screening is wide, ranging from testing for specific disorders like hemoglobinopathies and cystic fibrosis to broader panels with hundreds of genetic disorders. This scope demands that clinicians are well-informed about the available tests to enable them to advise patients accordingly. Finally, the emphasis on informed decision-making underlines the necessity to tailor screening approaches to suit specific circumstances, optimizing the possibilities for positive outcomes in prenatal care (Santoli et al., 2025). cfDNA screening is also a significant development, offering a non-invasive screening test for chromosomal abnormalities such as trisomies. The accuracy of cfDNA testing has made it a first-line choice for the majority of clinicians. With the endorsement from professional societies, patients are now routinely offered cfDNA screening for major aneuploidies at their prenatal visits. There is, however, controversy on whether microdeletion syndromes and rare autosomal trisomies should be included in screening guidelines. Whereas some organizations such as ACMG endorse cfDNA screening for certain microdeletions, others are conservatively opposed to screening for rare disorders. This continued argument underlines how healthcare providers must be adequately informed on the changing guidelines to allow better patient guidance and counseling (Koçbulut et al., 2025). Beyond the initial screening, diagnostic testing is also important to aid in evidence and clinical decision-making. The advocacy for chromosomal microarray analysis in the case of fetal structural anomalies and stillbirth has been given more recognition, with its established greater diagnostic yield than conventional karyotyping. Next-generation sequencing technologies such as fetal exome or genome sequencing are also being considered more by clinicians. However, the cautious support offered by ACOG for these new methodologies underscores the paramount significance of a considerable research foundation before their wide-ranging application in clinical practice. In conclusion, as these technologies evolve, a thorough understanding of the applicable guidelines and their implications is essential for healthcare providers to skillfully navigate the complexities involved in prenatal genetic diagnosis and screening (Santoli et al., 2025).

CLOSER LOOK

NONINVASIVE PRENATAL TESTING (NIPT)

NIPT is a revolutionary screening method used during pregnancy to detect certain genetic conditions in a fetus by analyzing small fragments of fetal DNA circulating in the mother's blood. First introduced in clinical settings around 2011, NIPT has quickly become a widely adopted tool due to its high accuracy, safety, and early applicability—typically available as early as the 10th week of gestation. Unlike traditional diagnostic procedures such as amniocentesis or CVS, which carry a small risk of miscarriage due to their invasive nature, NIPT poses no physical risk to the fetus since it only involves a simple blood draw from the pregnant person. The test works by examining cfDNA, which originates from the placenta and enters the maternal bloodstream. Using advanced genomic technologies, NIPT can assess the risk of common chromosomal abnormalities, most notably trisomies like Down syndrome (trisomy 21), Edwards syndrome (trisomy 18), and Patau syndrome (trisomy 13).

NIPT has demonstrated remarkable sensitivity and specificity, particularly for detecting Down syndrome, with detection rates exceeding 99% and very low false positive rates. This makes it a valuable tool for identifying pregnancies at high risk for genetic conditions early on, enabling families and healthcare providers to make informed decisions about further diagnostic testing and pregnancy management. In addition to the common trisomies, some versions of NIPT can screen for sex chromosome abnormalities, such as Turner syndrome (monosomy X) and Klinefelter syndrome (XXY), as well as determine fetal sex. More advanced or expanded panels may also include microdeletions and rare chromosomal conditions, although the accuracy of these extended screenings can be lower and may vary by provider.

Despite its many advantages, NIPT remains a screening—not a diagnostic—test. This means that while it can indicate a high or low risk for specific conditions, it cannot confirm a diagnosis. Any positive result should be followed up with confirmatory diagnostic testing, such as amniocentesis or CVS, to ensure accurate diagnosis. Furthermore, NIPT does not screen for all genetic disorders or birth defects, such as structural abnormalities or single-gene mutations, and its performance can be affected by factors like maternal obesity, multiple pregnancies, or low fetal DNA fractions. For this reason, pre-test and post-test counseling are essential components of NIPT, helping expectant parents understand the capabilities and limitations of the test.

The ethical and social implications of NIPT also warrant careful consideration. As the test becomes more comprehensive and accessible, concerns have arisen regarding informed consent, potential anxiety from uncertain results, and the societal impact of widespread genetic screening. In some countries, debates continue about how NIPT may influence perceptions of disability and reproductive choices. Nevertheless, NIPT represents a significant advancement in prenatal care, offering a safe, early, and highly accurate option for assessing fetal health. As technology continues to evolve, NIPT is expected to expand its diagnostic scope and become an even more integral part of routine prenatal screening worldwide.

REFERENCES

1. Allyse, M. A., Riggan, K. A., Bonhomme, N., & Michie, M. (2025). Rethinking the burden of traditional informed consent prior to prenatal genetic screening. *The Hastings Center Report, 55*(2), 29–38. https://www.semanticscholar.org/paper/0e81b10138f4179c99bd1aab2582b82a66bff4e5 (accessed on 27 May 2025).
2. American College of Obstetricians and Gynecologists. (2018). ACOG practice bulletin no. 190: Gestational diabetes mellitus. *Obstetrics and Gynecology, 131*(e49–e64). https://doi.org/10.1097/aog.0000000000002501.
3. Aragon-Martin, J. A., Child, A. H., & Sage, K. (2016). Genetic testing in Marfan syndrome. https://core.ac.uk/download/287649641.pdf (accessed on 27 May 2025).
4. Bilardo, C. M., Chaoui, R., Hyett, J., Kagan, K. O., Karim, J., Papageorghiou, A. T., Poon, L. C., et al. (2023). ISUOG practice guidelines (updated): Performance of 11–14-week ultrasound scan. *Ultrasound in Obstetrics and Gynecology, 61*, 127–143. https://doi.org/10.1002/uog.26106.
5. Blank, R., Barnett, A. L., Cairney, J., Green, D., Kirby, A., Polatajko, H. J., Rosenblum, S., et al. (2019). International clinical practice recommendations on the definition, diagnosis, assessment, intervention, and psychosocial aspects of developmental coordination disorder. *Developmental Medicine & Child Neurology, 61*, 242–285. https://doi.org/10.1111/dmcn.14132.
6. Boardman, F. K. (2013). Knowledge is power? The role of experiential knowledge in genetically 'risky' reproductive decisions. https://core.ac.uk/download/9562824.pdf (accessed on 27 May 2025).
7. Castaldo, G., Martinelli, P., Maruotti, G. M., Sarno, et al. (2013). Prenatal screening and counseling for genetic disorders. https://core.ac.uk/download/55118920.pdf (accessed on 27 May 2025).
8. Chacon-Camacho, O., Garcia-Montano, L. A., & Zenteno, J. (2017). The clinical implications of molecular monitoring and analyses of inherited retinal diseases. *Expert Review of Molecular Diagnostics, 17*, 1009–1021. https://www.semanticscholar.org/paper/4982939349d02cf69dccf4e2b4220f07ecdba361 (accessed on 27 May 2025).
9. Chan, K. C. A., Woo, J. K. S., King, A. D., Zee, B., Lam, W. K., Chan, S. L., Chu, S. W. I., et al. (2017). Analysis of plasma Epstein–Barr virus DNA to screen for nasopharyngeal cancer. *New England Journal of Medicine, 377*, 513–522. https://doi.org/10.1056/nejmoa1701717.
10. Chaukale, M. M., Waghmare, S. U., Kokate, S. A., & Kukar, K. A. (2024). Comprehensive overview of non-invasive prenatal testing (NIPT) and its ethical considerations. *Saudi Journal of Medical and Pharmaceutical Sciences*. https://www.semanticscholar.org/paper/872760e3515b3294c81985543052af1af4ffe51b (accessed on 27 May 2025).
11. Cools, M., Nordenström, A., Robeva, R., Hall, J. C., Westerveld, P., Flück, C. E., Köhler, B., et al. (2018). Caring for individuals with a difference of sex development (DSD): A consensus statement. *Nature Reviews Endocrinology, 14*, 415–429. https://doi.org/10.1038/s41574-018-0010-8.
12. Cunniff, C., & Bassetti, J. (2019). Advances in genetic medicine and shared-decision making. *Journal of Communication in Healthcare, 12*, 82–85. https://www.semanticscholar.org/paper/9132a8b765dbb492cd8adc415241bae88b6504e5 (accessed on 27 May 2025).

13. Cyto and Genomics Group of Medical Genetics Branch, Liu, N., Shi, P., Liu, L., & Kong, X. (2024). [Expert consensus on the prenatal diagnosis and genetic counseling for uniparental disomy-related imprinting disorders]. *Zhonghua Yi Xue Yi Chuan Xue Za Zhi = Chinese Journal of Medical Genetics, 41*(6), 685–695. https://www.semanticscholar.org/paper/ce6c27e4e913b27aa6cdb316f602bfd402456152 (accessed on 27 May 2025).

14. Daghsni, M., Sheehan, E., Madan-Khetarpal, S., Aarabi, M., Witchel, S. F., Rajkovic, A., & Yatsenko, S. (2024). Recurrent Xp22.31-Yq11 unbalanced translocations: Molecular diagnosis and clinical implications in three families. *American Journal of Medical Genetics. Part A*. https://www.semanticscholar.org/paper/743ea1bcec33de1a3cd462eadc1eec65b5aa513e (accessed on 27 May 2025).

15. De Smet, M., Dheedene, A., Grisart, B., et al. (2016). Implementation of non-invasive prenatal testing by semiconductor sequencing in a genetic laboratory. https://core.ac.uk/download/84040277.pdf (accessed on 27 May 2025).

16. Dileep, D., Karim, K., & Munim, S. (2020). Prenatal diagnosis of rare genetic conditions at a tertiary care hospital in Karachi. https://core.ac.uk/download/322820444.pdf (accessed on 27 May 2025).

17. Dorf, I. L. H., Lou, S., & Skakkebæk, A. (2025). Parental decision-making following a prenatal diagnosis of Turner syndrome: A systematic review. *American Journal of Medical Genetics. Part C, Seminars in Medical Genetics*. https://www.semanticscholar.org/paper/81430c24d2728ec094ae161092b2802761717723 (accessed on 27 May 2025).

18. Eltyeb, E., Alhazmi, S. A., Maafa, S. H. I., Mobarki, S. J., Sobaikhi, N., Sumayli, R. A., Alattas, K. K., et al. (2024). Public's perception and attitude toward genetic testing in Jazan region. *Journal of Family Medicine and Primary Care, 13*, 4715–4720. https://www.semanticscholar.org/paper/64c6e2b613a597dc7a927a4a1ec8b926229ae092 (accessed on 27 May 2025).

19. Freeman, K., Hyde, J., Osipenko, L., et al. (2005). Emerging prenatal genetic tests: Developing a health technology assessment (HTA) framework for informed decision-making. https://core.ac.uk/download/105293.pdf (accessed on 27 May 2025).

20. Gao, Y., Zhong, M. L., Dai, Y., Jiang, Y. H., & Zou, C. C. (2023). Overview of genetic testing in Prader-Willi syndrome. *Expert Opinion on Orphan Drugs, 11*, 16–25. https://www.semanticscholar.org/paper/37d39a4b3536d5972fb7754b6c0156a57a9a48a2 (accessed on 27 May 2025).

21. Garber, A. M., & Fenerty, J. P. (2025). Costs and benefits of prenatal screening for cystic fibrosis. https://core.ac.uk/download/pdf/6864455.pdf (accessed on 27 May 2025).

22. Ghazal, S. (2009). Chronic villus sampling and the risk of hypertensive disorders of pregnancy: A case control study. https://core.ac.uk/download/232768462.pdf (accessed on 27 May 2025).

23. Hong, M. K., & Ding, D. C. (2025). Early diagnosis of ovarian cancer: A comprehensive review of the advances, challenges, and future directions. *Diagnostics, 15*. https://www.semanticscholar.org/paper/3fda1b6758615cff957dbd3c3e3c0bf4e916d99b (accessed on 27 May 2025).

24. Howell, S., Davis, S. M., Carstens, B. J., Haag, M., Ross, J. L., & Tartaglia, N. (2024). Discordant prenatal cell-free DNA screening vs. diagnostic results of sex chromosome aneuploidies: Implications for newborn screening and genetic counseling. *International Journal of Neonatal Screening, 10*. https://www.semanticscholar.org/paper/a6fdc2a3fdd0de3a13a748bcc17a311df0c7d6ce (accessed on 27 May 2025).

25. Ijaz, M. R., Trepanier, A., Kleinert, H. L., Weiss, S. M., & Meredith, S. H. (2024). Parent-reported genetic counselor adherence to the NSGC practice resource for communicating a potential prenatal diagnosis: Impact on the Down syndrome diagnosis experience. *Journal of Genetic Counseling*. https://www.semanticscholar.org/paper/dc246bfdf04d0a66b50fc5f1ff20ce930382cd7e (accessed on 27 May 2025).

26. Jiang, X., Liang, B., He, S., Wu, X., Zhao, W., Xue, H., Wang, Y., et al. (2024). Prenatal diagnosis and genetic study of 22q11.2 microduplication in Chinese fetuses: A series of 31 cases and literature review. *Molecular Genetics & Genomic Medicine, 12*. https://www.semanticscholar.org/paper/7df29eed710b24d941cb14d3c0d36bb271077ffd (accessed on 27 May 2025).

27. Khalighi, S., Reddy, K., Midya, A., Pandav, K., Madabhushi, A., & Abedalthagafi, M. (2024). Artificial intelligence in neuro-oncology: Advances and challenges in brain tumor diagnosis, prognosis, and precision treatment. *NPJ Precision Oncology, 8*. https://www.semanticscholar.org/paper/96159eea50588975893787d2f13e21e38ed4615a (accessed on 27 May 2025).

28. Koçbulut, E., Kurt, A., Sarikaya Kurt, D., & Tolunay, H. (2025). Bibliometric analysis of publications on prenatal genetic screening using cell-free DNA. *Cureus, 17*. https://www.semanticscholar.org/paper/6028752f6b6bcc348dcd8d70213723dc5d256555 (accessed on 27 May 2025).

29. Liao, J., Xu, N., Gao, H., Hardy, T., Levy, B., Mehta, L., Choy, K., et al. (2025). Advances in prenatal cell-free DNA screening for dominant monogenic conditions: A review of current progress and future directions in clinical implementation. *Prenatal Diagnosis*. https://www.semanticscholar.org/paper/6f1df8d6fbd1cba62cdd5b76fb401bf188ff9807 (accessed on 27 May 2025).

30. Lugo, N. T. (2023). Ethical considerations in prenatal diagnosis and genetic counseling. *Seminars in Medical Writing and Education*. https://www.semanticscholar.org/paper/e8bb596e650a51df2bd6cc41b642aee9df25cf68 (accessed on 27 May 2025).

31. Maftei, A., & Danila, O. (2022). The good, the bad, and the utilitarian: Attitudes towards genetic testing and implications for disability. *Current Psychology (New Brunswick, N.J.)*. https://www.semanticscholar.org/paper/2ff0c7a7bea78843f3f9284d3d27302949581cb0 (accessed on 27 May 2025).

32. Mahalingam, S., Rasalkar, R., Lallar, M., Pradhan, A., Khairnar, S., Devanboo, A., Venkataswamy, E., et al. (2024). Mosaic embryo transfer after pre-implantation genetic testing for structural rearrangement: A case study. *Journal of Biochemical and Clinical Genetics*. https://www.semanticscholar.org/paper/9b5ec04ac9f5e01625d994db13cb03d698d305a8 (accessed on 27 May 2025).

33. Malasai, K., Jittikoon, J., Udomsinprasert, W., Talungchit, P., Youngkong, S., Sangroongruangsri, S., Mahasirimongkol, S., et al. (2025). Cost-benefit analysis of genetic testing as a prenatal diagnostic tool for thalassemia: A single-center study from central Thailand. *ClinicoEconomics and Outcomes Research: CEOR, 17*, 33–43. https://www.semanticscholar.org/paper/f1d60aaeb3ff88438b3828feeff701de334ab656 (accessed on 27 May 2025).

34. Melamed, N., Baschat, A., Yinon, Y., Athanasiadis, A., Mecacci, F., Figueras, F., Berghella, V., et al. (2021). FIGO (International Federation of Gynecology and Obstetrics) initiative on fetal growth: Best practice advice for screening, diagnosis, and management of fetal growth restriction. *International Journal of Gynecology & Obstetrics, 152*, 3–57. https://doi.org/10.1002/ijgo.13522.

35. Mladenović, T. (2024). Fundamental legal aspects of the prenatal genetic diagnosis. *Međunarodna Naučna Konferencija Izazovi I Otvorena Pitanja Uslužnog Prava–Tom1*. https://www.semanticscholar.org/paper/ebdd8d4a130d1d12e4bc4cfee3fe4db2c239c401 (accessed on 27 May 2025).

36. Mutti, G., Ait Ali, L., Marotta, M., Nunno, S., Consigli, V., Baratta, S., Orsi, M. L., et al. (2024). Psychological impact of a prenatal diagnosis of congenital heart disease on parents: Is it time for tailored psychological support? *Journal of Cardiovascular Development and Disease, 11*. https://www.semanticscholar.org/paper/353ecfa12f0cb3a1fa3a2ec1e701f13ea0c534af (accessed on 27 May 2025).

37. Palomaki, G. E., Chiu, R. W. K., Pertile, M. D., Sistermans, E. A., Yaron, Y., Vermeesch, J., Vora, N. L., et al. (2020). International Society for Prenatal Diagnosis position statement: Cell free (cf) DNA screening for Down syndrome in multiple pregnancies. *Prenatal Diagnosis, 41*, 1222–1232. https://doi.org/10.1002/pd.5832.

38. Pande, S., Bansal, V., & Sachdeva, G. (2025). Prenatal screening for genetic disorders: Updated guidelines, proposed counseling, a holistic approach for primary health care providers in developing countries. *Diagnosis*. https://www.semanticscholar.org/paper/7c044e0051ca01271fae5730c0b1e25e79c41d71 (accessed on 27 May 2025).

39. Peter, M., Baptiste, R., Buabeng, R., Islam, L., Fisher, J., Leeson-Beevers, K., Hill, M., et al. (2025). 'I have my beliefs, but then I have my reality': Reflections of Black and South Asian parents living in England on screening and genetic diagnosis in pregnancy. *Prenatal Diagnosis*. https://www.semanticscholar.org/paper/e664a1a3a0643fc1129806d6aa59dfbe82407513 (accessed on 27 May 2025).

40. Purwin, S., Młynek, M., Madej-Pilarczyk, A., & Zawadzka-Więch, U. (2024). The role of genetic techniques in prenatal diagnostics. *Diagnostyka Laboratoryjna*. https://www.semanticscholar.org/paper/0f321e18d862eda4ea6e582b795d2bf597c2abe4 (accessed on 27 May 2025).

41. Reddy, M. (2021). Ethical and medical implications of prenatal and preimplantation screening. *HPHR Journal*. https://www.semanticscholar.org/paper/1590fee8ef02b94ef33ef4866f73bbaade5f7563 (accessed on 27 May 2025).

42. Reproductive Health Branch of China Maternal and Child, Xu, C., Yin, C., Yin, A., Liu, S., Jiang, Y., Luo, Q., et al. (2024). Expert consensus on the clinical application strategy of NIPT2.0, a new-generation non-invasive prenatal screening technology. *Zhonghua yi xue yi chuan xue za zhi = Zhonghua yixue yichuanxue zazhi = Chinese Journal of Medical Genetics, 41*(10), 1155–1163. https://www.semanticscholar.org/paper/a1aeea4af3d11679e1b502ab2ab02008a74182f0 (accessed on 27 May 2025).

43. Roy, E., Malafa, S., Adwer, L. M., Tabache, H., Sheth, T., Mishra, V., Abouelmagd, M., et al. (2025). Artificial intelligence in healthcare: Medical students' perspectives on balancing innovation, ethics, and patient-centered care. *International Journal of Medical Students*. https://www.semanticscholar.org/paper/d2d3b920960d57edf2d41de605f6c274f6404f25 (accessed on 27 May 2025).

44. Santoli, C. M., Dotters-Katz, S., Sparks, T. N., & Kuller, J. (2025). An overview of current prenatal genetic screening and diagnosis guidelines. *Pregnancy*. https://www.semanticscholar.org/paper/7845b7672bc0495be00331f1959b105ced5b611d (accessed on 27 May 2025).

45. Shiekedien, E., Aljohani, K., Alsaidalani, R., Alatiyyat, N., Almarwani, G., Alali, R., Aljohani, S., et al. (2024). Prenatal diagnosis for congenital malformations and genetic disorders. *International Journal of Medicine in Developing Countries*. https://www.semanticscholar.org/paper/abb80c6609ac38e339585bb95badd75dd8e44675 (accessed on 27 May 2025).

46. Turrini, M., & Otín-Gavín, J. (2025). Let 'pregnant women choose the destiny for themselves and their child': How fertility clinic digital platforms frame preimplantation genetic testing (PGT) in Spain. *Sociology of Health & Illness, 47*. https://www.semanticscholar.org/paper/cecc6bbd85a19ea7647ad22f82ee538c1c2cb8ee (accessed on 27 May 2025).

47. Wittman, A. T. (2016). Patient perception of negative non-invasive prenatal testing results. https://core.ac.uk/download/46720404.pdf (accessed on 27 May 2025).

48. Yeganegi, M., Danaei, M., Azizi, S., Jayervand, F., Bahrami, R., Dastgheib, S., Rashnavadi, H., et al. (2025). Research advancements in the use of artificial intelligence for prenatal diagnosis of neural tube defects. *Frontiers in Pediatrics*. https://www.semanticscholar.org/paper/d98a1ac0a71d7578dd046413f6866d38852c09b7 (accessed on 27 May 2025).

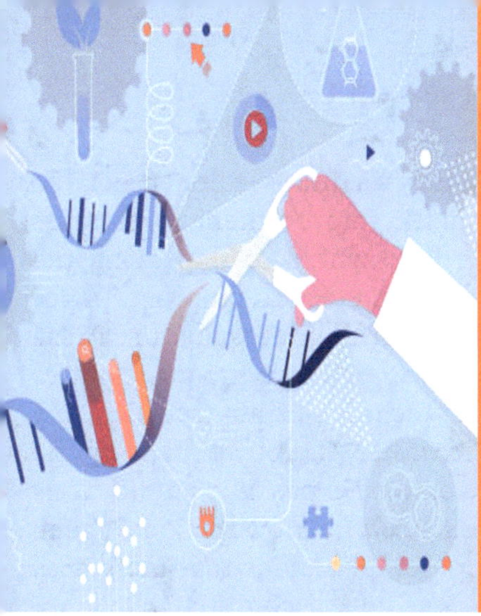

Chapter 11

GENE EDITING AND DEVELOPMENTAL RESEARCH

Contents

Introduction

The development of gene editing tools represents a landmark moment in the history of developmental science, and even more so with the advent of CRISPR-Cas systems. Such breakthrough tools enable researchers to edit genetic information with an unparalleled level of precision, thereby creating enormous potential for investigations across different biological settings. Of particular importance, model organisms like *Drosophila* have become the paramount choice for genetic investigation, given that they permit investigators to investigate complex genotype-phenotype interactions. The capacity to edit genes with precision using CRISPR not only informs our knowledge of gene processes but also offers potent means of visualizing and dissecting gene structure. With several applications already showing revolutionary potential, ongoing development of gene editing tools holds exciting possibilities for future research in developmental biology (Bier et al., 2018). One more promising field where gene editing meets development work is the manipulation of complex traits in trees and plants. Progress in CRISPR-based methods has particular importance in editing traits associated with wood composition, especially lignin, thereby facilitating dramatic improvement in biomass processing. Alteration of the composition and structure of lignin is essential to improving the processes of conversion of biomass into economically valuable products such as pulp and paper while minimizing the severity of chemical treatments that are necessary for their degradation. These changes, in addition to enhancing the efficiency of wood utilization, also enhance the possibilities for sustainable practice in the industry. By incorporating gene editing techniques into tree breeding programs, scientists envisage developing varieties with lower recalcitrance, thereby enhancing the valorization of cell wall polysaccharides. This inclusion is one of the extensive possible applications of gene editing in many fields of study (Chanoca et al., 2019). In essence, the introduction of gene editing technologies ushers in a new wave of innovation in developmental studies that integrates genetic analysis, agricultural advances, and industrial applications. As scientists continue to explore the genetic architecture of various organisms, the potential for achieving previously inaccessible characteristics and functions becomes more attainable. The concerted efforts aimed at leveraging CRISPR technologies across a wide range of biological sciences not only transform scientific research but also raise questions of genetic ethics and the potential environmental consequences of such advances. As the gene editing field develops, cross-disciplinary communication among scientists, ethicists, and policy-makers will be essential to ensure that the use of these powerful technologies is guided by ethics in developmental research. This nexus of scientific inquiry and ethical analysis will frame gene editing discourse in the future, with the challenge of sustainable innovation alongside tremendous scientific advancement (Figure 11.1).

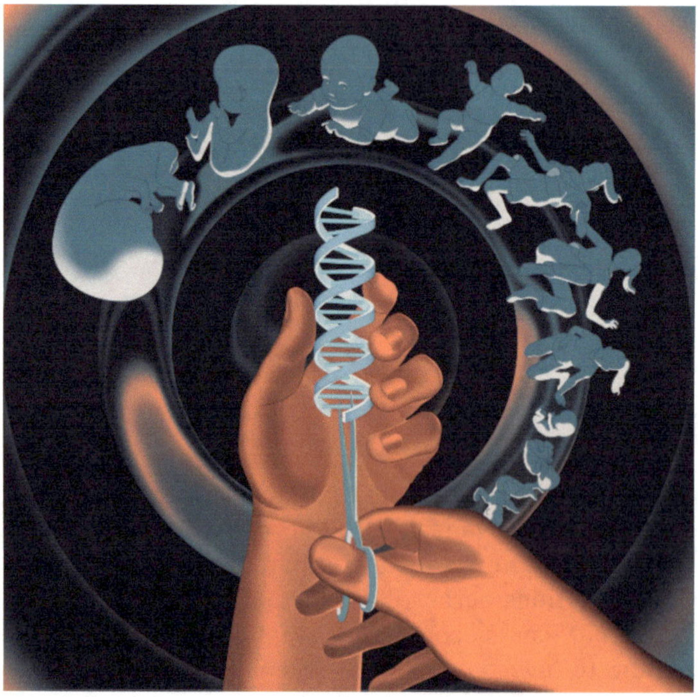

Figure 11.1. Overview of gene editing and developmental research.

Source: https://media.newyorker.com/photos/64ef779a8f63224180801ada/master/pass/230911_r42908.jpg.

Definition of Gene Editing

Gene editing is typically a collection of biotechnology methods that provide scientists with the capability to directly alter the gene make-up of living things. It entails the alteration of DNA codes in order to attain specific characteristics or functions, and it enables the unprecedented management of biological processes. Gene editing techniques, especially CRISPR-Cas9, have transformed the field in that they enable targeted and precise modification. These tools not only facilitate the removal, addition, or alteration of genetic elements but also enhance the efficiency and accuracy of genetic alterations compared to the previous approaches such as traditional gene therapy. As researchers strive to take advantage of the potential of gene editing, the implications for developmental biology are immense, offering possibilities to study genetic factors influencing growth, differentiation, and disease.

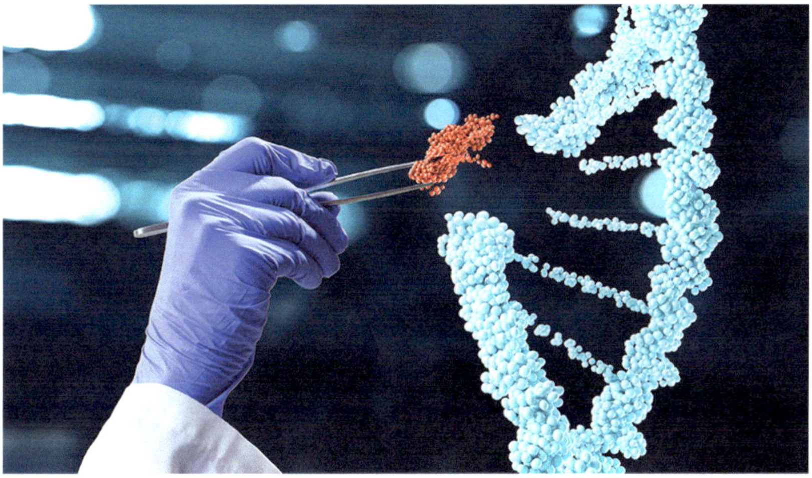

Figure 11.2. Gene editing.

Source: https://stmaaprodfwsite.blob.core.windows.net/assets/sites/1/2020/10/Gene_editing_AdobeStock_275702378_F_C_Adobe-Stock.jpg.

The expression gene editing represents a range of methods that have immense transformative potential in many areas of research, particularly in developmental research. By enabling targeted genetic alterations, researchers have the ability to examine the roles of individual genes in the development and functioning of organisms, hence defining clearer correlations between genotype and phenotype. This knowledge is paramount in fields such as embryonic development, where targeted genetic modifications enable scientists to investigate complicated pathways that regulate cellular differentiation. Secondly, gene editing techniques become valuable in the generation of genetically modified organisms (GMOs) for model systems, where one may investigate developmental defects and possible therapeutic strategies. The accuracy provided by modern techniques attests to remarkable advancement compared to the earlier techniques of genetic modification and is facilitating tremendous advancement in the biomedical field. Besides the technological component of gene editing, ethical and societal issues are raised as scientists continue to advance the frontiers of genetic manipulation. The capacity to edit genes presents new prospects for therapeutic intervention as well as scientific investigation; however, it also brings about concerns regarding the potential for unforeseen effects and the ethics of manipulating life at its very fundamental level. The explanation of gene editing should thus include not only the methods employed but also responsibility that comes with such immense powers. As research in developmental biology increasingly applies these technologies to comprehend gene expression complexity and interactions, it is important for both scientists and policymakers to deftly navigate the ethical terrain created by these innovations. It is essential to address these ethical issues to help ensure that gene editing progress meets societal values and public health objectives, thereby developing an ethical mindset in developmental research and applied practice (Figure 11.2).

Historical Context of Gene Editing Technologies

The history of gene editing technologies is an important milestone in our comprehension of molecular biology and genetics. Classical genetic work, dominated as it was by Mendelian inheritance, laid the foundation for biotechnology today. The advent of recombinant DNA technology during the 1970s was a watershed in enabling scientists to edit genetic material at will. This breakthrough paved the way for the creation of tools like restriction enzymes that could cut and rebuild DNA strands with precision. Concurrently with the evolution of these fundamental technologies, scientists initiated investigation into techniques for specific genomic modification, hence the emergence of more advanced gene editing instruments such as zinc-finger nucleases and transcription activator-like effector nucleases.

These findings facilitated intricate genome editing in various organisms, thereby broadening the range and possibilities within the genetic research field. The introduction of CRISPR-Cas9 technology in the early 2010s represented a significant turning point in the history of gene editing. Initially characterized as a microbial immunity system, CRISPR-Cas9 enabled the targeting of specific DNA sequences with unprecedented precision and ease. CRISPR-Cas9 technology consequently ushered in a quick expansion of research applications, especially in developmental biology and disease modeling, thereby creating a new era of scientific research. Scientists have also exploited the flexibility of CRISPR for generating more precise cell and animal models of diverse pathologic states, enabling a better insight into the genetic basis of diseases. Further, this new technology has initiated debate on the ethics and regulatory aspects of gene editing techniques. Accordingly, CRISPR introduction was a valuable step towards the future of gene editing, and it has been a core element in developmental studies to date (Frankish et al., 2020).

While there have been technological innovations, there has also been a great increase in the number of annotation projects that aim to enhance knowledge of gene functions and their interactions. One of the most important resources in this field has been the GENCODE project, which aims to create detailed annotations of mouse and human genomes and facilitate researchers in determining gene structures and functional elements that are at the core of developmental mechanisms. GENCODE is an attempt to bring together vast amounts of primary data, bioinformatics methods, and collaborative efforts to improve genome annotations and maintain consistency across reference databases. These tools have played a critical role in translating genomic data into practical applications in gene editing, aiding both basic research and clinical practice (Frankish et al., 2020). As gene editing technologies have evolved, the historical context relating to these innovations points to the tremendous interdependence of gene annotation and the effective application of gene editing technologies in diagnosing and treating genetic disorders (Figure 11.3).

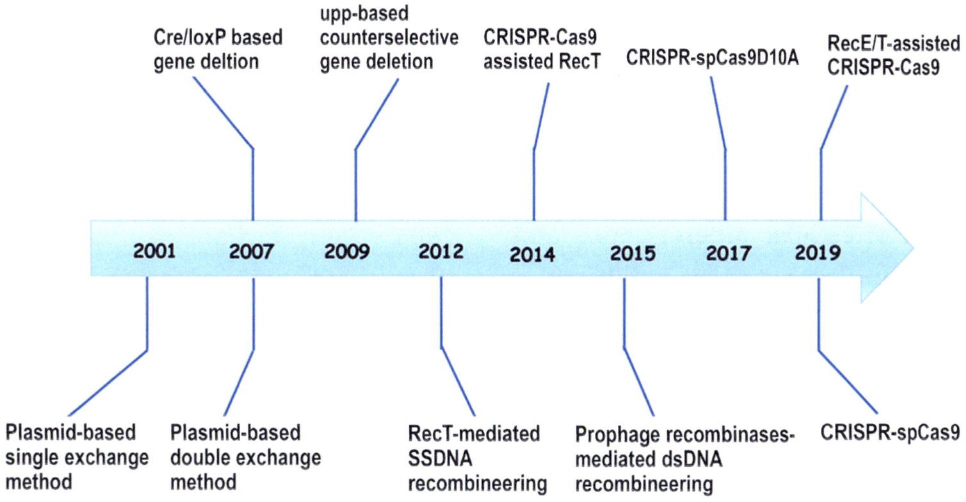

Figure 11.3. Historical context of gene editing technologies.

Source: https://www.researchgate.net/publication/355650849/figure/fig1/AS:1083389490798593@1635311591137/The-developmental-history-of-genome-editing-technology-in-n-butanol-tolerant-LAB.png.

Importance of Developmental Research in Gene Editing

Research targeting developmental processes is central to gene editing technology development as it offers crucial information on the genetic processes that regulate organismal development. Through such research, it becomes possible to identify key genes and regulatory pathways with significant functions during growth, differentiation, and morphogenesis. By deciphering these intricate biological processes, researchers can target particular genes for editing in a strategic manner, thereby improving the specificity and effectiveness of gene editing technologies such as CRISPR-Cas9. In addition, insights obtained from developmental studies help determine the likelihood of off-target effects, facilitating improved risk management in gene editing experiments. The scientific community remains engaged in the resolution of ethical issues concerning gene editing, whereas developmental research serves as an essential guiding roadmap. This roadmap provides the assurance that the application of these powerful technologies is in a manner that is responsible, with a complete awareness of their prospective influence on organism development and health. Developmental research further enhances the technical elements of gene editing and promotes interdisciplinarity between diverse fields, which include genetics, developmental biology, and bioethics. The interplay of these variables is of paramount importance because the stakes of gene editing reach outside the lab and into societal frameworks. For example, as the human population persists in its upward climb, there is a greater demand for sustainable farming methods. Research in plant biotechnology demonstrates the capabilities of gene editing to increase crop resilience and yield, thereby securing food sources and lessening the harm done to the environment. As highlighted in the discussion above, balance in agricultural innovations needs to be understood through the intertwinement of scientific progress, economics, and societal values. Such a complicated discipline demands continuous debate among various stakeholders on the environmental sustainability and ethical implications of gene editing. Moreover, the scope of research in development is not only limited to land use but also encompasses important progress in medical therapies as well. Gene editing holds great promise for the treatment of genetic disease but also comes with a set of challenges related to safety, off-target effects, and long-term ramifications. In such a context, knowledge from developmental biology is important, as it yields a better picture of cellular differentiation and the ultimate ramifications of gene modifications. By examining research that encompasses diverse biological systems, researchers are able to more accurately forecast the effects of gene editing in complicated organisms. The case of bacterial bio-communication, presented in Witzany (2008), demonstrates how the complex interaction of genetic components in various species enhances the knowledge of evolutionary processes and plasticity. Developmental biology studies thus not only shape the technique involved in gene editing but also dictate the general ethics and ecological paradigms that guide its use in both medical and biotechnology fields.

11.1. Overview of Gene Editing Technologies

Gene editing tools have transformed the arena of genetic research and application, with the potential for precise changes of DNA sequences in any organism. The emergence of CRISPR/Cas9, Zinc Finger Nucleases (ZFN), and Transcription Activator-Like Effector Nucleases (TALENs) technologies has made feasible genetic changes that were previously laborious or effectively impossible. Among these techniques, CRISPR/Cas9 stands out because of its comparatively straightforward architecture and effectiveness in enabling researchers to selectively target specific genes with unprecedented accuracy. This new tool not only enables gene editing but also significantly advances our knowledge of gene function, thereby propelling genetic medicines, agricultural innovations, and management of infectious diseases. As researchers keep pursuing innovation, the incorporation of such technologies into developmental biology presents unprecedented opportunities for successful manipulation of genetic pathways. Gene editing takes the center stage in developmental research in elucidating the mechanisms of both disease and development. Through the use of gene editing technology, researchers are able to construct models that replicate individual genetic disorders, thereby enabling them to develop a complete comprehension of disease development as well as therapy interventions. For instance, editing genes enables host-parasite interaction to be investigated, as can be observed through the growing application of systems biology that is made possible by NGS technologies. These technologies have increased the knowledge of complex biological systems, demonstrating the requirement for genomic information to be integrated with experimental approaches to drive research in developmental biology. This combination not only enables the exploration of fundamental biological questions but also addresses pressing problems, such as the emergence of drug-resistant microbes, due to its drastic implications for public health and therapeutic interventions (Jamshidi et al., 2015). Secondarily, the integration of CRISPR/Cas9 into vector control strategies highlights the applied significance of gene editing tools in disease combat against vector-borne diseases, e.g., mosquitoes. Recent research has demonstrated that transgenic lines of Aedes aegypti, which express Cas9, have been capable of efficiently editing their genomes, thus opening up new avenues for population control. These results highlight the promise that gene editing holds for generating triple mutants and enhancing gene drive systems for the purpose of interfering with the life cycle of disease-spreading vectors. This groundbreaking approach not only increases our ability to combat vector-borne disease but also establishes a benchmark for gene editing use in the control of ecological balance and crop pests. Therefore, the convergence of gene editing with development research not only expands the horizon of genetic investigation but also facilitates effective problem-solving in environmental control and public health (Akbari et al., 2017) (Figure 11.4).

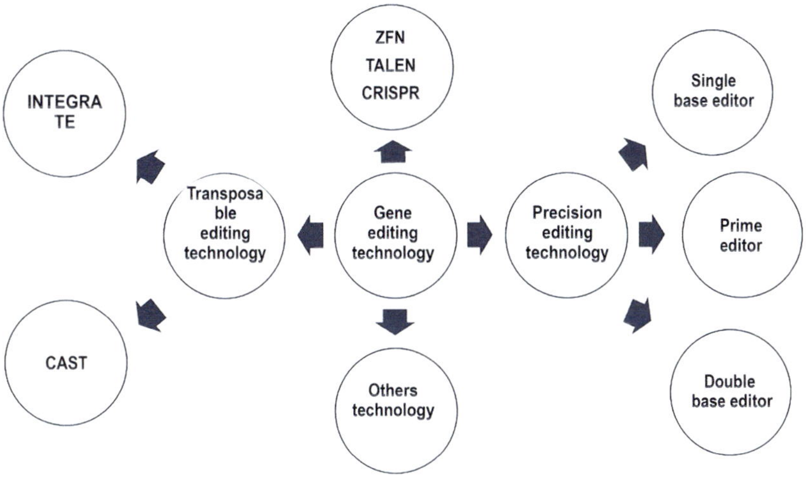

Figure 11.4. Gene editing technologies.

Source: https://article.imrpress.com/journal/FBL/26/10/10.52586/4997/4997/fig1.jpg.

11.1.1. CRISPR-Cas9: Mechanism and Applications

The CRISPR-Cas9 system is a significant improvement in gene editing, employing a natural bacterial immune system to edit genetic code with great accuracy. Central to this system is the employment of guide RNA (gRNA), which leads the Cas9 nuclease to a targeted position in the genome, thereby permitting the induction of a double-strand break. This disruption may be repaired by the mechanisms of non-homologous end joining or homology-directed repair, permitting precise alterations in the genome. The degree of specificity and flexibility that comes with CRISPR-Cas9 has enabled it to be a groundbreaking genetic engineering tool. By being able to edit genetic material in various organisms, scientists are empowered to explore basic biological inquiries and engineer novel applications, and in so doing, transform fields of regenerative medicine and developmental biology. The implications of CRISPR-Cas9 technology extend far beyond basic research, significantly impacting therapeutic strategies for genetic diseases. By creating faithful cellular and animal models, scientists can investigate the correlations between specific mutations and the onset of various diseases. Additionally, the therapeutic potential of this system is highlighted by its ability to correct genetic mutations at their source, thus offering hope for cures in diseases previously deemed uncontrollable by conventional treatments. Yet, as promising as the prospects of CRISPR-Cas9 for gene therapy are, there remain obstacles to its efficiency, specificity, and delivery to patient cells. The trajectory from laboratory findings to clinical application needs rigorous validation and optimization to ensure safety and efficacy in human medicine, so ongoing research is essential in this area (Ferreira et al., 2020). The CRISPR-Cas9 technology is also revolutionizing developmental research, especially in model organisms such as Drosophila. The aforementioned model organism has been a cornerstone of the investigation of genetics for a long while, and the introduction of CRISPR-Cas9 introduces an extra level of ease and precision to the manipulation of the genome.

The relative accessibility of the tool has allowed researchers to explore intricate inquiries into genotype-phenotype correlations and the overall arrangement of the genome itself. Furthermore, the CRISPR-Cas system enables visualization of RNA interactions and the development of new gene drive technologies that can alter populations over generations. As it continues to advance, many applications will emerge, resulting in a better understanding of genetic regulation and organism development (Bier et al., 2018). The range and breadth of CRISPR-Cas9 applications are a testament to its significance not only in gene editing but also in the investigation of biological systems in general (Figure 11.5).

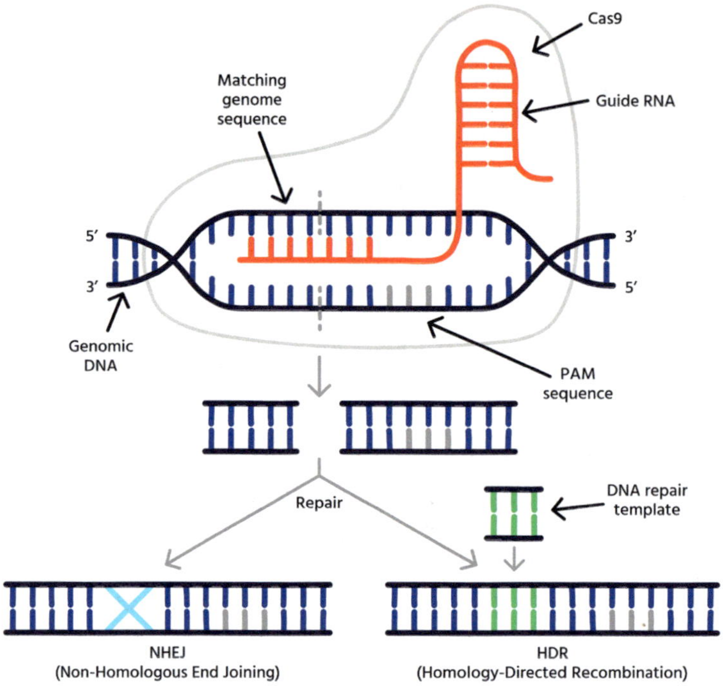

Figure 11.5. CRISPR-Cas9.

Source: https://iotasciences.com/wp-content/uploads/2024/06/CRISPR-Cas9_mechanism.jpg.

11.1.2. TALENs and ZFNs: Alternative Gene Editing Tools

The field of gene editing has been revolutionized with the development of tools like TALENs (Transcription Activator-Like Effector Nucleases) and ZFNs, which are equally vital alternatives to the more popular CRISPR/Cas9 system. These technologies utilize designed proteins to induce double-strand breaks at targeted genomic sites to facilitate precise changes in an organism's genetic composition. In contrast to CRISPR, which employs RNA-guided mechanisms, TALENs and ZFNs rely on protein-DNA interaction, with distinct advantages in some contexts. An instance is the modular nature of TALENs that can be readily modified to target a wide variety of genomic sequences with minimal optimization procedure. This level of specificity has the potential to increase their efficiency for use in developmental applications where precise genomic alterations are valuable for investigating gene function and regulation. One of the most important applications of TALENs and ZFNs in gene editing is their potential application in agricultural biotechnology and biomedical research. Through the facilitation of specific modifications, such tools can potentially allow the production of GMOs with desirable traits, such as enhanced disease resistance or improved nutritional value. As gene editing technologies become more common in agriculture, they could potentially be utilized to revolutionize crop production and sustainability. Moreover, TALENs and ZFNs have been shown to be important in the formulation of cellular models for the investigation of human diseases, thus enhancing our knowledge of genetic diseases.

These applications underscore the important contribution of these emerging methods in developmental studies as they equip investigators with a more extensive toolkit with which to study gene function and create new therapeutic approaches. Yet, the decision among ZFNs, TALENs, and CRISPR/Cas9 is more than a technological preference; it is an inherent function of the various objectives of the research. Although CRISPR has become very popular owing to its simplicity and efficiency, TALENs and ZFNs present attractive options in cases where precision and reduced off-target effects are of utmost importance. Besides, the ethical considerations of gene editing also point to the necessity of responsible use of these technologies. As debate continues on the ramifications of breakthrough gene editing advances, it becomes more necessary to discern the relative merits and drawbacks of each approach. The advances in TALENs and ZFNs serve to remind us of the variety of gene-editing reagents and their utility in the new science of developmental research, ultimately calling on researchers to select suitably based on their goals (Inada et al., 2019; Mariscal et al., 2016) (Figure 11.6).

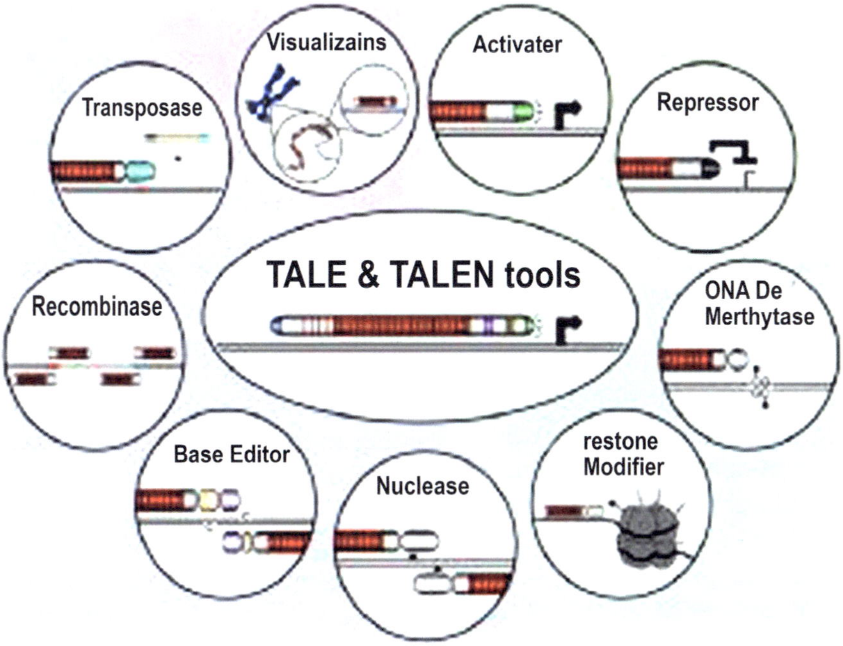

Figure 11.6. TALE and TALEN genome editing technologies.

Source: https://ars.els-cdn.com/content/image/1-s2.0-S2666388021000071-fx1.jpg.

11.1.3. Ethical Considerations in Gene Editing Technologies

As gene editing technologies like CRISPR/Cas9 become more utilized in medical and research environments, it is necessary to critically evaluate the ethical implications associated with their use. Despite the fact that these technologies hold great promise for treating genetic diseases, the implications of making genetic alterations are valid concerns regarding consent, justice, and the possibility of unintended consequences. Uncontrolled modification of the human genome may create societal divisions along the lines of access to such technologies, and hence further increase already present healthcare inequalities. Although such tools have revolutionary potential, the ethical questions they raise require a framework that can prioritize responsible application and fair access to ensure that progress is not at the expense of marginalized groups in society, which is at the core of gene editing bioethics today (Singh, 2024). The other critical element of gene editing ethics is the aspect of germline edits, which have implications extending beyond the individual. While somatic gene editing, which targets non-reproductive cells, is generally restricted to treatment, germline editing impacts future generations. The notion of playing God arises in the debate whether it is ethically right to introduce potentially heritable alterations to the human gene pool. A grave worry is that such interventions may unwittingly produce new types of social stratification because they can enable the enhancement or reduction of specific characteristics according to individual or societal desire. Therefore, the ethical considerations of gene editing technologies need to take into account the possible long-term results associated with germline edits and provide transparent and inclusive debates regarding these essential questions in developmental research (Stasi et al., 2024). Along with the equity and germline editing concerns, the new terrain of do-it-yourself (DIY) gene editing presents additional ethical concerns that cannot be overlooked. It is enabled by the availability of CRISPR technology and allows individuals beyond conventional scientific institutions to carry out genetic alterations. Though democratization of scientific research holds the promise of more innovation and public participation, it also presents serious biosecurity problems. Amateur scientists' unregulated gene manipulation can result in the development of dangerous organisms or the exploitation of biotechnological advancements for malicious intent. An ethical and regulatory framework for gene editing has to incorporate a complete set of control measures that weigh the urge for scientific investigation against the necessity to safeguard public health. Formulation of community-based regulatory policies and the integration of bioethical principles within the governance frameworks is crucial to promote responsible advancement in the area of DIY gene editing (Stasi et al., 2024).

11.2. Applications of Gene Editing in Developmental Biology

The use of gene editing in developmental biology research has revolutionized the research methodology so that researchers can now explore the complexities of genetic mechanisms underlying development. CRISPR-Cas9 is one such research methodology that has become an essential tool, as it has given researchers the ability to induce exact alterations in DNA sequences in organisms. This know-how forms the foundation of researching gene functions during development and modeling disease in vertebrate models. Through the generation of targeted insertions or mutations, developmental biologists can analyze resulting phenotypic alterations to understand the functions of particular genes in processes such as organogenesis and cell differentiation. Gene editing tools used in model organisms such as zebrafish and mice also improve our insight into developmental pathways and their relevance to regenerative medicine. Furthermore, gene editing has given researchers a tool with which to investigate complicated gene interactions and the control mechanisms involved in developmental processes. The recent developments take advantage of the capabilities of gene drive systems, which enable the biased transmission of edited genes to subsequent generations, hence speeding up the investigation of gene function across several generations. This approach underscores the potential of gene editing for following the inheritability of developmental traits and thereby gaining important insights into evolutionary processes. Moreover, being able to edit ESCs has important bearing on the generation of cell types involved in therapeutic uses, such as cell therapies and tissue engineering. Through the precise design of genetic modifications, researchers are able to access high-quality cell types with possibilities for regenerative applications in developmental biology, and this paves the way for future progress in the treatment of developmental disorders. Research into applications of gene editing tools also influences what is known regarding polygenic traits and environmental contributions to development. The integration of gene editing with advanced genomic approaches enables the detailed study of the interplay between genetic and environmental factors in developmental mechanisms. This integrated approach is important not only for understanding the functions of individual genes in determining phenotypic outputs but also the processes by which complex traits emerge over long time scales. In addition, the findings from such studies can provide insights into factors implicated in disorders that involve developmental disruptions, such as congenital defects and cancer. As technology evolves, the implications of gene editing continue to expand into ethical debates over the use of biotechnology for human enhancement and addressing genetic disease. The ongoing debate highlights the need for careful stewardship of these powerful tools within the field of developmental biology (Figure 11.7).

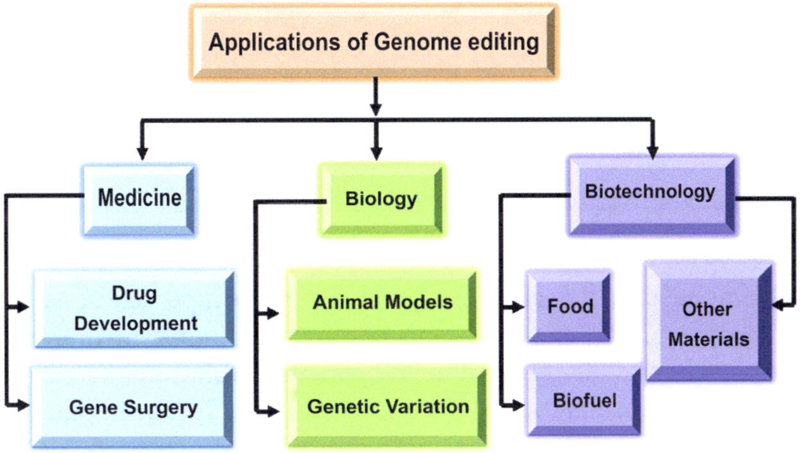

Figure 11.7. Applications of gene editing in developmental biology.

Source: https://www.researchgate.net/profile/Subbroto-Saha/publication/329449957/figure/fig4/AS:713741356265473@1547180608436/An-Overview-of-Applications-of-Genome-Editing-Genome-editing-can-be-used-in-various.png.

11.2.1. Gene Editing in Model Organisms

The incorporation of gene editing tools, more so CRISPR, in development studies presents unparalleled opportunities for the exploration of model organisms. *Drosophila melanogaster, Caenorhabditis elegans*, and *Mus musculus* have been the conventional paradigms for the study of genetic functions and developmental processes. Nevertheless, the inability of these models to capture the extensive biodiversity that exists in nature underscores the need to develop research on non-model organisms. This transition is not only necessary to improve our fundamental understanding but also to resolve applied problems such as invasive species control and disease, now feasible through the developments in genome editing technologies. This opening of research possibilities enables mechanistic investigations that improve our understanding at various scales of biological systems, thereby permitting improved understanding of developmental biology (Dickinson et al., 2020). As scientists investigate the application of gene editing on a wider range of species, a more nuanced understanding of the intricacies of phenotypic evolution can be achieved. Classical models of evolution, as embodied in the Modern Synthesis (MS), emphasize interactions among organisms, with heavy emphasis on gene transmission and exchange within populations. Yet scientists are contemplating an Extended Evolutionary Synthesis (EES) that accommodates more sophisticated interactions between epigenetic elements and intra-organismic processes.

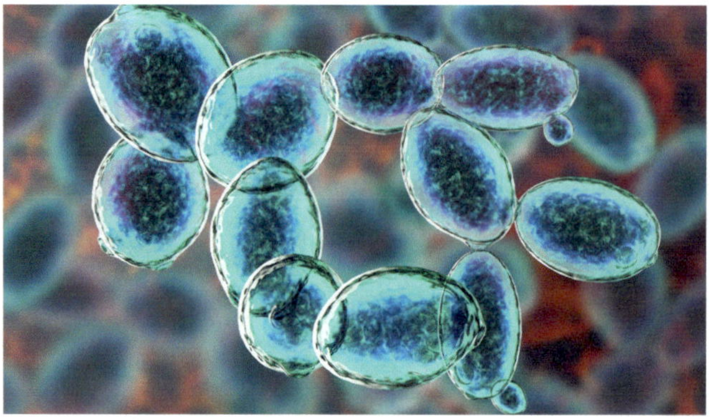

Figure 11.8. The Gene Editing in Model Organisms.

Source: https://images.contentstack.io/v3/assets/blte41c17d7f8dda379/bltb8b7fb5d4254b716/5d27794d8bcda8163689f101/Gene_editing_Using_CRISPR.jpg.

This viewpoint emphasizes the complex genotype-phenotype relations in model and non-model organisms. The possibility of using gene editing techniques in these organisms justifies investigations into epigenetic influences and developmental evolution and closes the gap between genetic determinism and organismal thought (Blancke et al., 2018). The implications of gene editing extend far beyond mere academic inquiry; they pose ethical questions, particularly the manipulation of living beings and natural systems. The ability to create chimeric organisms for the production of organs or to bring back extinct species raises both deeper questions of ethics and the environment. This therefore necessitates a careful consideration of the implications of gene editing within our framework in developmental studies. Furthermore, as gene editing becomes increasingly entrenched in a number of biological fields, cross-disciplinary partnerships will be necessary. By combining knowledge in genetics, ecology, and ethics, scientists can properly handle the complexities of gene editing, thereby satisfying responsible scientific practice. Lastly, though the potential of gene editing in model and non-model organisms is great, an approach to this powerful tool must be made with caution and a balanced ethical framework (Dickinson et al., 2020) (Figure 11.8).

11.2.2. Role of Gene Editing in Understanding Developmental Processes

The advent of gene editing technologies has greatly advanced the knowledge of developmental mechanisms in various organisms. Tools like CRISPR/Cas9 have made it possible for scientists to edit genes with high accuracy, and this has yielded crucial information on the genetic underpinnings of development. Using tools that target specific genes involved in morphogenesis, scientists are able to screen for alterations in phenotypes and infer the functions these genes have in the formation of structures and implementation of functions. Research on non-model organisms, including butterflies, illustrates the uses of these techniques in examining complicated evolutionary characteristics. The ability to make targeted manipulations in genes linked to wing patterns enhances knowledge of processes in morphological diversification, showing the interdisciplinarity of modern research that integrates genetics, developmental biology, and evolutionary studies (Ni et al., 2025). Furthermore, the use of gene editing extends beyond the simple alteration of phenotype; it includes the creation of accurate models of development that mirror complicated biological mechanisms. Through the use of CRISPR/Cas9 to introduce targeted mutations, researchers are able to develop models that recapitulate human disease or developmental defects. This particular use is of immense importance in neurodevelopmental disorder (NDD) research, where knowledge of gene function is essential for understanding the disease mechanism. For example, the use of gene editing has demonstrated tremendous utility in the generation of precise disease models for Alzheimer's disease, facilitating the ability to identify potential therapeutic targets as well as clarify molecular mechanisms involved in disease pathogenesis. These advances highlight the revolutionary nature of gene editing technologies, demonstrating their potential to advance research in developmental biology and open up critical paths to therapeutic interventions (Khan et al., 2025). As scientists refine gene editing techniques, the possibilities for understanding developmental processes are expanded.

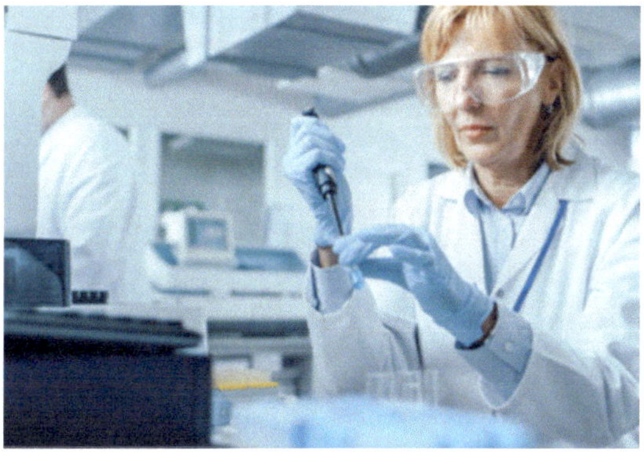

Figure 11.9. Gene editing technologies.

Source: https://vertassets.blob.core.windows.net/image/2a06cc69/2a06cc69-81ca-42a2-90aa-24d66cac7c86/375_250-istock_1140779660_drug_development_lab.png.

The combination of other sophisticated technologies like RNA interference and hybridization chain reaction with CRISPR/Cas9 improves functional verification and analysis of multi-factorial traits. For instance, recent studies on butterfly wing patterns illustrate how gene editing can unlock the interplay between genetic and environmental factors in complex phenotype development. These researches not only further the field of evolutionary developmental biology but also stimulate general debate on biodiversity and adaptation mechanisms. The prospects for the application of gene editing in developmental research look good, as current breakthroughs can allow greater insight into complex processes underlying life and maybe even hold the key to addressing pertinent biological issues (Ni et al., 2025) (Figure 11.9).

11.2.3. Potential for Gene Editing in Regenerative Medicine

The potential of gene editing in the field of regenerative medicine is increasingly recognized as a revolutionary technique for treating many diseases that currently do not have effective treatment modalities. Advances in genome-editing techniques, particularly CRISPR-Cas9, enable researchers to precisely edit DNA sequences in cellular components, thus providing unique avenues for correcting genetic defects that contribute to several diseases. Such specificity in regenerative medicine can be utilized to promote cellular regeneration through direct targeting of and alteration in the genetic bases causing dysfunction.

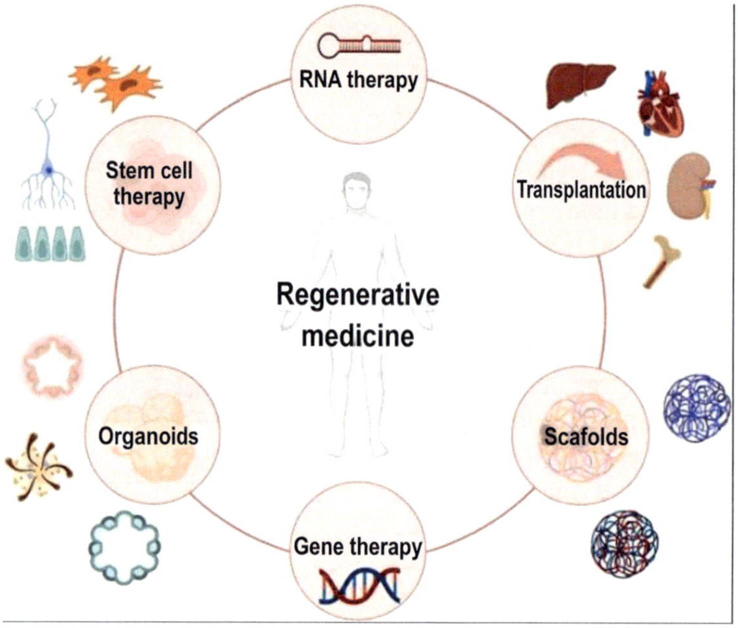

Figure 11.10. Potential for gene editing in regenerative medicine.

Source: https://ars.els-cdn.com/content/image/1-s2.0-S0753332222015207-gr1.jpg.

For instance, application of gene editing techniques in adult human intestinal stem cells (ISCs) has demonstrated potential towards treating monogenic and polygenic forms of intestinal failure, with the approach indicating that it would treat genetic disease at its etiological origin and pave the way for autologous ISC transplantation as a realistic treatment modality (Dunn et al., 2016). Moreover, gene editing holds much potential not only for the treatment of genetic disease but also for a variety of other uses in the arena of tissue regeneration. Studies on cardiovascular regeneration, for instance, describe how the editing of certain genes associated with cellular proliferation and differentiation can cause rejuvenation and restoration of cardiac tissues that have been compromised. Workshops and conferences have continued to stress the importance of elucidating cardiac lineage choices at a molecular level, showing how gene expression and tissue reaction interact (Schneider, 2016). The accumulation of this evidence indicates that the introduction of gene editing into regenerative paradigms is an important advancement, enabling the conception of strategies that augment the body's inherent ability for repair and regeneration. Yet, there are great hurdles along the way to the general application of gene editing for regenerative medicine. Key challenges are the enhancement of both the efficiency and accuracy of gene editing technologies, along with the necessity to confirm the safety of transformed cells before transplantation. Solutions to these issues entail ongoing research on optimizing gene delivery techniques, along with advances in integrating edited cells into target tissues. As shown in the case of induced pluripotent stem cell (ISC) study, large-animal models offer the essential bridge in spanning the gap between clinic and laboratory science in thereby substantiating the effectiveness and safety of novel therapies prior to testing through human clinical trials (Dunn et al., 2016). Overcoming these obstacles with further research and collaborative effort will be essential to unleashing the complete potential of gene editing within the realm of regenerative medicine (Figure 11.10).

11.3. Ethical Implications of Gene Editing

The ethical stakes of gene editing technologies are high and complex, encompassing both future uses and long-term consequences for society. While gene editing advances, especially CRISPR-Cas9, hold the promise of tremendous medical advances, such as the correction of genetic diseases, it also presents significant ethical issues. At the center of these arguments is the issue of consent, especially when germline treatments affecting future generations who cannot consent themselves are taken into consideration. Standards and protocols that safeguard not only individuals who are currently undergoing treatment but also guarantee the rights of unborn children should be established. The consequences of altering the genetic composition of individuals have repercussions within family and social systems and therefore require an expansive ethical framework considering the multifaceted dimensions of consent and responsibility. Above and beyond individual consent, the possibility that gene editing technologies may enhance prevailing social disparities presents important ethical hurdles. Access to gene editing therapies could be restricted to the wealthy segments of the population, and a divide may be created where only a part of the population can benefit from developments in medical technology. This can further lead to the creation of a divide between genetically modified and unmodified people and hence give rise to social tensions and discrimination on the basis of genetic traits. On top of this is the potential for designer babies, with the rich getting to choose the desirable characteristics for their offspring, locking in a vicious cycle of disparity that prioritizes genetic privilege over universal access to healthcare. Healthcare justice demands that gene editing be fashioned and shared in such a way that it does not add to the already existing societal rifts, demanding constant discussion and policy-making that follows the moral imperative of equity. Moreover, the long-term effects of gene editing on the trajectory of human evolution are a deep ethical question that remains partly unresolved. As gene editing technologies become more widespread, society needs to consider the possible changes to the human gene pool; the inadvertent creation of unexpected consequences or off-target effects can result in unexpected health problems or potentially destabilize ecosystems. These profound changes demand intense scrutiny and a more measured gene editing research and application agenda. Subjects such as microbiota modulation, as explored in pertinent studies such as those referenced in current reviews on microbiota health and dysbiosis (Hou et al., 2022; Swanson et al., 2020), highlight the necessity for comprehensive viewpoints in considering the effects of gene editing on broader biological systems. The moral implications of such long-term effects demand that we address the application of gene editing in developmental research in a responsive and responsible manner (Figure 11.11).

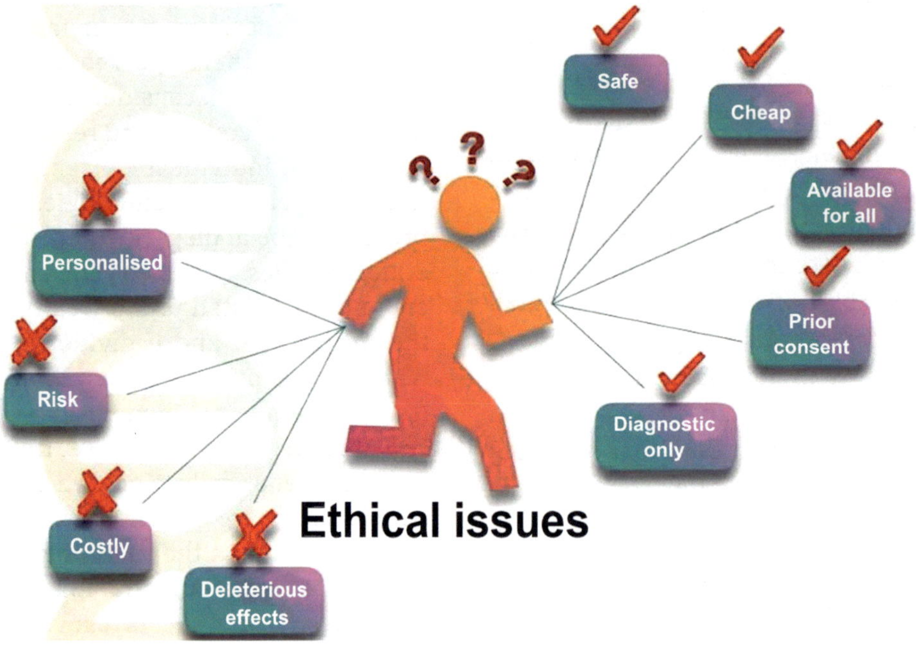

Figure 11.11. Ethical implications of gene editing.

Source: https://geneticeducation.co.in/wp-content/uploads/2018/12/gene-editing-.006-e1546088159980.jpeg.

11.3.1. Concerns Regarding Human Germline Editing

Problems of human germline editing have made more headlines with the rapid evolution of gene-editing tools, most prominently CRISPR-Cas9. While technology for precise genetic modification promises to eliminate inherited diseases, the implications of germline editing of the human genome are extremely complicated ethical concerns. A classic example of this is the alteration of embryos' genome, which will create unforeseen off-target effects that can result in potential health and developmental hazards, and the birth of so-called designer babies—genetically constructed children with particular characteristics deemed desirable by social or parental standards. The path outlined has the potential to make genetic inequalities worse and create a social gap between those who can purchase enhancements and those who cannot, thereby becoming an issue of equity and access to genetic healthcare (Doudna, 2025). The potential of germline editing to fundamentally transform human reproduction and identity thus serves to highlight the necessity for a comprehensive ethical scrutiny. Aside from the social ramifications, the worry of the long-term effect of germline editing underscores the intricacy of the matter. The alterations done on the germline can be heritable, which means that any modification may affect subsequent generations in a way that is hard to predict.

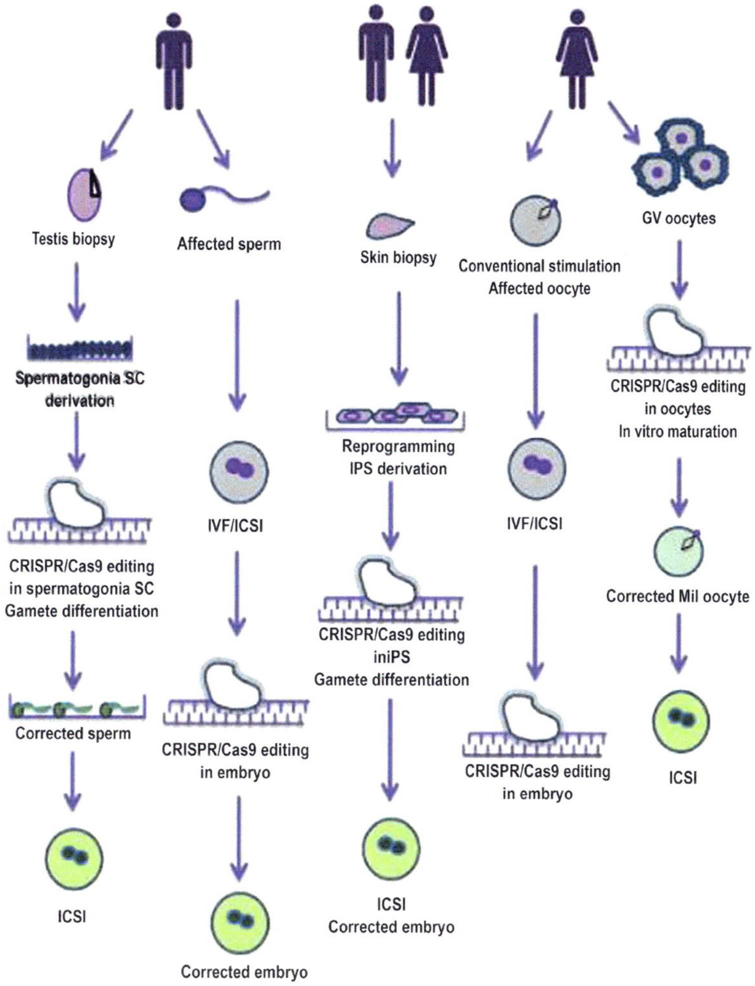

Figure 11.12. Responsible innovation in human germline gene editing.

Source: https://media.springernature.com/full/springer-static/image/art%3A10.1038%2Fs41431-017-0077-z/MediaObjects/41431_2017_77_Fig1_HTML.jpg.

The potential to cause unanticipated genetic aberrations or interfere with basic genetic processes warrants cautious consideration. Moreover, the ethical obligation to safeguard not just the individual on whom genetic editing is done but their offspring as well makes decision-making more complex because it extends beyond individual autonomy to include wider social repercussions. Debates around regulations on germline editing highlight the imperative for stringent regulatory frameworks that prioritize safety and ethical integrity (Allwardt et al., 2017). While the scientific community keeps extending the boundaries of genetic research, it is necessary that such ethical concerns are prioritized in the debate. The general public perception about germline editing is one of extreme fear, based usually on earlier experiences of eugenics and genetic testing. There have been concerns that germline manipulation might lead society down a problematic path characterized by genetic discrimination and the resumption of damaging ideas about genetic purity. These types of concerns are rightfully valid, in light of the past examples of ethical breaches that regularly disenfranchised certain groups based on arbitrary genetic or physical characteristics. It is important to conduct thorough public discourse, educational programs, and the spread of transparent research findings to reduce these fears. Ethical paradigms that include diverse perspectives from societies can lead to more inclusive policies and practices towards gene editing. In short, though scientific progress persists in reforming our knowledge of genetics, the prospective social implications of germline editing should always be at the front position of the current gene editing and developmental research discussion (Figure 11.12).

11.3.2. Societal Impacts of Gene Editing Technologies

The advent of gene editing technologies, more particularly CRISPR-Cas9, has transformed our approach to genetic modification, posing both tremendous opportunities and challenges to humankind. These technologies have the potential to drive huge breakthroughs in the field of medicine, agriculture, and nature conservation. Yet, their social implications are wide-ranging and complex. The prospect of editing genes brings about ethical considerations on how far human beings need to interfere with natural processes. Thus, there is a need for a new social contract that balances scientific advancement with societal and economic demands. This agreement must place ethical principles and public discussion at the forefront, making certain that technological innovation aligns with moral principles and fosters a beneficial impact on societal welfare (Montagu et al., 2020). As it is, the gene editing technologies are more than scientific instruments; they are potent forces of social transformation that demand adequate examination of the moral paradigms informing their application. Within agriculture, gene editing technologies offer hopeful resolutions to the problem of worldwide food insecurity by improving the resilience and nutritional value of crops. The technologies seek to resolve the urgency of feeding a rising population while, concurrently, preventing environmental damage (Montagu et al., 2020). Notwithstanding the appeal of these advancements to a broad audience, they concurrently raise significant apprehensions pertaining to biodiversity, food sovereignty, and the independence of conventional agricultural methods. As sectors increasingly embrace innovative biotechnological instruments, there arises an immediate necessity for comprehensive discussions that engage multiple stakeholders, encompassing farmers, consumers, and policymakers. Through the incorporation of varied viewpoints, society is positioned to develop regulatory structures that not only promote the adoption of technology but also protect against monopolistic tendencies that may marginalize small-scale agricultural producers. Thus, an understanding of the social implications of gene editing for agriculture is fundamental to developing sustainable strategies that align with both environmental goals and community needs. The implications of gene editing extend from the field of agriculture to the healthcare field, where advancements hold the potential to revolutionize the treatment of genetic diseases. The advent of gene therapy offers hope for conditions previously deemed incurable, with the potential to enhance the quality of life for many. But as the range of therapeutic possibilities grows, so does the demand for equal access to such innovations simultaneously. A danger exists that gene editing advances may widen the present health disparities unless such technologies are limited to only wealthy populations. In addition, the ethical dimensions of selective human genetic modification ignite a multifaceted discussion on designer children, with the debate revolving around future social hierarchies determined by genetic characteristics. For these issues to be addressed, there is a requirement that society promotes policies for guaranteeing that there is equitable distribution of gene editing technologies so that the concepts of justice and equality are upheld in scientific advancement (Figure 11.13).

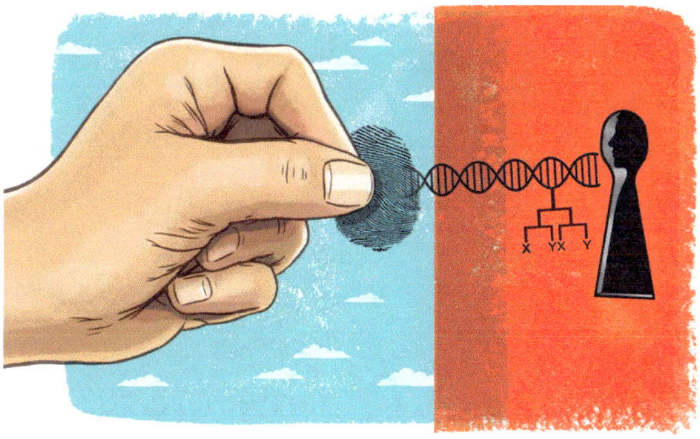

Figure 11.13. Societal impacts of gene editing technologies.

Source: https://news.harvard.edu/wp-content/uploads/2018/12/genefb.jpg.

1.3.3. Regulatory Frameworks Governing Gene Editing

The legal frameworks for regulating gene editing are multifaceted and diverse and are contingent upon a plethora of ethical, scientific, and social factors. As gene editing tools, especially CRISPR, become increasingly relevant, regulatory bodies must come up with legislation that is commensurate with swift scientific progress. These frameworks must cover not only the technical modalities of gene manipulation but also the ethical considerations surrounding possible applications. For example, controversy has emerged regarding the acceptable boundaries of germline editing, which induces inheritable alterations in human DNA. Bioethicists note that prominent considerations involve the danger of inducing unintended genetic effects as well as the wider social context, under which CRISPR can either be viewed as a precursor to dystopian futures or as a new mechanism for strengthening human health and resilience (Mariscal et al., 2016). Moreover, the formulation of regulatory frameworks needs interdisciplinary cooperation to be able to guarantee that a variety of viewpoints contribute to policy development processes. Scientists, ethicists, and legal scholars must collaborate to create standards that are both scientifically credible and ethically cautious. While regulations are being put in place, they must encapsulate the revolutionary possibilities of gene editing technologies, just like previous advancements have shaped public policy. Regulators need to take into account the possible long-term impacts of gene editing, alongside empirical evidence, together with societal perceptions and moral concerns. By placing CRISPR in the context of a technological advancement that has the potential to transform medicine and agriculture, regulators are in a position to align their management strategies and prudent application of editing technologies (Mariscal et al., 2016).

Also, the precision medicine concept demonstrates the prospective integration of gene editing into conventional healthcare systems. Precision medicine aims at making medical care personalized for individual patients according to their distinct genetic profiles and offers a hopeful pathway for the implementation of gene editing technologies. Nevertheless, the consideration of gene editing in practice depends on comprehensive regulatory frameworks that consider safety and efficacy. Difficulties regarding the use of precision medicine in a number of medical specialties are indicative of the requirement for precise definitions and systematic methodologies for assessing novel therapeutic approaches. Thus, regulatory frameworks as they continue to develop should be aimed at enabling the promotion of innovation while safeguarding patient interests and guaranteeing ethical considerations, thereby informing responsible application of gene editing in research in development and in the clinic (Figure 11.14).

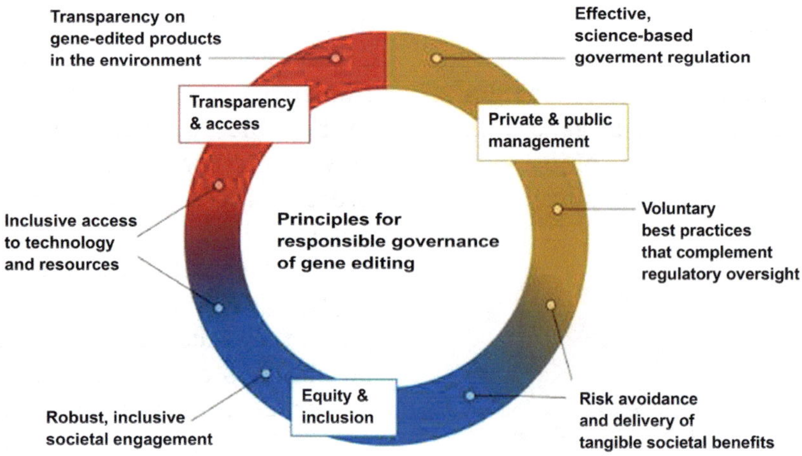

Figure 11.14. Regulatory frameworks governing gene editing.

Source: https://media.springernature.com/m685/springer-static/image/art%3A10.1038%2Fs41587-021-01023-1/MediaObjects/41587_2021_1023_Fig1_HTML.png.

11.4. Case Studies in Gene Editing Research

The advent of gene editing tools, and more especially CRISPR/Cas9, has accelerated advancements in a wide range of research fields. One of the most exemplary case studies demonstrating this is the application of CRISPR in agricultural biotechnology. Researchers have successfully edited the genomes of various crops to enhance traits like drought resistance and nutritional value. However, in spite of the promising results, the use of the technology faces a number of challenges. Scientists have raised concerns over indiscriminate cutting and cytotoxicity issues that may undermine the safety and effectiveness of genetic modification for use in agricultural purposes. These issues need to be resolved to pave the way for broader adoption and utilization of such innovations in the production of essential food staples. Significant advancement in predictive modeling with the use of deep learning technologies has been proposed to enhance the precision in targeting of CRISPR, representing the synergy of advanced technology and solving critical problems in gene editing techniques in agriculture (Cui et al., 2024). Aside from its agricultural uses, research on gene editing in medicine also presents other compelling case studies, particularly in the repair of genetic disorders. A notable case is the attempt to target the genetic mutation linked to sickle cell disease. Scientists were able to use CRISPR/Cas9 technology to edit the genetic material of cells from patients and thereby open a possible avenue of therapeutic intervention that may alleviate symptoms of this disease. The example not only demonstrates the potential of gene editing to transform therapeutic strategies but also provokes ethical debate regarding acceptable limits of germline manipulation in humans. Through ongoing research and development of gene editing technology with more depth, it invites important discussion on the ethical use of human genetic modification. Thus, a case study review on gene editing, particularly from a medical point of view, identifies the equilibrium that must be established between scientific development and ethical restraints on processes of research and development (Saluja et al., 2024). The application of gene editing technologies in medicine and agriculture fields is a twin tale of risks and promises. numerous empirical research papers demonstrate the revolutionary possibilities of CRISPR technology, yet simultaneously, they also highlight the necessity for rigorous ethical scrutiny to be applied to it. Science fiction literary works confront the ethical challenges of gene editing in a manner that resonates with public anxieties regarding human ability to manage these powerful technologies. Through reading literature that speaks to the ethical ramifications of genetic manipulation, scientists and ethicists alike are able to make informed conclusions regarding societal sentiment and possible consequences of gene editing. Thus, as advancements in developmental biology are achieved, it is ever more necessary to keep the discussion going, so that the quest for knowledge does not come at the expense of the ethical accountabilities inherent to it. Within the backdrop of this evolving landscape, case studies are integral elements for understanding the intricate dynamics between technological innovation, safety, and ethical oversight in the field of gene editing (Saluja et al., 2024).

11.4.1. Successful Gene Editing in Agricultural Development

In recent times, the use of effective gene editing tools has transformed agricultural innovations, making it possible to create crops with elite traits that address food needs on a global scale. A case in point is the genomic studies on sunflowers that have deciphered the intricate genetic composition responsible for important traits like oil production, disease resistance, and drought tolerance. Identification of particular genes relating to resistance to pests and environmental stresses is of great value to plant breeding programs. By utilizing the knowledge achieved through sunflower genomics, researchers can generate cultivars that not only are of nutritional value but also enhance sustainable agriculture by lessening the dependency on chemical controls and fostering biodiversity in farming systems. The focus on genomic data corroborates the view that gene editing is critical in elevating the productivity and climate tolerance of staple crops under climate change (Godara et al., 2024). Gene editing tools, especially CRISPR/Cas9, are a game-changer that amplifies agricultural genetic research. The capacity to create targeted mutations in legume crops, which are very important for sustainable agriculture production, is especially interesting. Recent developments have underlined the need to create precise gene editing technologies with the focus being on individual tissue types within legumes, more precisely those implicated in nitrogen fixation via rhizobial symbiosis. By employing a rhizobia-inducible and cell-type-specific CRISPR/Cas9 system, researchers have the ability to selectively knock out genes in root tissues without inhibiting the overall viability of the plant. Such precision not only enhances the effectiveness of the research process but also creates a more refined understanding of the genetic necessities needed for efficient nitrogen fixation, which is central to sustaining soil health and fertility in diverse cropping systems. In summary, the incorporation of effective gene editing techniques into agricultural innovations is central to tackling the contemporary issues related to food security and environmental sustainability. By leveraging genomic breakthroughs, researchers are identifying and breeding crops that can thrive in difficult conditions, a requirement for food security as the world grapples with increasing pressures from a burgeoning population. The potential offered by gene editing goes beyond mere yield improvement; it offers paths to developing crops that require less input while offering better nutritional profiles. As the discipline evolves, the coordination of academic research and agricultural practice is likely to provide new varieties that will assist in creating a more robust agricultural platform at a global scale. Such an assimilation and integration point to the importance of gene editing in influencing future agricultural systems and enabling developmental research (Godara et al., 2024) (Figure 11.15).

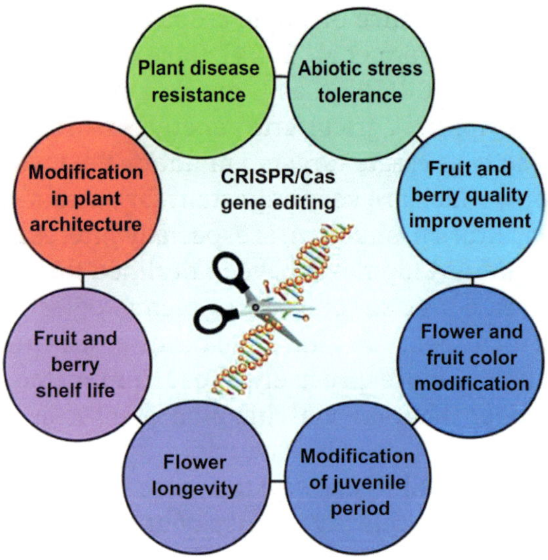

Figure 11.15. Successful gene editing in agricultural development.

Source: https://www.mdpi.com/horticulturae/horticulturae-09-00038/article_deploy/html/images/horticulturae-09-00038-g001-550.jpg.

11.4.2. Gene Editing in the Treatment of Genetic Disorders

Recent developments in gene editing technologies have significantly revolutionized the treatment of genetic disorder, especially with the use of methods such as CRISPR/Cas9. This groundbreaking tool enables the alteration of precise genetic sequences, thereby providing the possibility of targeted therapeutic intervention for hitherto treatment-resistant genetic disorders. One of the most important features of CRISPR technology is that it can generate accurate models of human disease, enabling researchers to study genetic mutations and their implications more conveniently. By enabling insights into the mechanism of disease and the development of possible therapeutic interventions, CRISPR is at the forefront of translational medicine, although there are still hurdles to its application in the clinic. Improving the efficacy, precision, and delivery modalities of CRISPR technology is also paramount for the advancement of this technology from laboratory settings to the clinical field, revealing the need for additional research and development for it to be fully harnessed (Ferreira et al., 2020). The possibility of using gene editing approaches in the management of neuronal channelopathies illustrates the potential of this technology for treating multifactorial genetic disorders. Various conditions of this type arise from mutations affecting ion channels, leading to cases of abnormal neuronal excitability. Methods involving gene therapy aimed at manipulating gene expression relevant to neuronal function have emerged as a promising avenue of research. Current trials for such conditions illustrate the urgent need for the establishment of new therapies that not only alleviate symptoms but also have the ability to cure these diseases. The latest advances in gene-editing tools, especially those related to the CRISPR-Cas9 system, present a new approach to the correction of harmful mutations directly, targeting the disorder's cause at the germline level. As such, gene editing has the potential to serve as an effective approach to shifting the therapeutic landscape of channelopathies and other genetic disorders (Lignani et al., 2017). The time at which therapeutic gene editing is done, as well as the intervention methods employed, can greatly determine the efficacy of the treatment. The selection of when to administer gene therapy—whether at germline, neonatal, or adult levels—can be immensely vital in driving developmental outcomes. Early treatments, especially at the neonatal level, could enhance possibilities for normal brain development and function because genetic defects that are not resolved can impair neural connectivity. Conversely, interventions in adults can remain effective, yet with a more complex scenario of likely compensatory mechanisms that may interfere with therapeutic benefit. Research in progress to ascertain the optimum time for gene editing interventions will further refine treatment protocols with the elucidation of the mechanisms in various genetic disorders. The convergence of gene editing with developmental studies has immense potential to overcome the issues of genetic disorders, ultimately making way for the introduction of innovative healthcare solutions (Figure 11.16).

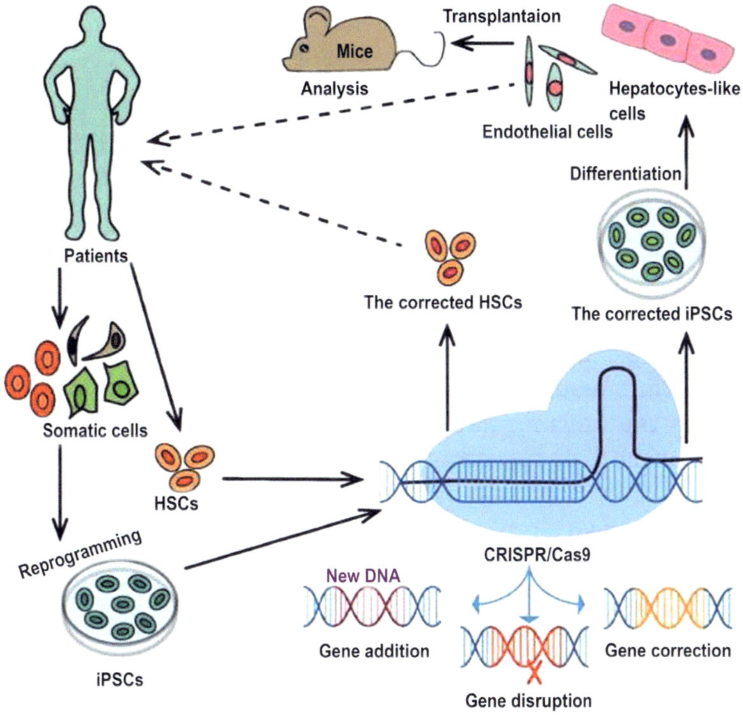

Figure 11.16. Gene editing in the treatment of genetic disorders.

Source: https://media.springernature.com/full/springer-static/image/art%3A10.1038%2Fs41434-021-00247-9/MediaObjects/41434_2021_247_Fig1_HTML.png.

11.4.3. Controversial Cases and Public Response

The intersection of gene editing and public opinion has been dominated by contentious instances that elicit strong emotional and ethical reactions. A particularly prominent instance is the application of CRISPR technology to genetically edit embryos. This innovation ignited strong public uproar as critics worried that it had the potential to bring about designer babies and exacerbate social disparities. As public faith in scientific institutions continues to reduce, such controversies can generate formidable resistance to the development of gene editing technologies. Ethicists call for public discussion of the possible consequences of gene editing, asserting that the public should be provided with some role within ethical deliberations concerning biotechnology. These discussions are vital since they connect scientific advancements and societal values, thereby making sure that innovations correspond to the ethical concerns and aspirations of the public, which is necessary for propagating responsible development in science (Ahmed et al., 2018). Further, the diverse responses of the public to contentious gene editing instances depict the sophistication of societal interaction with scientific research. For example, the revelation by the Chinese scientist He Jiankui that he had delivered twins whose genomes he had edited provoked outright upheaval within the international community of researchers, with controversy over the scientific limits of experimentation. Most researchers decried his actions as irresponsible and contended that not only did they threaten the welfare of the children, but they also tarnished the overall feasibility of gene editing technologies. The incident prompted calls for regulatory mechanisms that would dissuade abuse without inhibiting the advancement of scientific research. In the absence of appropriate regulation, gene editing activities can have adverse implications for research progress and undermine public confidence in potentially valuable innovations. As it is, institutional responsibility and ethical gravity are central issues that need addressing in the wider debate on gene editing and its societal repercussions (Mariscal et al., 2016). Secondly, the controversy around gene editing brings out the difficulty in navigating public opinion amidst fast-paced technological evolution. As the boundaries of genetic manipulation ever widen, both the rise of support and opposition are symptoms of profound social anxieties regarding what gene editing might herald. Detractors tend to cast the science as an imminent danger, arguing its misuse could have unintended effects, whereas proponents praise its potential to eliminate inherited diseases. This paradox makes legislative action challenging since policymakers must tread the tricky terrain of public opinion, scientific facts, and moral imperatives. To this end, stimulating informed public discussion and engaging various stakeholders is crucial to formulating effective policy. In conclusion, public response to these contentious cases is a key indicator for the future prospects of gene editing and therefore demands effective communication and adequate ethical guidelines in order to gain the technology's acceptance and adoption by society (Ahmed et al., 2018; Mariscal et al., 2016).

11.5. Future Directions in Gene Editing Research

The accelerated progress in gene editing technology, especially CRISPR/Cas9, is setting the stage for the development of novel therapeutic approaches in regenerative medicine. As the research keeps venturing into the possibilities of editing the human genome, one promising field of interest is the use of gene editing to treat genetic diseases at their source. The method entails the precision editing of genes whose malfunction causes inherited diseases, and this has the promise of transforming our therapeutic landscape. In addition, the development of organoid models derived from intestinal stem cells (ISCs) highlights the therapeutic implications of gene editing in addressing complex gastrointestinal diseases. By utilizing ex vivo human tissues for the exploration of disease mechanisms, researchers are in a position to develop targeted mechanisms that directly rectify genetic abnormalities, as evidenced in the study of adult human ISCs for therapy (Dunn et al., 2016). The merging of gene editing and stem cell technologies represents a profound advancement in the area of personalized medicine and patient outcome enhancement. Another imperative area for future gene editing research directions pertains to the optimization of current gene delivery systems. The current methodologies are often limited in terms of their efficiency and specificity, which may result in off-target effects or suboptimal gene expression. Overcoming these challenges is crucial for clinical application, especially for complicated diseases necessitating specific genetic modification. Viral vector development and the creation of novel delivery systems, including nanoparticles or electroporation methods, are among the most important research areas.

By working on these systems, scientists can make gene therapies safer and more effective, so these medications are not only effective but also safe for individuals. There is a great focus now on utilizing large animal models for preclinical studies as they provide a more pertinent physiological milieu to test the safety and effectiveness of these novel delivery systems (Dunn et al., 2016). Overall, these advances are poised to play a key part in the actual translation of gene editing to clinical practice. Further, as ethical dilemmas surrounding gene editing come to the forefront, it is important that future research prioritizes the development of comprehensive systems of governance. The repercussions of gene editing are not limited to personal health alone because they also generate enormous societal inquiries about genetic parity, consent, and the risks of unknown repercussions. Scientists and policymakers must collaborate on developing standards that ensure ethics without inhibiting progress in this area of science.

The involvement of various stakeholders, ranging from ethicists and public representatives to healthcare practitioners, is likely to facilitate a change in the gene editing discourse that reflects and represents societal values. In addition, more public engagement and education regarding gene editing technologies will be more likely to lead to increased understanding and acceptance of scientific advancements. These initiatives are crucial for steering through the complicated gene editing landscape effectively, ultimately resulting in the responsible and fair application of emerging technologies (Figure 11.17).

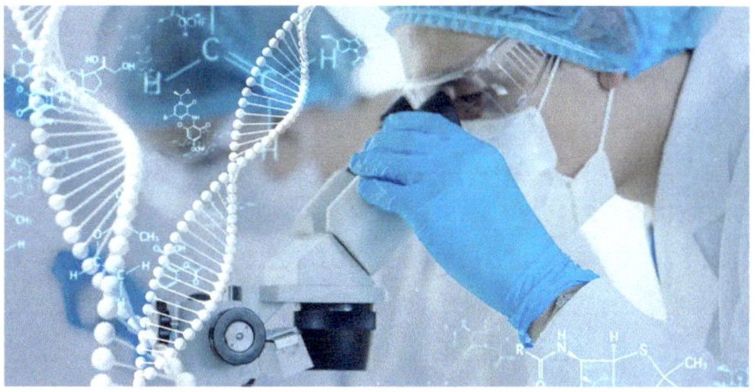

Figure 11.17. The emerging landscape of gene editing.

Source: https://blog.bccresearch.com/hubfs/mRNA-Therapeutics.webp.

11.5.1. Innovations in Gene Editing Techniques

Recent breakthroughs in gene editing tools embody a tremendous change in the field of biotechnology, leading to groundbreaking applications in development studies. Notably, the CRISPR-Cas9 system is described by its accuracy and efficiency in making specific changes in the genomes of any organism, including plants, animals, and humans. The above capability has far-reaching consequences for agricultural development, as gene editing can help develop crops that are more resilient to environmental stress and disease. As scientists are applying these sophisticated techniques to promote food security and sustainability, it is apparent that such practices are not merely scientific advancements but also carry ethical implications and societal concerns that need to be critically examined. The conflict between the potential of technology and the imperatives of ethics introduces the necessity of the establishment of a new social contract in genetic engineering, wherein scientific possibility is matched by ethical norms and societal needs (Montagu et al., 2020). The revolutionary nature of CRISPR technology is underlined by the fact that it can introduce fundamental changes in genetic designs with unprecedented ease and accuracy. The method enables scientists to edit individual genes by making double-strand breaks, which are then repaired using the cells' own machinery, either by adding new genetic information or modifying existing sequences. Not only does the technology speed up genetic research, but it also paves the way for novel therapeutic strategies for the treatment of genetic disease. Notwithstanding its potential benefits, the advent of CRISPR technology has provoked substantial ethical discussions regarding its ramifications for human health and the environment. Detractors articulate apprehensions that its possible misuse might result in unforeseen repercussions, including the emergence of designer babies or disruptions to ecological balance, thereby highlighting the necessity for comprehensive ethical guidelines to oversee its responsible utilization (Mariscal et al., 2016).

Apart from their therapeutic applications, the gene editing technologies hold great promise for the discipline of developmental biology, more specifically for studying gene function and regulation during organism development. Through the manipulation of gene sequences in model organisms, researchers can elucidate the pathways that regulate major developmental processes and provide insights into congenital disorders and their molecular etiology. Furthermore, gene editing technologies have spurred the development of new strategies in tissue engineering and regenerative medicine, where precision genetic manipulations can augment the capacity of stem cells for differentiation into desired cell lineages. Such convergence between gene editing and developmental biology not only advances the science but also signals the urgent need for inter-disciplinary research collaboration to address the complicated set of ethical, regulatory, and biological issues that will likely crop up in the future. Collectively, these technical developments recognize the bifurcated direction of gene editing development—possessing the potential for significant beneficial effects, but also representing ethical concerns necessitating serious consideration (Montagu et al., 2020) (Figure 11.18).

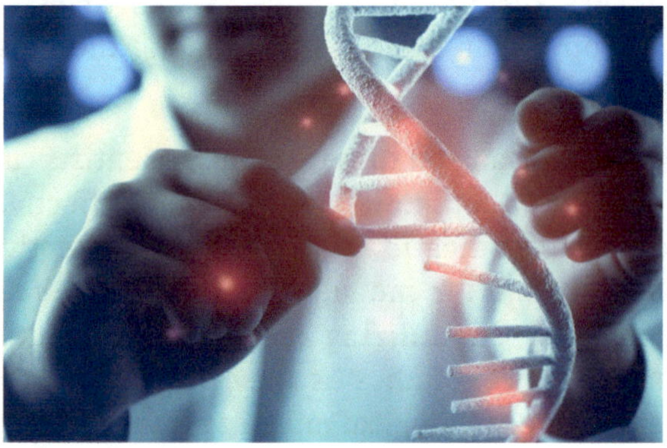

Figure 11.18. Innovations in gene editing techniques.

Source: https://proventainternational.com/wp-content/uploads/2023/07/m16ka7a_person_undergoing_genetic_testing_to_determine_their_ri_7c22f4f5-caf8-4e99-bd43-51479c78d1a5-1024x683.png.

11.5.2. Potential for Personalized Medicine

The development of gene editing technologies, in particular CRISPR-Cas9, has transformed the landscape of personalized medicine, holding unprecedented promise for individualized therapeutic approaches. With the ability to make specific changes in the genetic contents of individual patients, scientists are now more likely to decipher the genetic basis of countless ailments and edit them as appropriate. The degree of personalization afforded herein not only has immense potential for therapy of genetic inherited disorders but also offers a basis for targeted therapeutic approaches in multifactorial diseases, e.g., cancer. Through this capacity, clinicians are able to create therapy approaches that take into consideration precise genetic variation while also enhancing therapeutic effectiveness and limiting adverse effects, thereby rendering clinical therapy more effective and patient-centered (Sen et al., 2025). In the case of diseases such as hepatocellular carcinoma (HCC), the combination of gene therapy with personal medicine strategies holds great advantages. The conventional treatment modalities for HCC are not very effective due to the fact that they possess narrow therapeutic windows and unacceptable toxicities, and new modalities are sought. Gene therapy presents itself as a very appealing option in light of its ability to selectively target aberrant signaling pathways and immune evasion genes. This targeting enhances the possibility of successful intervention through the minimization of collateral damage to health tissues, one of the biggest drawbacks of conventional therapies. The application of new gene editing techniques, coupled with sophisticated gene delivery systems like nanomedicines, can further bridge the gap between clinical trials and treatment regimens, to the attainment of effective, Personalized approaches tailored to patient-specific characteristics (Younis and Harashima, 2024). Also, the creation of precision medicine using gene editing is not limited to the treatment of disease alone but also includes prevention strategies that may avert the development of genetic disorders. With the application of genome editing tools at the start of the healthcare continuum, one can not only treat but also prevent diseases well before they become clinically evident. The preventative aspect takes the idea of personalized medicine one step further by adapting treatment methods to align with an individual's genetic predispositions. As research continues in the field, it will be imperative to balance ethical concerns with the necessity of extensive clinical trials to guarantee safety and efficacy. The integration of ethical standards will be necessary to garner public trust and acceptance as this groundbreaking paradigm in health care evolves (Sen et al., 2025).

11.5.3. Challenges and Limitations in Current Research

The area of gene editing has experienced huge progress; however, it is confronted with significant challenges that hamper the advancement of basic in addition to applied research. Among the largest challenges is the use of typical model organisms, which are not very representative of the sophistication of natural evolutionary processes. As a result, when research identifies prospective loci by way of genome-wide association methods, such results struggle to demonstrate convincing causal links between genotype and phenotype. The validation experiments are typically narrow, and the majority of the studies using RNA interference (RNAi) and CRISPR approaches fail to fully capture ecologically important variations, resulting in constraints on functional tests (Gudmunds et al., 2022, p. 1104–1115). Such methodological limitations underscore the necessity of integrating a wide range of emerging model organisms in gene editing studies to enhance our knowledge of developmental processes and adaptive phenotypes. Alongside the issues intrinsic to model organism choice, technical sophistication presented by modern gene editing tools also hinders research efficiency. Despite the revolutionary impact of technologies such as CRISPR-Cas9 on genomic sequence manipulation, spatial precision and knock-in efficiency are still major challenges. Additionally, low throughput in functional verification is a hindrance, which makes it increasingly difficult to perform large-scale experimentation necessary for complex genetic interaction elucidation. In addition, with improvements in genome editing techniques, the necessity to create approaches that verify known gene function in ecologically relevant contexts becomes ever more urgent (Li et al., 2020). The difficulty is not only in the improvement of the techniques but also in confirming their usefulness in a wider assortment of biological systems. Hence, scientists need to be cognizant of such limitations in an attempt to explain the genetic foundations of phenotypes that are essential for evolutionary processes and developmental pathways. The significance of rectifying the methodological issues with respect to gene editing is amplified with the increasing number of studies that do not adequately confirm the functions of candidate genes. Most research is now motivated by the new potential of large data sets and not by meticulous testing of hypotheses to connect genotypes and phenotypes. As a result, academic literature has been flooded with speculative analyses, which have a tendency to obscure actual understanding of genetic functions and evolutionary processes. Such an event erodes the credibility of scientific arguments within molecular biology and allied disciplines. To address this issue, the focus in future research studies should be placed on the necessity of functional verification and the investigation of candidate genes regardless of their previous annotations or assumed biological functions. By implementing a more rigorous methodology for candidate selection and verification, researchers are able to encourage a more precise concept of gene function and its application in the fields of evolutionary biology and developmental studies (Gudmunds et al., 2022, p. 1104–1115; Li et al., 2020).

11.6. Public Perception and Acceptance of Gene Editing

Public perception of gene editing technologies, and CRISPR-Cas9 more specifically, is central to determining their rollout and uptake within the general public. As improvements in genome editing herald the era of improved agricultural methods and medical advancement, the reception of these technologies is closely tied to regulatory policies and popular opinion. Industry stakeholders in gene editing need to emphasize open and transparent communication to foster an improved understanding among laypersons. Research indicates that merely publishing information about the advantages of gene editing will not be enough; instead, there is a need to create a discussion in light of both the scientific facts and public concerns to facilitate acceptance (Fleischmann et al., 2019). It is only through this kind of comprehensive communication that scientists can expect to allay doubts and build up trust in communities that might have apprehensions regarding the meaning of genetic manipulation. Moreover, the findings of most surveys reveal that the acceptance of gene editing can differ greatly by cultural backgrounds and existing knowledge. A survey of European women's attitudes to predictive epigenetic testing for cancer susceptibility demonstrated diversity of opinions regarding new genetic technologies. A considerable percentage of the people expressed a wish to understand their cancer risks; however, fear of potential side effects overshadowed the perceived benefits, underlining the need for very well-informed discussions (Pashayan et al., 2019). The example shows that public acceptance of gene editing is far from uniform and can be highly variable based on personal experience, risk perceptions, and cultural contexts. Understanding such nuances will enhance policymakers' and researchers' capacity to tailor their communication approaches so that they tackle the specific concerns of different demographic segments. Further, the intersection of gene editing with ethical concerns raises questions about social responsibility and oversight. As the development of gene editing technologies advances, ethical dilemmas in relation to eugenics, informed consent, and the long-term consequences for future generations become more pertinent. The task is to make sure public discourse captures such complexities in a good way, thereby fostering informed decision-making on gene editing applications. Clear communication that brings out both the possible benefits and the ethical issues will be key in sustaining public trust and backing (Fleischmann et al., 2019). Researchers and policymakers must work together to develop guidelines that support ethical practice without hindering innovation. Involving the general public in conversation regarding the repercussions of gene editing will, by extension, define the future of this groundbreaking technology and how it pertains to developmental science (Figure 11.19).

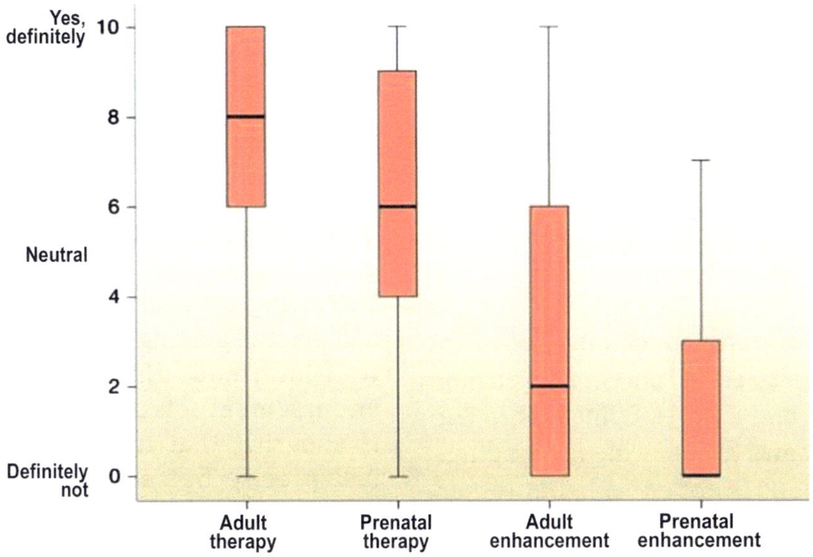

Figure 11.19. Public views on gene editing.

Source: https://media.springernature.com/m685/springer-static/image/art%3A10.1038%2Fnbt.3958/MediaObjects/41587_2017_Article_BFnbt3958_Fig1_HTML.jpg.

11.6.1. Surveys and Studies on Public Opinion

Empirical studies and surveys of public opinion are key to social attitudes regarding gene editing technologies, especially with new technologies such as CRISPR-Cas9 gaining increased attention. The fortunes of such technologies are not just a factor of scientific principles but also of the degree to which they are accepted and understood by the public and their meanings. Studies of public attitudes demonstrate a range of views, from skepticism to optimism, that can have profound effects on regulatory policies and research funding. Through the assessment of public opinions regarding the moral and ethical aspects of gene editing, key areas characterized by misinformation or lack of knowledge can be determined by researchers. Such knowledge is central to enabling properly informed discourse that can span the gaps between technological progress and societal concerns. With changing populations and technology, repeated surveys will be crucial in tracking variations in public opinions and adjusting communications accordingly. The relationship between regulatory gene editing decisions and public opinion is of significant interest. It is already determined through studies that regulatory agencies tend to consider the opinion of the public while designing their policies, particularly in contentious fields such as genetic modification. For example, the acceptance level of genetically edited products, such as crops and therapeutics, has a direct correlation with the investment and innovation level in the research sector. For gene editing to fulfill its promise in solving global issues, including food security and health inequality, there is a call to create awareness among the public through education and open discussion. The engagement enables the next generation of citizens to not only comprehend the scientific intricacies but also the ethical undertones that form the basis of their methodologies of gene editing. The inability to recognize the issues of society can lead to a regulatory stalemate and obstruct the potential gains of genetic technologies, thereby impacting their contribution towards sustainable practices.

The efficacy of communication measures on gene editing is also significant in influencing public acceptance and its development through time. Literature shows that sharing information on gene editing alone is not enough, but rather the public needs to be involved in effective dialogue that incorporates their values and fears. A critical part of such engagement entails responding to ethical issues confronting gene editing, as the public trust can easily be lost through misinformation or perceived failure of ethics. More effective communication strategies that combine narrative techniques, case studies, and public involvement can help achieve a more positive public perception of gene editing technologies. Research indicates that when scientists get involved in public deliberations and interact with individuals outside their field of expertise, they not only convey the scientific concepts but also create a sense of mutual responsibility when addressing ethical concerns. This cooperative strategy can be a powerful influence on public acceptance and help develop a more positive attitude toward gene editing progress in the future, thereby allowing new applications in agriculture as well as medical research.

11.6.2. Role of Media in Shaping Perceptions

The media have a significant part in shaping public attitudes towards gene editing and developmental science, affecting how the public perceives the technological development and ethical dimensions of these sciences. Through disseminating information via diverse mediums such as news sources, social media, and documentary films, the media shape narratives that can generate greater understanding or misunderstandings. Sensationalized portrayals of gene editing technologies, for example, may be prone to exaggerated fears among the public, thereby overshooting the promised gains, e.g., elimination of genetic diseases or enhancing agricultural resilience. Conversely, balanced reporting can facilitate an extremely well-informed discussion, enabling public endorsement of research efforts. The task is ensuring that the stories covered are not just precise but also representative of gene editing's complicated realities, thus equipping audiences with smart information rather than misinformation. Secondly, the way gene editing is portrayed in media accounts can significantly influence policy debates and ethical factors in development research. When media attention is on the revolutionary potential of gene editing, it may spur lawmakers to seek funding and regulatory frameworks that support cutting-edge research. In contrast, emphasizing risks, such as unforeseen long-term consequences or ethical dilemmas regarding "designer babies," may stir public outrage, ultimately affecting research trajectories and funding. This double pressure calls for a synergistic collaboration between scientists, ethicists, and media practitioners to create efficient communications strategies that convey a balanced perception of gene editing technologies. Through such a strategy, they are able to make sure that policies are able to reflect the intricacies associated with such fields, while also promoting public comprehension and involvement, an aspect underscored by the discrepancies evident in the wider discourse within the scientific community on animal diseases and health repercussions (Kappes et al., 2023). Last but not least, media coverage of gene editing has significant repercussions for the ethical and societal aspects of scientific inquiry. As social values change, media coverage can reflect and influence public opinion regarding matters of genetic privacy, consent, and access to gene editing technologies. This is especially observed when the media brings attention to conflicting opinions, most notably those promoting equal access as opposed to proprietary innovations. In this regard, media participation in these debates, adopting a responsible framework that prioritizes scientific literacy is paramount, as this allows the audience to thoughtfully deliberate on the ethical issues related to gene editing. In recognizing that emotional reactions and moral stances may be swayed by inaccuracies in media presentations, such as the misleading presentation of certain mental disorders as absolute adaptation failures, can also highlight the value of such public debates (Nesse, 2023). By facilitating informed discussion, media can contribute to enhancing a sophisticated appreciation of gene editing for fostering an societal ecosystem that balances innovation with ethical responsibility (Figure 11.20).

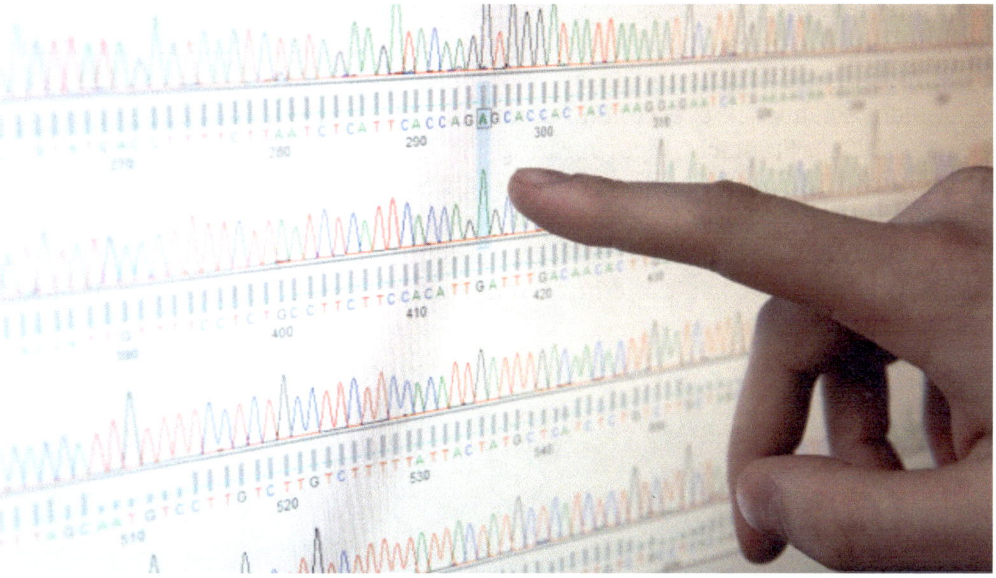

Figure 11.20. Media in Shaping Perceptions.

Source: https://www.pewresearch.org/science/wp-content/uploads/sites/16/2020/12/PS_20.10.08_internationalScienceAndReligion_featured.png?w=640.

11.6.3. Educational Initiatives to Inform the Public

Educational initiatives are key in influencing public perceptions of gene editing and its relevance to developmental science. With advances in genetic technologies happening at a faster rate, the necessity for competent communication strategies is also amplified. Public knowledge of gene editing must be extended from just the scientific methods employed to the ethical implications that follow with such advances. For example, activities like workshops, seminars, and public forums can establish an informed citizenry that is able to have thoughtful debates regarding the prospective advantages and boundaries of gene editing. Through simplification of intricate scientific principles and clarification of public concerns, such programs provide citizens with what they require to make thoughtful choices regarding genetic technologies and their implementation in different areas, including medicine, agriculture, and nature conservation. One other essential aspect of such education programs is the promotion of intersectoral collaboration among educational institutions, research institutions, and community leaders. Intersectoral partnerships can help improve the quality and reach of educational programs and ensure that gene editing-related information is not just accurate but also contextually applicable. For instance, the development of materials that link progress in gene editing to applicable local community concerns, including environmental health or food security, can render stakeholder engagement more effective. These efforts are enhanced by integrating outputs from developmental research that underscore the consequences of gene editing on human health and general well-being. By incorporating local knowledge and challenging community-specific issues, education campaigns can facilitate a strong discourse that enables the public to engage effectively in policy and practice for gene editing, towards an information-rich and participatory citizenry. Furthermore, incorporating interdisciplinary approaches in the education curriculum can foster a multidimensional understanding of gene editing. Through the inclusion of perspectives from biology, ethics, sociology, and law, such projects are able to more clearly depict the interconnectedness of gene editing technologies alongside their social effects. It then becomes imperative to focus on the creation of frameworks like the Plant Cell Atlas (PCA) that tackle the significance of plant sciences in overcoming environmental issues using gene editing, as proposed by Ahmed et al. (2021). Similarly, incorporating the principles of relational health can enhance educational efforts focused on the impacts of gene editing on childhood development and resilience. By putting interdisciplinary learning at the center of curriculum development, educators can give students a holistic appreciation of the potential applications of gene editing while empowering the public with the ability to solve the ethical and practical issues that are brought up within this fast-developing area.

SUMMARY

In summary, the gene editing research in developmental studies has illuminated the significant impacts of these kinds of technologies on both scientific success and ethical concerns. The CRISPR/Cas9 mechanism has transformed our capacity to edit individual genes, demonstrating key findings in essential developmental mechanisms. For example, the specific disruption of the POU5F1 gene in bovine embryos highlights the complex role played by this transcription factor in early embryo development. It was found that the disruption resulted in embryonic arrest at the morula stage; however, it also displayed residual functions which implicate the same mechanisms in humans, thus advancing our knowledge of developmental biology across species (Daigneault et al., 2018). The crossroads of genetic manipulation and developmental insights bring up questions regarding the direction of future research, especially in regard to ethical considerations that accompany such forays into fundamental biological mechanisms. Additionally, the topic of gene editing brings about the need to revisit evolutionary paradigms that have traditionally been centered on a gene-centric view. The Modern Synthesis, although a foundational framework, has been faulted for not being able to capture intra-organismic interactional dynamics and epigenetic influences on phenotypic expressions. The Extended Evolutionary Synthesis proponents believe in a more inclusive stance that is considerate of these intricacies, with recognition of the key role played by gene interactions and their evolutionary pathways (Blancke et al., 2018). By combining developmental biology and epigenetics, scientists can promote a better understanding of the ways in which gene editing technologies are capable of affecting evolutionary processes and the phenotypic diversity apparent among contemporary organisms. Such a view will eventually enable us to gain a better insight into the adaptive potential of species under extreme environmental changes. Lastly, ethical issues revolving around gene editing need to keep up with scientific progress. As scientists begin to realize the potential of gene editing technologies, their implications for human enhancement, agriculture, and biodiversity become increasingly urgent. To begin to resolve these ethical questions, one must know the developmental functions of individual genes and how they interact with the environment. For instance, what is learned from the application of gene editing in animal models can inform human applications, especially for such areas as genetic diseases and personalized medicine. It is imperative that the scientific community collaborates with ethicists, policymakers, and the public to navigate cautiously these multifaceted moral terrains and secure the responsible application of gene editing technologies. Moving ahead, the combination of stringent scientific research with ethical governance will be significant to enhance the utility of gene editing to the maximum and reduce the envisaged damages to society and the environment.

The discovery of gene editing technologies has transformed the field of developmental studies, offering researchers unprecedented tools for altering genetic sequences in eukaryotic cells. Techniques like CRISPR/Cas9, zinc finger nucleases (ZFNs), and TALENs have enabled the generation of extremely precise genetic edits. These sophisticated techniques allow the clarification of genes involved in a wide range of diseases, thereby advancing our knowledge of intricate biological processes. As scientists continue to push the limits of these technologies, the potential impact on biomedical research grows, including the creation of novel therapeutic approaches to treat genetic disease. The clinical translation of these editing technologies has the potential to revolutionize treatment regimens, moving us closer to the prospect of personalized medicine. The discipline of gene editing underscores the necessity for a comprehensive ethical framework to direct its applications, and especially that of developmental research. As researchers harness the ability to edit genomes, controversy erupts regarding what this means for human genetics, biodiversity, and the possibility of unintended consequences. The ethical concerns range from the danger of off-target effects, which have the potential to cause unexpected mutations and health consequences. Further, the societal impact of gene editing is contentious as it brings about concerns regarding access, equity, and the implications of creating GMOs. Any future studies need to be placed in the context of ethics for responsible scientific research with minimal risks. Solutions to these challenges will require collaboration among researchers, ethicists, and policymakers so that advancements are beneficial to society as a whole. Gene editing in developmental research also has a future that involves working in collaboration with interdisciplinary groups so that its potential can be fully harnessed. As recent consensus statements have pointed out, understanding interactions between genetic changes and their biochemical environments is critical so that therapeutic applications can be enhanced. This integration enables the creation of new approaches, such as the use of gene editing in synbiotics, where the health benefits from the synergistic utilization of prebiotics and probiotics can be further improved through genetic modifications in microbial communities. This is an example of how gene editing can move beyond traditional boundaries, in concert with various areas of research that also seek to improve human health. Through enabling interdisciplinarity linkages, gene editing has the potential to result in integrated solutions for complicated health disorders, thereby increasing our capacity in developmental research (Swanson et al., 2020, p. 687-701; Li et al., 2020).

CLOSER LOOK

GERMLINE EDITING

Germline editing refers to the genetic modification of germ cells—sperm, eggs, or embryos—in such a way that the changes are heritable and passed on to future generations. This powerful and controversial branch of genetic engineering has gained significant attention with the development of precise gene-editing tools like CRISPR-Cas9. Germline editing holds tremendous potential for eliminating inherited genetic disorders before birth, thereby preventing diseases such as cystic fibrosis, Huntington's disease, and certain forms of cancer. By directly altering the DNA in the earliest stages of development, scientists can theoretically ensure that not only the individual born from the edited embryo is free of a given condition, but also that the change becomes a permanent part of their genetic lineage. However, while the scientific prospects are promising, the ethical, social, and safety concerns surrounding germline editing have made it one of the most hotly debated topics in modern biotechnology.

The major advantage of germline editing lies in its preventive potential. Unlike somatic gene therapy, which treats an existing condition in a living individual and whose effects are not inherited, germline editing offers a one-time intervention with long-lasting generational benefits. In theory, it could eliminate certain genetic diseases from a family line permanently. However, this same heritability is the source of many ethical dilemmas. The most profound concern is the risk of unintended genetic consequences, often referred to as "off-target effects." These are unintended changes elsewhere in the genome, which could introduce new health problems or compromise genetic diversity. Since these edits affect not just one individual but all their descendants, even a small mistake can have far-reaching consequences. Additionally, there is concern about the long-term effects of such changes, which may not be fully understood until years or decades later.

Ethical concerns also extend beyond safety. Critics argue that germline editing could lead to a slippery slope toward "designer babies," where parents might seek to enhance traits like intelligence, physical appearance, or athletic ability, rather than preventing disease. This raises issues of social inequality, as access to such technologies might be limited to the wealthy, potentially exacerbating existing disparities. Moreover, altering the human germline touches on deep philosophical and moral questions about human identity, natural evolution, and the role of science in shaping our future. The scientific community has called for strict regulation and oversight, with many countries banning or heavily restricting germline editing in humans. In 2018, global attention focused on the case of a Chinese scientist who claimed to have created the world's first gene-edited babies, sparking widespread condemnation and reinforcing the need for global governance.

Despite these concerns, research continues in the area of germline editing, particularly in animal models, as scientists seek to improve the precision, safety, and ethical frameworks for future use. Many experts agree that if germline editing is ever to be used in humans, it must meet rigorous safety standards and be applied only in cases of serious genetic disease with no alternative treatments. As the science progresses, society must engage in thoughtful and inclusive discussions to balance innovation with responsibility and ethical integrity.

REFERENCES

1. Ahmed, A., Bruner, K., Gajewski, A., Kiraly, et al. (2018). *Triple Helix, Fall 2018*. https://core.ac.uk/download/211337566.pdf (accessed on 27 May 2025).
2. Ahmed, J., Alaba, O., Ameen, G., Arora, V., Arteaga-Vazquez, M. A., Arun, A., Bailey-Serres, J., et al. (2021). Vision, challenges and opportunities for a Plant Cell Atlas. *eLife*. https://doi.org/10.7554/elife.66877.
3. Akbari, O. S., Bowman, C. S., Bui, M., Li, et al. (2017). Germline Cas9 expression yields highly efficient genome engineering in a major worldwide disease vector, *Aedes aegypti*. eScholarship, University of California. https://pmc.ncbi.nlm.nih.gov/articles/PMC5724270/.
4. Allwardt, A. (2023). An exploration of the effects of gene-editing technology on human identity. *Voices in Bioethics*. https://www.semanticscholar.org/paper/f13f799da6fbd76e4b2bd714de17180921d22ad9 (accessed on 27 May 2025).
5. Alward, B. A., Ebling, F. J. P., Fernald, R. D., Kelly, et al. (2017). The value of comparative animal research: Krogh's principle facilitates scientific discoveries. *SAGE Publications*. https://core.ac.uk/download/131024966.pdf (accessed on 27 May 2025).
6. Balestrini, S., Guerrini, R., Mei, D., Sisodiya, et al. (2023). Steps to improve precision medicine in epilepsy. *Springer Science and Business Media LLC*. https://core.ac.uk/download/587390155.pdf (accessed on 27 May 2025).
7. Bier, E., Harrison, M. M., O'Connor-Giles, K. M., Wildonger, et al. (2018). Advances in engineering the fly genome with the CRISPR-Cas system. eScholarship, University of California. https://pmc.ncbi.nlm.nih.gov/articles/PMC5753851/.
8. Blancke, S., Braeckman, J., & De Tiège, A. (2018). *The Modern Versus Extended Evolutionary Synthesis: Sketch of An Intra-Genomic Gene's Eye View for The Evolutionary-Genetic Underpinning of Epigenetic and Developmental Evolution*. Publishing Press. https://core.ac.uk/download/187307814.pdf (accessed on 27 May 2025).
9. Chanoca, A., Boerjan, W., & de Vries, L. (2019). Lignin engineering in forest trees. *Frontiers Media SA*. https://core.ac.uk/download/227040193.pdf (accessed on 27 May 2025).
10. Chen, J. N., Geisler, R., Huang, J., et al. (2017). The Calcineurin-FoxO-MuRF1 signaling pathway regulates myofibril integrity in cardiomyocytes. eScholarship, University of California. https://pmc.ncbi.nlm.nih.gov/articles/PMC5576919/.
11. Costa, R. (2015). Book review: Gene H Bell-Villada and Nina Sichel (eds), (with Faith Eidse and Elaine Neil Orr), *Writing Out of Limbo: International Childhoods, Global Nomads and Third Culture Kids. International Sociology, 30*(2), 191–193. https://www.semanticscholar.org/paper/086b02acee6d53ea5a24303c7eaace0627a874fc (accessed on 27 May 2025).
12. Cui, Z., Lin, L., Zong, Y., Chen, Y., & Wang, S. (2024). Precision gene editing using deep learning: A case study of the CRISPR-Cas9 editor. *Applied and Computational Engineering*. https://www.semanticscholar.org/paper/051921a70398458bfdc3c64141738d0943830993 (accessed on 27 May 2025).
13. Daigneault, B. W., Rajput, S., Ross, P. J., et al. (2018). Embryonic POU5F1 is required for expanded bovine blastocyst formation. eScholarship, University of California. https://core.ac.uk/download/323071258.pdf.

14. Dickinson, M. H., Dow, J. A. T., & Vosshall, L. B. (2020). Genome editing in non-model organisms opens new horizons for comparative physiology. *The Company of Biologists*. https://journals.biologists.com/jeb/article/223/Suppl_1/jeb221119/224637/Genome-editing-in-non-model-organisms-opens-new.

15. Doudna, J. (2025). CRISPR and gene editing: Ethical and scientific perspectives. *International Journal of Innovative Computer Science and IT Research*. https://www.semanticscholar.org/paper/ab7766220260d30dd2db0a5f53e7407095ecff22 (accessed on 27 May 2025).

16. Dunn, J. C. Y., Hong, S. N., Martín, M. G., Stelzner, et al. (2016). Concise review: The potential use of intestinal stem cells to treat patients with intestinal failure. eScholarship, University of California. https://pmc.ncbi.nlm.nih.gov/articles/PMC5442796/.

17. Ferreira, B. I., Jacinto, F., & Link, W. (2020). CRISPR/Cas9-mediated genome editing: From basic research to translational medicine. *Wiley*. https://core.ac.uk/download/288958587.pdf (accessed on 27 May 2025).

18. Frankish, A., Diekhans, M., Jungreis, I., Lagarde, J., Loveland, J., Mudge, J. M., Sisu, C., et al. (2020). GENCODE 2021. *Nucleic Acids Research*, D916–D923. https://doi.org/10.1093/nar/gkaa1087.

19. Gao, J. P., Su, Y., Jiang, S., Liang, W., Lou, Z., Frugier, F., Xu, P., & Murray, J. D. (2024). Applying conventional and cell-type-specific CRISPR/Cas9 genome editing in legume plants. *Springer Science and Business Media LLC*. https://core.ac.uk/download/630301027.pdf (accessed on 27 May 2025).

20. Garner, A. S., & Yogman, M. W. (2021). Preventing childhood toxic stress: Partnering with families and communities to promote relational health. *Pediatrics*. https://doi.org/10.1542/peds.2021-052582.

21. Godara, S., Kalaiyarasi, R., Sasikala, R., et al. (2024). Advancements in sunflower genomics: Navigating the biotech revolution for crop improvement. *Horizon e-Publishing Group*. https://core.ac.uk/download/641609554.pdf (accessed on 27 May 2025).

22. Gudmunds, E., Wheat, C. W., Khila, A., & Husby, A. (2022). Functional genomic tools for emerging model species. *Trends in Ecology & Evolution*, 1104–1115. https://doi.org/10.1016/j.tree.2022.07.004.

23. Hou, K., Wu, Z. X., Chen, X. Y., Wang, J. Q., Zhang, D., Xiao, C., Zhu, D., et al. (2022). Microbiota in health and diseases. *Signal Transduction and Targeted Therapy*. https://doi.org/10.1038/s41392-022-00974-4.

24. Inada, E., Kawaguchi, H., Miyoshi, K., et al. (2019). Recent advance in genome editing-based gene modification in pigs. *IntechOpen*. https://core.ac.uk/download/322443699.pdf (accessed on 27 May 2025).

25. Jamshidi, N., Lewis, N. E., Swann, J., Winzeler, E., et al. (2015). Systems analysis of host-parasite interactions. *eScholarship, University of California*. https://pmc.ncbi.nlm.nih.gov/articles/PMC4679367/.

26. Kappes, A. J., Tozooneyi, T., Shakil, G. S., Railey, A. F., McIntyre, K. M., Mayberry, D., Rushton, J., et al. (2023). Livestock health and disease economics: A scoping review of selected literature. *Frontiers in Veterinary Science*. https://doi.org/10.3389/fvets.2023.1168649.

27. Khan, M. S., Qureshi, N., Khan, R., Son, Y. O., & Maqbool, T. (2025). CRISPR/Cas9-based therapeutics as a promising strategy for management of Alzheimer's disease: Progress and prospects. *Frontiers in Cellular Neuroscience*. https://www.semanticscholar.org/paper/c71d42516664ede11d12284a55372d730f40a013 (accessed on 27 May 2025).

28. Klatt, S., Konthur, Z., Maslov, D., Simpson, J., et al. (2019). Leishmania tarentolae: Taxonomic classification and its application as a promising biotechnological expression host. *PLoS*.

29. Lesci, G. F., Sereno, M., Radovich, M., Castignani, G., Bisigello, L., Marulli, F., Moscardini, L., et al. (2023). Euclid preparation. XXXVII. Galaxy color selections with Euclid and ground photometry for cluster weak-lensing analyses. *Astronomy & Astrophysics*. https://www.semanticscholar.org/paper/f05d5f4d48e16a2926cbc5e6e8d259cebe8bedcc (accessed on 27 May 2025).

30. Li, H., Yang, Y., Hong, W., Huang, M., Wu, M., & Zhao, X. (2020). Applications of genome editing technology in the targeted therapy of human diseases: Mechanisms, advances and prospects. *Signal Transduction and Targeted Therapy*. https://doi.org/10.1038/s41392-019-0089-y.

31. Lignani, G., & Wykes, R. C. (2017). Gene therapy and editing: Novel potential treatments for neuronal channelopathies. https://core.ac.uk/download/111013197.pdf (accessed on 27 May 2025).

32. Mariscal, C., & Petropanagos, A. (2016). CRISPR as a driving force: The Model T of biotechnology. https://core.ac.uk/download/131209784.pdf (accessed on 27 May 2025).

33. N/A. (2017). Compatibility of breeding techniques in organic systems. https://core.ac.uk/download/161988586.pdf (accessed on 27 May 2025).

34. Nesse, R. M. (2023). Evolutionary psychiatry: Foundations, progress and challenges. *World Psychiatry*, *22*(2), 177–202. https://doi.org/10.1002/wps.21072.

35. Ni, J. X., & Zhang, W. (2025). Progress and prospects on evolutionary developmental biology of butterfly wing patterns. *Yi Chuan = Hereditas*, 258–270. https://www.semanticscholar.org/paper/9f769a01cd7c44cf5d8d2c7d9f1543e54294da9b (accessed on 27 May 2025).

36. Pashayan, N., Rebitschek, F., Wegwarth, O., Widschwendter, M., et al. (2019). Women's perception, attitudes, and intended behavior towards predictive epigenetic risk testing for female cancers in 5 European countries: A cross-sectional online survey. *Springer Science and Business Media LLC*. https://core.ac.uk/download/219542630.pdf (accessed on 27 May 2025).

37. Saluja, M., & Khushi, K. (2024). Ethical contemplations in Indian science fiction: The case of gene editing. *Vantage: Journal of Thematic Analysis*. https://www.semanticscholar.org/paper/ccb825a29bbeef533b0363e411347c117d744b6c (accessed on 27 May 2025).

38. Schneider, M. D. (2016). Heartbreak hotel: A convergence in cardiac regeneration. *The Company of Biologists*. https://core.ac.uk/download/77011555.pdf (accessed on 27 May 2025).

39. Sen, A., Singh, V., Dwivedi, S., Agrawal, R., Bansal, A., Shekhar, S., & Kushwaha, S. S. (2025). Gene therapy and gene editing: Current trends and future prospects of molecular medicine. *Current Gene Therapy*. https://www.semanticscholar.org/paper/25fcf14d7421a285bda69cc ae261660da8cc8fcc (accessed on 27 May 2025).

40. Singh, S. (2024). Gene editing technologies: CRISPR/Cas9 and beyond for genetic disease therapy and research. *Universal Research Reports*. https://www.semanticscholar.org/paper/bdbe7a736460f042eaa6a1d2bb69cb21616d10c7 (accessed on 27 May 2025).

41. Stasi, A., & Thongpravati, O. (2024). Biotechnology innovation in do-it-yourself (DIY) gene editing: A call for a new regulatory framework. *OBM Genetics*. https://www.semanticscholar.org/paper/3d760d5a4fcab10e8490de8812eeb5591c97956c (accessed on 27 May 2025).

42. Swanson, K. S., Gibson, G. R., Hutkins, R., Reimer, R. A., Reid, G., Verbeke, K., Scott, K. P., et al. (2020). The International Scientific Association for Probiotics and Prebiotics (ISAPP) consensus statement on the definition and scope of symbiotic. *Nature Reviews Gastroenterology & Hepatology*, *17*(11), 687–701. https://doi.org/10.1038/s41575-020-0344-2.

43. Van Montagu, M. (2020). The future of plant biotechnology in a globalized and environmentally endangered world. *FapUNIFESP (SciELO)*. https://core.ac.uk/download/287941311.pdf (accessed on 27 May 2025).

44. Witzany, G. (2008). Bio-communication of bacteria and its evolutionary interrelations to natural genome editing competences of viruses. https://core.ac.uk/download/pdf/287751.pdf (accessed on 27 May 2025).

45. Younis, M. A., & Harashima, H. (2024). Understanding gene involvement in hepatocellular carcinoma: Implications for gene therapy and personalized medicine. *Pharmacogenomics and Personalized Medicine*, *17*, 193–213. https://www.semanticscholar.org/paper/f26f486812a98704478e7b8938ad266fa495a6c6 (accessed on 27 May 2025).

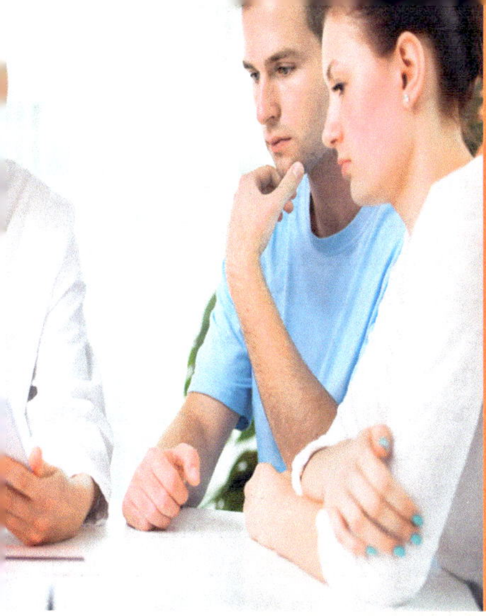

Chapter 12

TRANSLATIONAL EMBRYOLOGY AND GENETIC COUNSELING

Contents

Introduction

Translational embryology, as a new discipline, is employed to connect basic research in embryo development with practical strategies in genetic counseling. The point at which scientific information about human embryos and clinical practice meets has been advancing significantly, driven by developments in reproductive technologies, including *in vitro* fertilization (IVF). This collaboration not only enhances our understanding of embryonic health but also allows informed decision-making for prospective parents faced with genetic risks. Recent evidence suggests that the characterization of human embryo phenotypes with cohort-specific variables could optimize embryo selection in IVF therapy. Through the inclusion of such variables as overall embryo numbers, cleavage rates, and hormonal assessment, specialists are able to work out strategies that optimize the possibility of successful pregnancies and thereby guarantee that reproductive interventions are premised on sound scientific foundations (Behr et al., 2008). Genetic counseling is similarly relevant in addressing the intricacies involved in reproductive decisions as well as the prospects of hereditary abnormalities. This aspect is particularly crucial considering the elevated occurrence of infertility, which necessitates detailed understanding of the multifarious factors involved in this condition. Modern research in dermatoglyphics has established new avenues for explaining the potential genetic markers that could be linked to female infertility, as unique skin ridge patterns may serve as novel indicators of incipient reproductive issues. The integration of genetic counseling and data derived from dermatoglyphics can lead to a combined strategy in diagnosis and treatment of infertility disorders. However, a lot of research must be done to establish these correlations and also to facilitate inclusion in clinical practice (Anjankar et al., 2024). In total, the correlation between translational embryology and genetic counseling indicates that there is a requirement for a multidisciplinary strategy in reproductive health. By basing clinical practice in contemporary scientific research, health professionals are able to offer individualized, evidence-based information to individuals and couples struggling with the challenges of conception. As a discipline, future progress will require ongoing innovation and research to advance the combining of multiple diagnostic methods and therapeutic modalities. Its central priority is to maximize health outcomes for the next generation, while in parallel empowering individuals through knowledge and support during their reproductive lifetimes. This synergistic partnership of clinical practice and scientific research is expected to propel the field of reproductive medicine forward, and in so doing guarantee a healthier future for families globally (Figure 12.1).

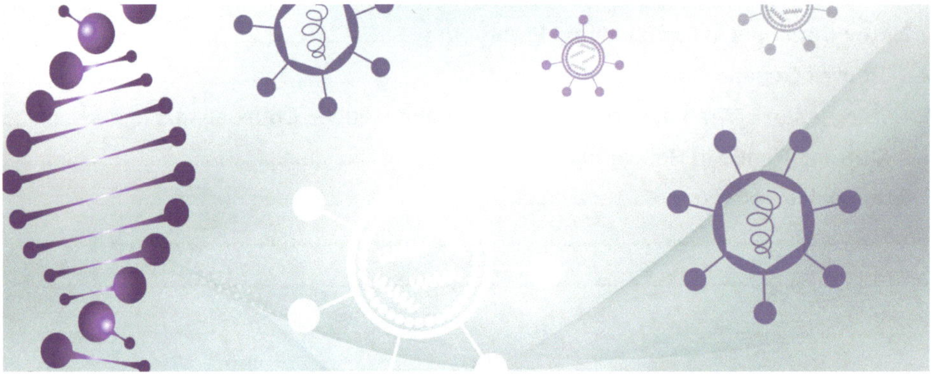

Figure 12.1. Translational embryology.

Source: https://external-content.duckduckgo.com/iu/?u=https%3A%2F%2Fwww.bio-rad.com%2Fsites%2Fdefault%2Ffiles%2Fstyles%2Fbrc_redesign_hero_desktop_1440_x_552_2_605_1%2Fpublic%2F2023-04%2Fspecialties-lsr-translational-research.png%3Fh%3D2d44e782%26itok%3DRwStSNOJ&f=1&nofb=1&ipt=588b125127379ff2fed2b09d5907e1044d94ec659007cae23622c8e512d044ce.

Definition of Translational Embryology

Translational embryology is an interdisciplinary science that connects basic embryological research to its clinical application, specifically through the vantage point of genetic counseling. Translational embryology involves the investigation of embryonic development with the ultimate goal of translating discoveries into the improvement of reproductive health outcomes. The overriding principle of translational embryology is its dedication to the translation of scientific discovery into practical health advantage, which has a profound impact on the comprehension of developmental disease, infertility, and prenatal diagnosis. As researchers learn more about the genes involved in embryonic development, this information emerges as a precious resource for genetic counselors assisting patients in making difficult decisions based on contemporary science. Consequently, translational embryology assists in complementing our understanding of developmental biology while simultaneously strengthening the practice of genetic counseling through the provision of better risk assessment and counseling strategies. Besides, translational embryology intersects with genetic counseling by allowing practitioners to use scientific breakthroughs in an attempt to meet patient demands successfully. With the use of new techniques, such as CRISPR gene editing and stem cell technology applications, genetic counselors have greater ability to discuss the implications of genetic results with their patients.

These understandings allow counselors to aid individuals and families who are affected by genetic disorders, thus creating an environment that fosters decision-making. Incorporation of genomics into genetic counseling curricula reflects the evolving nature of medical genetics, echoing the required competencies that match current practice in areas like risk assessment and patient education (Amanda et al., 2016). Hence, the application of embryological research into the clinic eventually leads to improved patient outcomes and insight into hereditary disorders. The effects of translational embryology go beyond individual cases, affecting broader healthcare policy and planning as it pertains to genetic counseling. In nations such as Spain, where genetic counseling has not yet been fully established as a standalone healthcare field, the role of translational embryology becomes essential. The field highlights the necessity for a strongly established genetic counseling infrastructure to deal with the psychosocial issues confronting individuals afflicted with rare diseases (Navas et al., 2021). By demonstrating how translational results can inform the provision of genetic services, various stakeholders are able to secure more appreciation of genetic counselors within the healthcare system. By so doing, the understanding and respect given to translational embryology enhance academic scholarship as well as affirm the integral position of genetic counseling in contemporary medicine, thereby guaranteeing holistic care for individuals with genetic intricacies.

Importance of Genetic Counseling

In current medical practice, genetic counseling is required to span the divide between complicated genetic information and patient comprehension, especially in the field of reproductive health. Genetic counselors offer expert guidance to patients and families about their genetic risks, which is of specific importance to those individuals who are dealing with the intricacies associated with IVF. As previously mentioned, a considerable proportion of embryos fail to survive the in vitro fertilization (IVF) procedure, thereby highlighting the contribution of counseling towards optimizing outcomes through informed choices (Behr et al., 2008). By empowering patients with knowledge regarding genetic aspects, possible results, and existing interventions, genetic counseling enables proactive action in dealing with reproductive issues while reducing the anxiety that comes with uncertainty. Also, genetic counseling is warranted for rare disease patients since they experience tremendous psychological and emotional stress from diagnostic delay and insufficient credible information. In certain nations such as Spain, where the acceptance of geneticists and counselors as part of the legitimate health professionals is still limited, patients tend to experience difficulties compounded by the intricacy of their diseases (Navas et al., 2021). Genetic counselors play a crucial role in the explanation of genetic diagnoses as well as in emotional support and counseling, thereby improving the quality of care overall. This comprehensive process helps to empower the patient by allowing them to make informed decisions regarding their health and navigate the healthcare system with greater ease. On a wider public health level, genetic counseling forms part of a larger public health initiative by raising awareness and knowledge of genetic disorders. The significance of this role is especially pronounced in the field of translational embryology, where developments in genetic testing and embryo selection techniques are transforming reproductive planning. Given that embryo cohort-specific variables have high predictive power, the acquisition of knowledge about such variables by means of genetic counseling can facilitate clinical practice and optimize treatment outcomes (Behr et al., 2008). By the integration of genetic information into reproductive medicine, counselors increase the probability of successful conception considerably and, at the same time, contribute importantly to the process of informed consent. They thereby ensure that patients are well informed about possible implications of genetic results on future family planning decisions (Figure 12.2).

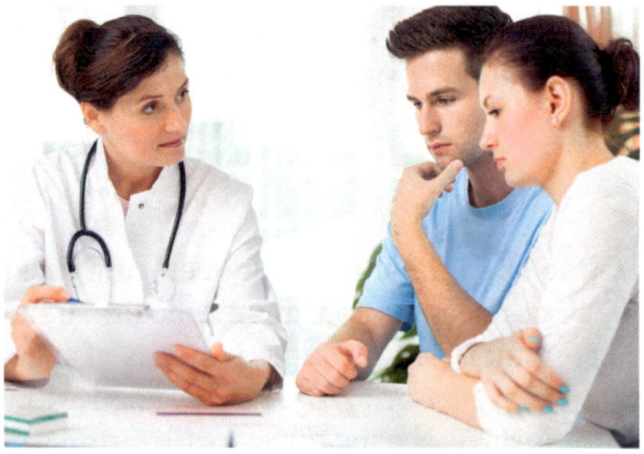

Figure 12.2. Genetic counseling.

Source: https://external-content.duckduckgo.com/iu/?u=https%3A%2F%2Fsharinghealthygenes.com%2Fwp-content%2Fuploads%2F2018%2F11%2Fdoctorconsultsayoungcoup_594370.jpg&f=1&nofb=1&ipt=408f68156d8018201205214a7b2eb126a198ce7ad49f4e422fd52b510c6c0bc3.

Overview of the Relationship Between the Two Fields

The coming together of genetic counseling and translational embryology is currently a key domain in the broad field of reproductive medicine and genetics. Translational embryology is dedicated to the translation of basic embryological research into everyday solutions, especially concerning assisted reproductive technologies. The discipline has made much progress in elucidating the multifaceted genetic and environmental determinants influencing embryonic development. Hence, genetic counseling forms the core of imparting essential information regarding the potential genetic risks involved with their reproductive decisions to prospective parents. Integrating competencies from both disciplines, practitioners are able to offer an integrated model of patient care that comprises the scientific foundation of embryology and the psychosocial dimensions of genetic information, thereby facilitating informed decision-making in the field of reproductive medicine. In addition, advances in omics technologies such as genomics, proteomics, and metabolomics have greatly enhanced the prospects of personalized medicine in the fields of translational embryology and genetic counseling. The ability to analyze genetic information at high accuracy enables the identification of genetic mutations and polymorphisms that may affect embryonic viability and overall health outcomes. Genetic counselors utilize this information to guide families through the intricacies of being faced with genetic testing, determining risk, and understanding the implications for future pregnancies. It has been noted in the literature that the application of these omic techniques into clinical practice has been slower for fields of study like dentistry than for more general medical specialties (Kabbashi et al., 2024). However, the possibilities for these technologies to reshape care within both fields are tremendous, with each challenging the other field to continue innovating in its practice. Moreover, the collective potential of translational embryology and genetic counseling to dramatically improve patient outcomes and inform research endeavors is great. For example, combining genetic counseling with pre-implantation genetic diagnosis (PGD) enables couples to make knowledgeable decisions in embryo selection, thus elevating the prospects of successful pregnancies and lowering the incidence of genetic disorders. These concerted efforts enable the comprehension of embryonic development in addition to genetic susceptibilities, ultimately leading to the formation of novel therapeutic approaches. Furthermore, as more research unfolds at the Institute of Basic Medical Sciences and other such institutions, the knowledge developed through their work is augmenting the clinical frameworks that connect these two disciplines (Wang et al., 2024). This development supports a model of patient-centered care that leverages scientific breakthroughs to tackle challenges in healthcare for reproductive medicine, thereby reinforcing the link between translational embryology and genetic counseling (Figure 12.3).

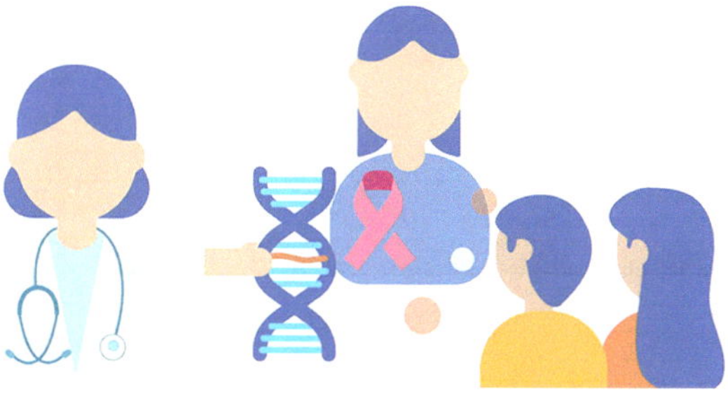

Figure 12.3. Relationship between translational embryology and genetic counseling.

Source: https://external-content.duckduckgo.com/iu/?u=https%3A%2F%2Fwww.drsupriyawakchaure.com%2Fimages%2Fgenetic-counselling.jpg&f=1&nofb=1&ipt=a819cf7b5f27d46f199394a672f8ab9786b2a66ab60af9dcb55eea0a0566b331.

12.1. Historical Context of Embryology

The embryological history provides the fundamental knowledge base that informs progress in translational embryology and genetic counseling. The field has evolved tremendously over the years, from initial philosophical inquiry into what life is to controlled scientific exploration. Pioneering minds like Aristotle formulated hypotheses regarding embryonic development, providing early perspectives that instigated interest in subsequent generations. By the 17th century, technological advances in microscopy enabled scientists like Leeuwenhoek and Harvey to examine embryonic development more closely, building a basis for observation and experimentation. These innovations laid vital foundations, highlighting the necessity of integrating observational and experimental approaches in embryology, thus influencing current genetic counseling practices that place embryo development within a paradigm of historical inquiry and scientific accuracy. With the advent of the 19th century, a new chapter opened in evolutionary biology when embryology was intimately linked with heredity and variation theories. Leading figures like Ernst Haeckel supported the theory of recapitulation, according to which the embryonic development of an organism is a mirror of its evolution. The theory put emphasis on interpreting embryonic development as not an isolated event but a complex phenomenon governed by genetic as well as environmental factors. These structures have persisted into modern discussions of genetic counseling, where the intricacies of embryonic development influence diagnostic and treatment plans. This developmental history not only illustrates the intersection of genetics and embryology but also enlightens current practice involved in genetic counseling, as practitioners seek to offer patients thorough understanding of hereditary disease and developmental anomalies on a historical basis.

At the end of the 20th century, embryology as a subject remained dynamic with developments in molecular biology, genetic engineering, and reproductive technologies. The dawn of the new millennium was marked by the cracking of the human genome, which linked the genetic data with embryonic development in ways unimagined before. This era demonstrated the promise inherent in early detection of genetic disease, as was evident in investigations of embryonal carcinomas, a model example of the application of embryologic knowledge directly to the clinical arena. Therefore, the historical development of embryology not only puts these advancements in perspective but also demonstrates the continued challenges, such as those delineated in the incorporation of omics technologies in medicine and dentistry. The call for a commitment to close the gap between research and clinical practice remains current, with unjustified gaps still present in the translational process of fundamental knowledge into accessible care (Kabbashi et al., 2024; Langner et al., 2024) (Figure 12.4).

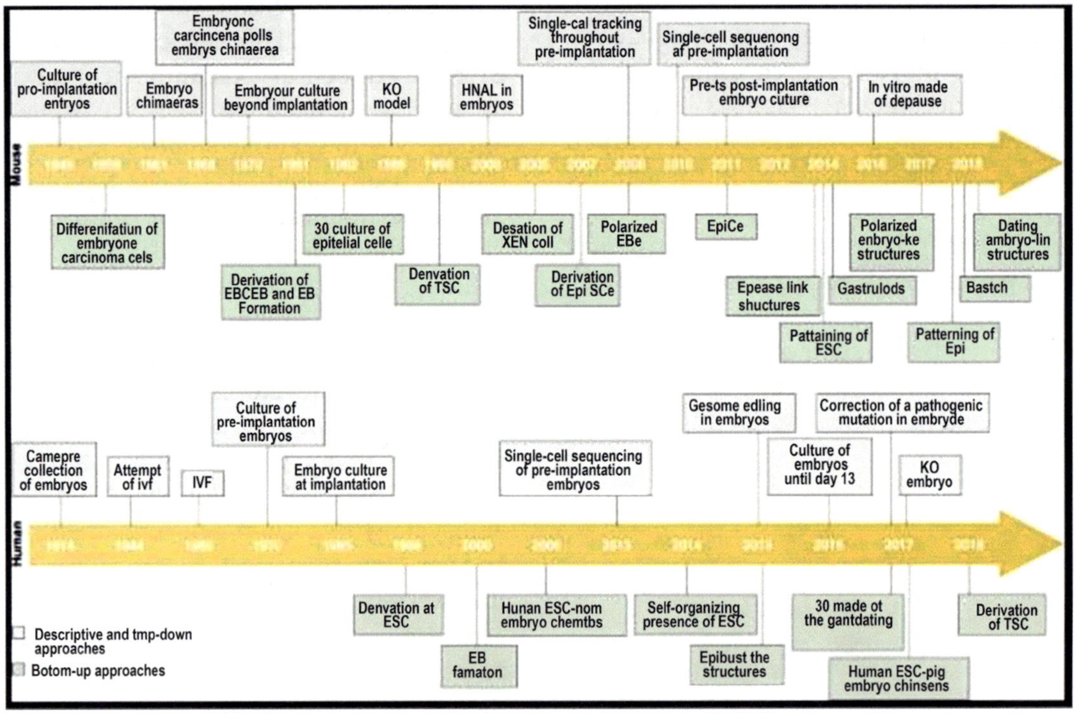

Figure 12.4. Historical context of embryology.

Source: https://media.springernature.com/m685/springer-static/image/art%3A10.1038%2Fs41556-018-0144-x/MediaObjects/41556_2018_144_Fig1_HTML.jpg.

12.1.1. Early Theories and Discoveries

The investigation of basic principles in genetics has also had a great influence on embryology development and genetic counseling practice. One milestone in the history of the discipline was the development of Mendelian laws of inheritance by Gregor Mendel in the mid-19th century. His exhaustive experimentation with pea plants explained simple patterns of inheritance, thereby highlighting dominant and recessive traits. Mendel's research, although not popular during his era, established the basics of genetics. This vital information set the stage for future findings that would continue to propel practices in translational embryology. As the discipline evolved, it became ever more apparent that this knowledge of such fundamental principles was required for genetic counseling because practitioners had to clarify intricate inheritance patterns to individuals and families afflicted with genetic disorders, thus bridging the gap between theoretical genetics and practical applications in the medical sector. The Human Genome Project completion in 2003 was the milestone moment in the merging of genetics and counseling practices in medicine. This breakthrough not only charted the whole human genome but also underscored the sophistication of genetic functions and variations. With this knowledge, medical professionals started to comprehend the effects of genetic susceptibility and aberrations on a wide range of diseases, thereby actually connecting initial theoretical frameworks to practical applications in medicine. This advancement demanded an advanced degree of genetic proficiency among medical teachers and counselors. Hence, an expectation has increased for practitioners to become extremely skilled at communicating genetic principles, thereby provoking inquiries on whether current education models are sufficient to address these needs, as reported in recent literature (Leblanc et al., 2009; Leblanc et al., 2012). Additionally, the incorporation of complex genetic information into curriculum models and clinical practices has also underscored the necessity for ongoing changes within the arenas of health education and counseling. As research within the genetics field continues to evolve, training initiatives have been slow to follow the changing dynamics. For instance, although a large proportion of graduate speech-language pathology programs have included genetic material in their curriculum, many clinicians report feeling inadequately prepared when confronted with genetic issues in the clinical environment (Leblanc et al., 2009). This inconsistency underscores the importance of reform in policy and graduate education, thereby equipping future generations of healthcare professionals with the requisite knowledge and confidence to manage the complex interface between embryology and genetics efficiently, thereby improving the quality of genetic counseling services provided to families affected by genetic disorders (Leblanc et al., 2012).

12.1.2. Advances in Reproductive Technologies

The advancement of reproductive technologies has truly shifted the field of fertility treatment, providing individuals and couples with revolutionary options for reproductive issues. Among this array of technologies, Preimplantation Genetic Testing for Monogenic Diseases (PGT-M) is a vital tool in translational embryology. This technique allows for the testing of embryos for specific genetic mutations before implantation, thereby reducing the chance of passing on inherited disease. Diseases such as Premature Ovarian Failure (POF), which are associated with fragile X mental retardation 1 gene (FMR1) mutations, can be diagnosed and managed proactively. Contemporary scholarly literature highlights that knowledge of the genetic foundations of diseases such as POF enables targeted interventions, and therefore, genetic counseling is an essential aspect of fertility treatment that not only empowers the patient but also optimizes clinical results (Persico et al., 2023). Moreover, emerging reproductive technologies have been developed to tackle the complex issue of female infertility, which plagues millions of people across the globe. Recent research announces possible associations between dermatoglyphic patterns—individual patterns of skin creases—and genetic predispositions to infertility-related conditions such as Turner syndrome and polycystic ovary syndrome (PCOS). This overlap of dermatoglyphics and reproductive medicine is one interesting area of research that could lead to the identification of novel genetic markers for fertility-related conditions. Preliminary results suggest some patterns to potentially have associations with the etiologies of infertility; large-scale research endeavors are, however, required for appropriate comprehension. Interdisciplinary strategies, besides genetic counseling, point to the necessity of expanding the diagnostic perspective from conventional methods to include new evaluations for a complete comprehension of fertility well-being (Anjankar et al., 2024). With progressing technological innovation, the application of genomic sequencing and artificial intelligence (AI) in reproductive medicine has great potential to revolutionize patient care. These advances enable better embryo selection and complete knowledge of the genetic profiles, thereby enabling clinicians to make knowledgeable choices regarding fertility treatment. As genetic sequencing technologies become more widely available and with the advent of personalized medicine, reproductive healthcare is poised to move in the direction of individualized patient care approaches. This development is in line with current objectives in genetic counseling, observing the need for adequately informed decision-making and ethical reflection. In total, such technological developments not only advance reproductive outcomes but also increase insight into the genetic components of infertility, thus ongoing discussion in translational embryology (Anjankar et al., 2024) (Figure 12.5).

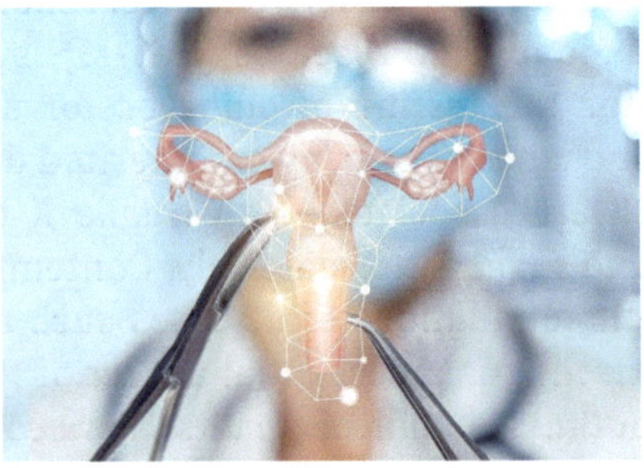

Figure 12.5. Advanced reproductive technology.

Source: https://www.rmia.com/wp-content/uploads/2022/09/rmia-Advanced-Reproductive-Technology-Why-eSET-Is-So-Revolutionary-For-Achieving-Pregnancy.jpg.

12.1.3. Impact of Genetic Research on Embryology

The ceaseless advances in genetics massively reconfigures the discipline of embryology, particularly as it relates to IVF and embryo selection protocols. Genetic testing has provided unprecedented possibilities for comprehending the viability and growth of embryos, allowing practitioners to forecast more precisely. For instance, studies have highlighted the significance of cohort-specific parameters that may influence the developmental potential of embryos, including the overall number of embryos and the proportion of cleavage arrest within a cohort. This direction has been based on observations that predictive variables of this nature may outperform conventional parameters in relation to individual embryos and thus improve embryo selection and transfer procedures in in vitro fertilization cases. The potential to annotate phenotypes of human embryos by genetic investigation offers tremendous possibilities for the advancement of clinical results in reproductive medicine, thereby assisting in the formation of more precise reproductive treatment and judicious strategies in genetic counseling (Behr et al., 2008). Furthermore, genetic investigation plays a significant role in overcoming the challenges faced in female infertility, offering information that goes beyond traditional knowledge. Because infertility is such a multifaceted condition, studies suggest that genetic markers can be informative regarding underlying etiologies and potential prognoses. Dermatoglyphics, for instance, has been examined for its purported association with genetic disease states affecting the reproductive health of women, such as Turner syndrome and PCOS. While intriguing correlations have been noted between dermatoglyphic patterns and etiologies of infertility, the field awaits more empirical research to clarify these observations. Through the incorporation of genetic information into the field of embryology, medical professionals are able to take an integrated approach that couples dermatoglyphic analysis with genetic testing and other diagnostic methods to promote improved detection and treatment of infertility (Anjankar et al., 2024). The synthesis between genetic research and embryological studies indicates the value of cross-disciplinary partnerships in the discipline of reproductive medicine.

As genetic technology continues to evolve, it offers clinicians and genetic counselors alike improved tools for the evaluation of embryos not on the basis of narrow phenotypic characteristics, but instead through an inclusive genomic perspective. Transnational embryology emphasizes that the incorporation of genetic data into clinical care has the potential to radically improve the decision-making frameworks of fertility treatment. This has especial significance in the counseling of future parents regarding their choices and the role of genetic information in reproductive outcomes. Thus, promoting a broad comprehension of the genetic foundations of embryonic development and infertility not only enhances clinical care but also enables families to make an informed choice regarding their reproductive well-being (Anjankar et al., 2024; Behr et al., 2008) (Figure 12.6).

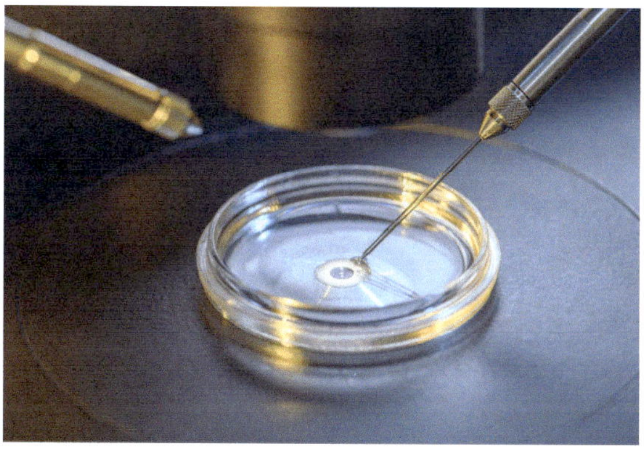

Figure 12.6. Impact of genetic research on embryology.

Source: https://www.openaccessgovernment.org/wp-content/uploads/2019/02/dreamstime_xxl_87277716.jpg.

12.2. Key Concepts in Translational Embryology

Translational embryology represents a critical juncture between basic embryological investigation and clinical practice, particularly as it relates to genetic counseling. Basically, the field seeks to convert scientific information pertaining to embryonic development and genetic disease into novel approaches that have the potential to improve patient outcomes. At the heart of translational embryology are ideas pertaining to the discovery of genetic markers for reproductive issues such as POF. As noted above, premature ovarian failure (POF) is also commonly linked to genetic determinants, namely abnormalities in the fragile X mental retardation 1 gene (FMR1), that directly affect reproductive potential and menstrual well-being. It is essential that genetic counselors understand these biomarkers, as they help facilitate informed decision-making among those pursuing fertility treatment or facing genetic susceptibility in their offspring. Consequently, a comprehensive knowledge of embryological principles enables counselors to advise patients more effectively through such challenging situations. The other crucial area in translational embryology is the application of preimplantantion genetic testing (PGT) to offer reproductive options to families at risk of genetic disorders, including those associated with POF. Through the use of PGT, clinicians are able to detect embryos with genetic mutations prior to implantation, allowing prospective parents to make educated choices in their reproductive health. This selection for genetically healthy embryos has major ramifications for the practice of genetic counseling because it affords families the opportunity to avoid the risks of inherited disease. The relevance of PGT is underscored by the increasing demand for personalized reproductive management based on individual genetic profiles and family histories. Genetic counselors are thus essential in communicating the complexities of PGT and its ethical, emotional, and practical nuances and establishing a supportive environment for the patients as they consider their family planning options. Also, the changing dynamics of genetic counseling highlight the need for professional competencies that facilitate the application of genomics and embryology in clinical practice. As noted by the American Board of Genetic Counseling (ABGC), newly created practice-based competencies (PBCs) highlight the relevance of genetic testing and counseling in a number of areas such as genetics knowledge, communication skills, and education competence. This holistic model equips genetic counselors with the ability to competently handle the technical components of genomic medicine and also strengthens their capacity to address complex genetic matters while building good patient relationships. By promoting effective communication and education regarding genetic concepts, the counselors enable patients to receive personalized care founded on scientific research. Thus, the integration of translational embryology and genetic counseling is a critical part of the evolution of reproductive health care, ultimately improving the standard of care for those who are involved in family planning and genetic risk determination (Figure 12.7).

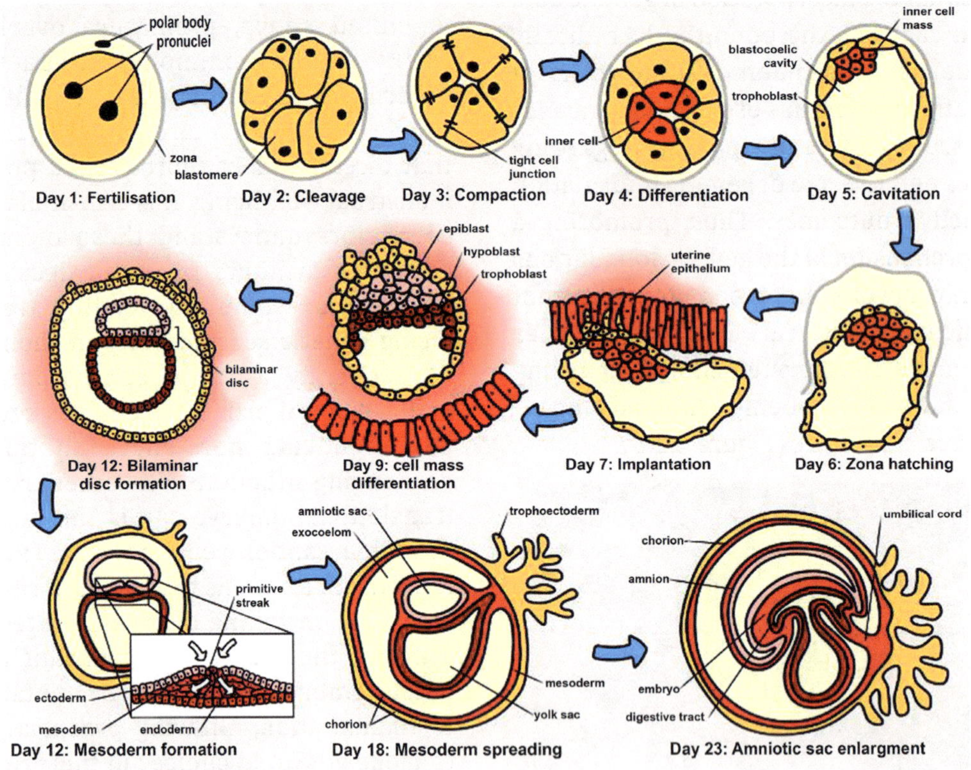

Figure 12.7. Key concepts in translational embryology.

Source: https://simplemed.co.uk/images/Human_Embryogenesis.png.

12.2.1. Stem Cell Research and Applications

The advances in the field of stem cell research have significantly impacted the field of translational embryology and genetic counseling, enabling a range of possibilities as well as challenges. Stem cells, particularly embryonic stem cells (ESCs), have the remarkable ability to differentiate into various cell types, thereby elevating the scope for the treatment of a wide range of disorders, including degenerative diseases and traumatic injuries. This potential for regeneration has fascinated scientists and clinicians alike, and therefore there have been discussions around ethical considerations and regulations over their use. States have addressed these issues variably; for example, the current discussion regarding mitochondrial transfer demonstrates a more complex public consultation procedure in the United Kingdom, which contrasts quite unfavorably with the lack of discussion of analogous topics in the United States, where a democratic deficit remains evident in the public health discourse around assisted reproductive technologies and their evolution (Lewis et al., 2019). As applications of stem cells grow, the ethical considerations warrant careful scrutiny. ESC harvesting is particularly a subject of concern as the cells are derived from human embryos. These activities introduce difficult ethical debates regarding the embryos' moral status and the consequences of experimenting with human life in its earliest form.

The requirement of informed consent and protection of patients' rights then becomes an essential part of this discussion, demanding an intentional balance between ethical values and scientific advancement. It is essential that the medical community, along with ethicists and policymakers, rise to these challenges to make certain that advancement does not undermine basic ethical values. The laws that regulate stem cell research can differ significantly, mirroring the diversity of cultural approaches to this delicate issue and highlighting the necessity for a cohesive framework that allows new technologies to function in an ethical and secure manner (Arda et al., 2020). In conclusion, the potential of stem cell research is genuine; it comes, however, with a host of ethical, legal, and societal issues that must be addressed through the creation of a general governance structure. As advances in translational embryology and genetic counseling evolve, these disciplines must put ethical arguments at the forefront in a manner that stimulates the public to take an active and open interest. By promoting open debate on stem cell research, scientists can ensure that innovative treatments and therapies remain grounded in respect for human life's dignity.

This sort of debate is essential not only for advancing scientific knowledge but also for establishing public trust. Engaging a range of stakeholders—patients, researchers, ethicists, and legislators—are all going to help shape the creation of a responsible approach to the promising, yet complex, area of stem cell research and its applications in medical practice (Arda et al., 2020; Lewis et al., 2019) (Figure 12.8).

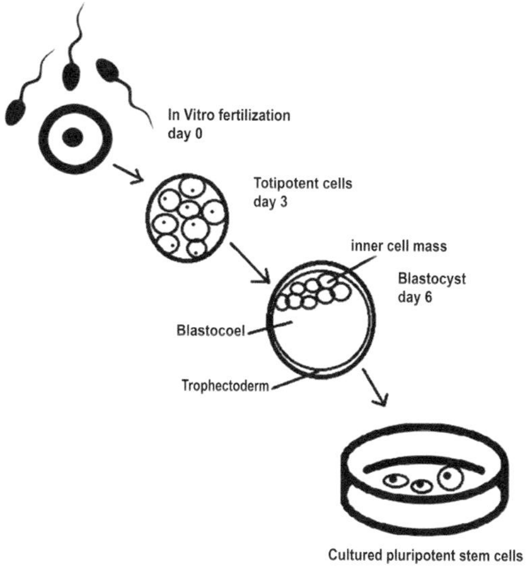

Figure 12.8. Stem cell research.

Source: https://media.springernature.com/lw685/springer-static/image/art%3A10.1186%2Fs13287-019-1165-5/MediaObjects/13287_2019_1165_Fig4_HTML.png.

12.2.2. In vitro Fertilization (IVF) Techniques

IVF treatments are a milestone in reproductive medicine that enables infertile couples to achieve successful pregnancies. The initial process is stimulating the ovaries using hormone medication to induce the development of multiple follicle-containing eggs. Upon maturity, they are subsequently harvested through a less complicated procedure. The initial process is the most critical since the number of healthy embryos developed directly affects the success rate. For instance, a case report of a 40-year-old male and a 32-year-old female highlighted that the couple experienced infertility for two years before attempting in vitro fertilization (IVF) after unsuccessful intrauterine insemination (IUI).

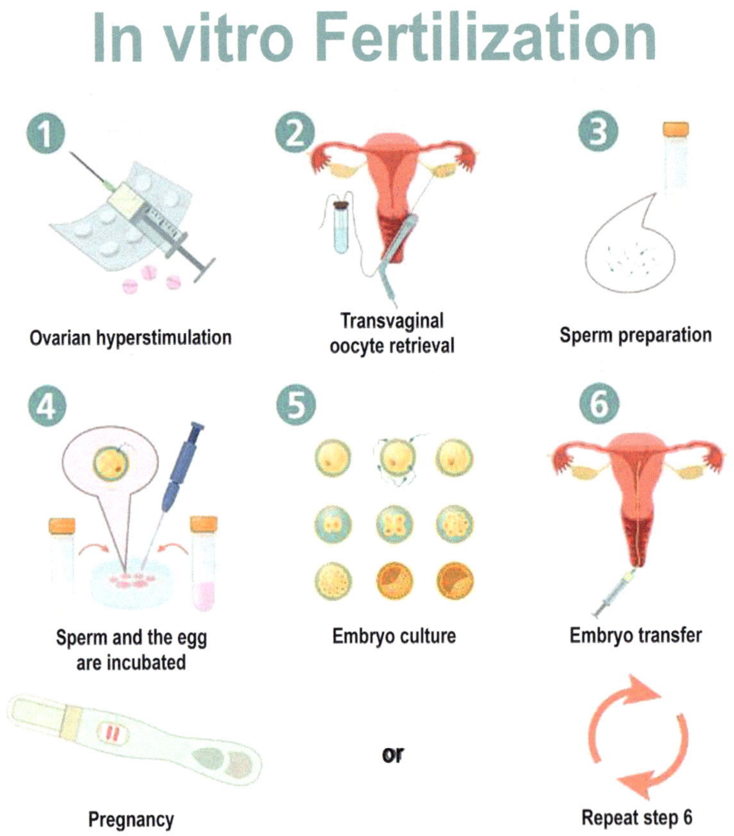

Figure 12.9. *In vitro* fertilization (IVF) techniques.

Source: https://www.esco-medical.com/images/upload/IVFPROCEDURE.png.

The situation highlights the imperative role of tailored protocols in assisted reproductive technology (ART), such as IVF/intracytoplasmic sperm injection (IVF/ICSI)46111612. The individualized situation of every couple emphasizes the requirement for informed decision-making throughout the IVF process. Following egg retrieval, fertilization is achieved either through regular insemination or ICSI, where a single sperm is actually injected into an egg. The procedure is best used in male factor infertility cases, including reduced sperm count and motility. The embryo culture stage is very critical, as embryos develop over the course of several days in a controlled laboratory environment. Assessment of embryo quality at this point is necessary to offer the optimal prospects for implantation. Recent advances in PGT allow for the embryos to be checked for some genetic disorders before transfer, which enhances the likelihood of a healthy pregnancy by a great deal. Through the development of genome-wide haplotyping techniques, the process of embryonic screening has been transformed, enabling the application of more rigorous selection criteria involving both the genetic composition and the general chromosomal health of the embryos, thereby unfolding a complex interaction between reproductive outcomes and technological advances (de Ravel et al., 2017). The inclusion of genetic counseling within the IVF process is significant in informing prospective parents of their options and the outcome of their choices. Genetic counselors can provide valuable information on the risks for hereditary diseases, particularly if they are confronted with genetic disorders. The couple will have an option of embryo selection based on certain genetic conditions, making them wiser reproductive decisions. Also, as technology improves in genetic testing procedures, continuous debate within the medical community and elsewhere seeks to improve the criteria for embryo selection. The debate is critical in informing patients and ensuring ethical standards among reproductive technologies. Thus, translational embryology not only signifies improvements in patient care but also reflects on the necessity of genetic counseling to address the multifaceted concerns of the use of assisted reproductive technologies, finally to enhance family planning strategy (Figure 12.9).

12.2.3. Genetic Modification and CRISPR Technology

With the progress in genetic modification, CRISPR technology has become a key tool offering unprecedented accuracy in genome editing. This novel approach takes advantage of an innate defense system in bacteria that employs RNA-guided enzymes to locate and modify targeted DNA sequences. The applications of CRISPR-Cas9 technology in general medical fields, such as translational embryology and genetic counseling, are nothing but revolutionary. By allowing for exact modifications to genetic codes, CRISPR can eradicate inherited diseases and improve desirable traits at the moment of conception. This feature calls for serious ethical considerations, and it underscores the necessity for rigorous genetic counseling to enlighten prospective parents about the risk and reward of genetic alteration in order to allow for well-informed reproductive decision-making. Within the field of personalized medicine, the integration of CRISPR technology is generating new opportunities for targeted therapeutic interventions, particularly with regard to complex conditions like cancer. Research has identified critical genes involved in tumor formation, thus making it easier to create more personalized treatment strategies. As a case in point, recent research has focused on ovarian cancer and has shown that genetic alterations, such as the overexpression of CARM1, can significantly influence therapeutic outcomes. The use of CRISPR technology at the embryonic stage offers the potential for utilizing genetic modifications in safeguarding future generations against inherited susceptibilities to various forms of cancer. This potential to alter the genetic blueprint of embryos highlights the promise of enhanced health outcomes; however, it also comes with challenges in comprehending the long-term implications of these alterations on the human genome. In addition, the application of newer therapeutic modalities requires a sophisticated genetic counseling infrastructure to help families understand the intricate relationship between disease and genetics. Additionally, the advent of CRISPR technology goes beyond traditional gene editing technologies, exploring territories such as somatic and inheritable alterations, thereby having significant implications for the field of genetic counseling. For example, advances in the understanding of myotonic dystrophy (DM1) highlight the potential of CRISPR to analyze precisely and intervene in genetic differences that affect the severity of disease. With new methods like No-Amplification targeted sequencing, researchers can better identify repeat expansions and their implications for disease manifestation. This heightened capacity enables genetic counselors to give informed counsel according to personal risk and genetic configuration, as for highly variable diseases such as DM1. The ramifications of such technology underscore the essential need for interdisciplinarity among geneticists, clinicians, and counselors to address the ethical and societal aspects of genetic modification responsibly in the furtherance of patient care within the arenas of translational embryology and genetic counseling (Figure 12.10).

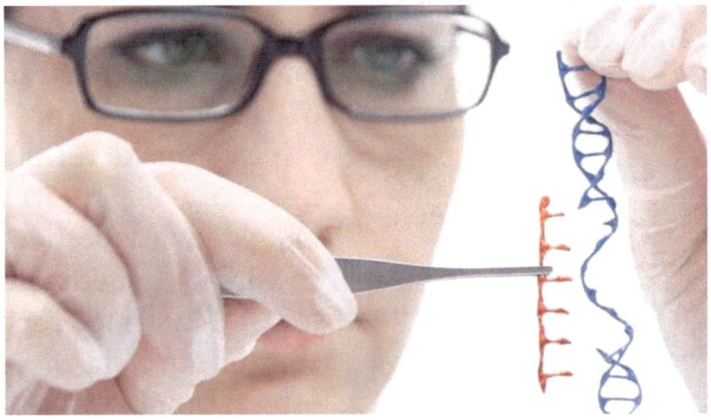

Figure 12.10. Genetic Modification and CRISPR Technology.

Source: https://external-content.duckduckgo.com/iu/?u=https%3A%2F%2Fgeneticliteracyproject.org%2Fwp-content%2Fuploads%2F2016%2F01%2Fgene-editing.jpg&f=1&nofb=1&ipt=2868fd71810ba89c85c7c2808496a6c884892d4735886b961631137ef13f43d0.

12.3. Role of Genetic Counseling

The role of genetic counseling has become increasingly important in the context of the present model of reproductive medicine, particularly in relation to translational embryology. As the field of embryology continues to evolve with newer techniques such as IVF and PGD, genetic counseling acts as an important bridge that interfaces patients with these complex scientific technologies. Genetic counselors provide important information related to genetic risk, inheritance patterns, and implications of genetic testing. Such assistance enables patients and couples to engage in informed reproductive decision-making in which their unique genetic vulnerability is taken into consideration. Being able to integrate genetic counseling into the IVF process effectively not only makes it less complicated to make decisions but also promotes patient comfort and confidence in emotionally charged contexts, thereby impacting reproductive procedure success rates as well as the psychological well-being of the patients. Recent advances in understanding embryonic development highlight the significant role embryo cohort variables—that is, total embryos and cleavage rates—are going to have to play in predicting outcome. This serves to highlight the need for genetic counseling in the application of assisted reproductive techniques. The results clearly point to an increased sophistication in our understanding of the ways in which genetic factors can influence embryonic viability and successful implantation rates. For those couples going through IVF, information gained from genetic counseling can clarify these elements, allowing them to have an enhanced understanding of their options for treatment. An inclusive genetic counseling strategy not only enables personalized care according to the couple's unique situation but promotes a collaborative decision-making process essential to managing the uncertainties and intricacies inherent in reproductive health. These findings assist in enhancing trust in the chosen treatment strategies and encourage multidisciplinary interaction among medical practitioners. Additionally, genetic counseling is at the forefront in the management of certain genetic disorders, including POF, which is indicated by premature age infertility occurring under the age of 40 and is usually associated with genetic components. The detection of abnormalities in individual genes, such as FMR1, holds great significance for individuals and couples pursuing fertility therapy. Genetic counselors can facilitate preimplantation genetic testing for monogenic disorders (PGT-M) when one of the couples is detected to have known genetic mutations. This prevention not only facilitates the avoidance of the transmission of genetic disorders to offspring, but it also focuses on the ethical considerations that come with reproductive decisions. Finally, genetic counseling plays a crucial role in improving patient experience and outcomes in the context of translational embryology. It provides individuals with the capacity to effectively deal with the complexities of genetic health in order to make informed reproductive choices and family planning (Figure 12.11).

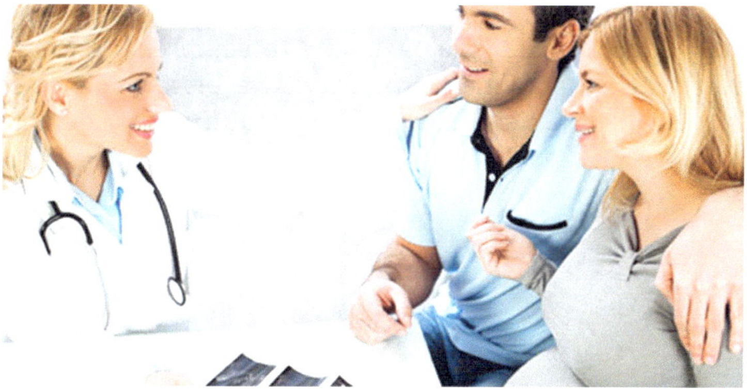

Figure 12.11. Genetic counseling.

Source: https://external-content.duckduckgo.com/iu/?u=https%3A%2F%2Fwww.healthbenefitstimes.com%2Fglossary%2Fwp-content%2Fuploads%2F2020%2F07%2FGenetic-counseling.jpg&f=1&nofb=1&ipt=1ab1b3af714cc599d1dfd68d3aff455d0e11a1181200bde1f7ba81157aa2581d.

12.3.1. Definition and Purpose of Genetic Counseling

Genetic counseling is a distinct discipline that arises at the interface between genetics, medical care, and psychosocial counseling. Its primary objective is to educate and empower individuals and families who are confronted with genetic disease or inherited risk. By evaluation of family medical histories, the genetic counselor assists patients in comprehending the risk of inherited disorders, thereby promoting fully informed decision making with respect to testing, management strategies, and possible interventions. As genetic technologies have evolved, genetic counselors' roles have expanded accordingly, demanding deep understanding of genomics and the sophistication of risk estimation. The American Board of Genetic Counseling (ABGC) has established practice-based competencies to equip professionals with these heightened complexities, delineating essential skills in genetic knowledge and interpersonal communication that are required to deliver holistic care to individuals impacted by genetic concerns (Amanda et al., 2016). Furthermore, the objective of genetic counseling is more than information giving; it involves the active addressing of the emotional and psychological aspects involved in genetic risk. Genetic counselors offer crucial information on inheritance patterns and test results while simultaneously offering emotional support to individuals uncertain about their genetic health. By utilizing effective interpersonal and counseling capabilities, practitioners create a secure space in which patients can share their fears, doubts, and hopes while simultaneously enabling them to understand the implications of their genetic information. This twofold role of education and support is the foundation of the holistic approach that is ingrained in genetic counseling in a bid to ensure that patients are not only educated but also psychologically equipped to handle the possible implications of their genetic condition (Amanda et al., 2016). Within translational embryology, genetic counseling takes on added significance as it acts as the interface between scientific progress and patient care. Breakthroughs in assisted reproductive technologies (ART) and genetic alterations initiate ethical and societal issues that must be discussed in the public domain with informed consent, which is frequently absent in contemporary America. Unlike the more consultative approach evidenced in the United Kingdom, where public consultation has been a hallmark of discussion of ART and genetic modification, there is a democratic deficit in the United States in this regard. The incorporation of genetic counseling within the context of translational embryology enhances individuals' ability to comprehend the meaning of what they are choosing and the interactive potential of reproductive biotechnology, once more calling for openness and active patient involvement in promoting health care (Figure 12.12).

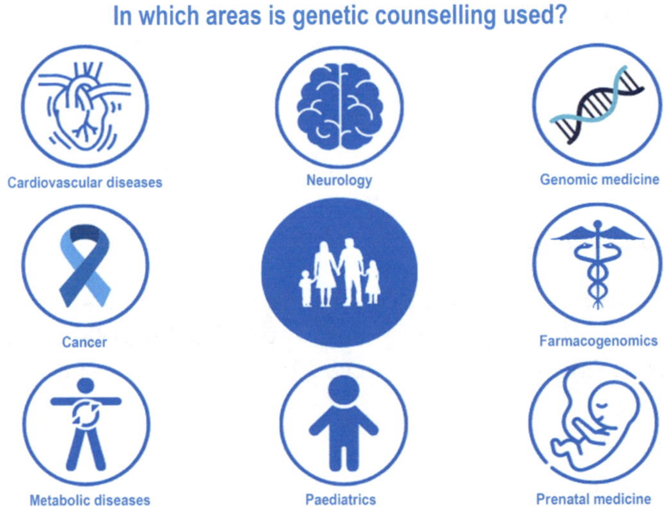

Figure 12.12. Purpose of genetic counseling.

Source: https://www.genosalut.com/wp-content/uploads/2022/05/Genosalut_Genetic_counselling_areas.png.

12.3.2. Types of Genetic Disorders Addressed

It is important to know the different kinds of genetic disorders in the practice of translational embryology and genetic counseling. Genetic disorders can be generally categorized into two large groups, namely chromosomal abnormalities and single-gene mutations. Chromosomal abnormalities encompass disorders such as Down syndrome, which is due to an additional chromosome 21 and has extensive effects on development, physiology, and intellect. On the other hand, those disorders that are due to a single gene, such as cystic fibrosis and sickle cell anemia, are caused by mutations in specific genes and are often inherited in Mendelian inheritance patterns. The intricacies involved in these disorders require genetic counseling because prospective parents may desire knowledge about the likelihood of transmission, possible health consequences, and available interventions, indicating the need for extensive genetic screening during the reproductive planning process. In understanding the complexities of genetic disorders, epigenetic factors have been a key focus of research. Epigenetic modifications, which influence gene expression without altering the DNA sequence itself, can have profound impacts on fetal development and are associated with several developmental disorders. Autism spectrum disorder (ASD) and specific congenital malformations have been associated with dysregulation of epigenetic processes during key stages of embryonic differentiation.

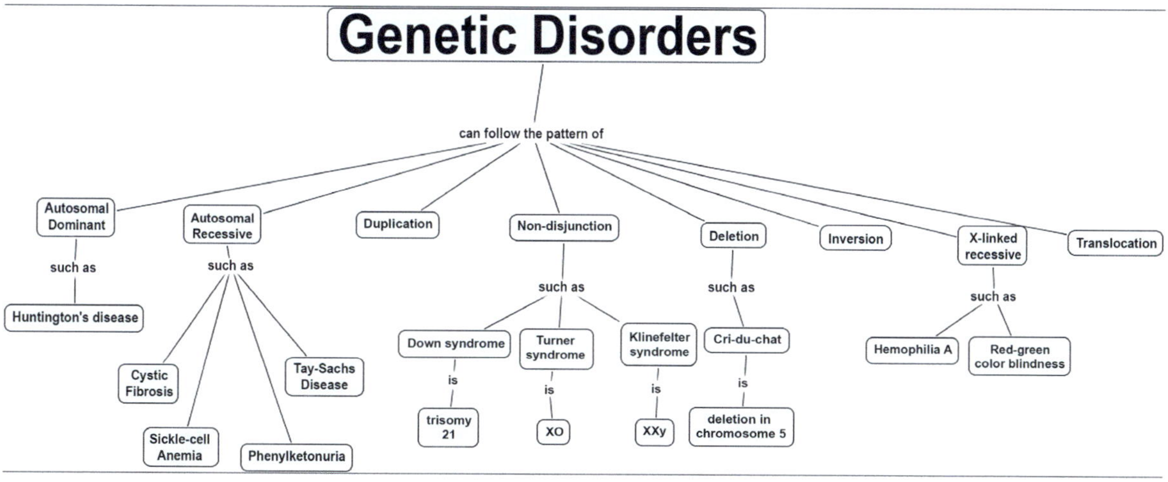

Figure 12.13. Types of genetic disorders addressed.

Source: https://miro.medium.com/v2/resize:fit:1184/1*s0ky9NQDOKwYuucqOpLXGA.jpeg.

For example, maternal dietary intake and exposure to xenobiotics are environmental factors that may induce epigenetic modifications of gene expression in the form of neurodevelopmental disorders. Such cross-talk between genetic counseling and epigenetics makes it an urgent requirement for practitioners to remain informed about the impact of environmental exposures and their possible implications on genetic disorders, thus being better equipped to provide personalized services to the affected families (Juga et al., 2022). Moreover, recent research has shown that dermatoglyphics, the study of fingerprint patterns, can reveal useful information about genetic predispositions to infertility along with some genetic diseases. Research has recently looked into associations between dermatoglyphics patterns and genetic disorders such as Turner syndrome and PCOS, in which there are severe difficulties in fertility and reproduction. Despite the results suggesting possible associations, the arena continues to lack extensive evidence to confirm direct cause-effect relationships, pointing to the need for more rigorous research approaches. By and large, insight into how various genetic disorders, including those manifesting in unique physical characteristics or problems with infertility, influence one another constitutes an essential aspect of translational embryology and genetic counseling. By incorporating interdisciplinarity, practitioners can more effectively assist families in navigating the intricate arena of genetic health (Anjankar et al., 2024) (Figure 12.13).

12.3.3. Ethical Considerations in Genetic Counseling

The practice of genetic counseling is inherently embedded with numerous ethical concerns that have to be carefully handled in order to uphold the rights and dignities of patients. As intermediaries, genetic counselors convey complicated genetic information with potential direct effects on reproductive choices, health care decisions, and family dynamics. Central to this function is the mandate of informed consent, which demands that patients be cognizant of the consequences of genetic tests, such as possible psychological effects and social stigmas linked with genetic disorders. There are ethical issues also in the provision of equal access to genetic counseling services, especially among marginalized groups. As translational embryology advances to improve the potential for genetic intervention, there is a likelihood that existing disparities can become exaggerated, leading to questions of the recipients of genetic technology and who might remain excluded. It is thus imperative to deal with these ethical concerns in order to promote equitable healthcare provision in genetics. Furthermore, a major ethical concern in genetic counseling is the control and storage of genetic information. Confidentiality is of utmost significance since genetic data has the potential to reveal personal information not only about an individual but also about his or her relatives, exposing them to discrimination and stigmatization. The fact that genetic information may be used by employers, insurers, and other third parties further complicates the resolution of these dilemmas. Genetic counselors must weigh these potentials against informing clients of the potential risks of sharing their genetic information.

Thus, it is important to have ethical models that safeguard the rights of patients and ensure that their data is handled in a way that values autonomy and confidentiality. Further, programs intended to foster trust between genetic counselors and clients are important, especially within the context of discussing the potential options for genetic testing and intervention through the application of translational embryology. As genetic counseling continues to develop with new technologies, ethical issues regarding the use of embryonic and stem cell research move to the center stage. ESCs have both spurred medical breakthroughs and ethical controversies, necessitating thoughtful examination of the consequences of such technologies. Recent studies have emphasized that the quest for knowledge with embryonic stem cell (ESC) research brings up queries regarding the ethical standing of embryos and the moral reasoning for their utilization in research along with therapeutic applications (Arda et al., 2020). Moreover, the Oncofertility Consortium's work is arguably the most eloquent demonstration of the value of interdisciplinarity in developing new choices for patients receiving fertility-limited interventions. Simultaneously, it testifies to the necessity of resolving the ethical considerations related to reproductive autonomy and decision-making models (Acharya et al., 2021). Generally speaking, the interplay between scientific development and ethics in genetic counseling is required for developing a practice that respects patient autonomy while successfully tackling the complicated moral landscape of contemporary biotechnology.

12.4. Integration of Translational Embryology and Genetic Counseling

The convergence of translational embryology and genetic counseling is an intriguing advancement in reproductive medicine and genetics. Translational embryology is primarily concerned with connecting laboratory findings to clinical practice, thus unraveling our comprehension of human development at the embryonic level. Such an understanding forms the basis of genetic counseling, whose ultimate goal is to offer individuals and families information regarding genetic disorders and hereditary ailments. Based on knowledge derived from embryology, genetic counselors are able to provide individualized risk assessments to facilitate family decision-making with respect to reproductive choices. Such an interdisciplinary methodology not only maximizes patient results but is also a testament to the value of interdisciplinary processes for the practice of healthcare today. Translational embryology and genetic counseling interaction also facilitates the creation of novel diagnostic modalities as well as therapeutic interventions. Through developments in techniques such as preimplantation genetic diagnosis (PGD) and next-generation sequencing (NGS), genetic counselors are able to use this information to advise patients on potential genetic risks of embryo selection. This integration is critical to the handling of inherited disease, as it provides medical practitioners with the tools required to detect and treat risks prior to conception or early during pregnancy. By integrating knowledge from embryology with genetic data, patients receive an individualized strategy that not only enhances their knowledge but also empowers them in the reproductive process. Furthermore, integration of these fields not only improves clinical practice but also is accompanied by ethical challenges that must be critically examined. As the possibilities offered by genetic testing increase, along with the growing availability of technologies such as gene editing, genetic counselors' roles will change to encompass the ethical dimensions of these advances. For example, the convergence of breakthroughs in embryology and genetic counseling calls for the revisit of current laws and policies on reproductive decisions and genetic alteration. It is critical that ethical frameworks promoting patient autonomy, fully informed consent, and equity in the face of this evolving environment be developed. Therefore, continued discussion and communication between professionals working in these areas are of the utmost importance in managing the complexity that comes with technological development in a manner that upholds human dignity and facilitates good practice, according to Pilyavsky (2024). Facing these multi-faceted challenges will finally shape the future of reproductive health care and genetic counseling in the 21st century.

12.4.1. How Embryology Informs Genetic Counseling Practices

The integration of embryological research and genetic counseling practice is now widely recognized as an integral part of managing reproduction issues. Detailed understanding of embryonic development provides essential information on the viability and genetic normalcy of embryos, which is essential in facilitating informed decision-making in genetic counseling. As an example, developments within the field of embryology have allowed for the development of a number of predictive markers for embryo quality, as one study of large data sets derived from in vitro fertilization (IVF) cycles has shown. In this study, it was determined that some cohort-level properties, including total embryos and cleavage arrest rate, are more predictive of successful pregnancy outcome than individual embryonic properties by themselves (Behr et al., 2008). The integration of these embryology discoveries allows genetic counselors to make evidence-based referrals and, by doing so, improve patient outcomes and promote a more comprehensive understanding of reproductive possibilities. Beyond contributions to embryo quality testing, embryology informs the understanding of genetic disease on fertility and embryonic development. The understanding relative to primary ovarian insufficiency (POF), for instance, has important implications for genetic counseling for the fragile X mental retardation 1 gene (FMR1). Abnormalities in the FMR1 gene, including POF, have a significant impact on the reproductive trajectory of a woman. Genetic counselors can use embryological studies and genetic screening to detect carriers of such abnormalities, thereby facilitate directed preimplantation genetic testing for monogenic disorders (PGT-M) for future parents (Persico et al., 2023). This measure not only serves to curb the incidence of genetic illness but also empowers patients by giving them holistic knowledge about their reproductive health choices. Furthermore, the application of embryological concepts to genetic counseling procedures significantly contributes to the entire patient experience by connecting scientific information to compassionate conversation. The intimate nature of reproductive health requires that genetic counselors clearly communicate intricate biological and genetic ideas to patients who might be confronted with emotionally significant choices. By basing discourse on current embryology research, counselors can assist patients in grasping the significance of their decisions regarding embryo viability and genetic results. This practice establishes a setting of informed consent in which patients feel supported in their reproductive choice, ultimately resulting in satisfaction with care. As a result, the ongoing expansion of translational embryology further supports the role of genetic counseling as an essential step forward in the practice of personalized reproductive medicine.

12.4.2. Case Studies of Successful Integration

In the past several years, case studies of successful integration in translational embryology have been instructive in the way that genetic counseling can be employed to optimize patient outcomes. A prime example involved a family who had a genetic predisposition to a difference in sex development (DSD). Parents were initially reluctant to share information about their child's status due to stigma. Nevertheless, through the use of individualized education that incorporated stakeholders' views, healthcare professionals managed to successfully promote open communication. Not only did this alleviate parental anxiety, but it also gave the child the awareness needed to have a complete grasp of their specific situation. The application of patient education, as evident in the research, showed the central position that knowledge occupies in enhancing psychosocial development and addressing the complex aftermath of DSD (Baskin et al., 2023). Yet another case study demonstrates how the incorporation of epigenetic data into genetic counseling routines can add to outcome measures in families that are at risk of neurodevelopmental disorders (NDDs). Here, prospective parents received holistic counseling in terms of epigenetic alterations that may influence fetal development. Through the application of advances in translational embryology, medical professionals enlightened such parents on the potential impacts of different environmental factors on gene expression during sensitive developmental windows. This empowers parents with the framework to make lifestyle decisions that pre-emptively reduce predicted risks. Emphasized in the available evidence, the exact timing of gene activation and silencing is fundamental in ensuring healthy fetal development, and as such, it is imperative to integrate epigenetic research into counseling procedures (Juga et al., 2022). This broad-spectrum approach not only ensures maternal health but also establishes a basis for the long-term health of the child. In addition, effective integration in the practice of genetic counseling can be evidenced by collaborative efforts of multidisciplinary teams comprising geneticists, psychologists, and social workers. In a case study, these specialists were brought together to create a concerted management plan for a child who was diagnosed with a genetic condition. By combining perspectives from different disciplines, they offered the family a comprehensive understanding of the implications associated with the diagnosis and the resources that they could access. This synthesis enhanced the child and parents' ability to cope with challenges, resulting in better overall family functioning. The success of this multidisciplinary practice underscores the importance of teamwork in genetic counseling, as it enables comprehensive discussion that incorporates medical, psychological, and social elements. The achievement in such instances foretells the future of translational embryology and its subsequent influence on genetic counseling approaches (Figure 12.14).

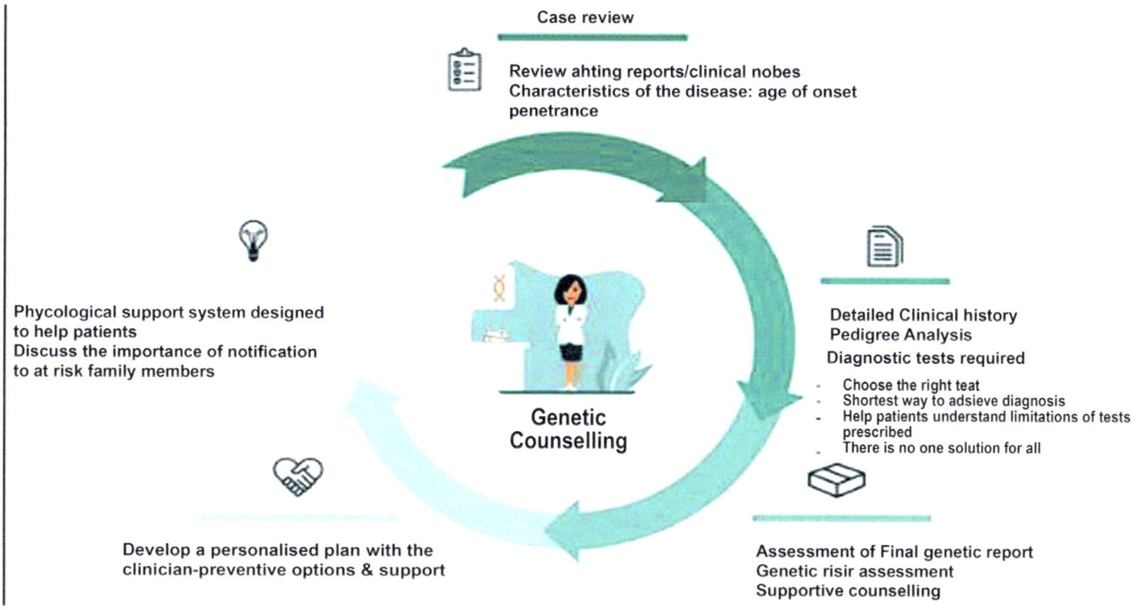

Figure 12.14. Embryology informs genetic counseling practices.

Source: https://media.springernature.com/lw685/springer-static/image/chp%3A10.1007%2F978-981-99-7028-5_19/MediaObjects/539776_1_En_19_Fig1_HTML.png.

12.4.3. Challenges Faced in Combining the Two Fields

The union of translational embryology and genetic counseling comes with numerous important challenges that workers in these areas must deal with. Foremost among these is the challenge of varied levels of knowledge and ability in genomic principles among workers. In spite of the developments in genetic science, a considerable percentage of workers, inclusive of genetic counselors, are usually tremendously insufficiently trained in the nuances of embryology. This inequality creates potential disparities in communication and understanding of information relating to genetic anomalies during the embryonic development process. Additionally, as noted in literature specific to nursing and genetics, the requirement is not just for maximizing knowledge but rather for an emphasis on the creation of comprehensive training programs incorporating both embryological information and genetic counseling practices, thereby preparing practitioners to provide more knowledgeable and consolidated patient care (Badzek et al., 2023). A further critical challenge arises from the dynamic nature of genomics by virtue of rapid scientific progress. To illustrate, the completion of the Human Genome Project has transformed the understanding of genetics, but in doing so, it has also raised, simultaneously, the demands on healthcare providers to remain current with developments. Many program directors and educators acknowledge the significant need for the incorporation of genetic literacy into educational curricula, yet there is a notable gap concerning the perceived readiness of today's graduates to translate this knowledge into effective use in clinical practice (Leblanc et al., 2009). Therefore, the integration of translational embryology and genetic counseling calls for continuous updates in the curriculum and in professional development activities to deliver more competencies for practitioners in effectively engaging their own patients in their own unique genetic stories. Further, the interprofessional framework that integrates translational embryology and genetic counseling is frequently faced with institutional and systemic obstacles in both education systems and healthcare organizations. Most programs concentrate on specialized expertise peculiar to their disciplines, unknowingly creating a disjointed educational process that may work to hinder collaborative practice. Additionally, the absence of general criteria and expectations regarding genetic competencies further complicates the issue, resulting in possible gaps in service provision. In order for these challenges to be addressed effectively, practitioners must make a concerted effort to develop collaborative training models that focus on mutual understanding and multidisciplinary practices in patient care. By overcoming these structural barriers systematically, the interface between translational embryology and genetic counseling can lead to improved patient outcomes and more efficient healthcare delivery (Badzek et al., 2023; Leblanc et al., 2009).

12.5. Current Trends in Research

Recent advances in the field of translational embryology have made an indelible mark on the field of genetic counseling, particularly in relation to rare diseases. Research emphasizes the vital role that genetic counselors play in providing specific information and emotional support to individuals faced with the complexities of rare disease diagnoses. In Spain, although geneticists and genetic counselors are not legally considered healthcare professionals, the demand for expert genetic care became increasingly evident. According to Navas et al. (2021), individuals who suffer from rare diseases also tend to suffer from not just the medical intricacies of their diseases but also psychosocial intricacies as a result of delayed diagnosis. This highlights the critical need for a more evolved framework as far as genetic counseling is involved, with a focus on the need for incorporating genetic specialists into the healthcare system for overall care and advice. Another important trend that has been observed in recent studies involves investigating epigenetic modifications in relation to embryonic development and the resulting health implications. These changes are vital processes that regulate gene expression at important phases of fetal development and growth, thereby rendering them instrumental in understanding a number of disorders. According to Juga et al. (2022), the regulation and timing of gene induction during embryogenesis could influence stem cell differentiation pathways. A new field of research emphasizes the interaction between environmental influences and epigenetic processes, which may lead to neurodevelopmental and psychiatric disorders. Elucidation of such intricate interrelations may advance genetic counseling practice through the identification of risk factors and the creation of personalized therapies for prospective parents regarding the effects on fetal well-being. The convergence of these lines of research highlights the shifting paradigms within the practice of genetic counseling and their relevance to clinical care. With the evolution of knowledge regarding the genetic and epigenetic determinants of health, genetic counselors are ever more so at the forefront of the interpretation of these data into meaningful recommendations for patients. The merging of personalized genetic data with knowledge derived from embryological studies enables the development of better counseling strategies and treatment therapies. As highlighted by Juga et al. (2022) and Navas et al. (2021), promoting multidisciplinary interaction among geneticists, embryologists, and counselors is crucial in eradicating the disparities in access to and equity in healthcare, and in improving the level of care offered to families affected by genetic disorders.

12.5.1. Innovations in Genetic Testing

Innovations in genetic testing have revolutionized the practice of translational embryology and genetic counseling, as well as our ability to diagnose and manage genetic disease. Through advances in genomic technologies, including NGS, physicians can now process large volumes of genetic data with unprecedented speed and accuracy. This enables the early detection of genetic abnormalities, with resultant proactive measures that can be instituted during pregnancy or even preconception. For instance, PGT identifies chromosome abnormalities in IVF-generated embryos, improving the chances of a successful pregnancy and reducing the risk of hereditary disease transmission to children. As we explore these developments, it's apparent that genetic testing is not only assisting individual health decisions but also has broader ramifications for public health and the future of reproductive medicine. Extending the discussion on genetic testing, its implications extend into the field of genetic counseling. This involves the provision of informed decision-making for future parents. Genetic counselors play an important role in interpreting test results, providing educational information on potential health effects, and guiding families through the intricacies of genetic information. The advent of advanced genetic testing has called upon counselors to engage in more serious discussions regarding ethical considerations, particularly in situations where reproductive choices are influenced by the outcomes of such tests. For instance, in managing sperm abnormalities linked to infertility, genetic counseling takes a central position, especially when cases of extreme oligoasthenozoospermia or azoospermia are identified. In this context, sperm aneuploidy testing can offer information that raises ethical issues related to assisted reproductive technologies, thereby ensuring families receive proper information on their available alternatives and the consequences of their choices (Dyulgerova-Nikolova et al., 2020). The connection between counseling and innovation highlights the sophistication of genetic services in the contemporary era. Moreover, the ethics of innovations in genetic testing cannot be overlooked. In the field of assisted reproductive technologies (ART), and more so in the United States, there is a robust democratic deficit in open discussion about regulatory choices as well as the ethical consequences of these innovations. It has been observed that the absence of extensive public consultation has complicated serious contemplation on the social and ethical concerns linked to the quick evolution of ART (Lewis et al., 2019). Conversely, some nations, like the United Kingdom, have initiated public consultations to consider intricate issues such as mitochondrial transfer, an indication of a proactive attitude toward dealing with ethical challenges. With ongoing development in the area of genetic testing, it is essential to maintain democratic discussion to provide transparency, accountability, and moral coherence to the evolving system of genetic counseling and reproductive medicine. This need for dialogue reaffirms the importance of embracing societal values in scientific innovation, thus shaping equitable policies that serve the interests of all stakeholders involved.

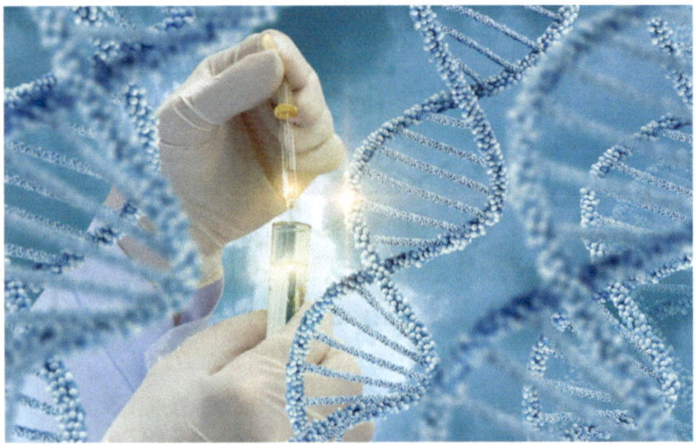

Figure 12.15. Innovations in genetic testing.

Source: https://external-content.duckduckgo.com/iu/?u=https%3A%2F%2Fwww.apdaparkinson.org%2Fwp-content%2Fuploads%2F2018%2F11%2Fgenetic-test.jpeg&f=1&nofb=1&ipt=b1bb817ad43b35eb3c99718e7d0e347fc6be9f5bab8b015db6231c60b985555e.

12.5.2. Advances in Embryonic Research Techniques

Recent developments in embryonic research techniques have had a major influence on the practice of translational embryology and genetic counseling, opening up new possibilities in studying infertility and genetic disorders. New methods, including genetic profiling and testing in the early stages of embryonic development, allow clinicians to determine if there are any genetic defects present prior to implantation. For instance, PGT developments allow embryos to be screened for some genetic diseases, significantly enhancing chances of successful pregnancy and reducing the risk of inherited diseases. Additionally, AI integration in embryonic research has improved embryo viability tests with increased accuracy, promising a future when personalized medicine can effectively and ethically guide reproductive choices, thus unlocking possibilities for infertile couples. One of the strongest points about these breakthroughs is that they have the potential to increase the precision of diagnostics. As noted by major professional societies, issues such as extended carrier screening and direct-to-consumer genetic testing have become prominent features in contemporary models of reproductive health (Abbott et al., 2017). The said techniques not only reveal individuals who have genetic disorders but also assist future parents in making wise reproductive decisions in light of their genetic profiles. Secondly, the development of non-invasive prenatal screening (NIPS) offers valuable information regarding the genetic well-being of the unborn, facilitating intervention processes that can be taken before birth. All these strategies signify a significant change in the paradigm of genetic counseling, wherein individualized information can educate and shape the experiences of prospective parents utilizing assisted reproductive technologies and thus reflect concepts of translational medicine. Further, the studies on embryonic development have determined associations with more extensive genetic and epigenetic influences. The analysis of dermatoglyphic patterns, according to recent research, offers possible correlations between these individualized skin ridge patterns and infertility in women, connecting embryonic development to genetic predispositions not necessarily apparent on the surface (Anjankar et al., 2024). The intersection of embryology and genetics here necessitates an acknowledgment of the requirement for a detailed diagnostic process involving the integration of several methodologies, such as genetic and epigenetic testing with conventional protocols. With the developments in the reproductive health sector, further delving into these interconnected domains is likely to improve our knowledge regarding infertility, too. Better genetic counseling procedures are bound to be outlined in turn. All of these developments represent not just the dedication of the scientific community to mitigate the advanced reproductive issues but also the possibility of novel solutions keeping in step with emerging technological advancements (Figure 12.16).

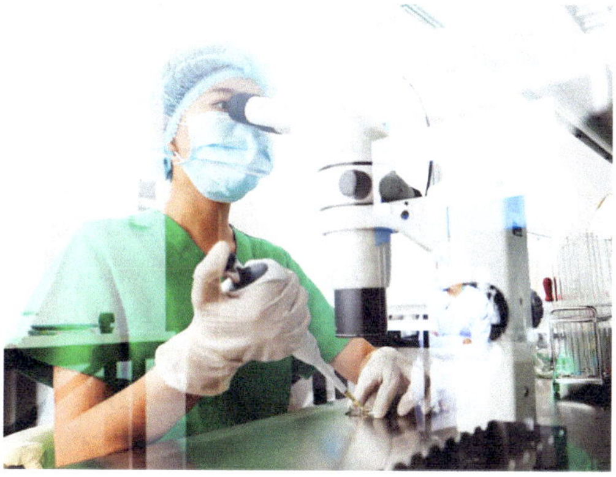

Figure 12.16. Embryonic Research Techniques.

Source: https://media.post.rvohealth.io/wp-content/uploads/2020/08/stem-cell-research_thumb.jpg.

12.5.3. Future Directions for Translational Research

As the field of translational research continues to develop, future directions are likely to focus on even greater interdisciplinarity to bridge basic scientific findings with their clinical uses. Such integration is vital to advancing translational embryology, as ongoing breakthroughs in genomics and biotechnology will continue to revolutionize the understanding of embryonic development and the mechanisms of inheritance. Through the utilization of knowledge produced from various areas including molecular biology, bioinformatics, and social sciences, researchers are able to develop concerted strategies for approaching intricate challenges like genetic disorders and infertility. For example, incorporation of dermatoglyphics studies in genetic counseling has the potential to provide novel information in female infertility through the selection of possible candidate genetic markers for diseases such as Turner syndrome or polycystic ovary syndrome (Anjankar et al., 2024). It will be essential that follow-up research not only examines these correlations but strives to apply the findings in the clinical environment to optimize patient outcomes. Further, the place of genetic counseling will be essential as translational research further adds layers to our knowledge regarding rare diseases and genetic disorders. Genetic counselors give personalized information and support to patients dealing with complicated genetic situations, a consideration of paramount significance to individuals dealing with rare diseases. In nations such as Spain, where geneticists and genetic counselors have no official recognition as healthcare providers, there is a critical demand for more genetic services for patients with rare diseases (Navas et al., 2021). Future translational directions should focus on developing frameworks that enable genetic counselors to facilitate patients in gaining the complete care required for accurate diagnosis and successful treatment. With more knowledge being unraveled about interactions between genetic determinants and embryonic formation, genetic counseling will play an increasingly significant role in assisting patients along their healthcare path, ensuring informed decisions and improved emotional support. Moreover, critical examination of ethical concerns in translational research involving embryology and genetic counseling is necessary for fostering public confidence and promoting responsible scientific progress. With advancing genetic technologies, it is critical that concerns regarding ethical issues surrounding gene editing and prenatal testing remain high on the priority agenda. Future studies need to prioritize not just the technological advancement but also the incorporation of ethical frameworks, policy requirements, and societal considerations to promote responsible practices in the field. The involvement of stakeholders like patients, families, healthcare professionals, and ethicists in the translational research will enable the creation of a more comprehensive model of genetic counseling that honors people's values and societal norms. As translational research embarks on more ambitious ventures, such as developing personalized medicine based on the genomic makeup of a person, it is essential that the ethical, legal, and social implications are carefully studied and resolved, thereby fostering a more equitable healthcare environment.

12.6. Ethical Implications

The translational embryology science has important ethical considerations that intersect and overlap with genetic counseling, especially as it pertains to the societal perception of infertility and assisted reproductive technologies. As practitioners grapple with how to describe the genetic cause of infertility, they are compelled to address the problematic concerns that come with new methods, for example, the examination of dermatoglyphics and its possible association with genetic disorders that influence fertility. Although the novel technique holds the potential of deciphering the myriad of causes of female infertility, the absence of large studies that provide a definitive causal link makes it ethically challenging to implement. The challenge lies in ensuring that the application of such research does not inadvertently spread misinformation or lead to the stigmatization of individuals experiencing reproductive challenges, while ensuring adherence to ethical standards that respect patient autonomy and informed consent. This highlights the need for responsible genetic counseling amidst a rapidly evolving scientific framework (Anjankar et al., 2024). Furthermore, the potential for preconception gender selection (PGS) raises more ethical questions that must be duly examined under the lenses of reproductive rights and societal gender biases. Although PGS is rationalized by its proponents as enabling parents to make informed decisions regarding their children, its effects on social norms and values are of concern. Critics also argue that the practice can lead to sex ratio imbalances and entrench gender biases that will arise from selective procedures enabled by PGS. The practice is, therefore, questioned in light of the consequences of genetic counseling practices that inadvertently promote some traits or genders, posing ethical issues on eugenic grounds. This balance of technological innovation and ethical accountability demands that genetic counselors negotiate the emotional vulnerabilities of future parents, thereby introducing the ultimate question of whether or not such decisions ultimately empower or exploit them (Sternke et al., 2010). Last but not least, the ethical concerns of translational embryology and genetic counseling are squarely significant and complicated. As research progresses and technological possibilities expand, it is crucial to create ethical frameworks that put the patients' welfare first while recognizing the risks involved in reproductive technologies. Employing novel approaches, such as the investigation of dermatoglyphics in the comprehension of infertility, requires a devotion to scientific precision and a full appreciation of the ethical landscape, thereby ensuring that the findings derived from such research are implemented wisely. Further, the current discussions on practices such as Participatory Guarantee Systems (PGS) must take into account the extended social implications and promote ethical standards that are conducive to equality and non-discrimination. Finally, there remains a necessity for a strong ethical framework to direct practitioners to create an inclusive and compassionate approach that promotes respect for the varied experiences that individuals endure in negotiating the complexities of reproductive health concerns (Anjankar et al., 2024; Sternke et al., 2010).

12.6.1. Ethical Dilemmas in Genetic Modification

As genetic modification technologies rapidly evolve, ethical issues are more pronounced in the field of translational embryology and genetic counseling. Among the most significant concerns is the classification of the embryo as a distinct entity from regarding them as simply biological material. The debate about this concern tends to accentuate the distinction between embryos created for reproductive goals and those created solely for research. Savulescu et al. believe that non-potentially reproductive embryos need not receive greater moral consideration than other tissues that constitute humans. This view opposes ingrained prejudices that single out reproductive cells, thus blocking research that may eventually result in great progress in the practice of reproductive medicine. By reframing ethical issues, society can create a more supportive environment for research that may help many patients and in the long run may benefit many patients; this strategy still provokes heated controversy among ethicists, researchers, and patients.

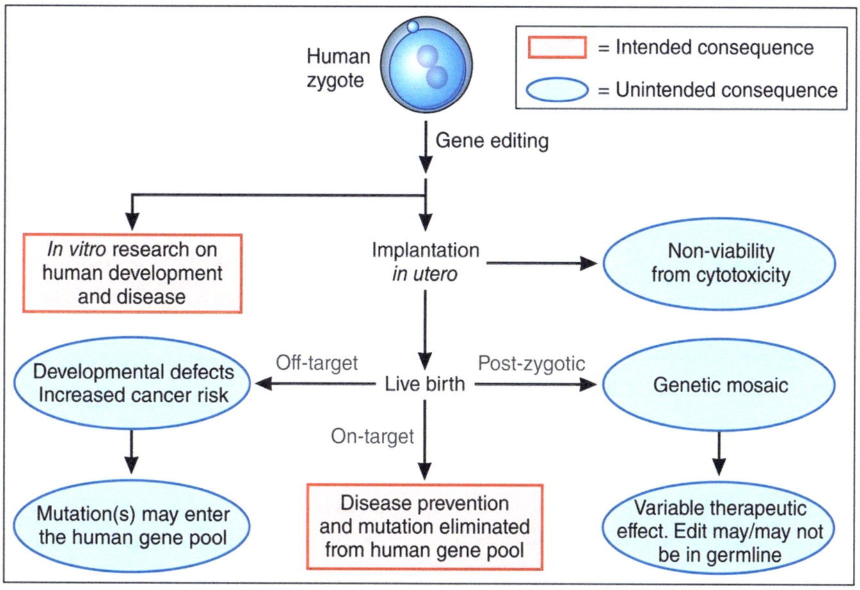

Figure 12.17. Ethical dilemmas in genetic modification.

Source: https://encrypted-tbn0.gstatic.com/images?q=tbn:ANd9GcS7r2FTGQhdLfejC9MLioxfuivVRbMMEwEkxA&s.

Furthermore, the ramifications of genetic modification reach into the realms of informed consent and patient autonomy. Diagnosis of genetic abnormality with the help of sophisticated karyotyping methods, particularly for microdeletions, points to the primary role of genetic counselors. The counselors must wade through complex ethical problems in managing results whose clinical significance may be uncertain. For example, when the fetus has an incidental genetic abnormality without apparent physical defects, cautious counseling is required about the possible outcomes and their implications in future pregnancies. As the literature dominates, genetic counseling is subjective in nature because personal attitudes toward normality and abnormality significantly influence patient attitudes. The principal dilemma, therefore, is the provision of objective information without imposing biases, which is essential in making informed reproductive decisions. Safeguarding patients' emotional welfare is a consideration at the same time. Finally, the moral framework for genetic modification involves not just the promise of benefit to better human health but also the risk of danger from unanticipated consequences. For instance, experimentation on future person embryos raises concerns about the potential long-term consequences of genetic alteration on successive generations. As Savulescu et al. have noted, incursions into embryology with the aim of improving clinical results, e.g., through enhanced viability in IVF, can potentially make negative contributions to both the embryo and future generations. This two-pronged sword of benefit and hazard calls for rigorous ethical examination to ascertain the balance between scientific advancement and moral responsibility. It is therefore imperative that the stakeholders remain in a state of vigilance and openness to the ethical dimensions at stake in genetic modification so that the quest for knowledge should not supplant significant aspects of human dignity and moral integrity. In this unstable situation, an interdisciplinary approach between scientists, ethicists, and society as a whole will be required to effectively deal with these ethical issues (Figure 12.17).

12.6.2. Informed Consent in Genetic Counseling

The theory of informed consent within the practice of genetic counseling is at the intersection of patient autonomy and ethical obligation. In this complicated landscape, genetic counselors are tasked with wading through a sea of information pertaining to genetic testing, risks posed by genetic disorders, and the possible impact on both patients and their families. Informed consent necessitates adequate communication to make sure that patients comprehend not just the technological facets of testing but also the potential emotional ramifications that may arise from disclosure of genetic information. The process is especially crucial given that most patients are likely to have a poor understanding of genetic principles. There is obviously a need for a comprehensive educational model, since disparities in comprehension may result in diminished levels of adherence to treatment regimens as well as heightened states of patient anxiety. It is therefore essential that counselors embrace an individualized approach, taking into consideration the individual circumstances and backgrounds of every patient to promote an educated decision-making process. Furthermore, the ethical aspects of informed consent in the context of genetic counseling are complex and, more often than not, contentious. Ethical issues frequently occur with regard to disclosure of genetic information to relatives and stigmatization that will follow inherited disorders. For example, whereas there is agreement by stakeholders on gradual release of information being advantageous, there is a considerable debate on criteria for revealing sensitive information, especially in the event of differences of sex development (DSD). Participants in pertinent research indicate that resistance by parents, as a result of shame or culture, may impede necessary education within the scope of genetic disorders, thus influencing the psychosocial growth of the children concerned. As such, it is the duty of healthcare professionals to surmount these barriers through family systems models by promoting candid communication and an atmosphere in which all members feel enabled to take an active role in the genetic counseling process. Finally, informed consent must also be considered in the context of additional developments in genetic technologies, such as stem cell research. The moral context of ESC research raises fundamental questions about patient rights and the formulation of consent. Arda et al. (2020) point out that the intricacy of informed consent is especially evident with regard to embryonic stem cells (ESCs) because of the ethical concerns of their derivation and the possible uses of such cells. Genetic counselors are charged with the duty of ensuring that patients possess a strong understanding not only of the scientific potential but also of the ethical concerns regarding genetic technologies that could influence their health-related choices. Thus, maintaining ethical integrity in genetic counseling entails ongoing education and facilitating discussion of the implications of new technologies, encouraging both patients and practitioners to critically consider the ever-changing landscape of genetic information.

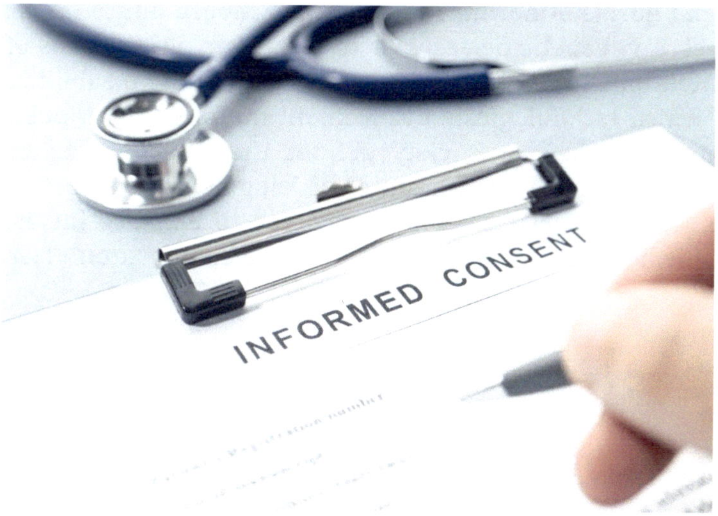

Figure 12.18. Informed Consent in Genetic Counseling.

Source: https://ciowomenmagazine.com/wp-content/uploads/2023/10/2.Informed-Consent.jpg.

12.6.3. Societal Impact of Embryological Advances

The development of embryological technologies, especially genetic testing and counseling, has significant social effects. Methods like PGT allow prospective parents to make an informed reproductive decision. Through genetic conditions such as hemoglobinopathies screening prior to implantation, PGT greatly lowers the incidence of specific inherited diseases, which could mean reduced burdens on the healthcare system in society. This proactive approach not only allows families to avoid the emotional and monetary costs of bringing up children who have serious genetic disorders but also fosters a broader discussion about reproductive rights and the moral responsibilities that come with these rights. The convergence of technology and reproductive decision-making incites a perpetual debate regarding the repercussions of such technologies on family life and societal norms, affecting how subsequent generations perceive genetic health and disease prevention (Kakourou et al., 2025). The development of non-invasive prenatal screening (NIPS) technology also highlights a significant advancement in prenatal care. As clinicians increasingly utilize NIPS for more genetic disorders on a more routine basis, the stakes for informed consent and parental autonomy are significant. NIPS enhances reproductive autonomy by allowing parents to make informed decisions regarding potential results for their children. However, this expansion of screening renders ethical issues surrounding the addition of late-onset conditions challenging, creating moral dilemmas for families. Consideration of these technologies highlights the imperative of clinical validity while simultaneously stimulating thoughts on equity and resource distribution in healthcare systems. Thus, with the increasing prominence of NIPS, it necessitates thoughtful deliberations on societal understandings of life-limiting conditions and the subsequent ethical obligations of healthcare providers to provide recommendations that are well-informed and empathetic (Tierry et al., 2025). Finally, the social ramifications of advances in embryology reach into the ethical realm in the manner in which these advances shape public attitudes toward disability and health. The capacity to conduct genetic screening prior to pregnancy routinely results in the exclusion of people with disabilities, thereby raising ethical concerns about societal values in relation to health and norms of normalcy. As families choose not to implant embryos that have been diagnosed with certain genetic diseases or to terminate on the basis of genetic information, society might be unintentionally reinforcing stigmas surrounding disabilities. This reality creates a complex context in which technological advancement intersects with public opinion and ethics, requiring a re-evaluation of the way society defines the value of human life. Engagement in continuous discussion and cautious application of developments in embryology is very important when handling these moral challenges. This is expected to enhance inclusiveness and preserve respect for all human beings, irrespective of their genetic composition (Tierry et al., 2025).

SUMMARY

This study of translational embryology and genetic counseling demonstrates that the crossroads of these disciplines has great potential for improving reproductive health. By combining sophisticated genetic testing methodologies along with an insight into embryonic development, clinicians are more capable of counseling patients regarding possible risks and results associated with fertility procedures and genetic disease. The fact that one is able to detect individual genetic markers using techniques such as genomic haplotyping enables more specific counseling and thus informed decision-making among potential parents. The interaction not only stimulates scientific progress but also the resultant complex emotions involved in planning a family, thus improving patients' overall experience. The study's implications reach beyond individual cases to encompass wider social influence. As embryology evolves, so do the ethical considerations of genetic counseling and testing. As the methods, like PGD, are refined, with genome-wide haplotyping being utilized to pick out embryos for selection on the basis of genetic health and chromosomal integrity, the need for rigorous guidelines amplifies. The results show how the practices of PGD guarantee the health and genetic soundness of embryos and, simultaneously, provide patients with essential information that facilitates decision-making and improves emotional outcomes. As highlighted, such discussions are necessary in order to put in place a solid framework that would guide clinicians and genetic counselors in their roles towards patients as well as society in general (de Ravel et al., 2017). In summary, the interface between translational embryology and genetic counseling is a virgin area that requires further scholarly studies and clinical innovations. The ability to connect dermatoglyphic patterns and genetic susceptibility presents a fascinating future research direction, one that may uncover additional vital links between embryogenesis and infertility (Anjankar et al., 2024). As these disciplines progress, it becomes more imperative for ongoing research to pursue comprehensive models that will synthesize genetic discoveries with conventional counseling interventions. This systematic knowledge will not only enable patients but also permit the development of a more aware and ethically accountable system of reproductive health care in the 21st century.

The complex interplay of genetic counseling and translational embryology is of paramount significance in the handling of modern reproductive disorders, including recurrent pregnancy loss (RPL). The literature indicates that a vast majority of RPL patients do not have definitive explanations, even with the evolution of evidence-based laboratory diagnostic testing, which has the potential to reveal diagnostic findings for close to 90% of them (Grant et al., 2024). Current practices among OBCPs reveal a remarkable lack of balance in the evaluation of RPL patients. Most practitioners order minimal laboratory tests, and this leads to a high percentage of evaluations being inappropriate. This lack of balance renders an already very sensitive and emotionally draining condition even more difficult, demonstrating the need for greater coordination and standardization in genetic testing for embryonic development and RPL outcome. In addition to the topics concerned with reproductive health, developments in the area of genetic science demand enhanced knowledge on the part of medical professionals. The Human Genome Project completion brought about a revolution in genetics education through its emphasis on the need for genomic literacy across different healthcare professions, including genetic counseling (Leblanc et al., 2009). A recent study conducted within the realm of speech-language pathology indicates substantial gaps in knowledge and skills, especially in the areas of genetics and its application to clinical practice. A considerable discrepancy exists between program directors' curricular demands and graduates' skills in applying genetic principles to effect. This mismatch highlights the necessity for education reforms targeting the incorporation of genetic principles into training programs, thus guaranteeing a manpower that is adequately capable of managing the intricacies involved in genetic counseling. The synthesis of translational embryology and genetic counseling represents a possibility for strengthening diagnostic expertise and intervention strategies within the field of reproductive health. Research on recurrent pregnancy loss (RPL) and genetic testing demonstrates that being able to explain genetic impacts based on embryonic development is vital to guide patient management (Grant et al., 2024). In addition, education aimed at developing genetic literacy, particularly in speech-language pathology, is essential to fill the gap between theoretical knowledge and clinical applications in genetic counseling (Leblanc et al., 2009). By enhancing healthcare providers' understanding of genetic concepts and their incorporation into models of comprehensive care, stakeholders can make diagnoses and treatment choices more precise and thus ultimately improved, lessening the emotional pain that frequently accompanies reproductive difficulty.

CLOSER LOOK

POLYCYSTIC OVARY SYNDROME

PCOS is a common hormonal disorder affecting individuals with ovaries, primarily during their reproductive years. Characterized by a complex interplay of hormonal imbalances, PCOS can present with a wide range of symptoms and health complications. One of the hallmark features of PCOS is the presence of multiple small cysts on the ovaries, which are often detected via ultrasound. However, the diagnosis is not solely dependent on imaging; it typically requires at least two of the following three criteria: irregular or absent menstrual periods, clinical or biochemical signs of hyperandrogenism (such as excess facial or body hair, acne, or elevated androgen levels), and polycystic ovaries. The exact cause of PCOS remains unclear, but it is believed to involve both genetic and environmental factors. Insulin resistance is a common underlying factor, contributing to elevated insulin levels that may stimulate the ovaries to produce more androgens, further exacerbating symptoms.

PCOS is estimated to affect 8–13% of reproductive-aged women globally, yet the presentation is so diverse that many cases are not detected. Among the most prominent symptoms is irregular periods, which can lead to ovulation and fertility issues. Weight gain or difficulty losing weight are also typical for women with PCOS, which further exacerbates the hormonal imbalance and insulin resistance. Other concomitant conditions, including type 2 diabetes, dyslipidemia, hypertension, sleep apnea, and an increased risk of cardiovascular disease, are also included. Moreover, psychological difficulties such as anxiety, depression, and low self-esteem have been commonly reported among women with PCOS and are believed to be influenced both by hormonal changes and the physically visible signs of the disorder.

PCOS diagnosis is often challenging due to the overlap with other conditions and the broad presentation of symptoms. Diagnosis typically includes a combination of blood work to evaluate hormone levels, inquiry about menstrual history, physical exams for signs of androgen excess, and imaging tests. Treatment of PCOS is individualized for the symptoms and health goals of the patient, namely whether or not fertility is a concern. Lifestyle changes, including diet, exercise, and weight loss, are usually the initial treatment and can lead to marked symptom and insulin sensitivity improvements. Medications, including hormonal contraceptives to control menstrual cycles and decrease androgen levels, and insulin-sensitizing medications like metformin, may be recommended to treat insulin resistance. Ovulation-inducing medication may be necessary for women who desire pregnancy.

Although there is no cure for PCOS, effective treatment can suppress the symptoms, avert long-term health-related complications, and improve quality of life. Ongoing research continues to determine the mechanisms underlying and potential treatments for PCOS. Awareness and early diagnosis are also necessary as an early intervention can avert many of the associated risks and allow individuals to live healthier lives. Multidisciplinary management, with the help of gynecologists, endocrinologists, nutritionists, and mental health professionals, is usually helpful in managing the complexity of PCOS.

REFERENCES

1. Abbott, A., Abulí, A., Amiri-Yekta, A., Bachelot, A., Bustamante-Aragones, A., Coates, A., Diez-Juan, A., et al. (2017). Recent developments in genetics and medically assisted reproduction: From research to clinical applications. https://core.ac.uk/download/157586216.pdf (accessed on 27 May 2025).
2. Acharya, K. S., Almeida-Santos, T., Anazodo, A., et al. (2021). A view from the past into our collective future: The Oncofertility Consortium vision statement. https://core.ac.uk/download/491172207.pdf (accessed on 27 May 2025).
3. Anjankar, V. P., Chimurkar, V., More, A., et al. (2024). Exploring dermatoglyphics as a potential indicator of female infertility: A review of current evidence and future directions. https://core.ac.uk/download/622174057.pdf (accessed on 27 May 2025).
4. Arda, B., & Gün, M. (2020). Embriyonik kök hücre araştırmaları hakkında etik açıdan ne söyleyebiliriz? https://core.ac.uk/download/492892686.pdf (accessed on 27 May 2025).
5. Badzek, L., Calzone, K. A., Dewell, S., et al. (2023). Current state of genomics in nursing: A scoping review of healthcare provider oriented (clinical and educational) outcomes (2012–2022). https://core.ac.uk/download/591678515.pdf (accessed on 27 May 2025).
6. Baskin, A., Fagerlin, A., Gardner, M., et al. (2023). It became easier once I knew: Stakeholder perspectives for educating children and teenagers about their difference of sex development. https://core.ac.uk/download/614875230.pdf (accessed on 27 May 2025).
7. Behr, B., Choi, B., Jun, S. H., et al. (2008). Defining human embryo phenotypes by cohort-specific prognostic factors. https://pmc.ncbi.nlm.nih.gov/articles/PMC2432022/.
8. Bergner, A. L., Greb, A. E., Fine, B. A., Baty, B. J., Walton, C. S., Franklin, C. R., Palmer, C. G., et al. (2016). 2013 review and update of the genetic counseling practice-based competencies by a task force of the Accreditation Council for Genetic Counseling. http://deepblue.lib.umich.edu/bitstream/2027.42/147172/1/jgc40868.pdf (accessed on 27 May 2025).
9. Chukov, V. S. (2024). The Sunni-Shia antagonism. https://doi.org/10.32591/coas.e-conf.10.22211c.
10. de Ravel, T., Debrock, S., Devriendt, K., et al. (2017). Principles guiding embryo selection following genome-wide haplotyping of preimplantation embryos. https://core.ac.uk/download/187732944.pdf (accessed on 27 May 2025).
11. Dyulgerova-Nikolova, D., & Milachich, T. (2020). The sperm: Parameters and evaluation. https://core.ac.uk/download/322445997.pdf (accessed on 27 May 2025).
12. Esteves, S. C. (2020). Are specialized sperm function tests clinically useful in planning assisted reproductive technology? https://core.ac.uk/download/326802071.pdf (accessed on 27 May 2025).
13. Garrido Navas, M. C., & Sánchez, S. (2021). Current status of genetic counselling for rare diseases in Spain. https://core.ac.uk/download/493007113.pdf (accessed on 27 May 2025).
14. Grant, E. (2024). Evaluation of the etiology of recurrent pregnancy loss (RPL): An explanatory mixed methods study exploring obstetrician gynecologist clinical provider behaviors and factors contributing to incomplete evaluations. https://core.ac.uk/download/622426618.pdf (accessed on 27 May 2025).

15. Juga, L. (2022). Epigenetic pathogenesis of neurological disorders *in utero* and considerations for genetic counseling. https://core.ac.uk/download/516439925.pdf (accessed on 27 May 2025).
16. Kabbashi, S., Roomaney, I. A., & Chetty, M. (2024). Bridging the gap between omics research and dental practice. *BDJ Open, 10*. https://doi.org/10.1038/s41405-024-00199-3.
17. Kakourou, G., Vrettou, C., Mamas, T., & Traeger-Synodinos, J. (2025). Reproductive choices in haemoglobinopathies: The role of preimplantation genetic testing. *Genes, 16*. https://www.semanticscholar.org/paper/c79ecf7b5aa10d8d93932b31101e59004b598ee9 (accessed on 27 May 2025).
18. Kumari, S., Gupta, S., Jamil, A., & Karakashev, S. (2025). Abstract 455: Targeting CARM1-expressing ovarian cancers with HSP-70 inhibitors. *Cancer Research*. https://www.semanticscholar.org/paper/d247314416921cf945f767e065e9991ffa7b6708 (accessed on 27 May 2025).
19. Laforce, T. M., Laberge, A., Malo, M. F., & Ravitsky, V. (2025). Blazing the trail of non-invasive prenatal screening expanded use: Healthcare providers' perspectives. *Prenatal Diagnosis, 45*, 163–170. https://www.semanticscholar.org/paper/37424290e1539e2dc2249987f0908a10fdad9304 (accessed on 27 May 2025).
20. Langner, J., Millard, F., Vavinskaya, V., Zhang, H., Yodkhunnatham, N., & Bagrodia, A. (2024). Evaluation and management of testicular cancer after late relapse. *Oncology*. https://doi.org/10.46883/2024.25921018.
21. Leblanc, E. M. (2009). Needs analysis of genetics and genomics in communication sciences and its disorders: Evidence for change. https://core.ac.uk/download/161440695.pdf (accessed on 27 May 2025).
22. Lewis, M. S. (2019). American democratic deficit in assisted reproductive technology innovation. https://scholarship.law.wm.edu/cgi/viewcontent.cgi?article=3000&context=facpubs (accessed on 27 May 2025).
23. Makrydima, S. (2016). Termination of pregnancy for an 11q terminal deletion incidentally diagnosed prenatally; Jacobsen syndrome penetrance and ethical dilemmas. *Volume 3*. https://www.semanticscholar.org/paper/24b0b548678306112070b579a8c61515b79004f2 (accessed on 27 May 2025).
24. Persico, T., Seracchioli, R., Sorrentino, U., et al. (2023). PGT-M for premature ovarian failure related to CGG repeat expansion of the FMR1 gene. https://core.ac.uk/download/611936251.pdf (accessed on 27 May 2025).
25. Pilyavsky, M. (2024). The effect of the Israeli Basic Law on human dignity and freedom on the use of incriminating evidence in Israeli courts. https://doi.org/10.32591/coas.e-conf.10.23225p.
26. Polyakov, A., & Rozen, G. (2022). Embryo research: Destiny is what counts. *Journal of Medical Ethics, 48*, 601–602. https://www.semanticscholar.org/paper/11d6a3ef78dbf595f2ef9b82be15227f037a2abb (accessed on 27 May 2025).
27. Sternke, L. M. (2010). Ethical considerations of nonmedical preconception gender selection research. https://core.ac.uk/download/301286795.pdf (accessed on 27 May 2025).

28. Tsai, Y., de Pontual, L., Heiner, C., Stojkovic, T., Furling, D., Bassez, G., Gourdon, G., et al. (2022). Identification of a CCG-enriched expanded allele in DM1 patients using amplification-free long-read sequencing. *bioRxiv*. https://www.semanticscholar.org/paper/a6d2fd91bc34870df8877246f23a066724570208 (accessed on 27 May 2025).

29. Wang, X., Wang, J., & Cheng, T. (2024). Development, growth, and future of the Institute of Basic Medical Sciences, Chinese Academy of Medical Sciences & Peking Union Medical College: 65 years tackling medical research paradigms. *Chinese Medical Journal, 137*, 883–886. https://doi.org/10.1097/cm9.0000000000003050.

INDEX

D

E

F

G

N

O

P

R